Clinician's Complete Reference to
Complementary/Alternative Medicine

CLINICIAN'S COMPLETE REFERENCE TO

Complementary/Alternative
MEDICINE

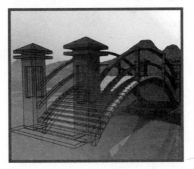

Donald W. Novey, MD

Medical Director
The Center for Complementary Medicine
Advocate Medical Group
Park Ridge, Illinois
www.advocatehealth.com/amgcompmed;
Instructor of Family Practice
Instructor of Medicine
Finch University of Health Sciences/The Chicago Medical School
Lecturer in Family Practice
Northwestern University School of Medicine
President, Medical Media Systems
Chicago, Illinois
www.medicalmediasystems.com

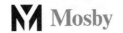 Mosby

A Harcourt Health Sciences Company

St. Louis   Philadelphia   London   Sydney   Toronto

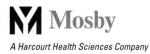

Mosby

A Harcourt Health Sciences Company

Editor in Chief: John Schrefer
Editors: Kellie White, Liz Fathman
Developmental Editor: Leslie Mosby
Project Manager: Linda McKinley
Production Editor: Ellen Forest
Designer: Judi Lang

Mosby, Inc.
A Harcourt Health Sciences Company
11830 Westline Industrial Drive
St. Louis, Missouri 63146

International Standard Book Number 0-323-00755-4

00 01 02 03 04 CL/FF 9 8 7 6 5 4 3 2 1

Contributors

John A. Astin, PhD
Complementary and Alternative Medicine Program at Stanford (CAMPS)
Stanford University School of Medicine
Palo Alto, California
Meditation

Judith Aston, MFA
Founder, Aston-Patterning
Incline Village, Nevada
Aston-Patterning

Leya Aum, MA, MFCC, MFT
Certified by the Feldenkrais Guild
Santa Rosa, California
Feldenkrais Method

M. Sue Benford, RN, MA
President and CEO
Public Health Information Services
Dublin, Ohio
Exploring the Concept of Energy in Touch-Based Healing

Dan Bienenfeld
Certified Hellerwork Practitioner and Trainer
Trustee, Hellerwork International, Los Angeles, California
Pacific Palisades, California
Hellerwork Structural Integration

Donald A. Bisson, MaR, CTR, CaR, CR, RR, CET, CCT
Dean and Chairman
Ontario College of Reflexology
New Liskeard, Ontario, Canada
Reflexology

Jeffrey S. Bland, PhD, FACN, CNS
CEO
HealthComm International
President
The Institute for Functional Medicine
Gig Harbor, Washington
Oxidative Stress

Keith I. Block, MD
Medical Director
Institute for Integrative Cancer Care
Evanston, Illinois
Clinical Assistant Professor
University of Illinois, College of Medicine
Adjunct Assistant Professor of Pharmacognosy
University of Illinois, College of Pharmacy
Chicago, Illinois
Nutritional Oncology and Integrative Cancer Care

Shane Boosey, BFA
Medical Student
The Ohio State University College of Medicine and Public Health
Columbus, Ohio
Exploring the Concept of Energy in Touch-Based Healing

David E. Bresler, PhD, LAc
Co-director
Academy for Guided Imagery
Associate Clinical Professor
UCLA School of Medicine
Los Angeles, California
Interactive Guided Imagery^{sm}

Shaun Brookhouse, PhD, DCH, PsyD
Director of Training and Research
The Washington School of Clinical and Advanced Hypnosis
Chorlton, Manchester, England
Neuro Linguistic Programming

Contributed topics are italicized.

Andreas Buchinger, MD
Medical Director
Klinik Dr. Otto Buchinger
D-31812 Bad Pyrmon, Germany
Fasting

Jane Buckle, RN, MA, B PH, Cert Ed
Hunter, New York
Aromatherapy

Stanislaw Burzynski, MD, PhD
Director, Burzynski Research Institute
Houston, Texas
Antineoplastons

Mary L. Chavez, PharmD
Director of Didactic Education
Associate Professor of Pharmacy Practice
Midwestern University College of Pharmacy–Glendale
Glendale, Arizona
Herbal Medicine

Pedro I. Chavez, PhD
Professor of Pharmaceutic Sciences
Midwestern University-College of Pharmacy–Glendale
Glendale, Arizona
Herbal Medicine

Nancy A. Corso, DC, DACBO, CAd
Hillsboro Beach, Florida
Macronutrients

Carolyn F.A. Dean, MD, ND
President
Holeopathic Pharmakeia
New York, New York
Acupuncture, Yoga

Therese M. Donnelly, RGN
London, England
Color Therapy

Catherine Downey, ND
Associate Dean of Clinical Education
The National College of Naturopathic Medicine
Portland, Oregon
Naturopathic Medicine

Douglas B. Drucker, PhD
Licensed Clinical Psychologist
Hellerwork Trainer
Co-founder, California Hellerwork Training
Los Gatos, California
Hellerwork Structural Integration

Jacqueline Fairbrass, ND
Reiki Master
Founder and Instructor, Fairbrass School of
Complementary Therapies
Gloucester, Ontario, Canada
Reiki

Jamie L. Feldman, MD, PhD
Assistant Professor
Department of Family Practice and Community Health
University of Minnesota
Minneapolis, Minnesota
Traditional Medicine in Latin America

Linda Kanelakos Fike, BA
Certified Hellerwork Practitioner
College Station, Texas
Hellerwork Structural Integration

Danielle L. Fraenkel, PhD, ADTR, NCC
Director, Kinections
Rochester, New York
Dance Therapy

Michael Reed Gach, PhD
Founder, Acupressure Institute
Berkeley, California
Acupressure

Mitchell J. Ghen, DO, PhD
Director, Biogenesis Medical Centers
Landrum/Columbia/Rockhill, South Carolina
Director, Millenium HealthCare
Atlanta, Georgia
Macronutrients, Micronutrients, Chelation Therapy

Jim Giorgi, MSEd, BCIA-C(EEG)
Director of Program Development
Biofeedback Consultants, Inc.
Suffern, New York
Biofeedback

Elliot Greene, MA, NCTMB
Past President
American Massage Therapy Association
Silver Spring, Maryland
Massage Therapy

Elson M. Haas, MD
Director, Preventive Medical Center
San Rafael, California
Detoxification Therapy

Marc Halpern, DC
Founder and Director, California College of Ayurveda
Center for Optimal Health
Founding Member and Facilitator, California Association
of Ayurvedic Medicine
Nevada City, California
Ayurveda

Daniel T. Hansen, DC, DABCO, FICC
Staff Chiropractic Provider
Coordinator, Quality Improvement
Texas Back Institute
Plano, Texas
Chiropractic

Kurt P. Heinking, DO
President, Osteopathic Sports Medicine S. C.
Adjunct Assistant Professor, Department of Osteopathic
Manipulative Medicine
Chicago College of Osteopathic Medicine
Midwestern University
Lombard, Illinois

Joseph Heller, BS
Founder, Hellerwork
Mt. Shasta, California
Hellerwork Structural Integration

Gloria Hessellund, MA
Practitioner, Senior Teacher, Rosen Method Bodywork
Director of Rosen Method Training Programs: California,
Scandinavia and Australia
Director of Teaching, The Rosen Institute
Berkeley, California
Rosen Method

Augustine Richard Hoenninger III, PhD, ND
Executive Director
International Association for Colon Hydrotherapy (I-ACT)
San Antonio, Texas
Colon Hydrotherapy

Ellen G. Horovitz, PhD, ATR-BC
Director of Graduate Art Therapy, Associate Professor
Nazareth College
Rochester, New York
Art Therapy

Bryan C. Hunter, PhD, MT-BC
Past President
American Music Therapy Association
Associate Professor and Coordinator of Music Therapy
Nazareth College
Rochester, New York
Music Therapy

Robert E. Kappler, DO, FAAO, FCA
Professor and Chairman, Department of Osteopathic
Manipulative Medicine
Director, Center for Osteopathic Research and
Educational Development
Chicago College of Osteopathic Medicine
Midwestern University
Lombard, Illinois

Ralf Kleef, MD
Center for Hyperthermia
A 1090 Vienna, Austria
Enzyme Therapy

Harold G. Koenig, MD, MHSc
Associate Professor of Psychiatry and Medicine
Duke University Medical Center
GRECC VA Medical Center
Durham, North Carolina
Spiritual Healing and Prayer

Edward V. Kondrot, MD
Adjunct Faculty
Desert Institute School of Classical Homeopathy
Phoenix, Arizona
Ophthalmologist
Pittsburgh, Pennsylvania
Homeopathy

Janneke Koole, BA, BEd
Medicine Director
D.T.M.M.F./Doorways
Scottsdale, Arizona
Shamanism

Leslie Korn, PhD, MPH, RPP
CWIS-Center for Traditional Medicine
Olympia, Washington
Polarity Therapy

Stuart Ledwith, PhD, RN
The Center for Therapeutic Touch
Baldwinsville, New York
Therapeutic Touch

Jack Liskin, MA, PA
Assistant Professor of Clinical Family Medicine
University of Southern California School of Medicine
Los Angeles, California
Trager Approach

Yuzeng Liu
Associate Professor, First Rank Police Officer
Director of the Chin'na and Fighting Teaching Section
Henan Police Academy
Zhengzhou, People's Republic of China
Tai Chi

Donald Londorf, MD, FRCPC
Qi Gong Therapist and Instructor
Chinese Healing Arts Center, Danbury, Connecticut
Under Master Tzu Kuo Shih
Rochester, New York
Qi Gong

Philip Maffetone, DC
MAF Group
Stamford, New York
Applied Kinesiology

Steve Meyerowitz, MS
Sproutman Publications
Great Barrington, Massachussetts
Juice Therapy

Theresa M. Morgan, BA
Wudang Research Association
Overland Park, Kansas
Tai Chi

Margaret Mullins, MD
President, Acupuncture Associates of Annapolis
Annapolis, Maryland
Acupuncture

Eileen Nauman, DHM(UK), FBIH, EMT-B
Core Faculty
Desert Institute School of Classical Homeopathy
Phoenix, Arizona
Homeopathic Medicine, Flower Essences, Quartz Crystal Therapy, Native American Medicine

Aline Newton, MA
Advanced Certified Rolfer
Chair, RI Board of Directors
Rolf Institute
Cambridge, Massachusetts
Rolfing

Donald W. Novey, MD
Medical Director
The Center for Complementary Medicine
Advocate Medical Group
Park Ridge, Illinois

Bret Nye, MD
Advanced Rolfer
Chair, Research Committee
Member, Board of Directors
Rolf Institute
Loveland, Colorado
Rolfing

Gary R. Oberg, MD, FAAP, FAAEM
Chairman, AAEM Continuing Medical Education Committee
American Academy of Environmental Medicine (AAEM)
Crystal Lake, Illinois
Environmental Medicine

Margo Jordan Parker, OMD, Lic Ac, Dipl Ac (NCCAOM)
Clinical Faculty Member, Program in Integrative Medicine
University of Arizona College of Medicine
Tucson, Arizona
Traditional Chinese Herbal Medicine

William Pawluk, MD, MSc
President
Advanced Magnetic Research Institute of the Delaware
Valley
Associate Clinical Professor
University of Medicine and Dentistry of New Jersey
Rancocas, New Jersey
Magnetic Field Therapy

Otto Pecher, MD
Manager, German Health Foundation
D 85653, Aying, Germany
Enzyme Therapy

Bonnie Prudden, MA
Founder and Director
Bonnie Prudden Pain Erasure and School
Founder, Board of Directors, Chairperson
International Myotherapy Association
Tucson, Arizona
Bonnie Prudden Myotherapy

Delia Quigley, BFA
President, Women for a Safe Future
Kushi Certified Chef
Newton, New Jersey
Yoga

Kenneth A. Ramey, DO
Adjunct Assistant Professor, Department of Osteopathic
Manipulative Medicine
Chicago College of Osteopathic Medicine
Midwestern University
Lombard, Illinois

Anne Rein, BA, CMP
Rosen Method Bodywork Practitioner
San Francisco, California
Rosen Method

Stephen Rojcewicz, MD
Past President
National Association for Poetry Therapy
Silver Spring, Maryland
Poetry Therapy

Marion Rosen, PT
Founder and Director, Rosen Method Bodywork
Rosen Method: The Berkeley Center
Berkeley, California
Rosen Method

Martin L. Rossman, MD, Dipl Ac (NCCAOM)
Co-director, Academy for Guided Imagery
Mill Valley, California
Interactive Guided Imagery^{sm}

Patrik Rousselot, PT (France), CMT, CBT
Member of the Bowen Therapy Academy of Australia
(BTAA)
The U.S. Bowen Therapy Instructor's Committee
Associated Bodywork and Massage Professionals (ABMP)
Certified Bowen Therapist and Registered Instructor for
the Bowen Therapy Academy
Oakland, California
Bowen Technique

Todd Rowe, MD, MD(H), CCH, DHt
Desert Institute of Classical Homeopathy
Phoenix, Arizona
Homeopathic Medicine

Theodore C. Rozema, MD, FAAFP
President-Elect, American College for Advancement in
Medicine (ACAM)
President, American Association of Alternative
Medicine (AAAM)
Secretary, American Board of Chelation Therapy
(ABCT)
Secretary, International Board of Chelation Therapy
(IBCT)
Past President and Director of the Great Lakes College of
Clinical Medicine (GLCCM)
Tryon, North Carolina
Chelation Therapy

Linda G.S. Russek, PhD
Clinical Assistant Professor of Medicine
Department of Medicine
University of Arizona
Tucson, Arizona
Exploring the Concept of Energy in Touch-Based Healing

Mary Jo Sabo, PhD
President CEO
Biofeedback Consultants Inc.
Suffern, New York
Administrator and Therapist
Pain and Stress Biofeedback Center
Spring Valley, New York
Biofeedback

Kenneth I. Saichek, FCH, PhD
Milwaukee, Wisconsin
Hypnotherapy

Gary E.R. Schwartz, PhD
Director, Human Energy Systems Laboratory
Co-facilitator in Energy Medicine, Program in
Integrative Medicine
University of Arizona, Department of Psychology
Tucson, Arizona
*Meditation, Exploring the Concept of Energy in Touch-Based
Healing*

Laura Servid, OTRL
Certified Aston Patterning Practitioner
Occupational Therapist
Seattle, Washington
Aston-Patterning

Shauna L. Shapiro, MA
University of Arizona
Tucson, Arizona
Meditation

Hector E. Solorzano del Rio, MD, DSc
Professor of Pharmacology
Centro Universitario de Ciencias de la Salud
Guadalajara, Jalisco Mexico
Enzyme Therapy, Orthomolecular Medicine

James Stephens, PT, PhD
Havertown, Pennsylvania
Feldenkrais Method

Judith C. Stern, MA, PT
Senior Faculty, American Center for the Alexander
Technique NY
Rye, New York
Alexander Technique

Russell Stolzoff
Certified Advanced Rolfer
Oakland, California
Rolfing

Phillip P. Sukel, BS, DDS
Past President (1988-1990), Chairman: Standards of
Care Committee
Vice-Chairman: Education Committee, Charter Member
International Academy of Oral Medicine and Toxicology
(IAOMT)
Accredited (AIAOMT) and Fellow (FIAOMT), Charter
Member
Bartlett, Illinois
Biologic Dentistry

Barry A. Sultanoff, MD
Founder and CEO
Healing Matters
Kensington, Maryland
Relaxation Therapies

John J. Triano, DC, PhD
Co-director, Conservative Medicine and Director,
Chiropractic Division
Texas Back Institute
Plano, Texas
Adjunct Faculty, Biomedical Engineering
University of Texas, Southwestern Medical Center
Dallas, Texas
Chiropractic

John E. Upledger, DO, OMM
President and Founder
The Upledger Institute
Palm Beach Gardens, Florida
CranioSacral Therapy

Larry B. Wallace, OD
Ithaca, New York
Light Therapy

Melvyn R. Werbach, MD
Assistant Clinical Professor
UCLA School of Medicine
Los Angeles, California
Micronutrients

Enid Whittaker, BS
Associate Director
Bonnie Prudden Pain Erasure and School
Member, International Myotherapy Association
Tucson, Arizona
Bonnie Prudden Myotherapy

Frank Wildman, CFT, PhD
Movement Studies Institute
Berkeley, California
Feldenkrais Method

Michael Winn, BA
President, National Qi Gong Association
Dean, Healing Tao University
Professor, Tao Arts and Sciences
Great Western University
Asheville, North Carolina
Qi Gong

Harri Wolf, MA
Director, Institute for Applied Iridology
Laguna Beach, California
Iridology

Jenna Woods, BFA, MsT
Member, Associated Bodywork and Massage Professionals
Boulder, Colorado
Aston-Patterning

Jeffrey Yuen, BS
Director, Acupuncture Program
Swedish Institute: School of Acupuncture and Oriental Studies
New York, New York
Acupuncture

Carlos P. Zalaquett, Lic., MA, PhD
Assistant Director, Counseling Center
Sam Houston State University
Huntsville, Texas
Relaxation Therapies

To all those who wish to take a step—simply the *openness* to considering the possibility that there is more . . . is enough

To the contributors of this text and their willingness to meet mainstream medicine halfway—we should only be as flexible . . .

To my own Teacher

And to my wonderful wife, Judy, who doesn't need a book to cure illness naturally

Preface

WELCOME TO THE WORLD OF COMPLEMENTARY MEDICINE. Learning about this field is a bit like raising teenagers. One does not exit from the process unaltered. This field is rich with experiences that enlighten and broaden one's horizons. Knowing that there is more than we thought, we can never be the same.

The overall purpose of this text is to simply lay out for the reader another set of options to consider. These options consist of therapeutic approaches and, even more fundamentally, additional ways to view health and healing. Mainstream medicine does not have to be rejected in favor of alternative medicine. They can both coexist as long as each is used appropriately. The burden is on us to learn of these additional methods so we can integrate them for the benefit of our patients and for ourselves as well.

You may have noticed that the cover of this text shows a bridge. In this case, the bridge symbolizes a means to go from one way of thinking to another, traversing a gulf of changing perspective. Human nature dictates that one can advance most easily when beginning from a safe and familiar setting. To provide this, I have structured this text along a mainstream medical perspective. Most therapies in the section on *Fields of Practice* follow an identical template that contains the information most medical personnel wish to know. This template is the *runway*, a starting point of stability. Within each chapter subsection, the contributors present their material and allow the reader to *lift off* into new ways of approaching illness and treatment. Some of these therapies are quite relatable and some are, frankly, way out there. But all are valuable options for individual situations.

This book presents an opportunity for exposure to many of the most common modalities in alternative medicine while imposing a sense of structure. The contributors of this book have graciously consented to fit their modalities into this structured model because it does provide that sense of familiarity while learning something entirely unfamiliar.

Section One gives an overview of the philosophy and basic concepts of complementary medicine. Use this section to gain a basic introduction to the field of complementary/alternative medicine.

Section Two, the largest section, reviews a number of alternative therapies, most of which contain a standardized structure. Because of this standard layout, you may look up specific information by turning to the desired subsection, regardless of the type of therapy. When subsections are missing, it is because no relevant information could be obtained. Use this section to read an authoritative review of individual therapies or to gain specific information about a particular therapy.

The template given to all contributors consists of the following:

Origins and History
Mechanism of Action According to Its Own Therapy
Biologic Mechanism of Action
Form of Therapy
Demographics
Indications and Reasons for Referral
Office Applications
Practical Applications
Research Base
   Evidence Based
   Basic Science
   Risk and Safety
   Efficacy
   Other
   Future Research Opportunities and Priorities
Druglike Information
   Safety
   Actions and Pharmacokinetics
   Warnings, Contraindications, and Precautions
   Drug or Other Interactions
   Adverse Reactions
   Pregnancy and Lactation
   Trade Products, Administration, and Dosage
Self-Help versus Professional
Visiting a Professional
Credentialing
Training
What to Look for in a Provider
Barriers and Key Issues
Associations
Suggested Reading
References

Section Three is a marvelous act of cooperation among the contributors. Where possible, they submitted similar lists of diagnoses, prioritizing them according to the applicability and effectiveness of their form of therapy. This extensive compilation shows the range of alternative therapies as they apply to a wide range of diagnoses. Use this section to gain a sense of this range as applicable to a particular diagnosis.

This book could offer so much more than it does, but size has presented its unavoidable constraints. Many of the therapies have been reduced from their original length to limit the text size to its present approximately 800 pages. Many other therapies were not included for the same reason of space limitations. This entire textbook is designed for a rapid-access approach. I hope it provides you with the information you need to begin your process of growth and understanding in this field. You, the reader, are a valuable contributor to the evolution of this text, and I welcome your comments on additions or changes for editions to come.

DONALD W. NOVEY, MD

Acknowledgments

THIS BOOK IS THE COMPOSITE EFFORT of over 90 individuals who saw the benefit of such a text. These individuals, the contributors to this text, worked long and hard to create chapters of consistent quality. Many of these contributors are leaders in their field, with little time to do one more project. To each of them I owe a debt of gratitude.

I also wish to thank the staff of Mosby, who helped me to publish this book on schedule despite the delays involved with a project as complex as this. In addition, I wish to acknowledge their vision in allowing this book to be published.

Even more than ever, this text was created electronically. Nearly all contact with authors was initiated and maintained by e-mail. Nearly all drafts of therapies, from start to finish, were transmitted over the Internet. Intensive spreadsheet support was required to keep track of the many authors and their various stages of production and communication. A very large database was created for the third section of this book. I thank my faithful laptop for not breaking down.

Finally, I wish to thank my wife, Judy, for her support as she watched me chained to my laptop for the six months it took to complete this text. To me, this was the world's biggest sandbox with all the toys in the world. To her, I was just a tired husband. Bless her heart.

DONALD W. NOVEY, MD

Contents

SECTION ONE

General Concepts, 1

Introduction, 2
DONALD W. NOVEY

Basic Principles of Complementary/Alternative Therapies, 5
DONALD W. NOVEY

The Dilemma of Evidence, 7
DONALD W. NOVEY

Leaving the Medical Model, 10
DONALD W. NOVEY

Integration, 13
DONALD W. NOVEY

SECTION TWO

Fields of Practice, 17

Mind-Body Interventions

Art Therapy, 20
ELLEN G. HOROVITZ

Biofeedback, 32
MARY JO SABO / JIM GIORGI

Dance/Movement Theory, 41
DANIELLE L. FRAENKEL

Hypnotherapy, 53
KENNETH I. SAICHEK

Interactive Guided Imagery^{sm}, 64
MARTIN L. ROSSMAN / DAVID E. BRESLER

Meditation, 73
JOHN A. ASTIN / SHAUNA L. SHAPIRO / GARY E.R. SCHWARTZ

Music Therapy, 86
BRYAN C. HUNTER

Neuro Linguistic Programming, 96
SHAUN BROOKHOUSE

Poetry Therapy, 105
STEPHEN ROJCEWICZ

Relaxation Therapies, 114
BARRY A. SULTANOFF / CARLOS P. ZALAQUETT

Spiritual Healing and Prayer, 130
HAROLD G. KOENIG

Yoga, 141
DELIA QUIGLEY / CAROLYN F.A. DEAN

Bioelectromagnetic Applications in Medicine

Light Therapy, 154
LARRY B. WALLACE

Magnetic Field Therapy, 164
WILLIAM PAWLUK

Alternative Systems of Medical Practice

Oriental Medical Practices

Acupressure, 178
MICHAEL REED GACH

Acupuncture, 191
CAROLYN F.A. DEAN / MARGARET MULLINS / JEFERY YUEN

Traditional Chinese Herbal Medicine, 203
MARGO JORDAN PARKER

Tai Chi, 219
YUZENG LIU / THERESA M. MORGAN

Qi Gong, 231
DONALD LONDORF / MICHAEL WINN

Professionalized Health Care Systems

Ayurveda, 246
MARC HALPERN

Homeopathy, 258
EDWARD V. KONDROT / EILEEN NAUMAN / TODD ROWE

Naturopathic Medicine, 274
CATHERINE DOWNEY

Community-Based Health Care Practices

Traditional Medicine in Latin America, 284
JAMIE L. FELDMAN

Native American Medicine, 293
EILEEN NAUMAN

Shamanism, 301
JANNEKE KOOLE

Manual Healing Methods

Chiropractic, 310
DANIEL T. HANSEN / JOHN J. TRIANO

Osteopathic Medicine, 325
ROBERT KAPPLER / KENNETH A. RAMEY / KURT P. HEINKING

Massage Therapy, 328
ELLIOT GREENE

Bodywork

Alexander Technique, 350
JUDITH C. STERN

Aston-Patterning®, 359
LAURA SERVID / JENNA WOODS / JUDITH ASTON

Bowen Technique, 371
PATRIK ROUSSELOT

CranioSacral Therapy, 381
JOHN E. UPLEDGER

Feldenkrais Method®, 393
FRANK WILDMAN / JAMES STEPHENS / LEYA AUM

Hellerwork Structural Integration, 407
JOSEPH HELLER / LINDA KANELAKOS FIKE / DAN BIENENFELD / DOUGLAS B. DRUCKER

Bonnie Prudden Myotherapy, 417
BONNIE PRUDDEN / ENID WHITTAKER

Polarity Therapy, 423
LESLIE KORN

Reiki, 435
JACQUELINE FAIRBRASS

Rolfing® Structural Integration, 444
ALINE NEWTON / BRET NYE / RUSSELL STOLZOFF

Rosen Method, 453
ANNE REIN / GLORIA HESSELLUND / MARION ROSEN

Therapeutic Touch, 462
STUART LEDWITH

Trager® Approach, 472
JACK LISKIN

Exploring the Concept of Energy in Touch-Based Healing, 483
M. SUE BENFORD / GARY E.R. SCHWARTZ / LINDA G.S. RUSSEK / SHANE BOOSEY

Pharmacologic and Biologic Treatments

Antineoplastons, 496
STANISLAW R. BURZYNSKI

Chelation Therapy, 508
MITCHELL J. GHEN / THEODORE C. ROZEMA

Enzyme Therapy, 517
RALF KLEEF / OTTO PECHER

Flower Essences, 535
IAN NAUMAN

Herbal Medicine, 545
JULIA CHAVEZ / PEDRO I. CHAVEZ

Diet and Nutrition in the Prevention and Treatment of Disease

Macronutrients, 566
MITCHELL J. GHEN / NANCY A. CORSO

Micronutrients, 576
MELVYN R. WERBACH / MITCHELL J. GHEN

Oxidative Stress, 595
JEFFREY S. BLAND

Orthomolecular Medicine, 606
HECTOR E. SOLORZANO DEL RIO

Nutritional Oncology and Integrative Cancer Care, 618
KEITH I. BLOCK

Unclassified Diagnostic and Treatment Methods

Applied Kinesiology, 638
PHILIP MAFFETONE

Aromatherapy, 651
JANE BUCKLE

Biologic Dentistry, 667
PHILIP P. SUKEL

Colon Hydrotherapy, 679
A.R. HOENNINGER III

Color Therapy, 690
THERESE M. DONNELLY

Detoxification Therapy, 702
ELSON M. HAAS / DONALD W. NOVEY

Environmental Medicine, 716
GARY R. OBERG

Fasting, 728
ANDREAS BUCHINGER

Juice Therapy, 741
STEVE MEYEROWITZ

Iridology, 756
HARRI WOLF

Quartz Crystal Therapy, 770
EILEEN NAUMAN

Reflexology, 779
DONALD A. BISSON

SECTION **THREE**

Health Conditions and Suggested Therapies, 791

Rapid Index, 792

Listing of Health Conditions, 794

SECTION **ONE**

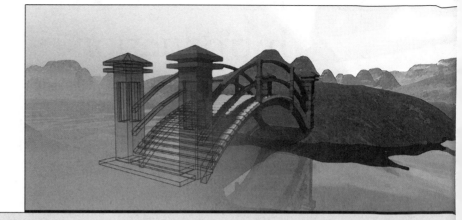

General Concepts

Introduction, 2

Basic Principles of Complementary/
   Alternative Therapies, 5

The Dilemma of Medical Evidence, 7

Leaving the Medical Model, 10

Integration, 13

Introduction

DONALD W. NOVEY

SINCE THE BEGINNING of time, there have been healers and their patients. The titles have changed with the era and with the culture, but the relationship has remained the same. In the absence of advanced technology, imaging, and pharmacology, medicine's state of the art remained variations of the same for most of human history. Treatments ranged from the extreme to the conservative, and the value of a therapy was based upon its word-of-mouth reputation. Until the last two or three centuries, therapies were predominantly what we would now call *alternative medicine,* with a heavy emphasis on herbal, energetic, and spiritual aspects of healing. Then, with the dawn of the scientific method, the healing arts diverged into two distinct directions: mainstream (allopathic), and alternative medicine.

In the United States, these alternative professions had a tremendous diversity of theory, practice styles, effectiveness, and quality of their practitioners. Regular (allopathic) medicine competed with at least two dozen other sects, including homeopathic, botanical, and hydropathic medicine. Although allopathy presented itself as the scientific branch of medicine and proclaimed the practices of the other sects to be quackery, its therapies were aggressive and toxic and had no proven advantage over the treatments used by competitors. Through the efforts of the American Medical Association (AMA), allopathic medicine eliminated its competition by promoting the reestablishment of licensure laws in the late 1800s. In a continuation of the same endeavor, the AMA sought to identify weak and inadequate medical schools and commissioned Abraham Flexner to write the famous Flexner report of 1910.[1] This report effectively reduced the number of nonallopathic medical schools in the U.S. to nearly zero. From that time forward, modern scientific medicine prevailed and flourished.

One would think this was the end of the story, but it was not. As a continuing tribute to human nature, some individuals continued to practice their alternative methods and to train others. Similarly, a proportion of patients continued to prefer nontraditional therapies to mainstream medicine. Much of the practice of alternative medicine went "underground," becoming a discreet enterprise. In parallel fashion, local and national medical associations imposed significant penalties on physicians who referred to nontraditional providers. Because of the philosophic and political rift between alternative and mainstream medicine, contact between them was strained at best, and professionally dangerous for both at worst.

The alternative medical perspective appeared radically different from that of mainstream medicine and so did its therapies. This occurred in part from a difference in theoretical approach, and in part from a need not to violate the licensure laws that gave mainstream physicians the authority to prescribe medications and perform surgery. To the mainstream community, alternative medicine seemed to become a "work-around," often attempting to bypass mainstream medicine to accomplish a similar goal. Without adequate support from allopathic practice, alternative medicine became, in essence, a counterculture. Isolationism, secrecy, an embattled persona, and poor communication with mainstream practitioners were features that reflected the protectiveness of its constituents. Nonetheless, many nontraditional therapies continued to be taught and sought after by the lay public.

In the 1970s alternative therapies became quite popular in the U.S. A resurgence of interest generated the appearance of new schools to teach some of the alternative therapies and an expanding clientele to use them. Interest in nontraditional therapies continued to grow steadily but quietly. The chiropractic profession embraced many of the tenets of alternative medicine early on and helped to generate significant interest among the general public. Some osteopathic physicians also took the opportunity to incorporate some naturopathic principles into their practice. Yet the majority of mainstream physicians continued to maintain their distance.

In 1993 Eisenberg's landmark study showed that a striking percentage of the general public were using or had used some form of alternative therapy and that equivalent dollars were spent out of pocket on alternative and mainstream medicine.[2] In 1998 Eisenberg's follow-up study showed even greater growth in the use of alternative therapies. Between 1990 and 1997 the likelihood of use of alternative medicine services increased from 36% to 46% and the number of total visits increased by 47%. By 1997 extrapolations for alternative therapy visits *exceeded* total visits to all U.S. primary care physicians, and estimated expenditures for alternative therapies increased by 45%. At the same time, out-of-pocket expenditures for alternative medicine professional services *equaled* those for all physician services and exceeded those for hospitalizations in the U.S.[3] Physicians knew that alternative medicine was used to some degree, but its true prevalence and economic impact was a revelation.

Our patients have moved ahead in their interest. We have stayed behind to see if the change was real. Now, we are like the tired parents lagging behind, while our patients, the excited child, scurries ahead, then stops and looks back, calling out, "Come on, Mom and Dad, hurry up!"

Today, a shift in focus is occurring. Rather than ignoring alternative medicine, health professionals have realized the need to learn more, because their patients want good counsel and even the safety of a supervised setting. With the increase in public interest, many health professionals have found themselves wanting in clear and accurate information. We now find ourselves playing educational "catch-up." Quality resources are only beginning to be available to assist the health professional in this new learning process, for this learning is not just an update in facts, but entirely new ways of thinking.

With this awakening comes the opportunity for integration. Alternative medicine and mainstream medicine no longer need be sparring partners. The proper use of these modalities lies simply in the statement, "What is the best for the patient?" Given a new and broader set of therapeutic tools, we have the opportunity to choose and to include.

Alternative medicine has tried to bypass mainstream medicine. Mainstream medicine has done the reverse. Now it is time to consider all the options.

Which is true, alternative medicine or mainstream medicine? The answer lies somewhere in the middle. Both are valuable perspectives, and each is incomplete without the other.

The definitions of complementary medicine vary. To some, the term is interchangeable with alternative medicine. To this author, complementary medicine is the best of both worlds. It is a blending of both mainstream and alternative medicine to provide a broader range of tools to assist the patient. It is an opportunity to look at illness from many viewpoints and therefore approach its treatment from many angles.

To assist the reader with this conceptual journey, several chapters follow in this first section to facilitate a shift in thought process and to provide practical information on integrating alternative therapies into a truly complementary medical perspective.

References

1. Ober KP: The pre-Flexnerian reports: Mark Twain's criticism of medicine in the United States, *Ann Intern Med* 126(2):157-163, 1997.

2. Eisenberg DM et al: Unconventional medicine in the United States. Prevalence, costs, and patterns of use, *N Engl J Med* 328(4):246-252, 1993.

3. Eisenberg DM et al: Trends in alternative medicine use in the United States, 1990-1997: results of a follow-up national survey, *JAMA* 280(18):1569-1575, 1998.

Basic Principles of Complementary/ Alternative Therapies

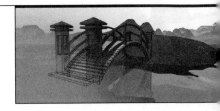

DONALD W. NOVEY

J UST AS MAINSTREAM MEDICINE has a fairly consistent approach to illness, so does alternative medicine. Most prevalent in alternative medicine are the six naturopathic principles. In one form or another, these principles are revisited again and again throughout Section Two of this text. The following principles are described by Dr. Catherine Downey and excerpted from her chapter on naturopathic medicine.

1. The Healing Power of Nature (*Vis medicatix naturae*)

   The body has the inherent ability to establish, maintain and restore health. The healing process is ordered and intelligent: nature heals through the response of the life force. The physician's role is to facilitate and augment this process, to act to identify and remove obstacles to health and recovery, and to support the creation of a healthy internal and external environment. In short, give the body the appropriate tools and it will heal itself.

2. Treat the Whole Person (The multifactorial nature of health and disease)

   Health and disease are conditions of the whole organism, involving a complex interaction of physical, spiritual, mental, emotional, genetic, environmental, and social factors. The physician must treat the whole person by taking all of these factors into account. The harmonious functioning of all aspects of the individual is essential to recovery from and prevention of disease and requires a personalized and comprehensive approach to diagnosis and treatment.

3. First Do No Harm (*Primum no nocere*)

   Illness is a purposeful process of the organism. The process of healing includes the generation of symptoms, which are, in fact, an expression of the life force attempting to heal itself. Therapeutic actions should be complementary to and synergistic with this healing process. The physician's actions can support or antagonize the actions of the *vis mediatrix naturae*; therefore methods designed to suppress symptoms without removing underlying causes are considered harmful and are avoided or minimized. Therapeutic actions are applied in an ordered fashion congruent with the internal order of the organism.

4. Identify and Treat the Cause (*Tolle causam*)

Illness does not occur without cause. Underlying causes of disease must be discovered and removed or treated before a person can recover completely from illness. Symptoms are expressions of the body's attempt to heal, but they are not the cause of disease; therefore naturopathic medicine addresses itself promptly to the underlying causes of disease, rather than symptoms. Causes may occur on many levels, including physical, mental-emotional, and spiritual. The physician must evaluate fundamental underlying causes on all levels, directing treatment at root cause rather than at symptomatic expression.

5. Prevention (Prevention is the best "cure")

The ultimate goal of naturopathic medicine is prevention. This is accomplished through education and promotion of lifestyle habits that create good health. The physician assesses risk factors and hereditary susceptibility to disease and makes appropriate interventions to avoid further harm and risk to the patient. The emphasis is on building health rather than on fighting disease. Because it is difficult to be healthy in an unhealthy world, it is the responsibility of both the physician and patient to create a healthier environment in which to live.

6. The Physician as Teacher (*Docere*)

Beyond an accurate diagnosis and appropriate prescription, the physician must work to create a health-sensitive, interpersonal relationship with the patient. A cooperative doctor-patient relationship has inherent therapeutic value. The physician's major role is to educate and encourage the patient to take responsibility for health. The physician is a catalyst for healthful change, empowering and motivating the patient to assume responsibility. It is the patient, not the doctor, who ultimately creates or accomplishes healing. The physician must strive to inspire hope as well as understanding. Physicans must also make a commitment to their personal and spiritual development in order to be good teachers.

A few clarifying points round out the complementary approach:

1. Alternative medicine does not suppress symptoms. It attempts to delve deeper than the symptoms and address their causes. This in turn diminishes or eliminates the symptoms.

2. Similar alternative treatment strategies are often applied to many unrelated disease and illnesses because the core alternative philosophy states that many illness manifestations stem from common root causes. There are no "off-label" indications for alternative medicine.

3. Alternative medicine is less interested in the manifestations of the disease and more interested in those elements that created the disease in the first place.

4. The patient is part of the healthcare team and has a strong say in planning for a future therapeutic approach. Patients are empowered to participate in the decision process and, in turn, have the responsibility to enact what they have agreed to do. In these scenarios, noncompliance is much less common.

5. The mind-body correlation is extremely important. Learning about the patient's social life, family life, and work life, and significant life events that predate the onset of illness can help immensely in understanding contributing factors in a patient's illness and in formulating a treatment plan. Even asking the question, "What happened to you around the time this illness began?" can be most revealing.

Many variations on this approach will be apparent through the pages of this text. The sense of facilitating a natural process or returning the patient to a natural state of balance is the common theme overall.

The Dilemma of Evidence

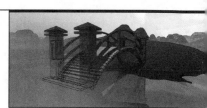

DONALD W. NOVEY

MANY HEALTH PROFESSIONALS, with a reserve that reflects the natural protectiveness for their patients, prefer to see well-designed studies documenting the effectiveness of any new or different therapy before adding it to their therapeutic repertoire. For many of the therapies listed in this text, this type of traditional evidence is lacking, and for several reasons.

1. The Finances of Research

A considerable portion of medical research is funded, either by National Institute of Health (NIH) grants, investors, or grants from pharmaceutic firms. Much available research revolves around substances or processes that can be patented and therefore marketed through a restricted channel. In other words, research dollars can eventually be recovered through product sales. Governmental grants are the most unrestricted, but also are in short supply.

Most alternative therapy modalities are in the public domain, as are common herbs and supplements. Without a patent, these services and products can be marketed through unrestricted channels. One company might fund research on its product and yet another company could sell a similar product under a slightly different formulation. This makes recapturing of research dollars much less likely and funded research for these products and services much more scarce.

With the dramatic increase in public and commercial interest in alternative medicine and services, more funding is likely. Sources may include national associations that represent a particular form of therapy, some of the larger supplement manufacturers, and NIH funding through the National Center for Complementary and Alternative Medicine. More funding will generate more well-designed research studies. This is likely to be a 5 to 10-year process.

2. Difficulties in Experimental Design

Well-designed research hinges on two standard expectations. The first is that the therapy under scrutiny is identical for each patient enrolled in the study. The second is that the study design includes at least two groups, a study group and a control group. Additionally, when placebo control is used, the test subjects should be unable to distinguish the placebo from the therapy.

The very nature of many alternative therapies make these types of trials difficult to design. Acupuncture studies, for example, require the use of sham needle insertion to give the effect of administering therapy to the control group. Although some researchers claim that sham acupuncture is truly a placebo,[1] others conclude that even sham acupuncture has a therapeutic effect beyond that of placebo.[2]

Homeopathy presents a different dilemma. In homeopathy, the chosen remedy is tailored to the individual patient. For example, 20 patients may have the same chief complaint. To the homeopath, the chief complaint is only a small factor in the patient's clinical picture, as the choice of remedy is often determined by more minor symptom nuances. These 20 patients likely would each receive a different homeopathic remedy. A single, identical remedy for all patients is contrary to the theory and practice of homeopathy. In this scenario, clinical research is often reduced to outcome studies.

Some modalities defy experimental design. A truly well-designed study creates an environment in which only one variable is manipulated, such as the treatment under study. Some forms of alternative medicine are so intertwined with culture and lifestyle that adjustment of study variables is virtually impossible. Some examples of this occur in therapies such as Native American medicine, shamanism, and detoxification. In certain energy medicine modalities such as Qi Gong, therapeutic touch, and quartz crystal healing, our ability to measure the human biofield and other emanations has not yet been successfully accomplished. For these modalities, present study design is often related to subjective as opposed to objective measurements.

Perhaps ingenuity is the answer. As more research is funded, study design can advance to include more alternative therapy modalities and methods created to "factor out" the diversity inherent in many alternative therapies.

3. Inexperience in Study Design

Many alternative therapies are only newly emerging from their counterculture. The creation of properly designed and controlled studies is a learned skill and requires the same degree of rigorous thinking for alternative therapies as for their mainstream counterparts. These skills simply are not learned overnight. Indeed, to learn these techniques requires interacting with mainstream medicine to learn these design techniques. This requires a professional self-image that allows practitioners to apply mainstream study criteria to their own alternative modality while retaining the unique perspective each alternative therapeutic approach provides.

What to Do until the Data Arrive

Health care professionals often practice one step ahead of available research. Practitioners congregate at meetings, in hallways, in hospitals, and in their own practice settings to share successful strategies for treatment of hard-to-manage conditions. Medical decisions are often made based on empiric data. Off-label indications are common in mainstream medicine until the indication makes its way onto the label through eventual research. Perhaps the greatest example of practice style based on empiric data is residency training or internship with a more experienced practitioner. Entire practice styles are modeled after that of the mentor without every item of decision-making being questioned for documentation. Learning from experience or from those with experience is a time-tested activity.

The decision to apply empiric thinking to alternative therapies is easier. These therapies often have fewer side effects and adverse reactions than their mainstream counterparts. Years of anecdotal reports, sometime centuries or even millennia in duration, support their usefulness. In a monitored setting where the risk of missed or delayed diagnosis is minimal, the application of these therapies can be most beneficial for the patient. The study-based documentation of their efficacy is valuable, but its absence need not delay their application for patient care.

References

1. Zaslawski C et al: Strategies to maintain the credibility of sham acupuncture used as a control treatment in clinical trials, *J Alt Complement Med* 3(3):257-266, 1997.
2. Ballegaard S, Meyer CN, Trojaborg W: Acupuncture in angina pectoris: does acupuncture have a specific effect? *J Intern Med* 229(4):357-362, 1991.

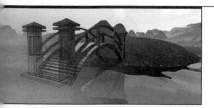

Leaving the Medical Model

DONALD W. NOVEY

Changing Paradigms

Changing paradigms is actually something we do everyday. When we leave home and go to work, we mentally shift gears from our household rules to our work-setting rules. We accept, and quite naturally, that different settings have different structures, where a change in approach applies.

Working with alternative therapies is no different. Traversing from one theory to another is just like "switching hats," something most health professionals know how to do quite well. Another example is shifting from one language to another; for example, from English to Spanish. Both say the same thing, but in different ways, and filtered through the culture of the mother tongue.

Perhaps the easiest way to reconcile the notion of alternative therapies and alternative perspectives is to use Venn diagrams as presented in the illustration.

The human body existed before allopathic medicine began. Allopathic medicine has made tremendous strides in explaining and manipulating the body's function, yet there is far more to know. The large circle symbolizes the body and all there is to know. The somewhat smaller circle symbolizes what we currently know in a mainstream medical framework. Given the current perspective of allopathic medicine, it is likely that all there is to know cannot be reached, as some aspects of its function lie outside of current theory. Current theory and knowledge therefore must expand.

Alternative medicine approaches the body from different theoretical perspectives. It is likely that it too has gleaned some understanding of the body. Some of its understanding intersects with the allopathic perspective and some lies outside of the bounds of allopathic theory. Some of this perspective is entirely outside the bounds of mainstream medicine, with no reconcilable bridge.

These are all subsets of the whole. Combining differing perspectives allow the whole to be perceived when one perspective alone cannot. Trying to explain the entire human body according to one theory is like attempting to explain particle physics by Newtonian mechanics. The nature of particle probabilities simply requires a different viewpoint because

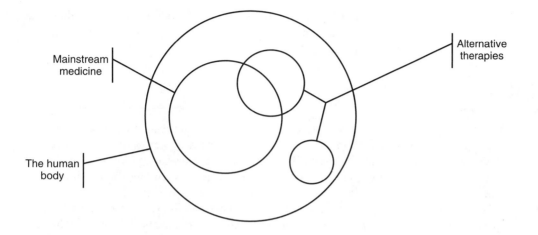

the behavior of real life exceeds the capabilities of one theory alone. In the same way, combining multiple health perspectives maximizes the opportunity to discern the problem and work towards its solution. A complementary medical approach has more to offer than either allopathic or alternative approaches alone. Physicists accept multiple theories. Psychologists work commonly with different theories. Why can't we?

Learning while Unlearning

Happily, many medical alternatives are well documented with allopathic model studies. The neophyte can enter the nontraditional world by clinging to the scientific model that is the basis for modern health care. Once aboard, the initiate can then branch out into other areas where there is less attachment to scientific basis.

Learning alternative medicine theory is both simple and difficult. The simplicity of alternative medicine theory lies in its fairly good internal consistency. As mentioned earlier, most of the therapies in this text touch on one or more of the fundamental naturopathic principles.

Learning alternative medicine is difficult because it is different from mainstream medicine. Concepts such as detoxification and energy are rather foreign to mainstream practitioners. At first, treating some ailments by alternative methods feels like scratching one's foot to relieve an itch on the nose. At first, it just does not compute! As the concepts sink in, and particularly when results are seen in our patients, openness develops. The internal dialogue usually sounds something like, "Holy cow, what if this stuff works?"

Unlearning means the ability to loosen perspectives and accept that there is more to learn, not only in facts, but in perspectives. The reader will find this a gratifying change, as it inherently embraces the humanity of the patient and forces us to look at the whole picture.

One of the easiest ways to unlearn is to ask plenty of questions. Physicians tend to ask questions when information challenges an existing paradigm. The visual analogy is that of rubbing a crayon on paper with a penny underneath. The boundaries become visible. The more clearly we can see the walls that restrict our perspective, the more easily we can see that they are merely self-imposed.

Taking a Step

Will peers, medical societies, and state boards of professional regulation frown upon this thinking? We as professionals may have great difficulty with answering these questions, but the patient consumer will demand our investigation into these uncomfortable, uncharted waters. This author recommends a dual-thinking approach. Consider the patient's problem from multiple perspectives, both allopathic and alternative. To avoid the allopathic perspective is to run the risk of missed or delayed diagnosis. To avoid the alternative perspective often is to miss the underlying cause, even *beneath* the medical diagnosis. Through readings, clinical experience, and through mentoring with trusted practitioners, this knowledge can be gained. If we are truly the patient's advocate, as our oath suggests, then we must sample the waters and lands that are presently foreign to us. Physicians of today now must become the Columbus and Magellan of yesteryear if they are to keep pace with the demands of modern health care.

Above all else, remember: alternative medicine is not magic. It is simply another set of useful tools to assist with patient care. Apply a balanced and thoughtful perspective and both the patient and the health professional will benefit.

Integration

DONALD W. NOVEY*

A LTHOUGH THIS DISCUSSION is written primarily for mainstream physicians, it can apply to any practice wishing to broaden its offerings to include complementary medicine.

Learning More

The incorporation of complementary medicine into regular practice can occur on several levels of involvement. Many physicians wonder where to begin. The best way is to survey the playing field, a vista this book hopes to provide.

The first question to ask is whether you wish to be involved with complementary medicine and to what degree. By virtue of the interest our patients have on the subject, and their questions on supplements and nontraditional therapies, we need to know enough to be at least conversationally literate on the subject.

The next decision is whether you wish to provide alternative therapies yourself or simply become knowledgeable in learning ways to refer to them. If you wish to learn a particular form of therapy and perform it within your practice, refer to the sections on training and credentialing in each therapy discussion, which will direct you to associations or resources for formal training. Learning a therapy effectively, however, can take years of study and practice. Even if you do learn one particular method, you will still need some literacy in others, at least enough to effectively refer when needed. One form of alternative therapy is not sufficient for complementary care.

Borrowing from the primary care-specialist model, the most practical way to learn effective alternative medicine referral is to build relationships with nontraditional practitioners. This often presents opportunities for firsthand observation and for frank discussion on patients seen and areas of particular success. A great deal of practical clinical information is learned during casual encounters with our medical colleagues. In the hospital environment, these brief conversations are often called "curbside consults." Building relation-

*The author wishes to express his thanks to Mitchell J. Ghen, DO, PhD, for his valuable input in the writing of Section One of this text.

ships with nontraditional providers will provide this same opportunity. When your alternative providers are only a phone call away, you can learn quickly and ask questions as they arise.

Working with the Medical Community

Before introducing alternative medicine modalities into a formal medical setting, this author would like to offer a few suggestions to smooth the process. Many difficulties that can potentially arise from a clash of cultures can be avoided by a few simple steps.

1. Perform a needs assessment. Are at least 25% of your colleagues open to the possibility of access to alternative therapy modalities? If there is no openness, such services can still be offered, but the setting in which they are offered will be isolated from the medical community.
2. Frankly discuss your colleagues' concerns. Most physicians' concerns fall into the following categories.

   - Delay in proper care: "My patients will risk missed or delayed diagnosis because they are not seeing a physician."
   - Poor communication: "How do I know what is happening to my patient?"
   - Lack of qualifications: "Who is doing this therapy? What is their training? How do I know if they are any good?"
   - Only in it for the money: "This practitioner keeps making my patient come back, and it's expensive."
   - Ineffective: "It's all placebo effect, anyway."

These are legitimate concerns, but are easily addressed with a properly structured set of services. A truly complementary approach offers the following answers, in order.

   - Complementary care is physician supervised. Reputable alternative practitioners know their limits and will quickly alert the physician if no improvement is made or the practitioner senses an unexpected outcome. Whether the alternative practitioners work in the same facility or separately, a closely-knit team of providers who are willing to learn from each other is the very safest option for the patient.
   - Alternative practitioners can communicate as effectively as other health care providers. Ideally, consultation and communication letters should be sent routinely from either a supervising physician or from the practitioner to the referring physician. In the author's own center, communication letters are sent to the patient's primary physician even if self-referred, as long as the patient consents.
   - If you are not qualified for a therapy, choose practitioners who are. The less you know, the more they need to know, and that translates into years of experience. Finding good alternative practitioners requires interviews, a thorough screening process, and reference checks. This is clearly one of the critical steps.

- Reputable practitioners, whether allopathic or alternative, perform care because it is indicated. When therapy is no longer needed or if it is ineffective, they stop. Many alternative therapists also set a time limit to evaluate the effectiveness of therapy and clearly communicate this time limit to the referring physician.
- Many alternative therapies are remarkably effective. A considerable body of literature is available to support their value. Watching these therapies succeed can be a humbling experience because this challenges the belief common to physicians that they understand the body.

3. Be very clear on the licensing laws of your state. Not all states license all modalities. Try to focus on therapies that are locally licensed or possess a national credentialing that is recognized locally.

Incorporating the Medical Model

A complementary medicine center can offer a great service to community physicians. Many physicians appreciate a reliable resource for questions on nontraditional therapies, and on details regarding herbs and supplements. Physicians and patients alike often feel more comfortable when these services are offered in a monitored setting. Building trust is essential to the success of such an endeavor. The incorporation of some essential features of the medical model can greatly assist in physician acceptance. The following sampling are some of the more valuable characteristics to include:

1. Provide an effective screening mechanism. Patients either should be seen initially by a physician, or discussed with the physician present through regular team meetings. A formal team approach allows practitioners to become more cross-literate in other modalities and also allows team members to discern if something has been missed by a treating practitioner. This screening process goes both ways. The physician inherently can overlook details important to other alternative practitioners and learn much from discussion in an environment of mutual respect.
2. If practitioners operate within the same center, perform an active chart review. Review the work done by other practitioners if possible. The fastest way to learn about their modality is through exposure to their terminology and treatment strategies.
3. Communicate diligently with area physicians. Communication letters are a powerful statement. They say "We are here, and we appreciate your input on the care we are providing." Such letters are also a powerful educational tool. Just as a physician looks to letters from consultants as an educational encounter, so can be correspondence with a complementary medicine facility. Such gentle education often raises interest or curiosity in the complementary medicine thought process. It initiates familiarity, which can lead to trust, and a more open referral stream.
4. Clearly delineate goals of therapy, its planned duration, and an alternative plan should initial treatment fail. State this in initial communications, whether in verbal or letter format, and provide a progress report on follow-up letters.

5. Ensure that patients receive realistic counsel. Such assurance begins with selecting the right practitioners who appreciate the strengths and weaknesses of their own profession. Many patients come to complementary medicine centers with unrealistic expectations or with magical thinking. Like any form of healing, alternative medicine has its limits. Patients must be asked clearly what they expect from alternative medicine and clearly but gently counseled on what is realistically possible.

6. Any center that offers complementary medicine should consider itself a community resource, not only for its patients, but also for all area health care professionals. An expanding file of literature and references on the subject provide a great service to local practitioners. Resources also can be made available to patients through a lending library. Additionally, education builds trust, which is a key element in the integration of complementary medicine.

7. Provide educational opportunities for area physicians and residency programs through training opportunities. Exposure to active, ongoing alternative therapies is a powerful educational stimulant and often accelerates the awareness of and curiosity about these modalities. Like many of the above measures, it also helps to build trust. In the author's center, residents rotate through the center regularly, and area physicians who express interest are invited to attend team meetings.

8. Refer back to mainstream colleagues when indicated. Truly complementary medicine is a two-way referral process. For some aspects of care, alternative approaches work best. For others, more mainstream approaches are more appropriate. This activity sends a powerful message to the medical community: the center and its practitioners are part of a larger team that includes area medical colleagues.

9. Consider becoming a research site. Only a handful of complementary medicine facilities perform research. Much improvement is needed in this area. Few activities strengthen the stature and therefore the longevity of a complementary medicine center better than education and ongoing research.

Integrating Yourself

As mentioned in the preface, contact with alternative medicine often results in personal experiences. Consider this a necessity. Personal exposure to alternative therapies greatly assists the new learner in understanding the modality, and in appreciating its strengths and weaknesses. Once past the initial shock of learning something completely different, the inquisitive mind can reengage and expand its perspective of the body and of healing.

As the walls of our thinking are challenged, they can reform. At least in medicine, what is real depends upon the chosen perspective. Each form of alternative therapy provides a different viewpoint on a larger whole. Thinking "outside the box" does not mean throwing away the box. It simply means having more ways than one to think about healing. Let your own process begin.

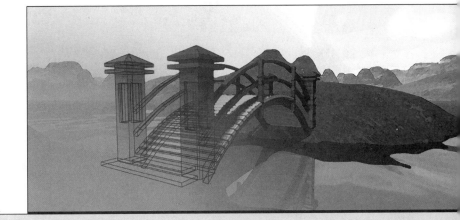

Fields of Practice

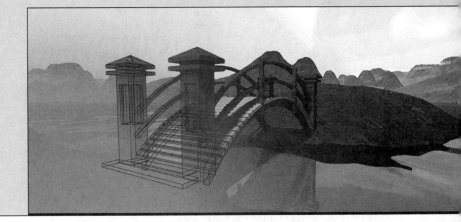

Mind-Body
Interventions

Art Therapy,   20

Biofeedback,   32

Dance/Movement Therapy,   41

Hypnotherapy,   53

Interactive Guided Imagery^{sm},   64

Meditation,   73

Music Therapy,   86

Neuro Linguistic Programming,   96

Poetry Therapy,   105

Relaxation Therapies,   114

Spiritual Healing and Prayer,   130

Yoga,   141

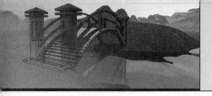

Art Therapy

ELLEN G. HOROVITZ

Origins and History

Although visual expressions have been basic to humanity throughout history, art therapy did not emerge as a distinct profession until the 1930s. At the beginning of the twentieth century many psychiatrists studied the artwork created by their patients in an attempt to understand the link between art and illness.[1,2] In the 1940s Naumburg ushered in the use of art materials as a psychodynamic tool to mediate psychotherapy. Naumburg believed that artwork constituted symbolic speech and used the art media to verbally engage her patients.[3,4] In the 1950s Kramer pioneered the idea of using "art as therapy."[5,6] She emphasized the art process as a way to stimulate sublimation and partially neutralize conflict among her patients. In 1967 Kwiatkowska introduced family art therapy and engaged her patients in a family systems orientation.[7]

Since then, the profession of art therapy has grown into an effective and important method of communication, producing a variety of cognitive, developmental, multicultural, and psychodynamically oriented art therapy assessments and treatment.[8-15]

Mechanism of Action According to Its Own Theory

The American Art Therapy Association (AATA)'s website (www.arttherapy.org) provides the following definition of *art therapy*:

> Art Therapy is a human service profession that uses art media, images, the creative art process, and patient/client responses to the created products as reflections of an individual's development, abilities, personality, interests, concerns, and conflicts. Art therapy practice is based on knowledge of human developmental and psychological theories that are implemented in the full spectrum of models of assessment and treatment including educational, psychodynamic, cognitive, transpersonal, and other therapeutic means of reconciling emotional conflicts, fostering self-awareness, developing social skills, managing behavior, solving problems, reducing anxiety, aiding reality orientation, and increasing self-esteem. Art therapy is an effective treatment for the developmentally, medically, educationally, socially, or psychologically impaired; and is practiced in mental health, rehabilitation, medical, educational, and forensic institutions. Populations of all ages, races, and ethnic backgrounds are served by art therapists in individual, couples, family, and group therapy formats.

Although the studio space may offer an outlet for joyous productivity, often the art does not. The art can be riddled with a litany of unwanted guests, each clawing to get out and be received, which can split the artistic temperament. The artwork may reflect this confusion. Nevertheless this confusion can yield to increased integration and produce healthy results. Although the work may be harrowing, the results can create a more harmonious human being.

Every line and erasure represent individual meaning. Therefore it is imperative to know the art, the materials used, its language, and its message to translate its meaning for each individual.[16] Self-examination and self-process becomes the railway to transformation of the self. The art medium becomes the taskmaster. The difficulty lies not in the message bearer but in the receiver. One must be art, otherwise the message is recursive and ill-received. According to Moon, this capacity to be an "imageorator" allows the art to be the healing agent.[17] This evocative power of art can transcend a powerful antidote and contribute to the wellness of another person's soul. The therapist merely becomes the messenger-orator; nothing more, nothing less. It is the art that becomes the catalyst for healing per force the language between patient and therapist.[18]

Biologic Mechanism of Action

Whenever a symbol operates, there is meaning. Depictions, no less than words, are forms of symbolic expression. Just as the writer uses words, the artist uses the plastic elements of form, space, line, texture, and color. Representation requires the review of experiences and clarification of impressions that call memory into play. Like words, visual symbols preserve ideas that might otherwise vanish. For the "linguistically challenged," pictures are a way of depicting the knowledge base while simultaneously sharing it with others. Many art therapists have claimed that art develops reasoning power by requiring organization and the constant exercise of judgment.

Art does more than reveal emotions. By providing release from emotional tension, art has proven to be both integrating and healing.*

For example, when working with imagery created by a sexually abused patient, the rendering often uncovers repressed memories and triggers discourse around the trauma. The art jolts every fiber of the collective being, bridging the gap between sight and smell, touch and sound. By unlocking the emotional playing field, art becomes purposeful and multilayered. The healing process affects every aspect of a person's being, from cognitive development to visual recall.

Forms of Therapy

As stated earlier, there are many different approaches to art therapy, but the following approaches are used most often by today's practitioner. One approach uses the process rather than product to lead the patient toward neutralization of conflict through sublimation. A

---

*References 3, 6, 10, 11, 16, 17, 19-24, 32.

second approach uses the art as a vehicle to moderate symbolic speech and moves the patient toward verbalization of inner conflicts. A third approach, Rhyne's Gestalt Art Therapy, is a group-oriented human potential movement. A fourth approach, family art therapy, uses a systems-oriented modality.[25] Although these areas created a template for art therapy, there have been a variety of theorists that have spun off from these categories. These theorists usually operate from an eclectic viewpoint and may borrow from several different theoretic constructs. The results have produced such interests as developmental art therapy,[26] cognitive-based art therapy,[14] studio art therapy,[16-18,27-30,40] and spiritual art therapy.[21]

Demographics

Between 1996 and 1997 the AATA conducted a survey compiled by Rauch and Elkins.[35] The result was a 42.3% return that represented 49 of the 50 states as well as the District of Columbia. North Dakota was the only state not represented by at least one art therapist. International membership in AATA was assembled from Canada, Israel, the United Kingdom, Switzerland, Japan, The Netherlands, New Zealand, Australia, Brazil, Guatemala, Indonesia, Korea, Norway, Saipan, Saudi Arabia, Thailand, and Taiwan. In the U.S., the largest membership demographics came from New York (298), followed by California (297), Illinois (137), Pennsylvania (127), and New Jersey (90).[39]

The majority of respondents (approximately 40%) were in private practice; 22% worked with mental health inpatients, 21% worked with mental health outpatients, and 17% worked in other settings, such as homeless shelters, physical rehabilitation centers, adult day care and senior care centers, correctional facilities, domestic violence shelters, hospices, group homes, skilled nursing homes, hospital medical units, drug and alcohol centers, art studios, public schools, community and social service agencies, mental health day treatment centers, and universities.

Indications and Reasons for Referral

Primarily, art therapy has been thought to serve as an auxiliary or ancillary treatment to verbal psychotherapy with emotionally disturbed populations of varying pathologies. Yet there have been many instances where art therapy has become the modality of choice. Multiple cases have been cited in the literature that span numerous diagnoses, such as autism, posttraumatic stress disorder, dissociative identity disorder, attention deficit hyperactivity disorder, and obsessive-compulsive disorder. Reasons for referral also can include physiologic conditions, such as developmental, cognitive, and enhancement of gross or fine motor coordination. For example, the repeated movements of an off-loom weaving activity can be both soothing and organizing for patients engaged in self-harming behavior, such as cutting or trichotillomania. Repetitive activities often regulate the self-harming maxim and replace injurious behavior with socially acceptable ones, such as knitting.

The following situations seem to be the main reasons for referral: 1) replacement for aggressive and socially unacceptable behaviors (ART—aggressive replacement therapy);

2) refusal to participate in traditional verbal psychotherapeutic interventions; and 3) generalized anxiety disorders, pervasive developmental disorders (for example, Asperger's syndrome and Rett syndrome), and mood disorders. The art therapist working with families needs to be well schooled in family systems dynamics and often needs to be prepared to involve community members such as clergy that are important contributors to a family's belief system.[19]

Office Applications

As previously stated, art therapy may be beneficial in certain diagnoses. As with all alternative therapies, the use of art therapy does not preclude the use of mainstream medical therapies. The following diagnoses are a guide for the medical or referring practitioner:

Adjustment disorder; antisocial behavior; agoraphobia; Alzheimer's disease; anxiety disorders; autistic disorders; bipolar disorders; borderline personality disorder; body dysmorphic disorder; cognitive disorders; depressive personality disorder; attention deficit and disruptive behavior disorders; eating disorders; elective mutism; impulse control disorders; learning disorders (specifically dyslexia); mood disorders; schizoaffective disorders; sexual abuse; sexual dysfunction; trichotillomania; and obsessive-compulsive disorders

The populations most often served by art therapy are behaviorally or emotionally disturbed individuals (32%); abused and neglected children (25%); and the general population (22%).[9] Other populations include runaways; homeless; gays, lesbians, and bisexuals; sex offenders; neurologic diseases and head injuries; AIDS and HIV; physical and sensory impairments; domestic violence; medical and chronic illness; eating disorders; Alzheimer and geriatric; developmentally delayed; and learning disabilities. With this list and a working knowledge of the *Diagnostic and Statistical Manual IV* (DSM-IV), a clinician can make an educated referral to an art therapist, knowing that such patients would most likely benefit from art therapy services.

Practical Applications

Art therapy has been effective when traditional forms of verbal psychotherapy have failed or been rejected by a patient. Additionally, art therapy can be effective with patients who have difficulty expressing feelings or use verbalization as a defense mechanism. This modality has been used with a variety of patient populations, ranging from inpatient psychiatric patients to community-based treatment. Art therapists are employed in schools, prisons, residential treatment centers, day treatment programs, community-based and group home placements, therapeutic foster care programs, geriatric facilities, AIDS units, pediatric hospital units, burn units, trauma and emergency units, outpatient treatment facilities, and private practice. These are just some of the multiple possibilities for art therapy treatment.

Research Base

Evidence-Based and Basic Science

In the recent text *Art-Based Research*, McNiff[32] covered the field of art therapy and discussed various research behaviors including practitioner research, artistic knowing, amplification of research as based on case studies, qualitative methods, heuristic and phenomenologic research, and empirically-based studies. Moreover, there recently has been a move toward using outcome-based measures to document the efficacy of art therapy–based treatment. Outcome-based assessment tools have been developed because measurement of outcomes in psychotherapy have presented a number of difficulties, such as somewhat high remission rates from patients with psychologic profiles and disorders,[33] diverse treatment approaches, different levels of psychotherapeutic interventions (for example, family, individual, intrapsychic, behavioral, and physiologic), the varying elements in each of these types of interventions (any of which can be typified as an outcome-based measure), and the lack of diagnostic agreement among clinicians.[34]

Risk and Safety

As previously stated, the medical clinician should use caution when referring patients to group art therapy. Although health maintenance organizations (HMOs) proclaim the efficiency of group treatment, it is *not* always the safest or most desirable method of treatment for various pathologies. Although individual treatment may proceed more slowly than group art therapy, Asperger's syndrome, for example, demands a more individualized approach. Also, it is preferable to group patients together that are working on specific issues, such as loss groups, eating disorder groups, and siblings of cancer victims.

Art therapy can be a relatively safe and noninvasive form of treatment. However, the art therapy clinician must be well versed in art materials and methods. For example, clay can work extremely well with aggressive antisocial personalities but can cause extreme regression in other disorders (such as obsessive compulsive disorder) and should be introduced slowly and cautiously.

Efficacy

Many art therapists question whether it is possible to "measure" art, and others propose that we begin to steep our outcome-based assessment in "art-based" research.[32] Many believe that the process of measuring art products is "reductionistic" and "overlooks the richness of the art." According to Rosal, the debate centers on *"how we know what we know* about art therapy." There appear to be two ways of approaching this dilemma. One approach purports that research would "uncover, document, and substantiate the efficacy of using art in therapy and psychological assessment."[35] The other approach states that using art therapy with patients is inherently a healing approach and that anyone who has experienced this firsthand (or even anecdotally) is aware of its medicinal properties.

Future Research Opportunities and Priorities

Art therapy services are needed in halfway houses and group homes, shelters, AIDS units and programs, and pay-for-service settings.[37,38] Creative arts therapists need to identify their unique contributions and articulate ways that this information can augment education and health care reform. There are also myriad applications involving forensic applications and wholesale use of the Internet. Conceivably, practitioners could provide services (on a consultant basis) online. Because of current communications trends and technological advances, the possibilities for providing service to patients are unlimited.[18] The use of empirical data to prove the efficacy of art therapy–based treatment would be welcomed by other disciplines. The reason for this preferential research is that most disciplines are used to receiving information that is presented along more scientific lines of inquiry. Therefore the emphasis on empirically based research, balanced by the efficacy of traditional methodology, might prove to be a useful determination of art therapy, its validity, and use in treatment.

Druglike Information

Safety

As stated earlier, art therapy is a relatively safe modality but when coupled with psychopharmaceutics, the clinician needs to be careful with the art media available for patient use. The reasons are multiple and quite obvious to educated art therapists. For example, when working with patients with tuberculosis or AIDS/HIV, the art therapy office needs to be well equipped with chemicals for clean up in case of blood spill or discharged sputum. When working with an AIDS or HIV patient, an experienced art therapist would not necessarily use linoleum or wood cutting tools because of the obvious risk of injury. The practitioner also needs to be aware that ventilation for certain kinds of materials requires solvents such as turpentine, mineral spirits, and others.

Warnings, Contraindications, and Precautions

Again, as previously described.

Drug or Other Interactions

As previously described, the art therapy practitioner needs to be careful with certain media if patients are on psychotropic medicine. Nevertheless, there are not exact rules per se that explain, for example, contraindications of haldol and the intervention of art therapy. As a generality, art therapists are advised to have a copy of the latest edition of *The Pill Book*.[42] This comprehensive book lists contraindications, food interactions, usual dose versus overdose of medication, and possible side effects. This book can aid the art therapy clinician in the use of specific art media with patients who are under medical or psychotropic care.

Adverse Reactions

Adverse reactions (other than those previously described) are not something that can be matter-of-factly listed, such as with pharmaceutic drugs. Nonetheless, the art therapy clinician needs to recognize that with certain populations, such as those suffering from post-traumatic stress disorder and the like, the art materials can unleash suppressed memories and emotions. As a result the art therapist always needs to proceed cautiously and be able to understand, interpret, and interact with patients experiencing abreactions to material that surfaces from the unconscious.

Self-Help versus Professional

Entrance into the field requires a masters's degree in art therapy with a minimum of 45 credits covering specific core competencies as outlined by the AATA. Although an art therapist may use art materials for self-actualization purposes, supervision by another art therapist or experienced clinician aids exploration of family of origin issues. While the medical clinician does not need firsthand experience to treat cancer, a therapist does need a certain degree of empathy to aid a patient with mental illness. Therefore it is highly recommended that all interns be engaged in their own therapy.

Visiting a Professional

If the identified patient (IP) is a child, it is recommended to meet with a parent to construct a three-generation genogram to gather psychosocial information and a timeline. From this baseline, symptomatic behavior can be charted visually and reveal psychologic IQ, global assessment according to the DSM-IV, descriptors according to the DSM-IV such as if Axis I-V (if known), and the strengths and weaknesses of the patient's personality. The genogram also can contribute considerable information to other practitioners and often has been heralded as invaluable. According to Horovitz,[10] a few art therapy assessments, such as the Kinetic family drawing test (KFD), reveal a baseline assessment of a patient's view of self within the family constellation. The cognitive art therapy assessment (CATA) requires that patients draw, paint, and create in clay whatever they wish.[10] From the CATA, developmental levels and emotive responses to art materials can be determined. The Silver drawing test of cognitive and creative abilities (STD) corroborates findings from the CATA and has been measured against such proven psychologic tests as the WISC-R and WAIS. Thus the developmental scores concluded from the SDT offer yet another profile for the referring practitioner. If preoccupation with spiritual and religious belief is suspected, the clinician might also administer the belief art therapy assessment (BATA) to rule out religiosity as a predictor of pathology.[19] Recommendations and conclusions for treatment and type of modality to be used (individual, group, or family art therapy) can be extracted from these batteries. From this point on, art therapy sessions for an individual might resemble the following scenario.

Johnny, an 8-year-old boy who has been severely sexually abused by his biologic father since age 3, arrives at the office. He decides to use the clay material. Working with the material, he fashions a large phallus and repeatedly shoves the phallus-shaped object into a mound with a hole. Depending on the verbal associations by the patient or his readiness to receive a gentle interpretation, a choice of two treatments may follow. Weeks might be spent allowing the patient to repeat the forming of such schema and nonverbally repeat the trauma in a safe, therapeutic, and supportive environment. If Johnny verbalizes such associations such as "Help, help!" then the clinician might gently aid him toward recovery of such feelings, reenactments of the experience, and neutralization of the conflict. Naturally, these variables depend on the patient's readiness for movement and the experience of the art therapy clinician. For detailed explanations of case studies such as these, see Horovitz 1983[43]; Horovitz-Darby 1991[11]; Horovitz-Darby 1992; Horovitz-Darby 1994[19]; and Horovitz 1999.[18]

Credentialing

As previously stated, at the national level the Art Therapy Credentialing Board (ATCB) has a yearly board certification (BC) examination that is offered to any art therapist registered (ATR). Applicants may apply for registration after meeting the educational requirements to enter the field plus having satisfied the criterion of undergoing 1000 hours of paid work with a patient population. (Note: Of the 1000 total hours, for 500 of them, the applicant must be supervised by an ATR.) After completion of the ATR application, the applicant may be allowed to sit for the BC exam.

Training

There are approximately 28 graduate schools in the U.S. approved by the AATA. There are also very specialized formats for supervision of students at all graduate programs approved by the AATA. These include 1 hour of supervision for every 10 hours of patient contact (individually) and group supervision with a 7:1 student-faculty ratio. For a more detailed breakdown of training programs as well as educational standards, brochures may be obtained from the AATA (E-mail: arttherapy@ntr.net, or visit the AATA website at www.arttherapy.org).

What to Look for in a Provider

Clinicians should choose art therapy practitioners that 1) have formal training in art therapy; 2) hold membership in the AATA (directories may be purchased from the national organization and are generally updated every 2 years); and 3) preferably have obtained the credentials of ATR (art therapist registered) from the ATCB (Art Therapy Credentialing Board).

Barriers and Key Issues

Licensing seems to be the key barrier that has kept art therapy from receiving the recognition that it so widely deserves. Nevertheless, this situation appears to be changing as more states have accepted the BC (board certification) exam as credentialing for licenses. For example, art therapists can qualify as licensed professional art therapists by taking the ATCB certification exam in New Mexico and in many more states. For a complete listing by state, the reader should visit the AATA website at www.arttherapy.org.

Associations

American Art Therapy Association (AATA)
1202 Allanson Rd.
Mundelein, IL 60060
Tel: (847) 949-6064
Toll-Free: (888) 290-0878
Fax: (847) 566-4580
E-mail: arttherapy@ntr.net
www.arttherapy.org

Art Therapy Credentials Board (ATCB)
3 Terrace Way, Suite B
Greensboro, NC 27043
Toll-Free: (877) 217-ATCB
Fax: (336) 547-0017
E-mail: info@atcb.org
www.atcb.org

Suggested Reading

1. Malchiodi CA: *Breaking the silence: art therapy with children from violent homes*, New York, 1997, Brunner/Mazel.

   Reviewed by Booknews, December 1, 1990: "Malchiodi, director of the Art Therapy Program at the University of Utah, demonstrates the power of art therapy as a tool for intervening with children from violent homes. The emphasis is on the short-term setting where time is at a premium and circumstances are unpredictable. Illustrated with 95 drawings by abused children." (Annotation copyright Book News, Portland, Or.)

2. Allen P: *Art as a way of knowing*, Boston, 1995, Shambala.

   With practical exercises, inspirational guidance, and the author's own experiences as an artist and art therapist, this book shows how creativity can be a path to self-discovery. Allen includes information on materials and methods, plus ideas for projects using art to help express emotions.

3. Horovitz-Darby EG: *Spiritual art therapy: an alternate path*, Springfield, Ill, 1994, Charles C. Thomas.

   In this practical text, the clinician is offered an assessment tool that rules out religiosity as a predictor of pathology that simultaneously taps into a patient's belief system. The text offers several vignettes of inpatient and outpatient emotionally disturbed children, adolescents, and adults with a variety of pathologies.

4. Kramer E: *Art as therapy for children*, New York, 1975, Schocken.
   This classic text walks the clinician through one of the leading theories in the field, using art materials for the purpose of sublimation and neutralization of conflicts. Several cases illustrate the author's approach to individual and group art therapies.

Bibliography

Allen P: Artist-in-residence: an alternative to "clinification" for art therapists, *Art Ther* 9(1):22-29, 1992.

Henley D: A consideration of the studio as therapeutic intervention, *Art Ther* 12(3):188-190, 1995.

Hillman J: *Revisioning psychology*, New York, 1975, Harper Colophon.

Horovitz EG: Preschool aged children: when art therapy becomes the modality of choice. *Arts Psychother* 10(2):23-32, 1983.

Horovitz-Darby EG: *Spiritual art therapy: an alternate path*, Springfield, Ill, 1994, Charles C. Thomas.

Johnson DR: Establishing creative arts therapies as independent professions, *Arts Psychother* 11:209-212, 1984.

Johnson DR: Envisioning the link among the creative arts therapies, *Arts Psychother* 12:233-238, 1985.

Julliard K: Outcomes research in health care: implications for art therapy, *Art Ther* 15(1):13-21, 1998.

Junge MB, Asawa PP: *A history of art therapy in the United States*, Mundelein, Ill, 1994, American Art Therapy Association.

Kramer E: We cannot look into the future, without considering the past and present, *Art Ther* 11(9):31-101, 1994.

Lambert M, Bergin A: The effectiveness of psychotherapy. In Bergin A, Garfield S, editors: *Handbook of psychotherapy and behavior change*, ed 4, New York, 1994, Wiley.

Lowenfeld V, Brittain WL: *Creative and mental growth*, ed 3, Hampshire, England, 1957, Macmillan.

Rauch TM, Elkins DE: AATA 1996-1997 membership survey, *Art Ther* 15(3):191-202, 1998.

Rosal ML: Research thoughts: learning from the literature and experience, *Art Ther* 15(1):47-50, 1998.

Silverman HM: *The pill book: the illustrated guide to the most-prescribed drugs in the United States*, ed 8, New York, 1998, Bantam.

Wadeson H: Question: will art therapy survive universal health coverage reform? *Art Ther* 11:26-32, 1994.

Williams G, Wood M: *Developmental art therapy*, Austin, 1977, Pro-Ed.

Wix L: The intern studio project: a pilot study, *Art Ther* 12(3):175-178, 1995.

References

1. Prinzhorn H: *Artistry of the mentally ill,* translated by von Brockdorff E., New York, 1972, Springer-Verlag. (Originally published in German, 1922).

2. Arnheim R: *Visual thinking,* Berkeley, Calif, 1969, University of California Press.

3. Naumburg M: *Dynamically oriented art therapy: its principles and practices,* New York, 1966, Grune and Stratton.

4. Naumburg M: *An introduction to art therapy: studies of the 'free' art expression of behavioral problem children and adolescents as a means of diagnosis and therapy,* New York, 1973, Teacher's College Press.

5. Kramer E: *Art therapy in a children's community: a study of the function of art therapy in the treatment program of Wiltwyck School for boys,* Springfield, Ill, 1958, Charles C. Thomas.

6. Kramer E: *Art as therapy for children,* New York, 1975, Schocken.

7. Kwiatkowska HY: Family art therapy, *Family Process* 6:37-55, 1967.

8. Cohen BM: *Multiple personality disorder from the inside out,* Lutherville, Md, 1991, Sidran.

9. Hiscox A, Calisch AC: *Tapestry of cultural issues in art therapy,* London, 1998, Jessica Kingsley.

10. Horovitz EG: Short-term family art therapy: a case study. In Watson D et al, editors: *Two decades of excellence: a foundation for the future,* Little Rock, 1988, American Deafness and Rehabilitation Association.

11. Horovitz-Darby EG: Family art therapy within a deaf system, *Arts Psychother* 18:251-261, 1991.

12. Landgarten HB: *Magazine photo collage: a multicultural assessment and treatment technique,* New York, 1993, Brunner/Mazel.

13. Rubin JA: *Child art therapy: understanding and helping children grow through art,* New York, 1997, Wiley.

14. Silver RA: *Silver drawing test of cognition and emotion,* Fla, 1996, Ablin.

15. Ulman E, Dachinger P: *Art therapy: in theory and practice,* New York, 1975, Schocken.

16. Allen P: *Art as a way of knowing,* Boston, 1995, Shambala.

17. Moon BL: *Art and soul: an artistic psychology,* Springfield, Ill, 1996, Charles C. Thomas.

18. Horovitz EG: *A leap of faith: the call to art,* Springfield, Ill, 1999, Charles C. Thomas.

19. Horovitz-Darby EG: *Spiritual art therapy: an alternate path,* Springfield, Ill, 1994, Charles C. Thomas.

20. Moon BL: *Existential art therapy: the canvas mirror,* Springfield, Ill, 1990, Charles C. Thomas.

21. Rubin JA: *The art of art therapy,* New York, 1984, Brunner/Mazel.

22. Silver RA: *Art and the deaf. Bulletin of art therapy,* Washington, DC, 1970, Ulman.

23. Silver RD: *Shout in silence, visual arts and the deaf,* Rye, NY, 1976, Silver Publications.

24. Silver RA: *Developing cognitive and creative skills through art,* Baltimore, 1978.

25. Kwiatkowska HY: Family art therapy, *Family Process* 6:37-55, 1967.

26. Williams G, Wood M: *Developmental art therapy,* Austin, 1977, Pro-Ed.

27. Allen P: Artist-in-residence: an alternative to "clinification" for art therapists, *Art Ther* 9(1):22-29, 1992.

28. Junge MB, Linesch D: Our own voices: new paradigms for art therapy research, *Arts Psychother* 21(1):61-67, 1993.

29. Henley D: A consideration of the studio as therapeutic intervention, *Art Ther* 12(3):188-190, 1995.

30. Wix L: The intern studio project: a pilot study, *Art Ther* 12(3):175-178, 1995.

31. Rauch TM, Elkins DE: AATA 1996-1997 membership survey, *Art Ther* 15(3):191-202, 1998.

32. McNiff S, Malchiodi CA: *Art-based research,* London, 1998, Jessica Kingsley.

33. Lambert M, Bergin A: The effectiveness of psychotherapy. In Bergin A, Garfield S, editors: *Handbook of psychotherapy and behavior change,* ed 4, New York, 1994, Wiley.

34. Julliard K: Outcomes research in health care: implications for art therapy, *Art Ther* 15(1):13-21, 1998.

35. Rosal ML: Research thoughts: learning from the literature and experience, *Art Ther* 15(1):47-50, 1998.

36. Kramer E: We cannot look into the future, without considering the past and present, *Art Ther* 11(9):91-101, 1994.

37. Wadeson H: Question: will art therapy survive universal health coverage reform? *Art Ther* 11:26-32, 1994.

38. Silverman HM: *The pill book, the illustrated guide to the most-prescribed drugs in the United States,* ed 8, New York, 1998, Bantam.

39. Horovitz EG: Preschool-aged children: when art therapy becomes the modality of choice, *Arts Psychother* 10(2):23-32, 1983.

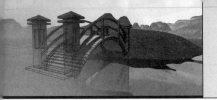

Biofeedback

MARY JO SABO

JIM GIORGI

Origins and History

Psychophysiology is the study of relations between psychologic manipulations and resulting physiologic responses measured in the body.

Biofeedback can be defined as the science of applied psychophysiology. The overall goal of biofeedback is to produce the desired psychophysiologic changes in the body. The long-term goal is the reduction or elimination of problematic symptoms and behaviors. Biofeedback's efficacy is based on a conceptually simple principle: awareness equals control. If a typically unconscious and involuntary physiologic response (for example, skin temperature, blood pressure, and brain wave activity) is amplified and fed back so that an individual can become aware of its presence and magnitude, the individual then can learn to apply a level of voluntary control over that response. This voluntary control guides the response toward a more balanced and salutary level of equilibrium.

Clinical biofeedback practice began with the use of simple electronic devices housed in bulky wooden boxes with an assortment of dials and gauges. The advent of the personal computer has both streamlined the appearance of biofeedback instrumentation and made possible the collection and analysis of extensive physiologic data. Such precision was heretofore undreamed of by researchers. Armed with this new instrumentation, practitioners in the late 1980s and 1990s have enormously expanded the scope of biofeedback's clinical applications. It is now used with a wide variety of medical and psychologic conditions, as well as to promote so-called peak athletic and mental performance states.

There is nothing new about physiologic self-regulation. Such feats, although rare in the Western world, are relatively common in societies with a more visible and long-standing mystic tradition. Meditation and yoga are two examples of low-tech self-regulation techniques that have been used in the Orient for centuries, if not millennia. At the Menninger Clinic in the 1960s, Swami Rama, an Indian yogi, astounded early biofeedback researchers Elmer and Alyce Green with his seemingly effortless ability to voluntarily control blood pressure, skin temperature, heart and respiration rate, brain wave activity, and other responses. He actually stopped his heart from beating for a full 17 seconds and restarted it without any outside intervention or apparent adverse effects. Of course, this swami had spent literally years in a cave in the Himalayas perfecting his technique. The beauty of biofeedback is that through the wonder of modern computer technology, this process can be both accelerated and accomplished in a much more hospitable environment than a mountaintop cave.

The level of control possible via biofeedback can be as exquisitely precise and subtle as it is dramatic. Biofeedback pioneer John Basmajian inserted a microelectrode into a single neuron in the optic tract and provided an audible "click" to the subject every time the neuron was fired. Not only did the subject quickly learn to fire that particular neuron at will (at a rate much more highly statistically significant than chance), but the subject also was able to isolate its activity from other neurons in its proximity, simultaneously firing the designated neuron and inhibiting the firing of surrounding ones.

The earliest researchers in the field of EEG biofeedback, such as Joe Kamiya, Elmer and Alyce Green, and Les Fehmi, were primarily interested in the relationship between particular brain wave patterns and states of consciousness. Their research focused on the brain wave frequency occurring between 8 to 12 Hz, called *alpha*. Subjects trained to produce these alpha brain waves at will reported entering states of deep relaxation, creative reverie, and meditative clarity.

Mechanisms of Action According to Its Own Theory

The physiologic mechanisms by which voluntary control is exerted are neither simple nor well understood. The fact that we know that biofeedback works, but are not totally clear about the way it works, has drawn more than a fair amount of criticism from the scientific community. It is a simple matter to connect a person to, say, a thermal biofeedback instrument and request the person to raise the temperature of the finger. Despite initial protests of ignorance and pleas for a tangible strategy to help achieve the desired goal, most people find that within a few sessions they are able to raise and lower their skin temperature at will. Ask them *how* they are accomplishing this, however, and you'll probably receive a puzzled expression, a shrug, and an "I don't know, I just do it." If a person consciously tries or expends mental effort to control the response in question, the result is typically the opposite of what is desired—much like the centipede, who, when asked by the ant he was able to coordinate all those legs, became so self-conscious that he tripped all over himself and fell flat on his face. However, by simply paying attention to a display that registers the measured level of the response, eventually the person "tunes in" to an intuitive type of control that can best be likened to maintaining balance when learning to ride a bicycle. It is more of a feeling than a consciously mediated thought process. Biofeedback researchers have labeled this type of control *passive volition*.

Attention and arousal levels as mediated by the thalamic and the reticular activating systems seem to play a pivotal role in this regulatory process. Biofeedback practitioners are undeterred by the criticism, however, and are confident that decades of clinical experience and cases of sometimes dramatic improvements in their patients' various conditions have supported a demonstrable, if mysterious, efficacy to this high-tech form of self-regulation. Although biofeedback practitioners have devised numerous strategies to assist in the learning process (notably relaxation, breath control, and imagery techniques) none of these are absolutely necessary for a person to master the appropriate self-regulatory skills. Simple attention to the task seems sufficient.

Forms of Therapy

Any physiologic response that can be monitored is amenable to intervention via biofeedback techniques. Some of the more common biofeedback modalities include muscle tension or electromyography (EMG), skin temperature (thermal), skin conductance (GSR or EDR), brain wave activity (EEG), blood pressure, respiration rate, and blood flow. Treatment programs may progress from more peripheral and voluntary responses (for example, EMG) to autonomic nervous system responses (for example, thermal and EDR) to central nervous system interventions (for example, various forms of EEG biofeedback).

Demographics

Biofeedback typically has been used by health care and mental health practitioners such as physicians, nurses, physical therapists, psychologists, social workers, and trained and supervised paraprofessionals. It has been used in research, hospital, and clinical settings. The majority of biofeedback clinicians in the U.S. are located in urban and suburban settings. Practitioners can be found in universities, colleges, hospital settings, and private clinics. Biofeedback was originally intended to be an adjunct to counseling, psychotherapy, and behavioral management techniques. With the advent of computers many other professionals such as hypnotherapists, marriage counselors, and stress management counselors have incorporated EEG biofeedback in their practices. Biofeedback's applicability as an appropriate treatment modality extends across all ages, genders, races, and diagnostic categories of patients.

Indications and Reasons for Referral

Biofeedback has multiple applications that are commonly divided according to the type of biofeedback technique applied, as presented in the table. As with all alternative therapies, use of biofeedback does not preclude the use of mainstream medical therapies.

Practical Applications

Biofeedback is usually used in a medical office where the physician is able to monitor the patient's treatment plan on a weekly basis. Many of the patients seeking this type of treatment have tried several other modalities to no avail. Physicians feel comfortable prescribing biofeedback because of its noninvasive technique. When used as an adjunct therapy in a private practice setting, biofeedback proves to be a procedure that works best when directed by a caring, supportive staff member. For this reason, physicians may train several

Type of Biofeedback Therapy	Examples of Diagnoses Treated
Electromyography	Tension headaches
	Muscle spasms
	Hypertension
	Back pain
	Urinary and fecal incontinence
	Muscle and motor rehabilitation
	Spinal cord rehabilitation
	Asthma
Thermal temperature	Migraine headaches
	Raynauds disease
	Hypertension
	Stress management
Electrodermal response	Stress management
	Chronic pain
	Anxiety disorders
	Panic disorder
Electroencephalography	Epilepsy and related seizure disorders
	Sleep disorders
	Closed head injuries
	Psychologic disorders (anxiety, depression, psychosis, conduct disorders)
	Attention deficit disorder
	Attention deficit hyperactivity disorder
	Learning disabilities
	Posttraumatic stress disorder
	Alcoholism and substance abuse disorders
	Endocrinological disorders
	Autoimmune disorders
	Sleep disorders
	Autism
	Chronic pain
	Headaches
	Muscle spasms
	Fibromyalgia
	Multiple chemical sensitivities

staff members to administer the treatment. In many instances, patients return in a timely fashion for their biofeedback sessions because the therapy is very calming and symptoms are often alleviated.

Research Base

Evidence Based

Scientific research in the field of biofeedback has been ongoing and expanding since the middle of the twentieth century. Basmajian[1] and Peper[2] have been major contributors in the field of EMG biofeedback. In the rapidly emerging field of EEG biofeedback, Kamiya,

Fehmi, Sterman, Lubar, Tansey, and Ochs have been in the forefront of the advancement of scientific research to validate biofeedback's efficacy.

Kamiya and Fehmi[3] led some of the earliest research in the field of alpha brain wave biofeedback and its relationship to states of consciousness and attentional orientation. Sterman performed the original research that demonstrated the effectiveness of sensory motor rhythm training as a treatment for epilepsy. Lubar[4] devised the first studies that showed success of EEG Biofeedback with attention deficit hyperactivity disorder (ADHD). Tansey[5] further extended this research using EEG biofeedback for attention deficit disorder (ADD) as well as specific learning disabilities. Ochs currently has developed an advanced form of biofeedback training that uses subthreshold photic stimulation correlated with real time EEG recordings to maximize brain wave flexibility.

Risk and Safety

Biofeedback is one of the safest treatment modalities among the healing repertoires. The history of biofeedback indicates practically no adverse reactions on record. No law suits have ever been successfully litigated for malpractice against biofeedback practitioners. This is because biofeedback simply is a noninvasive, painless learning technique that does not attempt to externally control normal metabolism or physiology. Nearly 70% of the patients using this modality achieve observable, clinically effective results and the average level of amelioration of frequency, intensity, and duration of symptoms is approximately 70%.

Future Research Opportunities and Priorities

Future research in biofeedback would include the following directions:

1. To scientifically validate its efficacy in large scale controlled studies in the conditions for which it is now being used clinically.
2. To identify with greater specificity treatment protocols in conditions for which it is currently being used.
3. To expand applications to other conditions that currently are not being treated with biofeedback.

Druglike Information

Biofeedback is nondrug and noninvasive, and would be considered one of the lesser-risk treatments a physician could prescribe for a patient.

Self-Help versus Professional

Biofeedback should be administered by a trained professional. Most biofeedback technicians are supervised by a medical clinician with a basic knowledge of biofeedback. It is always advisable to seek a trained person when using this type of therapy. Many physicians send their staff to training and certification programs. Insurance companies require training and ask for credentials before they will reimburse for services. Biofeedback is computerized and staff members must learn to use the software packages before they start to train patients.

Visiting a Professional

Patients first visit with the primary practitioner, who then prescribes a series of biofeedback sessions. For stress management, 10 sessions may be prescribed; some people may feel relief after the initial session. For ADD, 40 sessions may be prescribed in order to reach results. Patients are usually seen twice each week. Most biofeedback sessions are conducted by a trained professional who attempts to help the client feel relaxed.

The therapist instructs the patient as to what is expected during the sessions and usually shows the patient the way to achieve results. The computer feeds back the information to the patient in the form of visual and auditory feedback.

Some software packages include games that are programmed to feed back rewards when the patient achieves the desired results. The setting is friendly and the equipment is usually in a quiet room where the patient may sit and train privately. The biofeedback therapist stays in the room with the patient and gives verbal clues to let the patient know that the goals are being achieved. Music may be played in the background to help the patient relax. Positive reinforcement is an integral part of the training. With children, some small form of reward, such as stickers, may be given after the training if desired results are achieved. During the initial session the patient is taught diaphragmatic breathing to help with the relaxation response. Most patients leave the biofeedback room feeling more in control of their bodies.

Credentialing and Training

There are many private biofeedback schools throughout the U.S. that train and certify clinicians. There is no license needed to practice biofeedback in the U.S. but most insurance companies will only reimburse if a licensed practitioner prescribes and supervises the biofeedback technician.

The Biofeedback Certification Institute of America (BCIA), located in Wheat Ridge, Colorado, is presently the only certifying agency. However, it currently does not monitor practitioners and so many people rely on interviews or referrals to guide them in the selection process. BCIA has an examination and requires supervision hours for a therapist to be certified. At this time, BCIA only accept professionals in their credentialing process. Each state has a biofeedback society that is part of a national organization, the American Association of Psychophysiology and Biofeedback (AAPB). The AAPB is one of the largest organizations in the U.S. that holds annual seminars and conferences.

Futurehealth and SSNR (Society for Sensory and Neuronal Regulation) are two other organizations that hold annual EEG neurofeedback conferences. These organizations help inform the biofeedback community and present research at their meetings. They hold several training programs for interested practitioners, given throughout the U.S. and abroad.

The following organizations are useful sources of training:

American Biotec Corporation
24 Browning Dr.
Ossining, NY 10562
Tel: (914) 762-4646
www.mindfitness.com

Biofeedback Consultants
119 Rockland Center, Suite 411
Nanuet, NY 10977
Tel: (914) 369-7627
www.TheRippleEffect.org

EEG Spectrum
16100 Ventura Blvd., Suite 3
Encino, CA 91436
Tel: (818) 891-6789
www.eegspectrum.com

Futurehealth
3171 Rail Ave.
Trevose, PA 19053
Tel: (215) 364-4445
www.Futurehealth.org

What to Look for in a Provider

When visiting a professional it is best to seek out someone who has been certified by the BCIA, one of the few agencies with strict requirements for certification. A rigorous examination and supervised training is required before someone may receive BCIA certification.

Barriers and Key Issues

Exciting developments in the past 10 years of biofeedback therapy points to the potential for even more widespread applicability and effectiveness in the future. The advent of a medical philosophy that recognizes the innate healing potential of a person's own mind and body promises to become the ultimate medical breakthrough. With biofeedback and other self-regulation modalities, we hold the key to unlocking that potential. At the very least biofeedback represents an alternative first line response to a wide variety of conditions and symptoms. Such a response maintains a basic trust in the patient's innate healing potential and defers an automatic reliance on more invasive, pharmacologic, or surgical interventions.

Associations

Association for Applied Psychophysiology and Biofeedback
10200 West 44th Ave. #304
Wheat Ridge, CO 80033
Tel: (303) 422-8894

The Society for the Study of Neuronal Regulation (SSNR)
PO Box 160125
Austin, TX 78716
Tel: (512) 306-0406
www.ssnr.com

Biofeedback Certification Institute of America
10200 West 44th Ave. #304
Wheat Ridge, CO 80033
Tel: (303) 420-2902

Suggested Reading

1. Schwartz MS et al: *Biofeedback: a practitioner's guide*, New York, 1987, Guilford.
   Dr. Schwartz, with his extensive knowledge of biofeedback treatment as well as his vast clinical experience, offers readers an in-depth guide to biofeedback training. This book is a must for all new practitioners.

2. Andreassi JL: *Psychophysiology: human behavior and physiological response*, ed 3, Hillsdale, NJ, 1995, Lawrence Erlbaum Associates.
   Andreassi introduces the student to the field of psychophysiology. This book provides a comprehensive introduction for undergraduates, graduate students, or professionals seeking basic information about the field. This book is also useful for students of behavioral medicine, psychosomatic medicine, biofeedback, biomedical engineering, and other life sciences, including biology and physiology.

3. Sears W, Thompson L: *The ADD book: new understandings, new approaches to parenting your child*, New York, 1998, Little Brown and Company.
   This book is for parents, teachers, and medical professionals who wish to learn more about attention deficit disorder (ADD). It suggest ways to improve a child's attention and motivation and offers tips for helping children with frustration. It also offers advice on seeking professional help for children and adults with ADD. This book is clear and can be used as a comprehensive guide to help for ADD.

Bibliography

Abarbanal A: Gates, states, rhythms, and resonances: the scientific basis of neurofeedback training, *J Neuropath* 1:15-38, 1995.

Andreassi JL: Skin-conductance and reaction-time in a continuous auditory monitoring task, *Am J Psychol* 79(3):470-474, 1966.

Andreassi JL: *Psychophysiology: human behavior and psychological response*, Hillsdale, NJ, 1995, Lawrence Erlbaum Associates.

Fine AH, Goldman L: Innovative techniques in the treatment of ADHD: an analysis of the impact of EEG biofeedback training and a cognitive computer generated training. Paper presented at 102nd annual convention of the American Psychological Association, Los Angeles, August 12-16, 1994.

Linden M, Habib T, Radojevic V: A controlled study of the effects of EEG biofeedback on cognition and behavior of children with ADDs and learning disabilities, *Biofeedback and Self-Regulation* 21:35-50, 1996.

Penniston EG, Kulkosky PJ: A-k brainwave training and b-endorphin levels in alcoholics, *Alcohol Clin Exp Res* 13:271-279, 1989.

Rossiter TR, LaVaque TJ: A comparison of EEG biofeedback and psychostimulants in treating attention deficit/hyperactivity disorder. *J Neuropath* 1:489-459, 1995.

Schwartz MS et al: *Biofeedback: a practitioner's guide*, New York, 1987, Guilford.

Sterman MB: EEG biofeedback in the treatment of epilepsy: an overview circa 1980. In White L, Tursky B, editors: *Clinical biofeedback: efficacy and mechanisms*, New York, 1982, Guilford.

White L, Tursky B, editors: *Clinical biofeedback: efficacy and mechanisms*, New York, 1982, Guilford.

References

1. Basmajian JV, editor: *Biofeedback principles & practice for clinicians*, ed 2, Baltimore, 1983, Williams & Wilkins.

2. Peper E: *Mind/body integration*, New York, 1979, Plenum.

3. Sterman MD, Macdonald LR, Stone RK: Biofeedback training of the sensorimotor EEG rhythm in man: effects on epilepsy, *Epilepsia* 15:395-416, 1974.

4. Lubar JF et al: Evaluation of the effectiveness of EEG neurofeedback training for ADHD in a clinical setting as measured by changes in T.O.V.A. scores, behavioral ratings, and WISC—R performance, *Biofeedback Self-Regulation* 20:83-99, 1995.

5. Tansey MA: Righting the rhythms of reason. EEG biofeedback training as a therapeutic modality in a clinical office setting. *Med Psychother* 3:57-68, 1991.

Dance/Movement Therapy

DANIELLE L. FRAENKEL

Origins and History

For thousands of years indigenous societies have used elements of dance to heal and promote a sense of community. Fertility, productivity, and health were directly related to the community's ritual songs and dances. Whether the society was simple or complex, its members knew that shared rhythms, synchronous movement, and repetition altered affective states. Today, dance/movement therapy uses these and other aspects of dance and movement to prevent, assess, and treat psychologic and psychiatric disorders.

Treatment goals include awareness, expression, symptom reduction, mastery, insight, interpersonal communication, and intrapsychic reorganization. Patients achieve these objectives by working with natural elements of dance and movement. For example, breath provides a kinesthetic link to affect.[1] Rhythm integrates,[2] and qualitative changes in the flow of muscle tension provide information regarding basic needs.[3]

Because the fundamental elements of dance/movement are available to everyone, patients do not need training or talent in dance to benefit from dance/movement therapy. Treatment, affective, cognitive, and behavioral objectives are already in an individual's movement repertoire. The greater the repertoire (meaning the variety of movement, not skill) the better able a person is "to explore, to feel, and to express . . . Conversely, the emotionally restricted . . . display a narrower range, progressing downward to the catatonic schizophrenic with his immobile postures."[4]

In the United States, dance/movement was first used as a medical intervention in the early 1940s. Marian Chace at St. Elizabeth's Hospital's Department of Psychiatry in Washington, D.C., and Trudi Schoop at Camarillo State Hospital in California, used their experiences as performers to bring to seemingly unreachable patients new venues for communication and expression.[5]

Chace's innovative use of movement empathy and the therapeutic movement relationship embodied Stack's interpersonal theory of personality and basic counseling interventions. Movement empathy, sometimes called *kinesthetic identification* or *attunement*, has become a cornerstone of dance/movement therapy theory and practice, stimulating research in a wide variety of contexts.

Schoop discussed the ceaseless life-force, which is the value of taking on specific postures or attitudes for self-discovery, the power of humor, and the importance of structured movement activities that go beyond catharsis, toward self-reflection and insight. Many of these ideas permeate the contemporary interest in 12-step programs and spirituality.

In the 1960s Whitehouse identified the connection between *movement-in-depth* and Jung's active imagination. Those who teach Whitehouse's approach now refer to it as *authentic movement*. Some dance/movement therapists incorporate principles from authentic movement into their treatment plans.[6]

Evan and Espenak used dance as a vehicle for self-expression and a tool for diagnosis. Evan developed dance/movement/word therapy, a primary method of intervention that used dance as a projective technique. During her tenure at Flower-Fifth Avenue Hospitals in New York City, Espenak developed a series of concrete diagnostic movement tests to assess an individual's personality.

Currently, dance/movement therapists use a variety of diagnostic tools, most of which are grounded in Laban movement analysis and the Kestenberg movement profile. The parameters of these measures provide substance for treatment planning and nonverbal keys to understanding patients.

Mechanism of Action According to Its Own Theory

Dance/movement therapy works from the premise that the mind and the body are "inseparable," "mutual and bidirectional," such that a change in one effects a change in the other.[7] However, dance/movement therapy takes the body-mind connection further. As well as being the prime source of information, the body is also "the instrument of expression and the catalyst for change."[8]

According to the American Dance Therapy Association (ADTA), dance/movement therapy is the psychotherapeutic use of movement as a process that furthers the emotional, social, cognitive, and physical integration of the individual. Although there are many approaches to dance/movement therapy, the common understanding acknowledges the following principles:

- Dance communicates.
- Elements of dance and movement relate to culture, personality, mental status, and the healing processes in dance/movement therapy.
- Dance/movement therapy draws from the transformative processes and many levels of kinesthetic expression inherent in dance.[9]
- Movement empathy generates and supports the therapeutic alliance.

The inclusion of nonverbal and paralinguistic indicators in the therapeutic process provides keys to unlocking information unavailable to other forms of therapy. For example, a dance/movement therapist helped find that a 12-year-old girl had been sexually abused at a much earlier age than reports had indicated. The therapist also accurately predicted that the girl would start wetting her bed if conditions in the girl's life were not altered. The dance/movement therapist gathered her information through movement observation, movement analysis, and movement empathy.

Movement empathy requires that therapists consciously incorporate aspects of a patient's movement into their own expressions. By reflecting or "mirroring" the essence of the patient's movement, the dance/movement therapist is the kinesthetic equivalent of a conventional psychotherapist.

Biologic Mechanism of Action

Changes that occur in dance/movement therapy relate directly to the brain's interactive function, to physical exercise as a biogenic regulator that mediates mental states, and to the neural interplay between motion and emotion.[10] Dance and other forms of volitional movement constitute cortically-controlled responses and reflexive components that accompany purposeful acts. The cortex mediates the intention of an action "while the neuromuscular event is a function of the subcortical reflexes and servo-mechanisms." Intention affects the occurrence of neuromuscular actions and the expression of the ensuing feelings.[11-13] Thus, dance/movement therapists aim for meaningful expression characterized by levels of muscle tension and kinesthetic relationships to space, gravity, and timing that are conducive to the intention, affect, and event in which the action is embedded.

Demographics

Most of the 750 credentialed dance/movement therapists work on the East and West Coasts or in large urban areas and neighboring suburban areas. Dance/movement therapists can be found in most states. Contact the ADTA for the names of dance/movement therapists in your area.

Dance/movement therapists work with children and adults in psychiatric, rehabilitative, correctional, community, educational, hospice, and private practice settings. Patients come from all socioeconomic backgrounds. While men are generally less likely than women to use this modality, the men who do use dance/movement therapy tend to commit themselves to the process. Therapists, physicians, nurses, and other helping professionals often self-refer.

Indications and Reasons for Referral

Dance/movement therapy is both primary and adjunctive. As a primary therapy it is a specialized form of counseling. It engages psychotherapeutic procedures but also incorporates the body and nonverbal expression into the process. Thus patients with psychologic problems that stem from illness, injury, or developmental changes (for example, puberty and menopause) can use dance/movement therapy as a primary intervention. This also is true for individuals who use their body to express their emotional distress (for example, eating disorders, excessive clinging, anxiety attacks, and psychosomatic concerns).

Other reasons for referral include a reluctance or inability to communicate verbally, dysfunctional or unintegrated movement, disturbed responses to developmental stages (for example, autism, communication disorders, and identity disorders), mood disorders, and trauma. Research indicates that dance/movement therapy is highly effective as an adjunctive therapy in the treatment of psychiatric disorders.[14,15]

Practical Applications

Assessments usually require between two and four 30 to 60 minute sessions, depending on the patient's age and diagnosis. Although most patients have a *Diagnostic and Statistical Manual* IV (DSM-IV) diagnosis, patients in private practice also seek dance/movement therapy services for developmental concerns, such as empty nest syndrome, serious illness, relationship problems, and personal growth. Treatment for the latter concern may include building confidence, breaking creative blocks, addressing a weight preoccupation (non-eating disorder), and alleviating performance anxiety.

Dance/movement therapy is highly effective in the treatment of anxiety and for patients with psychiatric disorders such as schizophrenia. More specifically, rhythm and movement, grounded in basic biologic functions such as breath and pulse, have the power to organize individuals and groups,[16] and alter affect.[17] The rhythmic and synchronous characteristics of dance/movement reduce isolation, stimulate meaningful intrapersonal and interpersonal communication, promote group cohesion, alter moods, and organize thoughts and actions. Dance/movement therapy can enliven the depressed person and settle the manic person in the very same session. As with all alternative therapies, use of dance/movement therapy does not preclude the use of mainstream medical therapies.

Excellent candidates for dance/movement therapy include the following groups:

- Victims of physical and sexual abuse, men and women who have eating disorders, people who are struggling with serious illnesses such as asthma, cancer, AIDS, and heart disease
- Children and adults who express their problems somatically, for example, self-destructive behaviors, excessive involvement with real or feared bodily injuries, significant weight loss or weight gain, insomnia, promiscuity, poor hygiene, and others
- Children and adults with communication disorders, autistic disorder, learning disabilities, and other disorders first diagnosed in infancy, childhood, and adolescence
- Children who are suffering from separation anxiety or have reactive attachment disorder
- People with Alzheimer's disease

Healthy older adults also respond positively to awakening the body, activating muscles and joints, and reducing body tension. The dance/movement therapy session gives older adults the chance to reminisce and to preserve or reclaim their bodies.

Research Base

Evidence Based

Research investigating the efficacy of dance/movement therapy has focused on case studies and outcome studies examining, psychologic, performance, and motor-related variables. Subjects have included all ages, from infants to older adults. Although some studies have examined subjects without mental disorders, most subjects have DSM-IV diagnoses including pervasive developmental disorders,[18,19] schizophrenia,[20] eating disorders,[1,21] posttraumatic stress disorder,[22] learning disabilities,[23] and mental retardation.[24] Other subjects have had traumatic brain injuries,[25] neurologic insults such as strokes and Parkinson's Disease,[26,27] or life-threatening illnesses.[28,29] Still others have been blind or deaf.[30,31]

These studies have reported positive psychologic outcomes in a wide range of phenomena. These outcomes include reduced anxiety,[32-34] changes in self-concept or body image,[35-38] significant decreases in depression,[39] improved relatedness and social interaction,[30,40,41] and heightened levels of attention and improved cognitive processes.[42]

Dance/movement therapy also positively affects physical sequelae. This additional effect is especially important when emotional distress exacerbates conditions such as traumatic brain injury and heart disease.[41,43]

Metaanalyses examining effect size (ES) in an array of quantitative outcome studies show that dance/movement therapy is highly effective for psychiatric patients ($r = 0.37$) and the treatment of anxiety in general ($r = 0.70$[44]; $r = 0.54$[45]). ES estimates for dance/movement therapy, ranging from 0.15 to 0.54, are comparable to ES estimates of other psychotherapeutic and medical treatment modalities.[49]

Well-designed quantitative analyses have identified relationships between nonverbal phenomena and therapeutic processes such as echoed movements and empathy[46] and congruent posture and rapport.[47] Hypothesis-generating research suggests a relationship between the moments during appointments when a practitioner and a patient move in synchrony and the information the patient recalls later.[48]

Basic Science

The picture of the brain as a collective that requires neural communication between both hemispheres and among the various parts of the brain relates directly to dance/movement therapy's attention to the "neural interplay between motion and emotion."[10] As cited in Berrol, Marsden proposes that "the *motor loop* . . . concerned with control of movement and the *limbic loop* with the control of emotion . . . work together to *integrate* thought and emotion into behavior."[10] Similarly in dance movement therapy, feelings and thoughts generate movement, and movement in turn affects emotion and cognition.

Analyses of the limbic system (the part of the central nervous system that balances basic urges and reason through neuronal hookups to the cerebrum) link two of its components, the amygdala and hippocampus, to the processing of emotionally charged memories and posttraumatic stress disorder.[49] More specifically, recent brain imaging studies of patients who have undergone trauma suggest limbic abnormalities in this highly excitable part of the brain. Van der Kolk[50] therefore recommends that these patients receive body-based therapies to directly treat this part of the brain.

Future Research Opportunities and Priorities

Future research opportunities include outcome studies on work with patients who have undergone trauma, older adults at various stages of aging, patients with AIDS, heart disease, asthma, cancer, eating disorders, and bipolar disorder, and the use of dance/movement therapy in preventive medicine.

Druglike Information

Safety

Dance/movement therapists do not administer drugs; however, on rare occasions, some drugs may affect the degree to which a patient can engage in the dance/movement therapy process. Psychiatric patients may tire quickly if they are overmedicated or unaccustomed to the medication they currently are taking.

Warnings, Contraindications, and Precautions

The popular tendency to make interpretations based on a single movement parameter may be misleading or even dangerous. Movement must be assessed in terms of both the context and the patient's entire movement repertoire.

Some argue that exhibitionists, voyeurs, and adults with strong tendencies to act out violently are not appropriate referrals for dance/movement therapy unless the focus is on relaxation or "neutral" movements.[51] The patient's inability to distance from the modality is of concern to therapists.

Pregnancy and Lactation

Dance/movement therapy is safe and useful for pregnant and lactating women. It provides opportunities to exercise creatively and safely, attend to feelings associated with their conditions, and develop healthy nonverbal ways of relating to their newborn or *in utero* babies.[52,53]

Trade Products, Administration, and Dosage

Methods taught in dance/movement therapy sessions may require daily practice, which usually involves relaxation exercises, meditation, or sequential forms that may range from 5 to 60 minutes daily, with most requiring no more than 15 minutes.

Self-Help versus Professional

It is dangerous for patients to attempt in-depth dance/movement therapy on their own. Enlivening the body-mind connection and stimulating the unconscious is risky *without a trained witness*. It can halt rather than support a patient's progress. Patients who have undergone trauma must beware of overstimulating their limbic systems without supervision. Working with a dance/movement therapist is ideal for this population. Patients can practice techniques to help relax, reduce stress, counter symptoms, and engender feelings of self-confidence and well-being, but they first need a therapist's guidance.

Visiting a Professional

Typically, dance/movement therapists work in large offices, dance studios, or gymnasiums. Floors either are made of wood or are covered with a rug. Chairs are present for those patients who cannot sit on the floor or those who prefer not to stand. Both group sessions and individual sessions consist of three parts: the first is warmup, the second is development, and the third is closure.

Warmups that are set to music may include simple rhythmic steps, attention to individual body parts or developmentally based movement parameters, relaxation exercises, breath work, stretching, and verbal exchange. The dance/movement therapist directs the patient, dances with the patient, or witnesses the patient, moving among these leadership roles.

A patient's in-depth work occurs during the development phase. The dance/movement therapist and patient work as a team to seek creative ways to embody emerging themes and integrate motion and emotion.

Closure acknowledges the individual's process both nonverbally and verbally and ensures that the patient is oriented to the present. Follow-up may include the following: homework such as practicing new skills, making another appointment, deciding to join a group after a period of individual work, and communicating with referring health professionals.

Credentialing

The ADTA maintains a two-tier registry. Dance therapist registered (DTR) represents the completion of a master's degree and an internship. Academy of dance therapists registered (ADTR), which is the advanced level of registry, is a clinical credential. The ADTR credential represents completion of at least 3640 hours of supervised clinical work, plus a minimum of 48 hours of supervision by another ADTR, and also passing a written examination.

In certain states, dance/movement therapists may apply for licensure as licensed professional/mental health counselors. The discipline is defined as a *related area*.

Training

Dance/movement therapists require extensive training in dance and also a master's degree in dance/movement therapy, counseling, or another related field. Those dance/movement therapists with master's degrees in related fields must earn 30 additional credits (450 hours) in dance/movement therapy. Courses include theory, practice, movement observation and analysis, group processes, kinesiology, and internships in dance/movement therapy, for example.

What to Look for in a Provider

A preferred provider will have a minimum of a DTR, preferably an ADTR, and years of experience. Additional positive indicators include areas of specialization, publications, and positive endorsements.

Barriers and Key Issues

Dance/movement therapy works with the body and dance, two variables that often make others uncomfortable. With a small number of practicing dance/movement therapists and only five approved graduate programs, outcome research has tended to focus on qualitative rather than quantitative research. Increased referrals from physicians could stimulate growth in the field, in terms of both numbers of practitioners and quality of research.

Associations

The American Dance Therapy Association has more than 1100 members and individual state and regional chapters. It publishes the *American Journal of Dance Therapy*, releases compendia of academic theses and dissertations, sponsors an annual conference, fosters research, monitors standards for professional practice, and develops and upgrades guidelines for graduate education. The ADTA is a member of the National Coalition of Arts Therapies Association, and it provides continuing education for the National Board for Certified Counselors.

American Dance Therapy Association
2000 Century Plaza, Suite 108
10632 Little Patuxent Parkway
Columbia, MD 21044
Tel: (410) 997-4040
Fax: (410) 997-4048
E-mail: info@adta.org
www.adta.org

Suggested Reading

1. Chodorow J: *Dance therapy and depth psychology*, London, 1991, Routledge.
   An excellent discussion of the use of active imagination and affect theory in dance/movement therapy.
2. Espenak L: *Dance therapy theory and application*, Springfield, Ill, 1981, Charles C. Thomas.
   A clear description of Espenak's approach to assessment and intervention.
3. Levy F: *Dance movement therapy: a healing art*, Reston, Va, 1988, American Alliance for Health, Physical Education, Recreation & Dance.
   A well-researched introduction to dance therapy.
4. Sandel S, Chaiklin S, Lohn A: *Foundations of dance/movement therapy: the life and work of Marian Chace*, Columbia, Md, 1993, The Marian Chace Memorial Fund.
   Marian Chace's writings and thoughtful analyses of her contributions.

Bibliography

Chodorow J: *Dance therapy & depth psychology: the moving imagination*, London, 1991, Routledge.

Levy F: *Dance movement therapy: a healing art*, Reston, Va, 1988, American Alliance for Health, Physical Education, Recreation and Dance.

Sandel S, Chaiklin S, Lohn A, editors: (1993). *Foundations of dance/movement therapy: the life and work of Marian Chace*, Columbia, Md, 1993, The Marian Chace Memorial Foundation.

Schmais C: (1974). Dance therapy in perspective. In Mason K, editor: *Focus on dance vii*, Reston, Va, 1974, American Alliance for Health, Physical Education, Recreation and Dance.

References

1. Franks B, Fraenkel D: Fairy tales and dance/movement therapy: catalysts of change for eating-disordered individuals, *Arts Psychother* 18:311-319, 1991.
2. Schmais C: Healing processes in group dance therapy, *Am J Dance Ther* 8:17-36, 1985.
3. Loman S, Merman H: The KMP: a tool for dance/movement therapy, *Am J Dance Ther* 18:29-52, 1996.
4. Hunt V: Movement behavior: a model for action, *Quest* monograph (2):69-91, 1969.
5. Schoop T, Mitchell P: *Won't you join the dance?: a dancer's essay into the treatment of psychosis*, Mountain View, Calif, 1974, Mayfield.
6. Musicant S: Authentic movement and dance therapy, *Am J Dance Ther* 16:91-106, 1994.
7. Moyers B: *Healing and the mind*, New York, 1993, Doubleday.
8. Fraenkel D: The relationship of empathy in movement to synchrony, echoing, and empathy in verbal interactions, *Am J Dance Ther* 6:31-48, 1983.
9. Jacoby R: *Toward an integrated theory of dance/movement therapy*, master's thesis, Antioch New England Graduate School, 1993. Abstract in Chaiklin S, editor: *Dance/movement therapy abstracts: Doctoral dissertations, masters' theses, and special projects, Vol. 2, 1991-1996*, Columbia, Md, 1998, Marian Chace Foundation of the American Dance Therapy Association.

10. Berrol C: The neurophysiological basis of the mind-body connection in dance/movement therapy, *Am J Dance Ther* 14:19-29, 1992.

11. Laban R, Ullmann L: *The mastery of movement,* Estover, Plymouth, England, 1980, MacDonald & Evans.

12. Schilder P: *The image and appearance of the human body,* New York, 1950, International Universities Press.

13. Hunt V: Movement behavior: a model for action, *Quest* 69-90, 1969.

14. Cruz R, Sabers D: Dance therapy is more effective than previously reported, *Arts Psychother* 25:101-104, 1998.

15. Ritter, M, Low K: Effects of dance/movement therapy: a meta-analysis, *Arts Psychother* 23:249-260, 1996.

16. Schmais C: Healing processes in group dance therapy, *Am J Dance Ther* 8:17-36, 1985.

17. National Institutes of Health: *Alternative medicine: expanding medical horizons,* NIH Publication 94-066, Chantilly, Va, 1994, National Institutes of Health.

18. Costonis M: Case study of a puzzling child. In Costonis M, editor: *Therapy in Motion,* Urbana, 1978, University of Illinois Press.

19. Kalish B: Body movement therapy for autistic children, *Proceedings of the third annual conference of the American Dance Therapy Association* 49-59, 1968.

20. Leste A, Rust J: Effects of dance on anxiety, *Am J Dance Ther* 12:19-25, 1990.

21. Rice J, Hardenbergh M, Hornyak I: Disturbed body image in anorexia nervosa: dance/movement therapy interventions. In Hornyak L, Baker E, editors: *Experiential therapies for eating disorders,* New York, 1989, Guilford.

22. Gonzalez C: Dance/movement therapy with childhood posttraumatic stress disorder, master's thesis, Towson, Md, 1993, Goucher College. In Chaiklin S, editor: *Dance/movement therapy abstracts: Doctoral dissertations, masters' theses, and special projects,* Vol. 2, 1991-1996, Columbia, Md, 1998, Marian Chace Foundation of the American Dance Therapy Association.

23. Leventhal M: Dance therapy as treatment of choice for the emotionally disturbed learning disabled child. In Riordan, Fitts, editors: *Focus on dance ix: Dance for the handicapped,* Reston, Va, 1980, American Alliance for Health, Physical Education, Recreation & Dance.

24. Bertz J: (1995). A developmental comparison of body movement and mental age in children with Down Syndrome, master's thesis, Philadelphia, 1995, Hahnemann University. Abstract in Chaiklin S, editor: *Dance/movement therapy abstracts: Doctoral dissertations, masters' theses, and special projects,* Vol. 2, 1991-1996, Columbia, Md, 1998, Marian Chace Foundation of the American Dance Therapy Association.

25. Berrol C, Katz S: Dance/movement therapy in the rehabilitation of individuals surviving serious head injuries, *Am J Dance Ther* 8:44-46, 1985.

26. Berrol C, Ooi W, Katz S: Dance/movement therapy with older adults who have sustained neurological insult: a demonstration project. *Am J Dance Ther* 19:135-160, 1997.

27. Westbrook B, McKibben H: Dance/movement therapy with groups of outpatients with Parkinson's Disease, *Am Dance Ther Assoc* 11:27-38, 1989.

28. Hiller C: Dance therapy at the Momentum AIDS Project: a study of expected outcomes for an HIV+ group, master's thesis, New York, 1996, Hunter College of the City University of New York. Abstract in Chaiklin S, editor: *Dance/movement therapy abstracts: Doctoral dissertations, masters' theses, and special projects,* Vol. 2, 1991-1996, Columbia, Md, 1998, Marian Chace Foundation of the American Dance Therapy Association.

29. Dibble-Hope D: *Moving toward health—a study of the use of dance/movement therapy in the psychological adaptation to breast cancer,* unpublished doctoral dissertation, Berkeley, 1989, California School of Professional Psychology at Berkeley.

30. Cooper A: An exploratory look at the dance/movement therapist's role and practice with a group of deaf adolescents, master's thesis, Hunter College, NY. In Chaiklin S, editor: *Dance/movement therapy abstracts: Doctoral dissertations, masters' theses, and special projects, Vol. 2, 1991-1996,* Columbia, Md, 1998, Marian Chace Foundation of the American Dance Therapy Association.

31. Weisbrod J: Body movement therapy and the visually-impaired person. In Mason K, editor: *Focus on dance vii,* Reston, Va, 1974, American Alliance for Health, Physical Education, Recreation & Dance.

32. Brooks D, Stark A: The effects of dance/movement therapy on affect: a pilot study, *Am J Dance Ther* 11:101-112, 1989.

33. Kuettel T: Affective change in dance therapy, *Am J Dance Ther* 5:56-64, 1982.

34. Leste A, Rust J: Effects of dance on anxiety, *Am J Dance Ther* 12:19-25, 1990.

35. Loughlin E: "Why was I born among mirrors?" Therapeutic dance for teenage girls and women with Turner Syndrome, *Am J Dance Ther* 15:107-124, 1993.

36. Christup H: The effect of dance therapy on the concepts of body image. In Costonis M, editor: *Therapy in Motion,* Urbana, Ill, 1978, University of Illinois Press.

37. Heber L: Dance movement: a therapeutic program for psychiatric clients, *Perspectives in Psychiatric Care* 29:22-29, 1993.

38. Rice J, Hardenbergh M, Hornyak I: Disturbed body image in anorexia nervosa: dance/movement therapy interventions. In Hornyak L, Baker E, editors: *Experiential therapies for eating disorders,* New York, 1989, Guilford.

39. Brooks D, Stark A: The effects of dance/movement therapy on affect: a pilot study, *Am J Dance Ther* 11:101-112, 1989.

40. Adler J, The study of an autistic child. *Proceedings of the American Dance Therapy Association,* pp. 43-48, 1968.

41. Berrol C, Katz S: Dance/movement therapy in the rehabilitation of individuals surviving serious head injuries, *Am J Dance Ther* 8:44-46, 1985.

42. Berrol C, Ooi W, Katz S: Dance/movement therapy with older adults who have sustained neurological insult: a demonstration project, *Am J Dance Ther* 19:135-160, 1997.

43. Seides M: Dance/movement therapy as a modality in the treatment of the psychosocial complications of heart disease, *Am J Dance Ther* 9:83-101, 1986.

44. Ritter M, Low K: Effects of dance/movement therapy: a meta-analysis, *Arts Psychother* 23:249-260, 1996.

45. Cruz R, Sabers D: Dance therapy is more effective than previously reported, *Arts Psychother* 25:101-104, 1998.

46. Fraenkel D: The relationship of empathy in movement to synchrony, echoing, and empathy in verbal interactions, *Am J Dance Ther* 6:31-48, 1983.

47. LaFrance M: Nonverbal synchrony and rapport: analysis by the cross-lag panel technique, *Soc Psychol Q* 42:66-70, 1979.

48. Fraenkel D: The ins and outs of medical encounters: An interactional analysis of empathy, patient satisfaction, and information exchange, unpublished doctoral dissertation, 1986, University of Rochester. Abstract in Chaiklin S, editor: *Dance/movement therapy abstracts: Doctoral dissertations, masters' theses, and special projects, Vol. 2, 1991-1996,* Columbia, Md, 1998, Marian Chace Foundation of the American Dance Therapy Association.

49. van der Kolk B: *The body keeps the score: memory and the evolving psychobiology of posttraumatic disorder, Harvard Rev Psychiatry* 1:253-265, 1994.

50. van der Kolk B: Lecture at Strong Memorial Hospital, Rochester, NY, 1998.

51. Espenak L: *Dance therapy,* Springfield, Ill, 1981, Charles C. Thomas.

52. Loman S: Attuning to the fetus and the young child: approaches from dance/movement therapy, *Zero to Three* 15:20-26, 1994.

53. Kestenberg J, Buelte A: Prevention, infant therapy, and the treatment of adults 1: toward understanding mutuality, *Int J Psychoanal* 6:339-366, 1977.

Hypnotherapy

KENNETH I. SAICHEK

Origins and History

The days of misunderstanding hypnosis may be over. For centuries it seemed to be like a hologram, appearing organic and discrete, yet becoming a chimera at closer inspection and an illusion when one tried to grasp it. The only way that hypnosis could be understood was to encircle the problem, and in a climate of dichotomous thinking, this was impossible. Only in today's world of conjunctive thinking (*and* instead of *or*) and converging disciplines (*psycho* + *neuro* + *biology*) can the enigma be dissected. And what do we find? Not the histrionics of carnival sideshows, nor the intrinsic force of the operator willed upon the subject, but a marriage of language and psychology, of human nature and human aspirations, and, fundamentally, of the interaction of ideas and neurotransmitters. Modern scientific, clinical hypnosis conjoins the disciplines of psychotherapy and neurobiology. *Hypnosis* itself refers to any of three states: *trance*, the psychophysiologic phenomena that asserts itself during the state we call "hypnosis," *hypnosis*, the process of induction and the state subsequently experienced, and *hypnotherapy*, the clinical process of healing using the trance state, or simply, the therapy which follows the induction.

Hypnosis has been described numerous times throughout history, as follows:

Ancient peoples and shamans used trance states.[1] Many forms of divination, such as Delphic Oracle, geomancy, and I-ching, are early forms of hypnotic inductions.[2]

Paracelsus (1493-1541), a Swiss physician, believed all life is influenced by magnetic fields.

Jan Baptista van Helmont (1579-1644), a Flemish chemist, postulated that people emit *animal magnetism*.

Anton Mesmer (1734-1815), an Austrian physician, was the first historical hypnotist. He used animal magnetism to heal and produced a hypnotic state, but patients experienced convulsions or loss of consciousness. Investigated by dignitaries (including Franklin, Guillotine, and Lavoisier), his method was found to be dependent on imagination and therefore worthless and harmful.

Dr. James Esdaile (1808-1859), a Scottish surgeon, used *mesmerism* as the sole anesthetic in over 300 surgeries.

Dr. James Braid (1795-1860), an English physician, made hypnosis respectable to the medical community. He discovered that theories still held validity. He was incorrectly thought to have originated the term "hypnosis."[a]

Hippolyte Bernheim (1837-1919), a French neurologist, discovered the use of ideodynamic processes.[b,3]

Jean Charcot (1825-1893), a French neurologist, used hypnosis in the healing of hysteria and demonstrated its safety.[4]

Sigmund Freud (1856-1939), an Austrian psychiatrist, abandoned the use of hypnosis after initial enthusiasm, which damaged its credibility.

Clark Hull (1884-1952), an American psychologist, published accounts of controlled experimentation of hypnosis in a landmark textbook, making hypnosis a psychologic discipline.

Milton H. Erickson (1901-1980), an American psychiatrist, studied hypnosis under Hull, revived the medical application of hypnosis, and developed a new paradigm for the practice of hypnotherapy.[5,6]

The British Medical Society recognized hypnosis as a legitimate medical procedure in 1955, followed by the American Medical Association and the American Psychological Association in 1958.[7]

Mechanism of Action According to Its Own Theory

Hypnotherapy is a tool for both the physician and the psychotherapist. Psychotherapists are used to working with such intangibles as *the unconscious*, and *life scripts*, which might exasperate a physician used to trusting sense-oriented data. The author advises the reader to think of these terms not as "things" but as processes; for example, the term *the unconscious* refers not to a physical location but to sensory data not currently in consciousness. Not everything perceived is stored in memory, but we do store much more than we can consciously remember. Hypnosis promotes recall of data not easily accessed by the conscious mind. To do this, hypnotherapy dissociates the conscious, mediating ego from the unconscious self. This willful dissociation is therapeutic. However, life decisions, programs, or scripts may *dysfunctionally* dissociate themselves from the conscious mind and thereby create a frame of reference which, unless altered, forever limits the patient. Hypnotherapy alters that frame by providing a heuristic reassociation of the script content.[8]

By giving the unconscious *new learnings*, seminal perceptions that displace the existing restrictive messages, hypnotherapy helps the patient create a new attitudinal synthesis. Moreover, the original pathogenic messages fit the definition of hypnotic suggestion, whereby conscious sets are interrupted and new associations are formulated without cognitive analysis and reduction. Wherein the way in is the way out, the hypnotherapist may

---

[a]Braid named the process *neurohypnology* (nervous sleep), taking the name from Hypnos, the Greek god of sleep. Research has traced the term *hypnosis* to earlier sources.

[b]Processes such as ideomotor and ideosensory response, whereby the mental *idea* induces a physiological *dynamic*; for example, the therapist mentioning the smell of a good dinner causes alimentary peristalsis in the patient.

actually be dehypnotizing original hypnotic messages. This model is physiologic as well as psychotherapeutic. An individual's health is equally affected when a virus, autoantibody, or neurotransmitter provides the basis for the original pathologic script, instead of a parent or mentor.

Biologic Mechanism of Action

When an event is novel or continuous, the ascending reticular activating system (ARAS) transmits the message to the hypothalamus and limbic systems, including the amygdala and the hippocampus. This triggers the release of hormones and neurotransmitters that facilitate certain bodily functions, including messenger molecules affecting memory and learning. When an event is stored in the memory, it becomes encoded with the coexistent biochemistry. The information, including the resultant learnings and behavior, becomes *state-bound* or inseparable from the state in which it was first acquired.[9] It is believed that these state-dependent constructs are stored in the limbic-hypothalamic regions of the brain.

State-dependent memory, learning, and behavior theory is another way to understand conventional theories of neurosis, behavioral conditioning, and stress reactions. The information encoded in the brain during a stress-reaction (perhaps falling from a tree, being fired from a job, or having a heart attack) is synchronously encoded with the abnormal physiologic and emotional responses created to deal with the stressor. This is the defining moment. When the mind perceives a similar situation (usually an unconscious and illogical interpretation that distorts the perception), the original state-dependent construct emerges. The psychobiologic chemistry created to deal with the original stressor, which perhaps was functional at the time, becomes a dysfunctional re-creation of the absent stressor. This dynamic is seen in psychosomatic illness, where the patient suffers from a presently perceived but archaic reaction. To alter this dysfunction, we must help the patient experientially recall the defining moment. Hypnotherapy works by facilitating the re-creation of this psychophysiologic state, and through the eventual reconstruction of the defining moment, dissociates it along with the resulting diseases and maladaptations from its state-dependent matrix. Just as the original message seems to be stored in the limbic-hypothalamic regions of the brain, hypnotherapy likewise triggers the limbic-hypothalamic release of "information molecules" that apparently modulate activity in the autonomic nervous, endocrine, immune, and neuropeptide systems of the body.[9]

Forms of Therapy

The practice of hypnotherapy is divided into two groups, the paternal or authoritarian hypnotists, and the maternal or ericksonian hypnotists. The authoritarian hypnotist descends from the oldest schools of hypnosis, whereas the ericksonian or utilization hypnotist works from the teachings of psychiatrist Milton H. Erickson (1901-1980). Authoritarian hypnotists are the authority, imposing both the trance state and the resolution upon the subject. They believe that a person will accept any suggestion once in trance, although "boosters" are often needed. They use prepared inductions that are often the same for each pathology. Ericksonian hypnotists believe that the trance state alone will not create change. They do not seek to impose solutions on the patient. The patient remains the locus of power and possesses all resources needed for the desired change. Ericksonian hypnotists eschew prepared inductions, working *impromptu* and molding the induction and therapy to the unique variables of each moment.

The authoritarian hypnotists are further subdivided into the stage-show derivatives and the well-educated psychiatrists and psychologists who do not accept the ericksonian model.

In addition, most hypnotherapists are eclectic, merging the application of trance with other modalities.

Demographics

Hypnosis is practiced throughout the world. Major hubs for the study of hypnosis are Australia, Germany, Great Britain, Italy, Japan, Switzerland, and the United States. Patients are usually middle-aged adults, although ericksonian hypnotherapists (see "Forms of Therapy") often treat all age groups, including infants, as well as both sexes. Even the auditory- and visually-impaired can benefit from hypnotherapy (see "Druglike Information").

Indications and Reasons for Referral

The usual referral to a hypnotherapist is for an intractable condition that will not yield to conventional treatment. Hypnotherapists are commonly referred for habit alteration, easily treated biologic mechanisms such as hypertension or cardiac arrhythmias, and incurables, whether terminal or not. Patients who seek hypnotherapy for medical treatment on their own are usually those who disagree with a particular medical diagnosis, treatment, or regimen, or have found medicine to be ineffective. Many hypnosis patients are averse to prescription medicine, especially analgesics, or seek to avoid surgery. Many feel that hypnosis is more natural. A surprisingly large percentage of the population believe that their minds can simply be "reprogrammed" to expurgate mental or physical illness, often in a single session.

Hypnotherapy can be used medically in two ways. First, it may be employed to deal with the symptoms of disease and the patient's reaction to it, whether physiologic or emotional. Second, it may be used directly to affect the illness and its course through the body. By using hypnotherapy, physicians can reduce the dependence upon analgesics, offer an alternative to anesthesia especially in cases of respiratory compromise or allergy, avoid power struggles with patients, and have a plan of action should traditional medicine fail. The hypnotherapist should be called on as a consultant for pathologies that are known to have a psychologic component, an unknown organic etiology, a demonstrated response to hypnotic treatment, or a failed response to medical treatment; the hypnotherapist should also be referred at a patient's request. The placebo effect has been shown to exert a major role in healing.[10]

Office Applications

As with all alternative therapies, use of hypnotherapy does not preclude the use of mainstream medical therapies in addition. The diagnoses that respond well to hypnotherapeutic intervention are listed in the following order:

Top level: *A therapy ideally suited for these conditions*

Neuroses and some psychoses; some character disorders; stress; headaches; stomach aches; back aches; chronic pain; cardiac arrhythmias; hypertension; chronic fatigue syndrome; fibromyalgia; ciliary spasm; Meniere's disease; Raynaud's disease; insomnia; sleep disorders; periodic/restless leg movement syndromes; sleep paralysis; narcolepsy; tinnitus; habit management (smoking, obesity); torticollis; enuresis; paruresis; childbirth and postpartum care; vaginismus; dysmenorrhea; emotional amenorrhea; menstrual cramps; premenstrual syndrome (PMS); dyspareunia; neurodermatitis; and dental phobia

Second level: *One of the better therapies for these conditions*

Psychoses; asthma; cerebral palsy athetoid movements; constipation and chronic diarrhea; irritable bowel syndrome; GERD; gastritis; gastric ulcers; systemic lupus erythematosus; hemolytic anemia; Graves' disease; rheumatoid arthritis; myasthenia gravis; allergies; osteoarthritis; gout; AIDS; epileptic seizures; myoclonus; addictions (to prevent recitavism following detoxification); warts; psoriasis; herpes; fever; hyperreflexic bladder; sexual impotence (gender nonspecific); menopause; menorrhagia; uterine fibroids; ovarian cysts; fibrocystic breast disease; benign vocal cord nodules; myopia; and ptyalism

Third level: *A valuable adjunctive therapy for these conditions*

Many hyperplasias (benign or malignant); cervical, uterine, and ovarian cancer; colitis; Crohn's disease; prostatitis; sleep apnea; lazy eye; hemorrhoids; hay fever; sinusitis;, candidiasis; and diabetes mellitus

Practical Applications

In addition to the formal use of hypnotherapy, any health professional can learn to use simple hypnotic procedures to facilitate patient care. An example is the telling of metaphors designed to suggest positive results though imbedded implications.[11] Another example is the use of *hypnotic language*; instead of asking, "Where do you hurt?" the physician might ask, "What has gotten better since yesterday?" Hypnotic semantics can range from such simple usage to complex matching of the patient's linguistic patterns.

Research Base

Evidence Based

There is copious literature suggesting the effectiveness of hypnotherapy. Because each disease must be examined separately, the documentation of this effectiveness is well beyond the scope of this discussion. There are eight studies demonstrating the efficacy of hypnotherapy in treating venereal warts alone. For a discussion of key studies, this author recommends the reader see Banks' study of hypnotic suggestion for the control of bleeding in the angiography suite,[12] Erickson's collected papers,[13] and Udolf's *Handbook of Hypnosis for Professionals*.[7]

Risk and Safety

A major study was performed by Orne on the undesirable effects of hypnosis, concluding that hypnosis is safe.[14] Supporting studies by Erickson and Hilgard on the possible detrimental effects of experimental hypnosis and the sequalae to hypnosis, respectively, have supported this study.[15,16] Wineburg and Straker's study of self-limiting depersonalization following a first session of hypnosis, Rosen's studies of hypnosis, and Kleinhauz and Beran's study of misuses of hypnosis all have reported limited adverse reactions.[17-20]

Efficacy

The efficacy of hypnosis depends on the patient's psychology, pathology, history, the type of hypnosis being used, how it is used, and most importantly, the skill and experience of the clinician using it.

Other

Trance is a natural process that is occurring every 90 minutes or so as part of the ultradian rhythm.[21] A common complaint from patients who are first experiencing hypnosis is that they do not "feel hypnotized." This is because they actually experience this same state regularly each day. Trance subjects in EEG examination will demonstrate the patterns of the behavior that they are imagining, not the relaxed alpha rhythms of reclining comfortably with closed eyes.[22] This parallel seems to be indicative of the mimetic nature of trance.

Future Research Opportunities and Priorities

Candace Pert and colleagues at the National Institute of Mental Health are studying the role of neuropeptides and their receptors as a mind-body communication network.[23] Research needs to demonstrate the way hypnotherapy participates in this process. Specific targets can be assigned, such as the psychophysiologic process of hypnotherapy in turning off the autoantibody response in autoimmune disorders.

Druglike Information

Safety and Contraindications

Practiced by a clinically trained professional, is universally safe for all patients.[6] However, the paranoid patient may develop psychogenic reactions because of fear. Studies have demonstrated that most side effects to hypnosis occur because of ill-trained hypnotists. A stage hypnotist told a subject in trance to look in a mirror but not see herself. The woman was latently schizophrenic. Since the core issue of schizophrenia is the belief that one does not exist, her inability to see her reflection provoked the onset of a psychosis.

Precautions

Not everything recalled under hypnosis is valid. When the unconscious encounters memory gaps, it looks for patterns among bits of data, and when it cannot find them, it fabricates them. This is *confabulation*. It is neither conscious nor malicious.

Drug Interactions

Any resolution made in the trance state is bound to the coexistent inner chemistry. The use of a drug during trance may limit the effects of that trance to the administration of the same substance.[24] Therefore it is critical that the physician carefully consider prescription drugs for the patient in hypnotherapy. This argues strongly against the use of sodium amytal for age-regressive inductions.

Trade Products

No artificial devices or drugs are needed for the induction or clinical application of hypnosis.

Self-Help versus Professional

The patient should be taught to use the naturally occurring ultradian trance state. Illness has been shown to be correlated to the disruption of these cycles.[9] If the patient will take a brief break from ongoing activity when these trance states occur, it may aid in healing. The patient also should "practice" hypnotherapy at home. However, self-hypnosis for medical purposes should be under the supervision of a clinically-trained hypnotherapist.

Visiting a Professional

Except in cases of emergency, the hypnotherapist sees the patient in an office setting. A typical first visit is described in the following situation. The patient sits in a recliner opposite the hypnotherapist. The therapist asks what the patient wants of the therapy and expects the therapist to provide. The therapist answers all the patient's questions about both the treatment and hypnosis and gathers a history. The therapist will announce beforehand if there is to be a formal trance in this first session. The therapist simply talks to the patient. Drugs, "hypnodisks," flickering lights, and swinging pendulums are not used. The therapist offers permissions, not commands. The therapist informs the patient that the trance state may be entered with closed or open eyes. Relaxation is not necessary for anxious patients as it is not necessary to be comfortable when in trance. The patient is told to think and feel whatever is wanted.

The therapist may tell a simple story or ask the patient to perform simple tasks, such as sending attention out of the office or hearing as far as possible. The therapist may awaken the patient at the end of the trance or allow the patient to naturally awake. The therapist will discuss the signs of trance unconsciously demonstrated by the patient. In subsequent sessions, the patient and therapist may discuss the previous trance more thoroughly, and determine what changes occurred between sessions. The therapist will teach the patient to recognize and respond to messages from the unconscious. The therapist will give the patient numerous methods for accomplishing healing, including ideomotor signaling, arm levitation, and hypnotic catalepsy. Therapy continues until the problem is cured, successfully managed, or proves unresponsive to hypnosis.

Credentialing

Credentialing is a function of individual states or countries, and only a few require a terminal degree. Organizations also differ in their requirements. Some request a self-evidentiary statement of training. Others demand an examination. However, schools of hypnotherapy differ so greatly that a single examination cannot judge all applicants.

Training

There exists no consensus for the amount of training needed to practice hypnotherapy.

What to Look for in a Provider

The patient should seek a hypnotherapist with advanced training and experience, such as a psychotherapist or physician trained in psychotherapy. A friend's recommendation is extremely valuable. The patient should also feel comfortable with working with this therapist.

Barriers and Key Issues

Hypnosis has had poor publicity since the days of Mesmer. There are two obstacles to its respectability. First, there are so many poorly trained hypnotists that the discipline suffers through association. Many people still equate hypnosis with the stage-show variety.[c] Second, unscrupulous trainers have begun the practice of "selling" hypnotherapy to those without a proper background in medicine or psychology. The hypnotist who is unaware of the difference between a somatoform disorder and hypochondriasis is likely to commit many errors, embarrassing himself and the profession at the same time and harming the patient. Many patients come to hypnosis for the first time scared of treatment, concerned that they can be programmed to perform illegal or immoral acts or that they will remain in trance forever should the hypnotist die during the procedure. Because of these fears, many physicians and dentists use hypnosis without informing the client. The following is from a best-selling textbook on hypnosis:

> (The professionals) do not publish the fact . . . (that they use hypnosis) because so great is the public ignorance that if it were known that Hypnotism were the agent used for performing their painless operations their practice would seriously suffer and they would run some danger of being persecuted. Perhaps the day is not far distant when Hypnotism will take its rightful place among those whose mission it is to relieve suffering.

These words were published in 1900.

Associations

Among the many associations for the training and credentialing of hypnotherapists, the following are recommended only as beginning points of investigation. These in no way constitute endorsements.

American Association of Professional Hypnotherapists
PO Box 29
Boones Mill, VA 24065
Tel: (540) 334-3035

American Psychotherapy and Medical Hypnosis Association
210 South Sierra St. B-100
Reno, NV 89501
E-mail: psychhypno@powernet.net
http://members.xoom.com/Hypnosis

International Society of Hypnosis
Level 1, South Wing
A & RMC, Repat Campus
Locked Bag 1, West Heidelberg VIC 3081
Australia
Tel: +61-3-9496-4105
Fax: +61-3-9496-4107
E-mail: 100353.747@compuserve.com
www.ish.unimelb.edu.au

ᶜThe author once received this inquiry, "I have a question concerning stage hypnotists, as it has been my lifelong dream to become one. But, in my homecountry [sic] Sweden it has been forbidden by law . . . since 1906. I know that its forbidden in other countrys [sic] as well. Do you know if there is a way to avoid these laws?" (Saichek, 1998)

National Council for Hypnotherapy
Hazelwood Broadmead, Secretary
Sway, Lymington, Hants. SO41 6DH
United Kingdom
Tel: (01590) 683770

Society for Clinical and Experimental Hypnosis
2201 Haeder Rd.
Pullman, WA 99163
Tel: (509) 332-7555
Fax: (509) 332-5907
E-mail: sceh@pullman.com
www.sunsite.utk.edu/IJCEH

Suggested Reading

1. Saichek KI: *Hypnotherapy with resistant clients: an introduction to the Ericksonian method* (video-tape), Richmond, Calif, 1993, CommARTS.
   An instruction and demonstration of the use of clinical hypnotherapy and offers a paradigm for dealing with resistance.
2. Erickson MH, Rossi E: *Hypnotherapy, an exploratory casebook*, New York, 1979, Irvington.
   A thorough summary of Erickson's methodology and 16 case studies to explicate it.
3. Saichek KI: *Hypnosis: your questions answered!*
   www.hypnotherapy.com/ask/current
   An interactive monthly column on the nature and uses of hypnosis.
4. Erickson MH: *Mind-body communication in hypnosis: the seminars, workshops, and lectures of Milton H. Erickson* vol 3, New York, 1986, Irvington.
   Highly readable lectures by Erickson.
5. Udolf R: *Handbook of hypnosis for professionals*, Northvale, NJ, 1995, Jason Aronson.
   A thorough investigation of the science of hypnosis.

Bibliography

The perfect course of instruction in hypnotism, mesmerism, clairvoyance, suggestive therapeutics, and the sleep cure, New York, 1900, Sydney Flower.
Saichek KI: Hypnosis—your questions answered! Feb 1998, www.hypnotherapy.com/ask/02a98

References

1. Krippner S: Shamans: the first healers. In Doore G, editor: *Shaman's Path*, Boston, 1988, Shambhala.
2. Saichek KI: The relationship of the trance state to intuitive problem-solving techniques, *J New Dir Ed Psychother* Jan 1985.

3. Bernheim H: *Hypnosis and suggestion in psychotherapy* (1886), New York, 1973, Jason Aronson.

4. Gay P: *Freud: a life for our time*, New York, 1988, W.W. Norton.

5. Erickson MH: "Initial experiments investigating the nature of hypnosis," in Rossi E, editor: *The collected papers of Milton H. Erickson on hypnosis*, vol 1, New York, 1980, Irvington.

6. Connery DS: *The inner source: exploring hypnosis with Dr. Herbert Spiegel*, New York, 1982, Holt, Rinehart & Winston.

7. Udolf R: *Handbook of hypnosis for professionals*, Northvale, NJ, 1995, Jason Aronson.

8. Saichek KI: *Hypnotherapy with resistant clients: an introduction to the Ericksonian method*, Richmond, Calif, 1993, CommARTS (videotape).

9. Rossi EL: *The psychobiology of mind-body healing*, New York, 1986, W.W. Norton.

10. Levine J, Gordon N, Fields H: The mechanism of placebo analgesia, quoted in McMullin R: *Handbook of cognitive therapy techniques*, New York, 1986, W.W. Norton.

11. Rosen S: *My voice will go with you: the teaching tales of Milton Erickson*, New York, 1982, W.W. Norton.

12. Banks WO: Hypnotic suggestion for the control of bleeding in the angiography suite. In Lankton S, editor: *Elements and dimensions of an Ericksonian approach*, Ericksonian Monographs 1, New York, 1985, Brunner/Mazel.

13. Erickson MH: *The collected papers of Milton H. Erickson on hypnosis*, vol II, New York, 1980, Irvington.

14. Orne MT: Undesirable effects of hypnosis: the determinants and management, *Int J Clin Exp Hypn* 13(4):226-237, 1965.

15. Erickson MH: Possible detrimental effects of experimental hypnosis, in Rossi E, editor: *The collected papers of Milton Erickson on hypnosis*, vol. 1, New York, 1980, Irvington.

16. Hilgard JR: (1974) Sequalae to hypnosis, *Int J Clin Exp Hypn* 22(4):281-298, 1974; Ryken K, Coe WC: Sequalae to hypnosis in perspective. Paper presented at the annual convention of the American Psychological Association, August 1977.

17. Wineburg EN, Straker N: An episode of acute self-limiting depersonalization following a first session of hypnosis, *Am J Psychiatry* 130(1):98-100, 1973.

18. Rosen H: Hypnosis in medical practice: Uses and abuses, *Chicago Med Soc Bull* 62:428-436, 1959.

19. Rosen H: Hypnosis: applications and misapplications, *JAMA* 172(7):139-143, 1960.

20. Kleinhauz M, Beran B: Misuses of hypnosis: a medical emergency and its treatment, *Int J Clin Exp Hypn* 29(2):148-161, 1981.

21. Erickson MH: *Mind-body communication in hypnosis: the seminars, workshops, and lectures of Milton H. Erickson*, vol. 3, New York, 1986, Irvington.

22. Negley-Parker E: Physiological correlates and effects of hypnosis, in Zilbergeld B, editor: *Hypnosis questions and answers*, New York, 1986, W.W. Norton.

23. Pert C: Neuropeptides: the emotions and bodymind," *Noetic Sci Rev* 2:13-18, 1987.

24. Hilgard E: *Divided consciousness: multiple controls in human thought and action*, New York, 1977, Wiley.

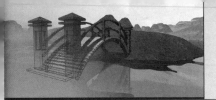

Interactive Guided Imagery^{sm}

MARTIN L. ROSSMAN

DAVID E. BRESLER

Origins and History

A mental image is a thought with sensory qualities. It is something we mentally see, hear, taste, smell, touch, or feel. The term guided imagery refers to a wide variety of techniques, including simple visualization and direct suggestion using imagery, metaphor and story-telling, fantasy exploration and game playing, dream interpretation, drawing, and active imagination where elements of the unconscious are invited to appear as images that can communicate with the conscious mind.

Once considered an alternative or complementary approach, guided imagery is now finding widespread scientific and public acceptance, and it is being used to teach psychophysiologic relaxation,[1] alleviate anxiety and depression,[2-4] relieve physical and psychologic symptoms,[5] overcome health-endangering habits,[6,7] and help patients prepare for surgery and tolerate procedures more comfortably.[8-11]

Mental images, formed long before we learn to understand and use words, lie at the core of who we think we are, what we believe the world is like, what we feel we deserve, what we think will happen to us, and how motivated we are to take care of ourselves. These images strongly influence our beliefs and attitudes about how we become ill, and what will or will not help us recover.

All healing rituals involve manipulation of these images, either overtly or covertly, and guided imagery thus can be considered one of the oldest and most ubiquitous forms of medicine. The healing rituals of various cultures that have persisted over time all have a certain level of clinical efficacy, and while we may attribute these therapeutic benefits to "placebo effects," they are real and measurable effects with important implications for our understanding of the healing process.

In the early 1970s, inspired by the pioneering work of Irving Oyle, Carl and Stephanie Simonton, Roberto Assagioli, and others, the authors began to develop and research contemporary imagery approaches for patients coping with chronic pain, immune dysfunction, cancer, heart disease, and other catastrophic and life-threatening illnesses.

By integrating techniques originating from Jungian psychology, Gestalt therapy, psychosynthesis, ericksonian hypnotherapy, object relations theory, humanistic psychology, and advanced communications theory, these approaches were constantly redefined, expanded, tested, and codified, giving birth to Interactive Guided Imagery (IGI), an extremely powerful yet remarkably safe and rapid therapeutic approach for mobilizing the untapped healing resources of the mind.

In 1989 the Academy for Guided Imagery[12] was established to provide in-depth training for clinicians, raise public and professional awareness about the benefits of imagery, and support research, professional communication, and the dissemination of imagery-related information. Since then the Academy has obtained professional accreditation, recruited an interdisciplinary faculty, sponsored and conducted research, and set contemporary standards for Professional Certification in IGI.

Mechanisms of Action According to Its Own Theory

Although no one really knows what *consciousness* is, it is critically related to the process of attention, for what we attend to and focus on is what we experience. There is an old saying that "whatever you give your attention to grows," whether it be your garden, your children, or your worries and fears.

Over the years, most of us learn to give our major attention to the conscious mind and the chatter of its little voice that narrates a linear, logical, rational, analytic monologue describing its perspective of the world and how we think about it. We quickly become lost in our thoughts, forgetting that any other parts of us exist.

However, we are much more than our conscious mind and what it thinks. We are also characterized by the richness of our unconscious mind and its intuitions, emotions, feelings, memories, drives, motives, goals, appetites, aspirations, ambitions, values, beliefs, attitudes, and perceptions, all of which are expressed more fully by our imagery experiences than by conscious verbal awareness. Yet in our Western culture, we tend to pay much less attention to these images and the feelings they convey than we do to the "little voice" of our conscious mind.

Therapeutic guided imagery allows patients to enter a relaxed state of mind and then focus their attention on images associated with the issues they are confronting. For example, a patient can invite the formation of an image that represents a particular medical symptom and then initiate an imaginary dialogue with the image to ask why it is here, what it wants, what it needs, where it is going, and what it has to offer. The information obtained from such a dialogue can often be more directly helpful than even the most sophisticated medical diagnostic tests.

Patients coping with chronic pain can be invited to visit and experience an "inner sanctuary" where there is no pain, and those facing difficult medical decisions can be introduced to a wise and caring "inner advisor" that can provide support and help them explore their feelings about the various options they are considering.

By using an interactive, nonjudgmental, content-free guiding style, experienced imagery practitioners can encourage patients to tap their latent inner resources to find new and creative solutions for their own problems. The consistent emphasis on inner resources and solutions leads to minimal transference, greater opportunities for effective self-care, an enhanced sense of self-efficacy, and the rapid development of patient autonomy.

Biologic Mechanism of Action

Imagery has profound physiologic consequences, and the body tends to respond to imagery as it would to a genuine external experience. For example, if you vividly imagine slowly sucking on the sour, tart slice of a fresh, juicy lemon, you will soon begin to salivate. Another example is sexual fantasy and its attendant physiologic responses. What happens to your body when you bring to mind something that makes you ferociously angry?

Imagery has been shown to affect almost all major physiologic systems of the body, including respiration, heart rate, blood pressure, metabolic rates in cells, gastrointestinal mobility and secretion, sexual function, cortisol levels, blood lipids, and immune responsiveness.

With respect to the production of specific physiologic changes that can promote healing, guided imagery represents an important alternative to pharmacotherapy with much greater safety and far fewer complications, precautions, and contraindications.

Demographics

Physicians, nurses, psychologists, social workers, and other health care professionals trained and certified in IGI are distributed internationally, with concentrations of practitioners currently in California, Washington, Oregon, and Arizona. Other practitioners are dispersed throughout the United States, and the Academy also has trained health professionals from Japan, England, Italy, Hong Kong, and Australia.

Forms of Therapy

The term *guided imagery* describes a range of techniques from simple visualization and direct imagery-based suggestion to metaphor and story-telling. IGI refers to the specific approach taught by the Academy for Guided Imagery in which imagery is used in a highly interactive format to evoke greater patient autonomy.

Rather than simply giving patients "better" images to imagine, IGI encourages patients to draw upon their own inner resources to support healing, make appropriate adaptations to changes in their health, and find creative solutions to challenges that they previously thought were unsolvable. IGI is particularly suited to our current health care climate, where cost-effective mind-body medicine, improved medical self-care, and briefer yet more empowering approaches to health care are valued by patients, providers, and insurers alike.

IGI is applicable as a self-care technique, in a group or class, or as part of an individual counseling relationship. Self-help imagery books and tapes are also an inexpensive option for many patients who are capable of learning and using these techniques on their own.

Indications and Referrals for Treatment

Because imagery has powerful physiologic consequences and also conveys important and otherwise inaccessible information from the unconscious mind, there are virtually an unlimited number of situations where it can be used in health care settings. For simplicity, however, it may be helpful to consider the following three major categories of use of this therapy:

1. **Relaxation and stress reduction:** This is easy to teach, easy to learn, and almost universally helpful to patients.

2. **Active visualization or directed imagery:** The patient is encouraged to imagine desired therapeutic outcomes in a relaxed, open state of mind. This affords patients a sense of participation and control in their own healing, which is of significant value by itself. In addition, visualization can be used to alleviate symptoms, stimulate healing responses in the body, modify health-endangering behaviors, and provide effective motivation for making positive life changes.

3. **Receptive or insight-oriented imagery:** Images are invited to enter conscious awareness, where they are interactively explored to gather more information about a symptom, illness, mood, treatment, situation, or possible solution.

Office Applications

Clinical applications of IGI in medicine are tremendously broad and include but are not limited to the following situations and medical conditions:

- Relaxation training
- Stress reduction and management
- Acute and chronic pain relief
- Chronic illness management and acute exacerbations prevention
- Preparation for surgery and medical procedures
- Medication compliance and adherence issues
- Cancer treatment and life-threatening illnesses
- Terminal illnesses and end of life care
- Fertility, birthing, and delivery
- Grief therapy
- Posttraumatic stress disorder
- Anxiety disorders
- Depression
- Sleep disorders
- Fitness training
- Smoking cessation and weight control

The Academy for Guided Imagery has developed IGI techniques applicable in the course of normal clinical interaction, brief medical office visits, or longer counseling and psychotherapy formats. Physicians may practice it themselves or employ an appropriate allied health professional to offer longer sessions.

Research Base

Clinical research studies on IGI have just been initiated with studies currently in progress at UCLA and UCSF-Mt. Zion Cancer Center. However, numerous studies in the literature document the effectiveness of guided imagery and visualization for the following situations: pain control,[13-16] cancer management,[17-20] irritable bowel syndrome,[21,22] arthritis,[23-25] menstrual irregularities,[26,27] eczyma,[28] fibromyalgia,[29] heart disease,[30-33] and even insomnia.[34,35]

Risk and Safety

Guided imagery is one of the safest complementary or alternative medical interventions. The primary danger in using imagery to augment healing in medical situations is when it is used instead of (rather than in addition to) more appropriate medical diagnosis and/or treatment.

Obviously, patients who are psychotic and patients with dissociative disorders or borderline personality disorders must be treated carefully by well-trained and experienced practitioners. Although these diagnoses do not represent absolute contraindications for imagery therapy, they require health professionals with specific expertise in these areas.

Efficacy

Imagery is the natural language of the emotions and the unconscious mind. It also has a profound controlling influence on our nervous, endocrine, and immune systems, so its potential uses in the healing professions are protean. Thus, with this in mind, imagery should be thought of as a way of working with the patient, rather than a way of treating a particular disease or symptom.

The efficacy of using imagery is extremely high in clinical situations classically considered psychosomatic or for conditions complicated by anxiety, stress, trauma, and loss of control. However, IGI is not a therapy that can be applied to an unwilling patient. Patients who do become engaged in the imagery process almost always receive some benefit from it and are grateful for the self-management skills they have learned in the process.

Future Research Opportunities and Priorities

There are many important research questions that currently remain unanswered. For example, can IGI actually slow the progression of a disease as well as enhance the well-being of the patient? How much is the healing process caused by engendering a sense of self-efficacy in the patient, and how much results directly from physiologic responses to imagery? Can patients self-diagnose more accurately if they use IGI? Does IGI lead to more effective and long-lasting lifestyle modifications in those patients with chronic illness? Can IGI be helpful toward the end of life in the reduction of distress and the prevention of care that may be futile?

Self-Help versus Professional

Although it is always advisable to seek care from a trained professional, many basic guided imagery techniques for simple relaxation, stress management, and related problems are commercially available on cassette tapes and may be helpful for minor, self-limiting problems. For more serious situations requiring IGI, appropriate care can only be provided by health professionals who have been trained and certified by the Academy for Guided Imagery.

Visiting a Professional

IGI is an easy-to-learn method of empowering the mind to enhance the process of healing. With the aid of a supportive, trained guide, patients will learn specific techniques designed to help relax, relieve stress, encourage physical healing, enhance body-mind communication, sharpen intuition and creativity, and become more effective at reaching goals.

Using a simple relaxation technique to help patients focus attention on their own personal inner world, the IGI guide teaches skills that will help improve effectiveness in problem-solving, conflict resolution, goal setting, stimulating healing responses in the body, and using latent inner strengths and resources to bring about emotional balance in daily life.

Credentialing and Training

The Academy for Guided Imagery has well-established standards of competence and ethical behavior that must be met as a prerequisite for Certification. The Academy is accredited by the American Psychological Association, the National Association of Social Workers, and the California Board of Nursing. Quality assurance is based on written examinations and direct observation of clinical work in small group and individual supervision sessions during the training program.

Candidates must satisfactorily complete 150 hours of academy-approved training, including direct observation of their guiding abilities. This direct observation is conducted by a team of four to six different faculty members during at least 52 hours of direct supervision to ensure the candidate has sufficiently mastered the methods of guided imagery. We know of no other such standards of quality assurance established for imagery practitioners.

What to Look for in a Provider

All providers of IGI should have a certificate from the Academy for Guided Imagery and should be listed with the Academy and on its website (www.healthy.com/agi) as a certified graduate.

Barriers and Key Issues

Clinicians have always been cognizant of the importance of attitudes, emotions, and mind/body relationships in medicine. Advances in the neurosciences, including peptide and receptor physiology, along with clinical studies of mind-body phenomenon, have renewed research interest in this field. With some research funds now being available to study this complex area, we will likely learn a great deal more in the next 10 to 20 years than ever before.

Associations

The Academy for Guided Imagery
PO Box 2070
Mill Valley, CA 94942
Tel: (800) 726-2070
Fax: (415) 389-9342
www.interactiveimagery.com

The International Association of Interactive Imagery
PO Box 124
Villa Grande, CA 95486
www.iaii.org

Suggested Reading

1. Achterberg J: *Imagery in healing*, Boston, 1985, Shambala.
   A classic history and overview of imagery in the healing arts, including many insights into how and why it works. Dr. Achterberg is a wonderful researcher, gifted writer, and genuine pioneer in the field.
2. Bresler D: *Free yourself from pain*, Mill Valley, Calif, 1999, Awareness Press.
   This is a reprint of Dr. Bresler's classic self-help book, first published by Simon and Schuster in 1979. It remains the most comprehensive and definitive guide available for helping people recover from chronic pain through mind-body and imagery methods, nutrition, bodywork, and other innovative self-help methods. Six cassette tapes accompany it.
3. Gurin J, Goleman D, editors: *Mind-body medicine*, New York, 1993, Consumer Reports Books.
   An in-depth text for professionals and laypersons alike examining the varieties of approaches to mind-body healing and how it can be used to treat common medical conditions.

4. Johnson R: *Inner work,* New York, 1986, Harper & Row.
A beautifully written book on inner work, the last third of which includes one of the best written treatises on the use of "active imagination" that currently exists.

5. Nucho A: *Spontaneous creative imagery: problem-solving and life-enhancing skills,* Springfield, Ill, 1995, Charles C. Thomas.
A thorough professional review of the uses of imagery in stress reduction, creativity, and healing, the research that supports it, and resources that provide training.

6. Oyle I: *The healing mind,* Millbrae, Calif, 1975, Celestial Arts.
A brilliant, classic work, but long out of print and now hard to find. If you can obtain a copy, it is a very worthwhile read, written by one of the first contemporary medical practitioners to see the enormous potential of imagery for healing.

7. Rossman M: *Healing yourself: a step-by-step program for better health through imagery,* Mill Valley, Calif, 1999, Awareness Press.
This award-winning book by Dr. Rossman is still the most thorough, user-friendly guide to using imagery for self-healing. It is especially effective when used with the companion set of six tapes.

8. Samuels M, Samuels N: *Seeing with the mind's eye,* New York, 1975, Random House.
A fascinating and thorough look at imagery through the ages, with a special emphasis on applications for healing.

References

1. Zahourek RP, editor: Relaxation & imagery: tools for therapeutic communication and intervention, Philadelphia, 1988, W.B. Saunders.

2. King JV: A holistic technique to lower anxiety: relaxation with guided imagery, *J Holistic Nurs* 6(1):16-20, 1988.

3. McDonald RT, Hilgendorf WA: Death imagery and death anxiety, *J Clin Psychol* 42(1):87-91, 1986.

4. Schaub BG, R; The use of mental imagery techniques in psychodynamic psychotherapy, *J Ment Health Counsel* 12(4):405-415, 1990.

5. Prendergast D: The use of relaxation and imagery in the treatment of rheumatoid arthritis, thesis, 1984, National Library of Canada.

6. Ahsen A: Imagery treatment of alcoholism and drug abuse: a new methodology for treatment and research, *J Ment Image* 17(3-4):1-60, 1993.

7. Krystal S, Zweben J: The use of visualization as a means of integrating the spiritual dimension into treatment: II. Working with emotions, *J Substance Abuse Treatment* 6(4):223-228, 1989.

8. Blankfield RP: Suggestion, relaxation, and hypnosis as adjuncts in the care of surgery patients: a review of the literature, *Amer J Clin Hyp* 33(3):172-186, 1991.

9. Enqvist B, von Konow L, Bystedt H: Pre- and perioperative suggestion in maxillofacial surgery: effects on blood loss and recovery, *Int J Clin Exp Hypn* 43(3):284-294, 1995.

10. Holden-Lund C: Effects of relaxation with guided imagery on surgical stress and wound healing, *Res Nurs Health* 11:235-244, 1988.

11. Tusek DL et al: Guided imagery: a significant advance in the care of patients undergoing elective colorectal surgery, *Dis Colon Rectum* 40(2):172-178, 1997.

12. Academy for Guided Imagery, Mill Valley, Calif. Internet site: www.healthy.com/agi.

13. Achterberg J et al: Severe burn injury: comparison of relaxation, imagery, and biofeedback for pain management, *J Ment Imagery* 12(1):71-87, 1988.

14. Raft D et al: Selection of imagery in the relief of chronic and acute clinical pain, *J Psychosomat Clin Res* 30(4):481-488, 1986.

15. Krueger LC: Pediatric pain and imagery, *J Child Adolescent Psychiatry* 4(1):32-41, 1987.

16. Newshan G: Use of imagery in a chronic pain outpatient group, *Imagination, Cognition, and Personality* 10(1):25-38, 1990/1991.

17. Caudell KA: Psychoneuroimmunology and innovative behavioral interventions in patients with leukemia, *Oncol Nurs Forum* 23(3):493-502, 1996.

18. Bridge LR et al: Relaxation and imagery in the treatment of breast cancer, *BMJ* 297(6657):1169-1172, 1988.

19. Brigham DD: The use of imagery in a multimodal psychoneuroimmunology program for cancer and other chronic diseases. In Kunzendorf R, editor: *Mental imagery*, New York, 1991, Plenum.

20. Troesch LM et al: The influence of guided imagery on chemotherapy-related nausea and vomiting, *Oncol Nurs Forum* 20(8):1179-1185, 1993.

21. Blanchard EB et al: Relaxation training as a treatment for irritable bowel syndrome, *Biofeedback and Self Regulation* 18(3):125-132, 1993.

22. Francis CY, Houghton LA: Use of hypnotherapy in gastrointestinal disorders, *Eur J Gastroenterol Hepatol* 8(6):525-529, 1996.

23. Prendergast D: The use of relaxation and imagery in the treatment of rheumatoid arthritis, National Library of Canada, Thesis, 1984.

24. Bennett AK: Rheumatoid arthritis: effects on the disease process utilizing a behavioral approach to treatment, *DAI* 46(3-B):993, 1985.

25. Rider MS: Treating arthritis and lupus patients with music-mediated imagery and group psychotherapy, *Arts Psychother* 17(1):29-33, 1990.

26. Tasto D: Muscle relaxation treatment for primary dysmenorrhea, *Behav Ther* 5(5) 668-672, 1974.

27. Torem M: Hypnotherapeutic techniques in the treatment of hyperemesis gravidarum, *Amer J Clin Hypn* 37(1):1-11, 1994.

28. Ehlers A, Stangier U, Gieler U: Treatment of atopic dermatitis: a comparison of psychological and dermatological approaches to relapse prevention, *J Consult Clin Psychol* 63(4):624-635, 1995.

29. Albright GL: Effects of warming imagery aimed at trigger-point sites on tissue compliance, skin temperature, and pain sensitivity in biofeedback-trained patients with chronic pain: a preliminary study, *Perceptual Motor Skills* 71(3):1163-1170, 1990.

30. Ulmer D: Stress management for the cardiovascular patient: a look at current treatment and trends, *Progress Cardiovasc Nurs* 11(1):21-29, 1996.

31. Ornish D: *Dr. Dean Ornish's guide to reversing heart disease*, New York, 1990, Random House.

32. Thomas SA et al: Psychological factors and survival in the cardiac arrhythmia suppression trial (CAST): a reexamination. *Amer J Critical Care* 6(2):116-126, 1997.

33. Mandle CL et al: The efficacy of relaxation response interventions with adult patients: a review of the literature, *J Cardiovasc Nurs* 10(3):4-26, 1996.

34. Morin CM: Stimulus control and imagery training in treating sleep-maintenance insomnia, *J Consult Clin Psychol* 5(2):260-262, 1987.

35. Lichstein KL, Johnson RS: Relaxation for insomnia and hypnotic medication use in older women, *Psychol Aging* 8(1):103-111, 1993.

Meditation

JOHN A. ASTIN*

SHAUNA L. SHAPIRO

GARY E.R. SCHWARTZ

Origins and History

This discussion reviews evidence for the efficacy of meditation as a complementary medical approach to the treatment and prevention of health-related problems. For purposes of this review, we define *meditation* as the intentional self-regulation of attention, a systematic focus on particular aspects of inner or outer experience.[1-3] Unlike many approaches in behavioral medicine (for example, biofeedback and relaxation), most meditation practices were developed within various religious/spiritual contexts. However, as a health care intervention, meditation can be effectively employed regardless of a patient's cultural or religious background.[1,4]

Over the past 3 decades, there has been considerable research examining the psychologic and physiologic effects of meditation,[5] and meditative practices are now being used within a variety of health care settings. Meditation can generally be divided into two broad types: *concentration* methods, which emphasize the stabilizing of attention on a specific object or focal device, such as the breath; and *mindfulness* practices, in which attention is not restricted to any one object but rather attends to any and all sensations, perceptions, cognitions, and emotions as they arise moment to moment in the field of awareness. It should be noted that mindfulness practices presuppose a certain degree of ability to focus or direct attention and often include concentrative elements.[6]

The scientific study of meditation and its applications in health care has focused on three specific approaches: 1) transcendental meditation (TM)[7]; 2) the elicitation of the "relaxation response," a generic approach to meditation formulated by Benson[8]; and 3) mindfulness meditation, specifically the mindfulness-based stress reduction program developed by Kabat-Zinn.[9] These techniques, along with several other related forms of meditation, are being incorporated into various health care settings.

*We would like to thank Dr. W. R. Van Nostrand for his contribution to this discussion and his insight regarding a physician's perspective on integrating meditation into health care.

It is now estimated that the mindfulness meditation program developed by Kabat-Zinn is available in more than 250 hospitals and medical clinics throughout the United States.

Biologic Mechanism of Action

The research on meditation suggests several possible mechanisms of action.[4,9-12] These center on four primary areas: 1) attenuation of stress reactivity; 2) effects on neuroendocrine function; 3) enhancement of sense of control or self-efficacy; and 4) prevention of relapse. However, the mechanisms outlined as follows are not mutually exclusive; for example, altering one's cognitive response to stress results in beneficial changes in neuroendocrine function.[13]

1. **Stress reactivity:** Chronic stress appears to contribute significantly to declines in physiologic function and health. These effects include suppression of immune function; cognitive impairment, including atrophy of brain structures; hypertension; cardiovascular disease; and loss of bone mineral density.[14] It is estimated that up to 80% of health-related problems have a significant stress component. Psychologic stress is also a frequent concomitant or consequence of disease and may also aggravate disease activity and exacerbate medical symptoms, such as chronic pain.[15] Meditation may reduce stress and its associated health consequences in several ways. First, through training in meditation, individuals become more aware of their characteristic cognitive-emotional patterns and habitual ways of reacting to stress. The recognition of the automatic and largely unconscious nature of stress reactivity may in turn facilitate the development of greater control over such reactivity and expand the range and repertoire of possible responses to stressful life events.

   Second, according to Schwartz's system's model of disregulation, stress may contribute to diminished health and well-being when individuals disattend to critical cognitive-emotional or physiologic feedback, resulting in a breakdown in communication between the organism's various subsystems.[16] Meditation emphasizes the development of greater awareness of proprioceptive, affective, and cognitive processes and states and therefore may be particularly effective in reducing stress and its negative health consequences by increasing the amount of communication or information in the "system," thereby leading to greater psychophysiologic regulation and balance.[3]

2. **Effects on neuroendocrine function:** The attenuation of sympathetic arousal that often accompanies meditation[8,17] may be a particularly effective approach for addressing the negative health consequences associated with chronic and acute stress reactivity.[18] Meditation may result in beneficial changes in physiologic parameters such as levels of adrenal hormones, platelet aggregation, autonomic tone and balance, blood pressure, and brain biochemistry and cerebral blood flow.

3. **Enhancing self-efficacy:** Studies suggest that having a sense of personal control can have profound physiologic effects, including altering immune and cardiovascular function, increasing longevity, and improving quality of life.[19] *Self-efficacy*, the subjective assessment that one has the resources to cope with a given or hypothetical sit-

uation,[20] is associated with a number of positive health outcomes and the adoption of healthy behaviors.[21,22] Studies with clinical and nonclinical populations suggest that meditation can increase feelings of self-efficacy and sense of control.[4,10,23]

4. **Relapse prevention:** Patients participating in meditation interventions for disorders such as chronic pain and anxiety have been able to maintain treatment gains for up to 4 years postintervention.[24,25] Meditation may facilitate the maintenance of such gains for several reasons. First, meditation is a generic skill that can be practiced on a range of experiences in addition to those specifically related to a given disease. Therefore patients can continue to practice and use the attentional skills of meditation in the period following a successful intervention, even in the absence of initial disease-related symptoms.[4,12] Second, meditation training emphasizes attending to thoughts and feelings, whether pleasant or unpleasant. This orientation reflects "turning toward" (accepting or acknowledging) rather than "looking away from" (denying) problems and difficulties that may facilitate early detection of signs of symptom relapse and thereby increase the likelihood of taking proactive steps to address them.[12]

Forms of Therapy

As noted, although there are a wide array of meditation practices, they generally fall into one of two broad categories: those that emphasize *concentration* (such as TM) and those that emphasize *mindfulness* (such as Vipassana). Some meditation traditions also combine elements of both concentration and mindfulness.[6]

Demographics

Individuals who use relaxation techniques in general (of which meditation is one subtype) tend to be younger, more educated, and subscribers to a holistic philosophic orientation that emphasizes the importance of body, mind, and spirit in treating health-related matters.[26] In a recent study of Medicare patients, those who reported practicing meditation were more likely to be women and tended to be younger and more educated, have a higher income, and be more likely to exercise.[27] Based on the research examining consumer use of complementary/alternative medicine, the practice of meditation, although potentially more concentrated in certain geographic regions, can be found across most demographic groups and areas.[26,28]

Indications and Reasons For Referral

The majority of patients are referred to meditation-based interventions for the following conditions: 1) those in which *stress* is implicated as a major causal factor, such as hypertension; 2) those involving chronic pain, such as headaches and musculoskeletal disorders; and 3) those in which emotional distress (anxiety and depression) is a frequent concomitant, such as cancer and other chronic diseases.

Office Applications

The following list provides a guide to medical conditions for which meditation would be most likely to have therapeutic value. As with all alternative therapies, use of meditation does not preclude the use of mainstream medical therapies. In general, we believe that meditation may be a potentially important complementary therapy in both the treatment and prevention of a number of conditions because of its demonstrated psychologic and physiologic stress-reducing effects. Therefore the following list focuses primarily on those illnesses in which stress has been implicated as an important causal factor or major consequence of the disease. In most cases, the recommendations and rankings are based on current empiric evidence. However, in some instances in which there is less of an evidence base, we have still included the condition if there is good theoretic support for the use of meditation. We have indicated next to each condition the primary rationale for its inclusion: evidence (E), theory (T), or both (ET).

Top level: *A therapy ideally suited for these conditions*
None

Second level: *One of the better therapies for these conditions*
Panic disorder (ET); generalized anxiety disorder (ET); psoriasis (ET); substance dependence and abuse (ET); ulcers (T); colitis (T); dysthymic disorder (T); and chronic pain conditions (ET)

Third level: *A valuable adjunctive therapy for these conditions*
Moderate hypertension (ET); prevention of atherosclerosis (ET); prevention of cardiac arrest (T); arthritis (including fibromyalgia) (ET); neoplastic disease (cancer) (T); insomnia (T); migraine (T); and prevention of stroke (T)

Practical Applications

As noted, referral for meditation may be particularly appropriate for patients with health-related problems and diseases in which stress has been implicated as an important causal factor or major consequence. Referral for meditation also can be applied to both mental and physical health problems. In terms of mindfulness meditation, which is one of the more popular forms of meditation employed in medical settings, there are currently more than 240 mindfulness-based stress reduction programs offered at health care settings around the world, modeled after the program at the University of Massachusetts.[58] Of these, the majority (in the U.S.) are located at teaching hospitals, large medical centers, and health maintenance organizations.[59] Patients are referred to these clinics by their physicians for training in mindfulness meditation as a complement to traditional medical care in the treatment of diverse illnesses and stress-related disorders.

Research Base

Evidence Based

CARDIOVASCULAR DISEASE

Murphy et al found strong evidence that meditation can lower blood pressure in normotensive or moderately hypertensive individuals.[5] However, results are equivocal with respect to more acute hypertension and essential hypertension.[29]

Meditation may also be an effective treatment for coronary artery disease (CAD). In a study of 21 CAD patients, those practicing TM meditation for 8 months evidenced significant increases in exercise tolerance, maximal workload, and delay in onset of ST-segment depression compared to controls.[30] Meditation is also a central component of the lifestyle intervention developed by Ornish that has been shown to reverse coronary artery disease.[31]

CHRONIC PAIN

Meditation may be particularly effective in the treatment of chronic pain.[9,24] Significant reductions have been observed in pain symptoms, inhibition of activity by pain, psychologic symptoms, and pain-related drug use.[9] In a 4-year follow-up, the majority of patients in the mindfulness program reported "moderate to great improvement" in pain status at all follow-up time points.[24] In a nonrandomized trial, positive changes were observed in pain, functional status, and psychologic symptoms among fibromyalgia patients practicing meditation.[32] Meditation may be an effective adjunct to pain treatment for two reasons: 1) the state of hypoarousal may serve to diminish pain and its related symptoms; and 2) through the cultivation of detached or "bare attention," cognitive-emotional alarm reactions to painful sensations (such as "I'll never survive this," "This pain will probably go on forever") become less all-consuming or overwhelming.[9] Although the physical (nociceptive) experiences of pain may remain largely unchanged among patients trained in meditation, the emotional and cognitive components of the pain experience appear to be significantly diminished, resulting in less suffering and distress.[24]

ANXIETY

Findings suggest that meditation is effective in reducing symptoms of anxiety and treating anxiety-related disorders.[33,34] In comparison with other approaches such as biofeedback and progressive muscle relaxation, meditation has demonstrated equal if not greater effect sizes, particularly for trait anxiety. In an observational study of 22 patients with anxiety disorders, 90% of those receiving training in mindfulness meditation showed improvement in anxiety and depression scores postintervention and at 3 months[35]; 82% showed maintenance of gains at 3 years.[36]

SUBSTANCE ABUSE

Research suggests that meditation is particularly effective in the treatment of chemical dependency.[5] Gelderloos et al[37] reviewed 24 studies and reported that all showed significant positive effect of the TM program on smoking cessation as well as drug and alcohol abuse.

DERMATOLOGIC DISORDERS

In a recent study, 37 psoriasis patients were randomized to standard UV light treatment with or without mindfulness meditation.[38] Patients received approximately 40 treatments over the course of 13 weeks. Those practicing meditation evidenced more rapid clearing (3.8 times faster) of their dermatologic condition than nonintervention controls.

DEPRESSIVE SYMPTOMS

We are aware of no randomized trials examining the effects of meditation on clinical depression. However, studies suggest that meditation can lead to reductions in depressive symptoms in nonclinical populations[10,11] or when such depressive symptoms are comorbid with anxiety disorders.[36] Preliminary work suggests that meditation may be a particularly effective cognitive strategy for preventing depressive relapse.[39]

ADJUNCT TO PSYCHOTHERAPY

Meditation may also be useful as an adjunct to psychotherapy. In an observational study, improvements in psychologic function were found among psychotherapy patients undergoing training in mindfulness meditation.[40] Bogart[41] suggests that meditation may facilitate greater calmness, acceptance of self and others, access to unconscious material, insight into cognitive-emotional processes, and changes in personal identity. Along these lines, there is evidence that meditation can lead to improvements in measures of positive psychologic health[42] such as empathy,[11,43] sense of coherence and "hardiness,"[4] control,[10] self-actualization,[44] and spirituality.[10,11]

OTHER DISORDERS

Little research has been carried out examining the efficacy of meditation in the treatment and prevention of a number of conditions, including cancer, arthritis, allergies, and asthma. However, because of the likely role of psychologic stress in their etiology and because stress is frequently a major consequence or concomitant of these diseases, meditation may be a particularly useful complementary therapy for these conditions.

Basic Science

Although some of the physiologic changes observed during meditation may vary as a function of the type of meditation being practiced,[4,5] some overall trends have emerged. Most forms of meditation can generally be characterized by a hypometabolic state evidenced by reductions in heart rate, oxygen consumption, respiratory rate, and carbon dioxide production by muscle.[45,46] Reductions have also been observed in cholesterol and blood lactate levels.[5] Cardiac output typically shows increases while blood flow to the liver and kidneys is reduced.[46] Electroencephalographic (EEG) changes have also been reported with increased alpha and theta wave production in both waking and sleeping.[47] Meditation (TM) is also associated with increased cerebral blood flow in the frontal and occipital regions coupled with decreased cerebrovascular resistance.[48]

Although a majority of studies have shown decreases in cortisol levels following meditation,[49,50] others have failed to do so.[51] Several studies have shown increases in plasma norepinephrine[52]; others have found lower levels of the norepinephrine metabolite vanillylmandelic acid (VMA) in meditators. Other effects include increased plasma renin, prolactin, phenylalanine, and argenine vasopressin.[46] Benson suggests that meditation may reduce end-organ responsiveness to norepinephrine, which would explain the corresponding reductions in heart rate and blood pressure that have been observed.[53]

A recent study examined physiologic differences brought about by the long-term practice of TM meditation (minimum of 8.5 years).[13] Compared to a matched group of nonmeditators, long-term meditators evidenced lower levels of cortisol and aldosterone and were higher in dehydroepiandrosterone sulfate (DS) and the serotonin metabolite 5-hydroxyindoleacetic acid (5-HIAA). Excretion of sodium, calcium, zinc, and the norepinephrine metabolite (VMA) was also lower in the meditation group, as well as the Na+/K+ ratio.

Preliminary research has shown that the practice of mindfulness meditation is associated with increased levels of melatonin, suggesting a potential role for meditation in the prevention and treatment of breast and prostrate cancer.[54]

Risk and Safety

Meditation appears to be a safe treatment for most individuals. However, there are case reports and descriptive studies documenting some adverse effects. Among individuals participating in silent mindfulness meditation retreats (lasting 2 weeks to 3 months),[55] between 33% and 50% of participants reported increased tension, anxiety, depression, and confusion. However, most of these subjects also reported very positive effects from the meditation practice. Similar results were found in a study of TM practitioners.[56] As Kabat-Zinn et al[1] note, these studies failed to differentiate between serious clinical or psychiatric disturbance and normal variability in emotional mood states. They suggest, however, that meditation may require concurrent psychotherapy for certain individuals who are at high risk for emotional flooding or uncovering of repressed material (such as those with post-traumatic stress disorder and suicidal ideation). It has also been suggested that meditation may be contraindicated for those with psychotic or borderline personality disorders.[57]

Efficacy

See "Evidence Based."

Future Research Opportunities and Priorities

Although there has been considerable research examining the health benefits of meditation, there is a need for larger controlled trials comparing these techniques with one another, with other relaxation and cognitive-behavioral strategies, and with usual medical care. We are aware of several large clinical trials that have been proposed or are now underway. One is an ongoing examination of the effects of meditation on patients with breast cancer at the University of Massachusetts Medical Center. Another is a large trial comparing meditation with usual care in the treatment of arthritis at Stanford University. Further studies are also needed to examine the psychophysiologic mechanisms underlying meditation's health-promotive effects and the role of intention in coordinating these effects.[3]

Self-Help versus Professional

Individuals can certainly learn meditation on their own. There are numerous books and tapes that provide a sound introduction to these practices (see "Suggested Readings"). However, it can often be helpful to have the guidance of a trained meditation instructor, particularly when meditation is used as a complementary therapy for a health-related problem.

Visiting a Professional

Because there are a variety of approaches to meditation in medical settings, we briefly summarize here what visiting a professional would involve for one such therapy: mindfulness meditation. The meditation-based stress reduction (MBSR) program developed by Kabat-Zinn is typically taught in a group format. Patients with an array of medical conditions are referred to these groups by their health care practitioners and receive weekly instruction in a variety of meditation techniques. MBSR requires a high degree of commitment; participants are asked to practice the meditation techniques on a daily basis for between 45 and 60 minutes. However, research suggests that the duration of meditation practice and program specifics can be tailored to meet the particular needs and motivational levels of individuals and groups.[10] For example, an MBSR intervention offered to medical students required only 20 minutes of practice per day and still found significant decreases in stress-related symptoms.[11]

Credentialing

Although the Center for Mindfulness in Medicine, Health Care, and Society currently does not offer any type of certification or licensing process, certain guidelines are suggested for teachers to work toward. For example, the guidelines proposed by the Northern California Advisory Group on Mindfulness and Medicine include both "qualifications" and "qualities." Qualifications include a minimum of 5 years mindfulness meditation experience, extensive mindfulness meditation retreat experience, an ongoing affiliation with a community of mindfulness practitioners, and most importantly, a personal daily mindfulness meditation practice. The list of qualities includes an ability to create a safe environment for participants and an ability to empathize while maintaining a neutral perspective. As for the Transcendental Meditation program, the organization does formally recognize TM instructors. To receive a list of credentialed TM instructors, contact the TM organization's headquarters (see "Associations").

Training

Different schools of meditation vary in terms of what they consider adequate training. For example, individuals need to undergo fairly extensive training in order to be formally recognized instructors of Transcendental Meditation. The Center for Mindfulness in Medicine, Health Care and Society at the University of Massachusetts Medical Center also offers training and workshops for health professionals and others interested in teaching mindfulness-based stress reduction; however, there is no formal credentialing. The Center's offerings include an intensive 7-day retreat for health professionals, intensive weekend workshops, and a 10-week internship program.

What to Look for in a Provider

As noted, meditation providers/instructors ideally should have a regular meditation practice of their own. This is particularly important because properly viewed, meditation is less of a technique to address specific health-related problems or diseases and more of a general way of orienting the self to the world and life experiences.[1,4] Instructors who are teaching meditation in a group context ideally should also have experience working with diverse groups of people and well-developed interpersonal and communication skills.

Barriers and Key Issues

There are two key issues that have served as obstacles to the integration of meditation into conventional medical practice. First, despite decades of rigorous scientific research documenting the important role that psychosocial factors (such as emotional stress and hostility) play in the development, treatment, and prevention of health-related problems, the prevailing biomedical paradigm has been slow to change. The reductionist notion that physical disorders have purely or even primarily physiologic, biochemic, and genetic causes can no longer be supported by the available research. Evidence from fields such as health psychology and behavioral medicine points to the need for a bio-psycho-social-spiritual[60,61] rather than biomedical model, yet the latter remains the dominant paradigm. A second issue is the inaccurate perception that meditation practices are the exclusive province of esoteric religious or Eastern schools of thought and therefore are simply too strange or unfamiliar to be accepted by mainstream health care practitioners and their patients. The work of clinician-researchers such as Kabat-Zinn have done much to move meditation beyond its esoteric and mystical trappings, while at the same time remaining true to its original roots and spirit as a contemplative discipline with the ultimate purpose of fostering spiritual and personal growth, insight, and wisdom and reducing suffering.

Associations

Center for Mindfulness in Medicine, Health Care, and Society
University of Massachusetts Medical Center
Worcester, MA 01655
Tel: (508) 856-5849
www.mbsr.com

The Transcendental Meditation Program
Tel: (800) LEARN TM
www.tm.org

Mind-Body Medical Institute
Beth Israel Deaconess Medical Center,
One Deaconess Rd
Boston, MA 02215
Tel: (617) 632-9525
www.mindbody.harvard.edu

Suggested Reading

1. Kabat-Zinn J: *Full catastrophe living: using the wisdom of your body and mind to face stress, pain, and illness*, New York, 1990, Dell.

   This book describes the 8-week meditation-based stress reduction program developed by Kabat-Zinn. It also reviews some of the literature linking psychologic factors (including stress) to various health outcomes.

2. Benson H: *The relaxation response*, New York, 1975, Morrow.

   Herbert Benson's landmark work details the nondenominational meditation technique he labeled the "Relaxation Response," a term that refers to the research suggesting that meditation produces a hypometabolic state counter to the fight-or-flight mechanism.

3. Murphy M, Donovan S: *The physical and psychological effects of meditation: a review of contemporary research with a comprehensive bibliography 1931-1996*. Sausalito, Calif, 1997, Institute of Noetic Sciences.

   The most comprehensive review to date of scientific studies examining the psychologic, physiologic, and health effects of meditation.

4. Shapiro DH: *Meditation: self-regulation strategy and altered state of consciousness*, New York, 1980, Aldine.

   One of the first comprehensive reviews of meditation and its potential applications in psychology and behavioral medicine.

References

1. Kabat-Zinn J et al: Meditation. In Holland JC, editor: *Textbook on psycho-oncology*, Oxford, 1998, Oxford University Press.

2. Goleman DJ, Schwartz GE: Meditation as an intervention in stress reactivity, *J Consult Clin Psychol* 44:456-466, 1976.

3. Shapiro SL, Schwartz GER: The role of intention in self-regulation: toward intentional systemic mindfulness. In Boekaerts M, Pintrich PR, Zeidner M, editors: *Handbook of self-regulation*, New York, 1999, Academic Press (in press).

4. Kabat-Zinn J: Mindfulness meditation: what it is, what it isn't, and its role in health care and medicine. In Haruki Y, Suzuki M, editors: *Comparative and psychological study on meditation*, Delft, 1996, Eburon.

5. Murphy M, Donovan S, Taylor E: *The physical and psychological effects of meditation: a review of contemporary research with a comprehensive bibliography*, Sausalito, Calif, 1997, Institute of Noetic Sciences.

6. Shapiro DH: *Meditation: self-regulation strategy and altered state of consciousness*, New York, 1980, Aldine.

7. Orme-Johnson DW, Farrow JT: *Scientific research on the transcendental meditation program: I. Collected papers*, New York, 1977, Mount Meru Press.

8. Benson H: *The relaxation response*, New York, 1975, Morrow.

9. Kabat-Zinn J, Lipworth L, Burney R: The clinical use of mindfulness meditation for the self-regulation of chronic pain, *J Behav Med* 8:163-190, 1985.

10. Astin JA: Stress reduction through mindfulness meditation: effects on psychological symptomatology, sense of control, and spiritual experiences, *Psychother Psychosom* 66:97-106, 1997.

11. Shapiro SL, Schwartz GER, Bonner G: The effects of mindfulness-based stress reduction on medical and pre-medical students, *J Behav Med* 21(6):581-599, 1999.

12. Teasdale JD, Segal Z, Williams JM: How does cognitive therapy prevent depressive relapse and why should attentional control (mindfulness) training help? *Behav Res Ther* 33:25-39, 1995.

13. Walton KG et al: Stress reduction and preventing hypertension: preliminary support for a psychoneuroendocrine mechanism, *J Altern Complement Med* 1:263-283, 1995.

14. McEwen BS: Protective and damaging effects of stress mediators, *New Engl J Med* 338:171-179, 1998.

15. Shearn MA, Fireman BH: Stress management and mutual support groups in rheumatoid arthritis, *Am J Med* 78:771-775, 1985.

16. Schwartz GE: Psychobiology of repression and health: a system approach. In Singer J, editor: *Repression and dissociation: implications for personality theory, psychopathology, and health*, Chicago, 1990, University of Chicago Press.

17. Wallace RK: Physiological effects of transcendental meditation, *Science* 167:1751-1754, 1970.

18. Friedman R, Steinman M, Benson H: The relaxation response: physiological effects and medical applications. In Haruki Y, Suzuki M, editors: *Comparative and psychological study on meditation*, Delft, 1996, Eburon.

19. Shapiro DH, Astin JA: Control therapy: an integrated approach to psychotherapy, health, and healing, New York, 1998, John Wiley.

20. Bandura A: Self-efficacy: toward a unifying theory of behavioral change, *Psychol Rev* 84:191-215, 1977.

21. Taylor SE: *Health psychology*, ed 3, New York, 1995, McGraw-Hill.

22. Lorig K, Holman H: Arthritis self-management studies: a twelve-year review. Special Issue: Arthritis health education, *Health Ed Q* 20:17-28, 1993.

23. Shapiro DH: A mode of control and self-control profile for long term meditators, *Psychologia* 35:1-11, 1992.

24. Kabat-Zinn J, Lipworth L, Burney R: Four-year follow-up of a meditation-based program for the self-regulation of chronic pain: treatment outcomes and compliance, *Clin J Pain* 2:159-173, 1987.

25. Miller JJ, Fletcher K, Kabat-Zinn J: Three-year follow-up and clinical implications of a mindfulness meditation-based stress reduction intervention in the treatment of anxiety disorders, *Gen Hosp Psychiatry* 17:192-200, 1995.

26. Astin JA: Why patients use alternative medicine: results of a national study, *JAMA* 279:1548-1553, 1998.

27. Astin JA et al: Complementary and alternative medicine use among the elderly, *J Gerontol* (under review).

28. Eisenberg DM et al: Trends in alternative medicine use in the United States, 1990-1997: results of a follow-up national survey, *JAMA* 280:1569-1575, 1998.

29. Eisenberg DM et al: Cognitive behavioral techniques for hypertension: are they effective? *Ann Intern Med* 118:964-972, 1993.

30. Zamarra JW et al: Usefulness of the transcendental meditation program in the treatment of patients with coronary artery disease, *Am J Cardiol* 77:867-870, 1996.

31. Ornish D et al: Intensive lifestyle changes for reversal of coronary heart disease, *JAMA* 280:2001-2007, 1998.

32. Goldenberg DL et al: A controlled study of a stress-reduction, cognitive-behavioral treatment program in fibromyalgia, *J Musculoskeletal Pain* 2:53-66, 1994.

33. Eppley KR, Abrams AI, Shear J: Differential effects of relaxation techniques on trait anxiety: a meta-analysis, *J Clin Psychol* 45:957-974, 1989.

34. Edwards DL: A meta-analysis of the effects of meditation and hypnosis on measures of anxiety, *Dissert Abstr Int* 52(2B):1039, 1991.

35. Kabat-Zinn J et al: Effectiveness of a meditation-based stress reduction program in the treatment of anxiety disorders, *Am J Psychiatry* 149:936-943, 1992.

36. Miller JJ, Fletcher K, Kabat-Zinn J: Three-year follow-up and clinical implications of a mindfulness meditation-based stress reduction intervention in the treatment of anxiety disorders, *Gen Hosp Psychiatry* 17:192-200, 1995.

37. Gelderloos P et al: Effectiveness of the transcendental meditation program in preventing and treating substance misuse, *Int J Addict* 26:293-325, 1991.

38. Kabat-Zinn J et al: Influence of a mindfulness meditation-based stress reduction intervention on rates of skin clearing in patients with moderate to severe psoriasis undergoing phototherapy (UVB) and photochemotherapy (PUVA), *Psychosom Med* 60:625-632, 1998.

39. Teasdale JD, Segal Z, Williams JMG: How does cognitive therapy prevent depressive relapse and why should attentional control (mindfulness) training help? *Behav Res Ther* 33:25-39, 1994.

40. Kutz I et al: Meditation as an adjunct to psychotherapy: an outcome study, *Psychother Psychosom* 43:209-218, 1985.

41. Bogart G: The use of meditation in psychotherapy: a review of the literature, *Am J Psychother* 45:383-412, 1991.

42. Gelderloos P et al: Transcendence and psychological health: studies with long-term participants of the transcendental meditation and TM-Sidhi program, *J Psychol* 124:177-197, 1990.

43. Lesh TV: Zen meditation and the development of empathy in counselors, *J Humanist Psychol* 10:39-74, 1970.

44. Alexander CN, Rainforth M, Gelderloos P: Transcendental meditation, self-actualization, and psychological health: a conceptual overview and statistical meta-analysis. Special issue: Handbook of self-actualization. *J Soc Behav Personality* 6:189-248, 1991.

45. Wallace RK, Benson H: The physiology of meditation, *Sci Amer* 226:84-90, 1972.

46. Jevning R, Wallace RK, Beiderbach M: The physiology of meditation: A review. A wakeful hypometabolic integrated response, *Neurosci Biobehav Rev* 16:415-424, 1992.

47. Mason LI et al: Electrophysiological correlates of higher states of consciousness during sleep in long-term practitioners of the transcendental meditation program, *Sleep* 20:102-110, 1997.

48. Jevning R et al: Effects on regional cerebral blood flow of transcendental meditation, *Physiol Behav* 59:399-402, 1996.

49. Jevning R, O'Halloran JP: Metabolic effects of transcendental meditation: toward a new paradigm of neurobiology. In Shapiro DH, Walsh RW, editors: *Meditation: classic and contemporary perspective*, New York, 1984, Aldine.

50. MacLean CRK et al: Effects of the transcendental meditation program on adaptive mechanisms: changes in hormone levels and responses to stress after 4 months of practice, *Psychoneuroendocrinology* 22:277-295, 1997.

51. Werner OR et al: Long-term endocrinologic changes in subjects practicing the transcendental meditation and TM-sidhi program, *Psychosom Med* 48:59-65, 1986.

52. Benson H: The relaxation response and norepinephrine, *Integrat Psychiatry* 1:15-19, 1983.

53. Benson H: The relaxation response and norepinephrine: a new study illuminates mechanisms, *Austral J Clin Hypnother Hypn* 10:91-96, 1989.

54. Massion AO et al: Meditation, melatonin and breast-prostate cancer: hypothesis and preliminary data, *Med Hypoth* 44:39-46, 1995.

55. Shapiro DH: Adverse effects of meditation: a preliminary investigation of long-term meditators, *Int J Psychosom* 39:62-67, 1992.

56. Otis L: Adverse effects of transcendental meditation. In Shapiro DH, Walsh R, editors: *Meditation: classic and contemporary perspectives*, New York, 1984, Aldine.

57. Wilber K, Engler J, Brown DP: Transformations of consciousness: conventional and contemplative perspectives on development, Boston, 1986, Shambhala.

58. Kabat-Zinn J: News, views and musings, *Indra's Net: bulletin of the mindfulness-based stress reduction network* 3:3, 1998.

59. Roth B, Creaser T: Mindfulness meditation-based stress reduction: experience with a bilingual inner-city program, *Nurse Pract* 22:150-176, 1997.

60. Schwartz GE: Testing the biopsychosocial model: the ultimate challenge facing behavioral medicine, *J Consult Clin Psychol* 50:1040-1050, 1982.

61. Shapiro DH, Schwartz CE, Astin JA: Controlling ourselves, controlling our world: psychology's role in understanding positive and negative consequences of seeking and gaining control, *Am Psychol* 51:1213-1230, 1996.

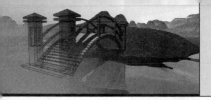

Music Therapy

BRYAN C. HUNTER

Origins and History

Bruscia[1] defined *music therapy* as "a systematic process of intervention wherein the therapist helps the client to promote health, using music experiences and the relationships that develop through them as dynamic forces of change." Although the profession of music therapy began in 1950 with the founding of the National Association for Music Therapy (NAMT), the ideas for the discipline of music therapy date to antiquity, including the writings of Plato and Aristotle and the often quoted biblical story of David playing the harp for Saul to ameliorate the king's depression. Throughout recorded history, musicians, physicians, psychiatrists, and special education teachers have written about the power of music to influence people physically, psychologically, and socially. From the sixteenth century music theorist Zarlino, who advocated music training as a part of medical education, to the writings of psychiatry's founder Benjamin Rush, noted professionals in music and medicine have advocated the use of music as therapy.[2,3]

However, it took the human devastation of World Wars I and II to create an overwhelming demand for the birth of a new profession. As thousands of war veterans suffering physical and mental illness filled Veterans Affairs and other hospitals across the country, volunteer community musicians came to perform for them. The patients' physical and psychologic responses were so remarkable and consistent that hospitals began to hire musicians to play for them. In time, the hospitals wanted musicians to have some training with regard to hospital procedures, and this eventually led to the first college curricula in music therapy at the present Michigan State University in 1944 and the University of Kansas in 1946. The NAMT began shortly thereafter to establish education and clinical training guidelines and eventually established a registration procedure to certify trained music therapists. In the early years a number of physicians, including Ira Altschuler in Michigan and Karl Menninger in Kansas, advocated music therapy and supported the new profession.[2]

In recent years the scientific basis for music therapy practice has been greatly expanded, allowing for new and exciting applications of music therapy in neonatal units to programs in geriatric medicine, from psychiatric units to oncology units, from neurology units to obstetrics, and throughout the rest of medicine. Its long-standing history and current research base have positioned the profession to be an important part of the current developments in integrative medicine.

Mechanism of Action According to Its Own Theory

Ethnomusicologist Alan Merriam[4] stated in a bold proclamation regarding music, "There is probably no other human cultural activity which is so all-pervasive and which reaches into, shapes, and often controls so much of human behavior." A music therapist's ability to effect positive physical, psychologic, and social change through music stems from the functions of music that have been observed in societies worldwide. Merriam identified the following ten primary functions of music:

1. Provides for emotional expression
2. Facilitates aesthetic enjoyment
3. Provides entertainment
4. Serves as a mode of communication
5. Allows for symbolic representation
6. Promotes physical response
7. Enforces conformity to social norms
8. Validates social institutions and religious rituals
9. Contributes to the continuity and stability of culture
10. Contributes to the integration of society

Refining Merriam's ideas into a theory of music therapy, Sears[5] outlined a set of processes in music therapy that centered on three categories in which music allows for experience within the structure of the music itself, in self-organization, and in relating to others.

If mental and physical health are considered as representing a state of desirable order in life, then the opposite end of the continuum would be the disorder experienced in disease or disability. Music therapy engages the client in one or more music experiences such as listening, singing, playing, improvising, writing, and moving to music in an attempt to facilitate change toward the positive end of the continuum. Underlying all of music therapy practice are three important music traits. First is the element of rhythm, which sustains the temporal existence of music and holds the potential to energize and bring order, something often missing or weakened by illness or disability.[6] Second is the nonverbal nature of music, which allows communication and responses at levels otherwise not accessible. Third is music's flexibility and adaptability, which in large part explains the diverse applications of music therapy, along with the fact that patients do not require music training to benefit from it.

Biologic Mechanism of Action

Taylor[7] articulated perhaps the first attempt at a biologic explanation of music's influence on behavior. His biomedical theory of music therapy is founded on one general conclusion and four correlated hypotheses.

Basic premise: "Music influences human behavior by affecting the brain and subsequently other bodily structures in ways that are observable, identifiable, measurable, and predictable, thereby providing the necessary foundation for its use in treatment procedures."

Hypothesis 1: "Because all sound stimuli are accessed by all parts of the brain, sound as music affects pain perception through its direct effect on the ability of the somatosensory cortex to receive pain sensations ascending through the spinothalamic tract following reception by sensors in the peripheral nervous system."

Hypothesis 2: "The normal neurological pathway for sound sensation allows music to have an effect on those structures in the human brain most responsible for emotional behavior, the hypothalamus and limbic system, thereby inhibiting negative emotional reactions which can delay or otherwise interfere with the treatment or recovery process."

Hypothesis 3: "Active participation in expressive musical activities provides structured movement behaviors necessary for maintenance or recovery of physical function, and for development of the skills necessary for interpersonal communication."

Hypothesis 4: "Music has direct effect on specific physiological processes whose functional variations are indicators of anxiety, tension, or stress."

There is mounting evidence to support much of Taylor's theory. At the very least, his model provides an excellent framework against which research can be evaluated and applied to clinical practice.

Forms of Therapy

Music is an extraordinarily rich, diverse, and multifaceted phenomenon that allows the therapist a choice of sounds and interventions such as listening, singing, playing, improvising, writing, and moving to music, depending on the patient's physical, psychologic, or social needs. Because of the diversity of music, patients' needs and cultures, and therapists' philosophic orientations, a number of distinct music therapy approaches have evolved. Some approaches focus on one of the above interventions and also may rest primarily on one of the traditional philosophical orientations to treatment or education such as psychodynamic, behavioral, cognitive, humanistic, and biomedical.[2,3] The following examples are not exhaustive but represent widely recognized music therapy approaches.

Behavioral music therapy focuses on using music to increase nonmusical adaptive behaviors and decrease maladaptive behaviors. Classical and operant conditioning is often (but not always) a part of this approach.[8] As the name implies, this approach grew out of behavior modification theory, but it also draws on cognitive and social learning theory, as well. Any of these interventions may be used in this approach.

Guided imagery and music (GIM) uses only music listening in a deeply relaxed state to evoke images for the purpose of exploring unconscious thoughts and feelings, along with different levels of consciousness. Therapists with advanced clinical training serve as facilitators to help patients process their experiences, which may include resolving conflicts, and integrating creative fantasies, memories, and positive aspects of the self.[9] GIM draws heavily from humanistic and psychodynamic theories.

Nordoff-Robbins improvisational music therapy (creative music therapy) focuses on music improvisation to connect with the "musical intelligence" or aesthetic response in people, which even in a person with severe disabilities often remains available for stimulation and development as an ego-strengthening force for self-actualization.[10] This approach also uses humanistic and psychodynamic theories.

Eclectic model recognizes that although diversity exits in music therapy practice, there is an important shared phenomenon of music and its influence on human beings. Consequently, it is common for music therapists to be eclectic in their approach depending on patients' ages, needs, and cultural backgrounds. However, it is important for music therapists using primarily psychodynamic approaches to have advanced clinical training beyond the bachelor's level.

Demographics

The AMTA estimates that there are 5000 credentialed music therapists in the United States. Its annual sourcebook contains demographic data based on surveys returned by music therapists who choose to be members of AMTA. The *1998 AMTA Member Sourcebook* demographics, based on a 56% return rate of the member surveys, indicated that there were music therapists in every state except Alaska. The top four states were New York, California, Pennsylvania, and Texas. In addition, there were member surveys returned from 24 foreign countries, some of which also have their own music therapy associations. Health care professionals and consumers needing assistance in locating a music therapist should contact the AMTA directly at (301) 589-3300.

The same sourcebook lists the following populations assisted by music therapy: abused and sexually abused, AIDS, Alzheimer's and dementia, autistic, behavioral disorder, cancer, chronic pain, comatose, developmentally disabled, dual diagnosed, early childhood, eating disorders, elderly persons, emotionally disturbed, forensic, head injuries, hearing impaired, learning disabled, medical and surgical, mental health, multiply disabled, neurologically impaired, nondisabled, Parkinson's disease, physically disabled, posttraumatic stress disorder, Rett syndrome, school-age population, speech impaired, stroke, substance abuse, terminally ill, visually impaired, and others. Music therapists work with male and female patients from diverse cultural backgrounds across the entire age span, from newborns to older adults. However, demographic data on these parameters is not available.

Indications and Reasons for Referral

People are referred to music therapy when they have conditions that demonstrate needs in the following areas:

1. Receptive communication: attention and concentration, auditory discrimination and sequencing, and short-term auditory memory
2. Expressive communication: vocal manipulation and inflection, language delay, and expression of feelings

3. Physical: stress reduction and relaxation, pain management, and perceptual-motor coordination
4. Socialization: establishment or reestablishment of personal relationships
5. Mental health: schizophrenia, mood disorders, personality disorders, and anxiety disorders

Office Applications

As with all alternative therapies, use of music therapy does not preclude the use of mainstream medical therapies in addition. A simple ranking of conditions responsive to music therapy is as follows:

Top level: *A therapy ideally suited for these conditions*
Autism and Retts syndrome

Second level: *One of the better therapies for these conditions*
Alzheimer's disease; developmental disabilities; mental health; palliative care; pregnancy and childbirth

Third level: *A valuable adjunctive therapy for these conditions*
Cancer; chronic pain; hearing loss; heart disease; physical disabilities; neurologic impairment; addictions; AIDS; and traumatic brain injury

Practical Applications

Music therapists work with individuals and small groups in a variety of settings. These include general hospitals, schools, mental health facilities, clinics, group homes, nursing homes, day treatment programs, correctional facilities, state facilities, Veterans Affairs hospitals, rehabilitation facilities, hospice settings, music stores, wellness programs, and private practice. Health care and education professionals, as well as parents, may refer patients to music therapy. A physician referral is often helpful in receiving third party reimbursement, which is growing on a case-by-case basis across the U.S.

Research Base

Evidence Based

Research regarding the effectiveness of music therapy has been accumulating since at least 1964 with the establishment of the peer-reviewed *Journal of Music Therapy*. Expansion of the research base has occurred in publications such as *Music Therapy, Music Therapy Per-*

spectives, *The Arts in Psychotherapy*, foreign music therapy journals, and other music and medical publications. In recent years a number of compilations of music therapy research have been published.[11-15] Furman's *Effectiveness of Music Therapy Procedures: Documentation of Research and Clinical Practice*[16] summarizes music therapy research in a variety of clinical and educational settings.

Basic Science

Hodges[17] reviewed the neuromusical research extensively and offered the following tenets in consideration of music and the brain.

1. All human beings are born with a musical brain and can demonstrate and improve musical behaviors, which has implications for education.
2. The human musical brain is different from other animal brains.
3. The musical brain is in operation in infancy and perhaps even in the later fetal stages of development, which has implications for prenatal care and stimulation.
4. The musical brain consists of an extensive neural system (or systems) involving widely distributed but locally specialized regions of the brain.
5. The musical brain has cognitive components.
6. The musical brain has affective components, which likely play a role in psychoneuroimmunology.
7. The musical brain has motor components.
8. The degree to which the musical brain is lateralized is still debated, but music is clearly not solely a "right brain" function.
9. The musical brain is a very resilient system, which has implications for music therapy.
10. Early and ongoing musical training affects the organization of the musical brain, which also has implications for education.

In a series of studies focusing on auditory-motor response to rhythm in music, researchers have demonstrated that muscles fire more effectively in the presence of a rhythmic cue than in its absence.[18] The research further suggests that the brain quickly forms a template with regard to the beat interval and then uses the template to synchronize and entrain coordinated motor movements.[19,20]

Bartlett[21] summarized the research on music's effect on heart rate, skin conductivity, respiration, blood pressure, muscular tension, motor-postural response, peripheral skin temperature, blood volume, and biochemical response. The research indicates that music can affect these physiologic parameters without question. What is not definite is the nature or cause of the change. Despite the difficulties in interpreting the research, Bartlett notes that of the 190 hypotheses tested, 62% demonstrated results in the predicted direction. For example, heart rate increased in response to stimulative music and decreased in response to sedative music. Bartlett also notes, along with Hodges,[17] that a small but growing body of literature indicates that music can increase endogenous opioids and IgA and decrease stress-related hormones, such as cortisol.

Risk and Safety

Music therapy is considered a noninvasive and virtually risk-free intervention.

Efficacy

Standley's[22] metaanalysis of 92 studies revealed that the application of music vs. nonmusic conditions enhanced the medical objectives on at least one dependent variable in every study, whether measured by physiologic, psychologic/self-report, or behavioral observation. A total of 233 dependent variables across diverse diagnostic categories were reviewed. To date, this is the only such efficacy study in the literature. The potential for immediate and cost-effective results was demonstrated in Lane's[23] study in which the levels of salivary immunoglobulin A (sIgA) in hospitalized children were significantly higher after just one 30-minute music therapy session, as opposed to children who did not receive music therapy.

Future Research Opportunities and Priorities

Management and psychoneuroimmunology should remain high priorities for future research.

Druglike Information

Safety

Music therapy is considered a noninvasive and virtually risk-free intervention.

Warnings, Contraindications, and Precautions

Music therapists, as per the AMTA's "Standards of Clinical Practice," should not expose patients to prolonged music or sounds that exceed 90 decibels because of the potential for damage to the ear.[24] In addition, extreme caution is needed in using Guided Music and Imagery with some mental health diagnoses, particularly those involving psychoses.

Self-Help versus Professional

Initial music therapy interventions should be with a certified practitioner. There are applications that can be taught and carried out by the individual patient.

Visiting a Professional

A visit to a music therapist will vary widely depending on the age and needs of the patient. The initial visit may likely include some type of assessment that gathers information about the person, including past music experiences and preferences. Subsequent music therapy sessions, which could last between 15 minutes and 1 hour or more, may involve some aspect of music experiences such as listening, singing, playing, improvising, writing, or moving to music.

Credentialing

Credentialed music therapists are identified with one of the following designations.

MT-BC (*music therapist-board certified*) from the Certification Board for Music Therapists. The credential is awarded based on completion of education and clinical training requirements and passing a national examination. Continuing education is required for recertification. As of January 1, 1998, the MT-BC is the only available credential for new music therapists.

CMT (*certified music therapist*) from the former American Association for Music Therapy, awarded based on completion of education and clinical training requirements. New designations are not available. Music therapists choosing to maintain the designation remain on the National Music Therapy Registry.

ACMT (*advanced certified music therapist*) from the former American Association for Music Therapy, awarded based on advanced education and clinical experience. New designations are not available. Music therapists choosing to maintain the designation remain on the National Music Therapy Registry.

RMT (*registered music therapist*) from the former National Association for Music Therapy, awarded based on completion of education and clinical training requirements. New designations are not available. Music therapists choosing to maintain the designation remain on the National Music Therapy Registry.

Training

The AMTA lists 70 approved schools that train music therapists at the bachelor's, master's, and doctoral level. Although the majority of music therapists practice at the bachelor's level, 26% of the members surveyed in 1998 held advanced degrees, which is necessary for practicing music psychotherapy.

What to Look for in a Provider

The patient should only procure music therapy services from someone holding one of the designations listed in "Credentialing."

Barriers and Key Issues

The main barrier keeping music therapy from mainstream medical practice is third-party reimbursement. Progress in this area slowly is being made, including the designation of music therapy as reimbursable under Medicare's partial hospitalization guidelines. Physicians willing to refer patients to music therapy for specific outcomes can be of great assistance on a case-by-case basis in music therapy reimbursement.

Associations

American Music Therapy Association
8455 Colesville Rd., Suite 1000
Silver Spring, MD 20910
Tel: (301) 589-3300
Fax: (301) 589-5175
E-mail: infor@musictherapy.org
www.musictherapy.org

Suggested Reading

1. Bruscia KE: *Defining music therapy,* ed 2, Gilsum, NH, 1998, Barcelona.
   A thorough treatment of the evolving process in defining music therapy, including what does and does not constitute music therapy.
2. Bruscia KE, editor: *Case studies in music therapy,* Gilsum, NH, 1991, Barcelona.
   Forty-two case studies by numerous music therapists representing the breadth and depth of music therapy practice.
3. Davis WB, Gfeller KE, Thaut MH: *An introduction to music therapy: theory and practice,* ed 2, Dubuque, Iowa, 1999, W.C. Brown.
   A thorough yet accessible overview of the music therapy profession.
4. Furman CE, editor: *Effectiveness of music therapy procedures: documentation of research and clinical practice,* ed 2, Silver Springs, Md, 1996, National Association for Music Therapy.
   A summary of music therapy research in medical treatment, physical rehabilitation, acute mental health care, gerontology, special education, hearing impairment, traumatic brain injury, and developmental disabilities.
5. Taylor DB: *Biomedical foundations of music as therapy,* St Louis, 1997, MMB Music.
   A well-articulated theory of biomedical foundations for music therapy practice based on interdisciplinary music/brain research.

Bibliography

American Music Therapy Association: *Member sourcebook,* Silver Spring, Md, 1998, The Association.

References

1. Bruscia KE: *Defining music therapy*, ed 2, Gilsum, NH, 1998, Barcelona.

2. Davis WB, Gfeller KE, Thaut MH: *An introduction to music therapy: theory and practice*, ed 2, Dubuque, Iowa, 1999, W.C. Brown.

3. Peters JS: *Music therapy: an introduction*, Springfield, Ill, 1987, Charles C. Thomas.

4. Merriam AP: *The anthropology of music*, Chicago, 1964, Northwestern University Press.

5. Sears WW: Processes in music therapy. In Gaston ET, editor: *Music in therapy*, New York, 1968, Macmillan.

6. Gaston ET: Man and music. In Gaston ET, editor: *Music in therapy*, New York, 1968, Macmillan.

7. Taylor DB: *Biomedical foundations of music as therapy*, St Louis, 1997, MMB Music.

8. Hanser S: *Music therapist's handbook*, St Louis, 1987, Warren H. Green.

9. Bonny HL, Savary LM: *Music and your mind*, ed 2, Barrytown, NY, 1990, Station Hill Press.

10. Nordoff P, Robbins C: *Creative music therapy*, New York, 1977, John Day.

11. Froehlich MA, editor: *Music therapy with hospitalized children: a creative arts child life approach*, Cherry Hill, N.J., 1996, Jeffrey Books.

12. Loewy J, editor: *Music therapy and pediatric pain*, Cherry Hill, NJ, 1997, Jeffrey Books.

13. Maranto CD, editor: *Applications of music in medicine*, Washington, DC, 1991, National Association for Music Therapy.

14. Pratt RR, Spintge R, editors: *Music Medicine*, vol 2, St Louis, 1996, MMB Music.

15. Tomaino CM, editor: *Clinical applications of music in neurologic rehabilitation*, St Louis, 1998, MMB Music.

16. Furman CE, editor: *Effectiveness of music therapy procedures: documentation of research and clinical practice*, ed 2, Silver Spring, Md, 1996, National Association for Music Therapy.

17. Hodges DA: Neuromusical research: a review of the literature. In Hodges DA, editor: *Handbook of music psychology*, ed 2, San Antonio, 1996, IMR Press.

18. Thaut MH, Schauer ML: Weakly coupled oscillators rhythmic motor synchronization, *Proceedings of the Society for Neuroscience* 298:20, 1997.

19. Thaut MH, Miller RA: Multiple synchronization strategies in tracking of rhythmic auditory stimulation, *Proceedings of the Society for Neuroscience* 146:11, 1994.

20. Thaut MH, Miller RA, Schauer ML: Multiple synchronization strategies in rhythmic sensorimotor tasks: phase vs. period corrections, *Biological Cybernetics* 79(3):241-250, 1998.

21. Bartlett DL: Physiological responses to music and sound stimuli. In Hodges DA, editor: *Handbook of music psychology*, ed 2, San Antonio, 1996, IMR Press.

22. Standley J: Music research in medical/dental treatment: an update of prior meta-analysis. In Furman CE, editor: *Effectiveness of music therapy procedures: documentation of research and clinical practice*, ed 2, Silver Spring, Md, 1996, National Association for Music Therapy.

23. Lane D: Effects of music therapy on immune function of hospitalized patients, *Quality of Life* 3:74-80, 1994.

24. American Music Therapy Association: Standards of clinical practice. In *Member sourcebook*, Silver Spring, Md, 1998, The Association

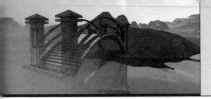

Neuro Linguistic Programming

Origins and History

Neuro Linguistic Programming (NLP) is a model of therapy that focuses on resolving problems by identifying the way that individuals create and also maintain their problems through the way they think and what they believe. The problem then can be resolved by changing the patients' thought patterns and mental strategies in order to give the patients more—and better—choices. NLP uses patterns of thought that can influence individuals' behavior as a means of improving the quality and effectiveness of their lives.[1] NLP offers a paradigm of how the brain works (neuro), how language interacts with the brain (linguistic), and how individuals sequence their actions in order to obtain the desired results (programming). *Programming* has nothing to do with computers.[2] Instead, the idea of neuro linguistic programming is an effective and proven vehicle for accelerated human change—a vehicle that radically alters the perceived need for lengthy psychotherapy.

NLP was initially created by linguist John Grinder, along with computer scientist and Gestalt therapist Richard Bandler, along with their associates, principally Robert Dilts. Together, they produced a linguistic model based on the language patterns of a few gifted psychotherapists, principally the work of the following people: hypnotherapist Milton Erickson; Fritz Perls, who was the originator of Gestalt therapy; anthropologist Gregory Bateson; and Virginia Satir, who was a pioneer of family systemic therapy. The one common factor among the people who were originally modeled was their individual success in their respective fields. Their findings were partly published in the two volumes of *The Structure of Magic* in 1976.[3,4] The synthesis of their findings, which are a blend of cognitive science and behavioral science, resulted in the technology that is now known as Neuro Linguistic Programming. Although the original research and work relating to NLP was performed more than 20 years ago, the NLP model continues to develop and to evolve.[5]

*A special note of appreciation goes to Joseph O'Connor for his contributions to this discussion.

Mechanism of Action According to Its Own Theory

NLP is defined as the study of the structure of subjective experience; in other words, how we make sense of our experiences and construct our mental world. When used in therapy, NLP uses these principles to give patients more choices in their own frames of reference. It does not seek to impose a theory or practice that the patient must accept in order to proceed.

According to NLP, thought is a representation of sensory experience. The five senses (visual, auditory, kinesthetic, olfactory, gustatory) are known in NLP as the five main *representational systems*. NLP proposes that the way we think is shown by our words, body language, and eye movements. It instructs in ways to use the mind to achieve specific and desired outcomes consistently.[6] The practitioner *models* how the patient produces the presenting problem by listening to the patient's spoken language, watching the patient's body language, and asking specific questions to identify the patient's values and beliefs. When the patient and practitioner both understand how the problem is produced, they then can work together to resolve it.

Because NLP began from modeling excellent communicators, it is heavily based in communication theory. Unlike many other forms of psychotherapy, NLP also can be used in nontherapeutic contexts, such as business, sales, sports, education, and training.

NLP shares many aspects of solution-oriented therapy and cognitive brief therapy. The patient's goals are carefully considered and evaluated. Additionally, NLP uses some approaches and language patterns from ericksonian hypnotherapy. Many hypnotherapists also train in NLP to help them to become more effective with trance work. NLP has its roots firmly in clinical hypnosis, but NLP therapists do not usually perform formal hypnotic inductions or use trance explicitly. However, as in many other forms of therapy, NLP uses the naturally occurring trance states of the patient to explore the inner experience of the problem.

Forms of Therapy

There is really only one type of NLP therapy. However, there can be a difference in the ways practitioners use it, according to their sources of training. The main "schools" of NLP are led by Richard Bandler, Tad James, Wyatt Woodsmall, John Grinder, Robert Dilts, Judith DeLozier, and Connierae and Steve Andreas. This is not to say that these are the only sources for NLP training, but most of the world's certified NLP trainers were trained by one or more of these persons.

Demographics

NLP practitioners originally practiced primarily in the United States on the West Coast, where NLP originated. However, NLP is now practiced worldwide, and many countries have national NLP associations. Europe, especially the United Kingdom, has a great number of NLP practitioners. NLP is used by many types of patients. Most conform to the usual psychotherapeutic criteria of being reasonably well educated, between 20 and 50 years of age, and with a fairly even split between men and women.

Indications and Reasons for Referral

Persons who tend to seek out NLP therapy tend to fit the same profile as those who seek any other form of psychotherapy. NLP can be used for the treatment of a variety of psychosomatic conditions. NLP is also used in behavioral modification treatments as well as stress management.

Office Applications

NLP has been useful in treating the following conditions, beginning with those most likely to respond and progressing to those less likely to respond. As with all alternative therapies, use of NLP does not preclude the use of mainstream medical therapies.

Phobias: The NLP model has been used to treat most identified types of phobia. The success rate is high because NLP helps the patient to rationalize and resolve the phobia, thus allowing the patient to release the unrequired fear. It is also a short procedure and lasts no longer than half an hour in most cases.

Limiting beliefs (feelings of inadequacy): NLP is very effective in these conditions by bringing limited beliefs into awareness so they can be resolved.

Smoking cessation: NLP allows patients to change their response to cigarettes, thus allowing them to cease smoking. This is not done through substitution but through values and belief changes. Through these changes, secondary issues related to smoking cessation, such as weight gain and irritability, can be reduced if not totally eliminated.

Stress management: Through strategy elicitation, patients are taught how to recognize stress causation and manage its effects in a more healthy way. In some cases, this can induce a modest reduction in blood pressure.

Assertiveness: NLP deals with assertiveness by linking the specific situations and interactions with identified intrapsychic resources.

Neurosis: NLP helps patients to recognize the causes of their neurosis. By getting patients to acknowledge and take ultimate responsibility for the causes and take ultimate responsibility for it, NLP gives patients the necessary tools to use their own resources to overcome the neurosis.

Weight control: NLP can be used to teach patients about changes in their behavior in quite ways unrelated to dieting alone.

Performance enhancement: NLP allows patients to reach their maximum potential in sports and other areas.

Gender dysphoria: NLP is used to reconcile patients' "parts" so that they cease to be in conflict with each other, thus allowing patients to accept who they are without some of the destructive tendencies related to this condition. *Parts* refers to different personality elements. An example of this could be that part of me wants to smoke while another part of me wants to quit. Through a process known as *chunking* both parts are taught that they have the same ultimate purpose so that there is no need for conflict.

Schizophrenia: NLP also has been used to help schizophrenics to improve. This is not to say that NLP has cured psychosis, but it has in some cases helped to alleviate some symptoms associated with these conditions.

Practical Applications

NLP is used primarily either within hypnotherapeutic interventions or as a stand-alone therapy. NLP is a rapid form of therapy, with a series of techniques that are very easy to understand. NLP can be used by a variety of practitioners who need to elicit information from patients and use forms of suggestion therapy. Use of NLP techniques can help therapists make more effective suggestions to their patients.

NLP is a rapid form of therapy. Furthermore, the linguistic model (Meta Model) is extremely useful in eliciting problems and also getting patients to become clear about their desired outcome for the treatment. The model of hypnotic language (Milton Model) is very useful in eliciting resources of which the patient has been unaware.

Research Base

Evidence Based

One of the most common arguments against NLP as a therapy is the lack of formal research.[7] There is a great deal of informal research and case histories on the effectiveness of NLP in journals, such as *Anchor Point* in the U.S., *Rapport* in the U.K., and *NLP World*. The situation outlined by Eric Einspruch and Bruce Foreman in their 1985 review of research on NLP is changing. "Many skilled NLP practitioners have a wealth of clinical data indicating that this model is highly effective. Clearly these practitioners would provide a service to the field by presenting their data in the literature so they may be critically evaluated."[8]

Much research into NLP has been performed primarily at the master's level. Studies in clinical hypnosis or the other models of therapy that were used to design NLP could be used as a basis to prove the efficacy of NLP. The early books written by Bandler and Grinder, such as like *Frogs Into Princes, Trance-Formations, Patterns 1 and 2*, and *Structure of Magic 1-2* provide a strong research basis for the effectiveness of NLP. However, these works are, on average, 20 years old.

However, more research is being performed as NLP becomes more widespread. Research has indicated that NLP training increases individual self-actualization.[9] There have been many studies on specific eye movement patterns. An early study supports the claim that specific eye movement patterns exist and that trained observers can reliably identify them.[10] Research indicates that NLP is effective in reducing anxiety and depression in patients with phobias[11,12] and is as successful for longer behaviorist desensitization.[13] Studies indicate that the NLP allergy process can be effective with certain conditions.[14,15]

Risk and Safety

NLP has risk factors similar to hypnotherapy and other forms of psychotherapy. Unless they are a registered medical practitioner, psychologist, or mental health professional, practitioners should not attempt to treat psychosis with NLP. NLP has a procedure for treating allergies that should not be used without medical supervision if the possible allergic response is dangerous or life-threatening.[16]

Efficacy

As with other forms of psychotherapy, the effectiveness of NLP therapy is linked directly to the skill of the practitioner. However, in the opinion of the authors, some 73% of the patients who come for therapy achieve their desired outcome. That may not necessarily mean that patients are "cured" of the condition. It simply means that they achieved a good therapeutic outcome and were able to go back to living a more effective life with new skills and resources. Practitioners do vary in their success rate, but as long as the practitioner is competent, some form of therapeutic change should occur.

Future Research Opportunities and Priorities

The need for NLP research is vital. The existing research is reasonable but not as extensive as clinical hypnosis, for example. For NLP to move into a more "respectable" position in the therapeutic and medical world, more research needs to be done. The most important research that needs to be undertaken is the efficacy of the treatment with a variety of conditions. This is the first and only priority in the future of research in NLP. NLP must be proved to be effective for it to become more widely practiced.

Druglike Information

Safety

NLP is a safe form of therapy. However, it is important that practitioners confine their activities to the treatment of conditions within their sphere of competence. This is especially relevant in the treatment of psychosis.

Warnings, Contraindications, and Precautions

See "Safety."

Drugs or Other Interactions

As previously stated, NLP is very useful in conjunction with clinical hypnosis and cognitive psychotherapy. NLP is useful to help a hypnotherapist be more effective with hypnotic language patterns.

Adverse Reactions

There are very few reported cases of adverse reactions associated with NLP. The most likely adverse reaction is the possibility of abreaction. An *abreaction* occurs when a patient is in a flooded emotional state. This state not dangerous per se, but it is problematic for therapists that perhaps are not accustomed to high emotional states.

Pregnancy and Lactation

There are no contraindications to patients who are currently pregnant or breast-feeding.

Self-Help versus Professional

Ideally, NLP will not only help patients with their problems but also change the thought patterns that gave rise to the problem situation. Therefore part of the treatment involves teaching the patient to recognize and deal with the problem if it recurs. It is advisable in the first instance to seek out a professional. Thereafter, part of the intervention is to enable the patient to use these techniques on a self-help basis. NLP is something that a lay person can master with practice.

Visiting a Professional

A patient should expect a consultation with an NLP therapist to be similar to any other counseling service. Therapists tend to be casually dressed, which helps to establish a comfortable environment for the patient to achieve the desired change. Sessions usually begin with a detailed personal history, which can take an hour or more. Some therapists tend to use a 2-hour session, in which case therapy would commence after the case history. Otherwise, a patient would return the following week for therapy. Depending on the condition, therapy can be a single session or a series of sessions. Follow-up sessions would depend upon the success of the intervention.

Credentialing

The only licensure issues relating to NLP are in areas where legislation restricts psychotherapeutic practices, such as hypnotherapy. However, there are distinct levels of certification, which are outlined in "Training." In Europe, legislation is pending that may limit the practice of complementary/alternative therapies to licensed practitioners.

Training

There are three standard levels of certification for practitioners, as well as one level that is not considered traditional. Level one is a certified practitioner of NLP. This level usually consists of 125 hours of training. Level two is a certified master practitioner of NLP. This level is usually an additional 125 hours of training after certified practitioner training. Level three is a certified trainer. This level can include up to an additional 165 hours after completing master practitioner training.

There are also specialized NLP therapy trainings. The nontraditional level is that of certified master trainer, which is usually a personal development program. The certified master trainer program generally consists of 1 to 4 years of apprenticeship at the trainer level.

What to Look for in a Provider

The most reliable way to choose a provider is to see if the person is certified through one of the main certifying bodies or trained by one of the accepted developers of NLP. Additionally, the practitioner should belong to an existing professional body for NLP, such as a national association.

Barriers and Key Issues

There are five main reasons why NLP has not received the credibility it deserves. The first reason is that when Bandler and Grinder began teaching NLP, they used a deliberate confrontational and iconoclastic style, which had the result of alienating some medical professionals. In fact, however, NLP has a solid intellectual basis in systemic theory that is now being recognized.

The second reason is that NLP early acquired an unfortunate reputation for being manipulative. Any powerful communication skills can be misused by short-sighted practitioners. The effectiveness or morality of any branch of medicine or psychotherapy should not be judged by the activities of a few nonprofessional practitioners.

The third reason is that NLP has yet to acquire a solid peer-reviewed research base. The medical profession would be more likely to refer to NLP practitioners if there were more scientific research as to the efficacy of NLP as a therapy. Such a research base is now being developed.

The fourth reason is that there has been some confusion that NLP is trademarked or that the term is restricted. There are no restrictions on the term NLP, and there are no special entry restrictions to using NLP, apart from the normal entry requirements of learning the skills in an accredited training.

The fifth reason is that medical practitioners may see only the more visible, nonmedical applications and conclude that NLP has nothing to offer them. In fact, NLP began by studying the work of arguably the three greatest psychotherapists of the time, and it is well grounded in psychotherapeutic practice.

Associations

American Board of NLP
16842 Von Karman Ave., Suite 475
Irvine, CA 92714
Tel: (949) 261-6400
www.hypnosis.com

Association for NLP (UK)
PO Box 78
Stourbridge
West Midlands, UK
DY8 4ZJ
Tel: +44 (1) 384-443935
www.anlp.org

International NLP Trainers Association
1201 Delta Glen Ct.
Vienna, VA 22182
Tel: (703) 757-7945
www.inlpta.com

Society of NLP
44 Montgomery St., 5th Floor
San Francisco, CA 94104
Tel: (415) 955-0541
www.purenlp.com

Suggested Reading

1. Bandler R, Grinder J: *The structure of magic,* vol 1-2, Palo Alto, Calif, 1976, Science and Behavior Books
   The first published books on NLP, the results of modeling Virginia Satir and Fritz Perls. The precision model of language, known as the Meta Model, is first outlined here as a tool for therapy.
2. Grinder J, Bandler R: *Patterns of the hypnotic techniques of Milton H. Erickson, MD,* vol 1, Cupertino, Calif, 1975, Meta.
   The results of modeling Milton Erickson. This volume is very accessible and gives the language patterns in a structured way.
3. Grinder J, Bandler R, DeLozier J: *Patterns of the hypnotic techniques of Milton H. Erickson, MD,* vol 2, Cupertino, Calif, 1977, Meta.
   A more academic consideration of the issues surrounding language patterns in hypnotherapy.
4. O'Connor J, Seymour J: *Introducing NLP,* London, 1990, Thorsons.
   A thorough introduction to all main patterns of NLP and the theory behind them.

Bibliography

Ader R: *Psychoneuroimmunology*, San Diego, 1981, Academic Press.

Ader R: Behavioral conditioning and the immune system. In Temoshok L, Van Dyke C, Zegans L, editors: *Emotions in health and illness*, London, 1983, Gruner and Stratton.

Bateson G: *Steps to an ecology of mind*, New York, 1972, Chandler.

Grinder J, Bandler R: *Patterns of the hypnotic techniques of Milton H. Erickson, MD*, vol 1, Cupertino, Calif, 1975, Meta.

Grinder J, Bandler R, Delozier J: *Patterns of the hypnotic techniques of Milton H. Erickson, MD*, vol 2, Cupertino, Calif, 1977, Meta.

O'Connor J, Seymour J: *Introducing NLP*, London, 1990, Thorsons.

References

1. Bandler R, Grinder J: *Frogs into princes*, Moab, Utah, 1979, Real People Press.

2. *American Board of NLP prospectus*, Irvine, Calif, 1995, ABH Press.

3. Bandler R, Grinder J: *The structure of magic*, vol 1, Palo Alto, Calif, 1975, Science and Behavior Books.

4. Bandler R, Grinder J: *The structure of magic*, vol 2, Palo Alto, Calif, 1976, Science and Behavior Books.

5. Washington School of Clinical and Advanced Hypnosis prospectus, Manchester, England, 1998, Brookhouse Publications.

6. James T: *NLP practitioner's manual*, Honolulu, 1998, Advanced Neuro Dynamics.

7. Yapko M: Pain control, lecture, Manchester, England, 1997, Withington Hospital.

8. Einspruch E, Foreman B: Observations concerning research literature in neurolinguistic programming, *J Counsel Psychol* 32(4):589-596, 1985.

9. Duncan R, Konefal J, Spechler M: Effect of neurolinguistic programming training on self-actualization as measured by the personal orientation inventory, *Psychol Report* 66:1323-1330, 1990.

10. Buckner M et al: Eye movement as an indicator of sensory components in thought, *J Counsel Psychol* 34(3):283-287, 1987.

11. Einspruch E: Neurolinguistic programming in the treatment of phobias, Psychother Private Pract 6(1):91-100, 1988.

12. Koziey P, McLeod G: Visual kinesthetic dissociation in treatment of victims of rape, *Prof Psychol Res Pract* 18(3):276-282, 1987.

13. Allen K: An investigation of the effectiveness of neurolinguistic programming procedures in treating snake phobias, *Dissert Abstr Int* 43:861b, 1982.

14. Swack J: A study of initial response and reversion rates of subjects treated with the allergy technique, *Anchor Point* 6(2):16-20, 1992.

15. Lund J, Lund H: *Asthma management*. Research study presented to the Congress of the European Respiratory Society, Vienna, October 14, 1994.

16. O'Connor J, McDermott I: *NLP and health*, London, 1996, Thorsons.

Poetry Therapy

STEPHEN ROJCEWICZ*

Origins and History

Poetry therapy, or bibliotherapy, is the intentional use of poetry and other forms of literature for healing and personal growth. It may be traced back to primitive humans, who used religious rites in which shamans and witch doctors chanted poetry for the well-being of the tribe or individual. As far back as 4000 BCE in ancient Egypt, words were written on papyrus and then dissolved in a solution so that the words could be physically ingested by the patient and take effect as quickly as possible. It is also recorded that around 1030 BCE, the music (and lyrics) of a shepherd boy named David soothed King Saul.

The ancient Greeks and Romans laid the foundation for poetry therapy. The Sicilian Greek philosopher Gorgias (ca. 485-375 BCE) is quoted by Socrates as saying he could convince the noncompliant patients of his brother, a physician, to submit to medicine or surgery after they had refused medical advice to do so, by using only the art of rhetoric. Gorgias relied on poetic rhythm, organizing his sentences into short symmetrical clauses, and poetic figures of speech. One of the first poetry therapists on record was the physician Soranus, born in Ephesus but practicing in Rome around 125 AD, who prescribed tragedy for his manic patients and comedy for those who were depressed. It is not surprising that Apollo is the god of poetry as well as medicine, since medicine and the arts historically were entwined.

The Pennsylvania Hospital, the first hospital in the U.S., founded by Benjamin Franklin in 1751, employed many ancillary treatments for its mental patients, including reading, writing, and publishing their poems and other writings in their own newspaper. Dr. Benjamin Rush, the "Father of American Psychiatry" and a signer of the Declaration of Independence, introduced music and literature as effective ancillary treatments for psychiatric patients.

In 1928 Eli Greifer, a poet who was a pharmacist and lawyer by profession, began a campaign to show that poetry has healing power. In the 1950s he became a volunteer to test his theories and started a "poem therapy" group at Creedmore State Hospital, and later, a

---

*In addition to the author's own views, this discussion relies on the work of many poetry therapists, and summarizes "Poetry Therapy: Testimony on Capitol Hill,"[18] as well as portions of *The Guide to Training Requirements for Certification/Registration as a Poetry Therapist*.

105

poetry therapy group at Cumberland Hospital with two supervising psychiatrists, Jack Leedy and Sam Spector. He passed along his love of "poem therapy" to Leedy, who continued to explore the therapeutic benefits of poetry at Cumberland Hospital and the Poetry Therapy Center in New York.

Additional pioneers in the 1960s included Ann White at the Nassau County Recreation Department and Gil Schloss at the Institute for Sociotherapy in New York. In 1969, they joined with Leedy to found the Association for Poetry Therapy. The 1970s also saw the development of several groups and training institutes. Arthur Lerner founded the Poetry Therapy Institute in California; Arleen Hynes, a librarian at St. Elizabeth's Hospital in Washington, D.C., founded the Bibliotherapy Roundtable; and Morris Morrison founded the American Academy of Poetry Therapy in Austin, Texas.

By 1980 the field was represented by different institutes with their own training certificates, but uniform requirements for training poetry therapists had not been established. In 1980 Sherry Reiter called a board meeting of the Association for Poetry Therapy, which invited leaders in the field to deal with issues that were impeding the profession's growth as a viable, national creative arts therapy group. This meeting led directly to the formation of the National Association for Poetry Therapy (NAPT) as the national organization representing the field, as well as the ongoing process of developing uniform training requirements.

Principles

Poetry therapy or bibliotherapy is the intentional use of poetry and other forms of literature for healing and personal growth. Poetry therapy works with participants toward the following therapeutic and developmental goals:

- To promote change, increase coping skills, and improve adaptive functions to work through underlying conflicts
- To heighten participants' reality orientation
- To enable participants to ventilate overpowering emotions and release tension
- To encourage positive thinking and creative problem solving
- To strengthen participants' communication skills, especially their willingness to listen carefully and speak directly
- To enhance participants' self-understanding and accuracy in self-perception
- To encourage participants' awareness of personal relationships
- To encourage participants' capacity to respond to vivid images and concepts and the feelings aroused by them
- To encourage and balance participants' creativity and self-expression and their greater self-esteem
- To help participants experience the liberating and nourishing qualities of harmony and beauty
- To increase participants' spontaneity and capacity for playing with words and ideas

- To help participants find new meaning through new ideas, insights, and information
- To help participants integrate the different aspects of the self for psychologic wholeness

Mechanism of Action According to Its Own Theory

Poetry and poetry therapy enable individuals to express what they may be unable to say in other ways. Poetry therapy promotes an integration of basic raw emotions, freedom of expression, and a highly organized poetic structure. It allows primitive feelings and impulses to be placed in perspective, mastered, and expressed in a more constructive manner. The therapist does not directly assault defenses and masks but uses them creatively. Through poetry therapy, the patient develops self-worth, handles some critical conflicts nonverbally and symbolically, and increases overall functioning.

Poetic structures, such as stanza form, rhythm, meter, rhyme, metaphor, simile, and phonetic associations contribute to the overall therapeutic effect.

The use of meter in poetry is intrinsically connected with human biology, with the rhythms of the body, the heart, sleep, respiration, and the life cycle, and the dictates of human neurophysiology. Poetic rhythm is a neurophysiologic command, brought into being by the brain's demand for familiarity and unambiguity on the one hand, and the brain's need for controlled novelty on the other hand. The use of rhythm and of poetic techniques, however rudimentary or vague, helps the poetry therapist gain access to basic human emotions.

Forms of Therapy

Poetry therapy is practiced within individual psychotherapy, marital, and family psychotherapy formats; however, group psychotherapy forms the bulk of poetry therapy experience.

Poetry therapy is an interactive process with three essential components: the literature, the therapist or facilitator, and the patient. The trained poetry therapist selects a poem or other form of written or spoken media to serve as a catalyst and evoke feelings and responses for discussion. A published poem may be chosen by the therapist or group members, a collaborative poem may be created by the group members as a whole, or a new poem may be created by an individual patient or the therapist. The focus is on the person's reaction to the literature, not on literary merit per se. A basic principle in choosing a poem for use is that the poem's emotional tone should match the clinical situation or the mood of the individual patient, but it should not be excessively negative or depressing or glorify suicide or antisocial behavior. The poem is chosen primarily not for its literary merit but for its usefulness as a tool for awareness, self-discovery, and therapeutic change.

Demographics

Practitioners include psychiatrists, psychologists, physicians, social workers, nurse practitioners, mental health counselors, addiction counselors, pastoral counselors, and marriage, family, and child counselors.

Users include individuals with mental illness and adjustmenst disorders, acute grief reactions, reactions to diagnoses of severe medical illnesses (such as cancer or AIDS), addictions to drugs and alcohol, and eating disorders; veterans; survivors of violence, abuse or incest; families with problems; adolescents; older adults; the learning disabled; individuals in jails and prisons; persons with sexual dysfunctions; and the homeless.

Indications and Reasons for Referral

Poetry therapy is used in a variety of mental health, medical, geriatric, therapeutic, educational, and community settings. It has a broad range of application with people of all ages and is used for health, maintenance, and populations requiring treatment for a variety of illnesses and conditions. As with all alternative therapies, use of poetry therapy does not preclude the use of mainstream medical therapies in addition. Therapeutic rankings for specific indications include the following:

> Top level: *A therapy ideally suited for these conditions*
> Acute grief reactions; life review in the elderly; and survivors of violence, abuse, or incest

> Second level: *One of the better therapies for these conditions*
> Addictions to drugs and alcohol; adjustment disorder with depressed mood; adolescent identity issues; family and marital dysfunction; and reactions to diagnoses of severe medical illnesses

Practical Applications

In addition to its use as part of a treatment plan for mental illnesses, grief reactions, adjustments to acute stressors, and others, poetry therapy can be used for individual personal growth in both patients and practitioners. Physicians have been writing poetry for centuries as a way to maintain their connection with the broad humanistic tradition, achieve the inspiration to continue healing, and deal with the issues of medical practice that call for more than a purely mechanical, technologic solution.

Research Base

The professional literature has demonstrated that poetry therapy is an effective and powerful therapeutic tool for the following groups:

Adults with mental illness[1]; adolescents with mental illness[1]; children with mental illness[1]; prison inmates[2]; forensic psychiatric patients[3]; youths incarcerated in jail[4]; adults with acute grief reactions[5]; children with acute grief reactions[6]; persons with adjustments to severe medical illnesses such as cancer[7]; emotional problems in persons with AIDS[8]; persons with eating disorders[9]; persons with addictions to alcohol or drugs[2]; families with problems[1]; older adults[10]; survivors of violence, abuse, and incest[11]; the homeless[12]; the learning disabled[13]; patients with posttraumatic stress disorder[14]; the hearing impaired[2]; patients who are not fluent in English[15]; and women /who have miscarried.[16]

Druglike Information

Safety and Adverse Reactions

Inappropriate use of poetry therapy may lead to worsening of mental illness and medical illnesses. The literature[17] warns against excess practitioner zeal and inappropriate application of poetry therapy as a panacea. Worsening of depression or psychotic symptoms can occur if there are premature or unwarranted attempts to break down needed defenses. Worsening of symptoms of schizophrenia can occur if poetry therapy is used in an aggressive, intrusive fashion. Symptoms of any medical illness can worsen if poetry therapy is used inappropriately and in isolation to treat illnesses such as asthma or ulcers.

However, it is not likely that harm will occur from poetry therapy or that poetry therapy would be applied indiscriminately or inappropriately as a panacea. Trained poetry therapists have sensible, realistic expectations. They are not likely to become fanatics, applying poetry therapy to any and all clinical situations. As the late Arthur Lerner, a distinguished practitioner of poetry therapy, pointed out, poetry therapy is a "tool, not a school." As a tool, it is used only when clinically indicated. Harm is prevented by assuring that poetry therapists are well trained and adhere to the highest ethical standards.

Visiting a Professional

A typical session would be in the format of a weekly poetry therapy group, led by a certified poetry therapist. The session begins with a warm-up exercise, consisting of a word game, a song or chant, or some other comfortable icebreaker. Prior to the meeting, the group leader would have chosen a preexisting poem, based on knowledge about the group members; in more advanced groups, each participant would be asked to write a poem during the session. If the group members have been working on difficulties with anger, the poetry therapist may choose, for example, the first stanza of "A Poison Tree" by William Blake (1794):

I was angry with my friend:
I told my wrath, my wrath did end.
I was angry with my foe:
I told it not, my wrath did grow.

Each participant is given a copy of this poem to read. In addition, a volunteer is asked to read the poem out loud, so that rhythm, rhyme, and alliteration can be experienced.

Eventually, all group members will have the experience of reading aloud. The therapeutic use of the poem proceeds through the following four general stages:

1. Recognition: The group members recognize and identify with the selection.
2. Examination: The patients explore specific details through questions and dialogue. One person, for example, may deny ever feeling any anger, or another person may describe his reactions to the phrase "my wrath did end," giving a personal experience of a marital conflict in which he felt less depressed after finally telling his wife about a sensitive issue.
3. Juxtaposition: This process explores the significant interplay between contrasts and comparisons. If an individual who characteristically never "tells his wrath" hears the experiences of those group members who "told my wrath" and the "wrath did end," that individual may develop a new awareness that can be very useful. For those individuals who have had experiences of violent acting out, this poem emphasizes the value of talking about the anger, as well as the value of expressing feelings in general.
4. Application to the self: The therapist encourages the feelings to emerge and become integrated with cognitive concepts and deeper self-understanding. A group member then may be able to say, "I understand why I felt more depressed after not telling my husband about my anger," or "I understand why I still have difficulties with anger."

The poetry therapist concludes the session with a formal closure, summarizing some of the key points, always making sure to end in a positive and mutually affirming way. Sessions often end with a group recitation of a favorite poem.

The next scheduled session usually provides immediate follow-up, as participants recapitulate themes from the earlier meeting.

Credentialing

The NAPT Certification Committee awards the designations of registered poetry therapist (RPT) and certified poetry therapist (CPT) to those who have fulfilled all applicable training requirements.

The registered poetry therapist (RPT) has a master's degree or doctorate in a clinical field, appropriate knowledge of psychology and literature, 975 hours of specialized training, and appropriate clinical supervision. The RPT is trained to facilitate groups and work with individuals in clinical or remediational settings such as inpatient and outpatient medical and mental health, geriatric, and special education facilities.

An RPT can practice independently. The certified poetry therapist (CPT) has a bachelor's degree, 440 hours of specialized training, and appropriate clinical supervision. The CPT is trained to facilitate groups and work with individuals in a developmental setting such as a school, library, or recreational facility. In a clinical setting, the CPT must work under the clinical supervision of an RPT or other qualified mental health professional.

Training

The heart of the training program is individualized supervision through an approved mentor or supervisor. Training institutes are active in many states, including California, the District of Columbia, Maryland, and New York. Academic courses in poetry therapy are available at universities, and the American Psychiatric Association has sponsored continuing medical education courses on poetry therapy at its annual meetings. Vermont College of Norwich University in Montpelier, Vermont, offers two degree programs in poetry therapy: a master's of arts in fine arts, specializing in poetry therapy; and a master's of arts in counseling psychology, with a specialization in poetry therapy.

What to Look for in a Provider

A provider should have credentials as a psychotherapist or physician, as well as the designation of registered poetry therapist (RPT) or certified poetry therapist (CPT) from the NAPT Certification Committee. Individual practitioners are listed in the Membership Directory, available from the NAPT at (202) 966-2536.

Poetry therapy services are provided at selected hospitals, psychiatric facilities, and rehabilitation centers. As examples of referrals, an inpatient psychiatrist may refer a patient to a poetry therapy group in a psychiatric hospital, or a psychotherapist in an community mental health center may refer a patient to a poetry therapist in private practice.

Barriers and Key Issues

One barrier to the use of poetry therapy is the fact that the field is still young, although it is growing. Geographical distribution of poetry therapists is uneven. As more psychotherapists complete training as registered or certified poetry therapists, this therapeutic tool will become more readily available.

Key issues for the future include further scientific outcome studies and greater integration of all creative arts therapies.

Associations

The National Association for Poetry Therapy
#280, Connecticut Ave. NW
Washington, D.C. 20015
Tel: (202) 966-2536

Suggested Reading

1. Fox J: *Finding what you didn't lose: expressing your truth and creativity through poem-making*, New York, 1995, Jeremy P. Tarcher/Putnam.

   Containing numerous consumer-friendly exercises to help any individual write, this book emphasizes the therapeutic value of creating poetry. An added bonus are the wonderful quotations scattered throughout the margins.

2. Lerner A, editor: *Poetry in the therapeutic experience*, St Louis, 1994, MMB Music.

   This collection of essays includes an overview of general principles, specific case studies, and concrete examples of interventions such as warm-up activities and action techniques.

3. *The Journal of Poetry Therapy* (Fall 1987 to present) is the primary source for current articles, resources, news, abstracts of articles from other journals, dissertation abstracts, and original poetry.

Bibliography

Longo P: "If I had my life to live over"—Stephanie's story: a case study in poetry therapy, *J Poetry Ther* 10:55-67, 1996.

Mazza N, Prescott B: Poetry: an ancillary technique in couples group therapy, *Am J Fam Ther* 9:53-57, 1981.

Reiter S: Enhancing the quality of life for the frail elderly: Rx: the poetic prescription, *J Long-Term Home Health Care* 13:12-19, 1994.

References

1. Hynes AM, Hynes-Berry M: *Biblio/poetry therapy: the interactive process*, Boulder, Co, 1986, Westview.

2. Leedy JJ, editor: *Poetry as healer: mending the troubled mind*, New York, 1985, Vanguard.

3. Rojcewicz S: No artist rants and raves when he creates: creative art therapies and psychiatry in forensic settings. In Gussak D, Virshup E, editors: *Drawing time: art therapy in prisons and other correctional settings*, Chicago, 1997, Magnolia Street.

4. Stino Z: Writing as therapy in a county jail, *J Poetry Ther* 9:13-23, 1995.

5. Bowman DO, Sauers RJ, Halfacre D: The application of poetry therapy in grief counselling with adolescents and young adults, *J Poetry Ther* 8:63-73, 1994.

6. Davis SL: Poetry as the hidden voice: adults with developmental disabilities speak out, *J Poetry Ther* 8:143-148, 1995.

7. Hodges D: For every season . . . art and poetry therapy with terminally ill patients, *J Poetry Ther* 7:21-43, 1993.

8. Grayson DE: The bride of hope: the use of the creative arts therapies in group treatment for people with AIDS and HIV infection, *J Poetry Ther* 8:123-133, 1995; and Grayson DE, Johnson DB: Living on the moon: persona, identity, and metaphor in Paul Monette's *Borrowed Time: an AIDS memoir*, 9:3-11, 1995.

9. Place F: A tale of eating: writing as a pathway out of an eating disorder, *J Poetry Ther* 7:189-195, 1994.

10. Silvermarie S: Poetry therapy with frail elderly in a nursing home, *J Poetry Ther* 2:72-83, 1988.

11. Sartore RL: Poetry and childhood trauma, *J Poetry Ther* 3:229-233, 1990.

12. Alschuler M: Finding our way home: poetry therapy in a supportive single room occupancy residence, *J Poetry Ther* 9:63-77, 1995.

13. Stiles CG: How to make a hill: a narrative perspective in special education, *J Poetry Ther* 9:89-91, 1995.

14. Belli A: Poets in combat: muse of fire, *J Poetry Ther* 6:87-94, 1992.

15. Rojcewicz S: Multilingual poetry therapy, *J Poetry Ther* 8:3-15, 1994.

16. Heninger OE: Poetry generated by stillbirth and livebirth: transgenerational sharing of grief and joy, *J Poetry Ther* 1:14-22, 1994.

17. Lauer R: Abuses of poetry therapy. In Lerner A, editor: *Poetry in the therapeutic experience*, St Louis, 1994, MMB Music.

18. Reiter S: Poetry therapy: testimony on Capitol Hill, *J Poetry Ther* 10:169-178, 1997.

Relaxation Therapies

BARRY A. SULTANOFF

CARLOS P. ZALAQUETT

Origins and History

Nearly 100 years ago, Dr. Walter B. Cannon, then chairman of the Department of Physiology at Harvard Medical School, conducted a series of experiments on cats. A substance extracted from the adrenal glands of one group of cats was injected into other cats, who responded physiologically with increased heart rate, blood pressure, and breathing rate. Blood flow to the skeletal muscles also increased markedly. Cannon recognized that this was an integrated physiologic response geared to preparing the cats to respond to danger. This "syndrome" of physiologic changes came to be known as the *fight-or-flight* response, as it seemed to be preparing the animals to respond to a potentially life-threatening emergency, either by fighting or by running away.

In humans there is a physiologically similar fight-or-flight response, which is most typically brought on by stressful situations and characterized by feelings of anxiety and fear. Its opposite, often referred to as the *relaxation response,* can be invoked in a wide variety of ways. Bringing forth or awakening the relaxation response is central to most relaxation techniques and approaches. The relaxation response is characteristically opposite to the fight or flight response. It is associated with a slowing of metabolism, lowered heart rate and blood pressure, slower, calmer breathing, and a feeling of well-being. Thus, invoking it serves as an antidote to stress in many life circumstances.

In the mid-twentieth century, Canadian researcher Hans Selye used the terms *disstress* and *eustress* to distinguish between "good stress" (eustress) and the more destructive stress that can lead to illness and imbalance. By making this distinction, he underscored the point that too much stress can undermine health. An optimal level of stress—in other words, just the right life challenges, at the right time—can move us to expand our horizons in healthy ways. Everyone needs challenges in order to grow, and such challenges generally can be viewed as good or healthy for the individual. But to be healthy, individuals must learn to balance the excess of stressors or life challenges that they face with their capacity to nullify the effects of those stressors with a variety of stress-managing tools.

It is the circumstance of feeling or being overwhelmed by stress that can disable, immobilize, and even kill. It is this chronic malignant stress that is at the core of many chronic diseases. In the last quarter-century, as modern living has become more and more intense, there has been an accelerating interest in stress-management and relaxation approaches. A wide variety of such approaches have emerged. In this discussion the emphasis will be on approaches to alleviating stress and achieving relaxation that clinicians can employ without the use of special equipment; in other words, approaches that they "always have with them."

Mechanism of Action According to Its Own Theory

The techniques in this discussion are of three main varieties: refocusing techniques, conscious breathing, and body awareness. Each type is discussed separately.

Refocusing Techniques

These techniques are based on the principle "What you focus on is what you get," or "Energy follows attention." There are an unlimited number of ways that any of us can choose to tell the story of our life or any part of our life. How we choose to frame that story—what we tell ourselves about how we are, how life is, and how the world is—actually has a major impact on our health and well-being. The relevance of perceived meaning can be summed up in the following short verse:

> All that there is
> is what you tell yourself
> about all that there is.

It is useful to listen to patients' reports in the perspective of the reports are really stories about how they have chosen to view their current circumstances and that the practitioner's role is to help patients select alternative stories that would better support them in getting the results that they truly want.

Conscious Breathing and Meditation

Conscious breathing is a way of reducing stress by reintegrating mind and body. It is a time-tested method of achieving profound relaxation. Concentration on the breath, with or without the use of a specific sound or *mantra*, is central to many meditation practices.

To benefit from relaxation and meditation techniques of conscious breathing, patients must learn to turn their attention away from the mental flow of ordinary thinking and focus it instead on the breath or mantra. What ensues is a self-generated vacation from the clatter of "monkey mind" and a "tuning in" to the naturally calming flow of breath.

In meditation techniques, the goal often is to develop a fuller awareness of the individual's self and place in the universe. Relaxation is a byproduct of meditation. However, many relaxation techniques that are not meditations in the strictest sense (for example, the relaxation technique that is presented in this discussion) also serve as an antidote to stress.

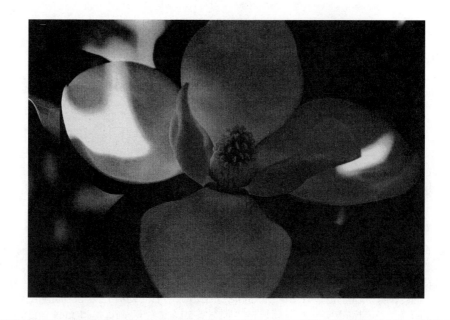

Courtesy Barry Sultanoff, 1999.

Body Awareness

Our culture is excessively focused on the mind. Every day we are expected to figure things out, make sense of things, and come up with ideas. In school, at work, and even in our personal relationships, we are acknowledged and rewarded for coming up with the right answers and the correct solutions to problems.

We spend much of our waking lives "lost in thought"—worrying, planning, judging, daydreaming, and second-guessing ourselves. Effective stress management must then include ways of reconnecting or coming home to our bodies again.

When we do come home consciously—when we learn to integrate mind and body—we feel calmer and more relaxed, steadier, and safer. When we learn to consciously feel the body that is our earthly home, we can tap into the innate wisdom of our bodies and feel more balanced and at peace in our daily lives.

As patients achieve greater mastery with these techniques, they develop a greater sense of self-empowerment and self-sufficiency. They feel safer as active participants in life and more connected with the living earth. In essence, they develop a more comfortable, harmonious relationship with other people and with all of life.

Biologic Mechanism of Action

The techniques in this discussion primarily work through their capacity to activate the relaxation response. This is a physiologic response or healthy syndrome in which the autonomic nervous system becomes balanced, blood supply to muscles becomes normalized, and brain wave activity shifts to include more alpha and theta waves. In its simplest form, when the conscious attention is focused on something interpreted as neutral or positive for the organism's well-being or safety (in other words, the organism concludes that all is well), impulses from the forebrain influence the autonomic nervous system in a general shift toward relatively more parasympathetic activity.

Rather than feeling anxious, fearful, and insecure, patients shift toward feeling more calm, centered, and steady. Self-esteem and self-confidence increases as patients learn that they can shift their mood and physiology at will toward a state of well-being.

Forms of Therapy

Relaxation can be described as a cluster of physiologic and psychologic changes that can be evoked by a wide variety of techniques. Thus there are many ways to achieve relaxation and bring on the relaxation response.

This discussion only provides a small sampling of these approaches. Practitioners are encouraged to select techniques found in this chapter or elsewhere (see "Suggested Reading") that, for whatever reason, seem compatible with their own personal style.

The best results are generally achieved when practitioners choose approaches with which they resonate. This is particularly so with the techniques presented here, as they are most effectively taught when the practitioner is practicing alongside the patient at the same time.

A Refocusing Technique
STOP/LOOK/LISTEN/CHOOSE

This is a reframing technique that patients can use as needed anytime they find themselves in a life situation in which they feel upset, stressed, or out-of-balance because things are not going the way that they want.

This is cognitive first aid that, once learned, patients will always have with them and can use in the trenches of everyday life. It is an antidote to feelings of powerless over life circumstances.

This cognitive technique uses the power of choice and intention. It has the following five steps.

Instructions to Clinician   Teach this technique to patients by having them recall a recent example of a time when they were in a situation where things were not going the way that they wanted. Though this can certainly be used with major life events, it is most helpful in learning the technique to have patients choose an example that is less monumental, such as getting stuck in traffic, losing track of some important item (such as car keys), a disagreement with a friend, and others.

Guide patients through each step of the process, and at the end of the session give them a written description of the steps involved so that they can remember how to practice on their own.

Exercise Life sometimes has moments that are problematic. At those times, we may find ourselves at a crossroads.

This is something like approaching a crossing where a speeding train is about to pass through. If we choose, we can stop, look, and listen so that we will not be hit by the approaching train.

The speeding train represents an old habit, an old way of processing information that has led to distressed feelings and thoughts. We need not be run over or overwhelmed by these old habitual ways that no longer serve us.

This is a simple but effective exercise that uses your capacity to stop, look, listen, and also choose the path that you desire. You can use it anytime you want to change course, whenever things are not going the way you want and you find yourself behaving "on automatic."

This is a way of using your power of choice and intention to redirect the course of your life at that moment. So whenever you find yourself at a crossroads, some glitch in your day where things are not going well, feel out of control, etc . . .

1. *STOP.* Call "time-out"; blow the whistle; if you like, make the letter *T* with your hands, as if you were the referee of your own game of life (as, of course, you are!).
   Remember that you are the one who calls the shots. You are in charge!
   Remind yourself that there are many options other than "being on automatic" with old patterns of behavior, and thought. The way you are proceeding is not the only way to go. There are many others that may work better.

2. **LOOK.** Take an honest look at what is going on. Ask yourself the question, "What's going on here?" and answer that question for yourself by giving yourself a brief "news report" (include the news of what is going on inside of you as well as externally).

3. **LISTEN.** Take a few moments to feel the earth beneath you.
   Bring your attention to your chest, especially in the area in the center of your chest, near your heart. (You don't have to be anatomically precise. Anywhere in the general vicinity of your heart will do.) This is a way of listening to the heart's wisdom and sensing what it may have to say. It is a way of listening "deeper" than the place where information is stored in the "rational" brain, to a place in you that knows the truth about what you really want.
   Notice whatever feeling (or lack of feeling) is in your chest. Ask yourself, "What do I *really* want?" and answer that question for yourself, letting what you *feel* in your chest guide you. This is your way of finding out what is your heart's desire, right in that moment.

4. **CHOOSE.** Make a one-sentence statement of choice for what you want and how you want to be feeling or experiencing the situation. Begin with the words "I choose to enjoy" (for example, "I choose to enjoy feeling balanced and confident.")
   This choice reflects what you *really* want, right here, right now.

5. **LET IT GO!** Now, proceed with your day.

What you have effectively done, using a golfing analogy, is to gently retrieve your ball (you) from the rough and gently place it on the fairway (of life) again.

A Breathing Technique
CONSCIOUS BREATHING

Instructions to Clinician Have patients sit in a comfortable position with their eyes closed. Instruct them to bring their awareness to the breath, simply watching the flow of breath in and out, without trying to change the breathing in any way—just observing. Remind the subject that there is nothing to accomplish here, no particular right way to do it. "All that is necessary is your willingness to explore . . . and your choice to participate and be available to any benefits that may be here for you."

Remind the patient that the mind may be very active, so that focusing just on the breath may be difficult. "But that's OK. If your attention drifts, just bring your mind back to the breathing."

The following is a model script for instructing the patient in conscious breathing.

(Please note: Your success in assisting the patient will depend upon how well you yourself do the exercise. It is essential that you establish, by your own conscious breathing while you guide the exercise, an "energy template" or context for the patient to follow.)

Exercise (approximately 5 minutes) First, find a comfortable relaxed position, with legs uncrossed and feet flat on the floor.

Acknowledge yourself for being willing, right now, in this moment, to explore something that will be of benefit to your health and well-being . . . your choice to participate, to explore is what counts here . . . there is no specific "something" to accomplish . . . there is no particular "right way" to do this . . . just allow yourself to be available to whatever benefits may come forth . . .

Now bring your attention to your breathing . . . notice the flow of breath in and out . . . without trying to change your breathing in any way, just observe the breath . . . you may find that you become distracted by thoughts generated by the busy mind . . . that's fine . . . just bring your attention back to the breath . . . and continue . . .

. . . As you watch the flow of breath, you may notice that you become calmer, more relaxed . . . as you notice yourself feeling calmer, allow that calmness to spread throughout your body . . . let the easy flow of breath teach the rest of you how to be easy too . . . notice how effortless this all can be . . . nothing to accomplish . . . nowhere to go . . . nowhere else to be but right here, right now . . . just allowing the gentle rhythm of the breath calm and relax you . . . (longer pause) . . .

So now, take one full easy breath, letting the breath out with a little sigh, if you wish . . . and gently allow your eyes to open . . . returning fully to present time and place.

A Body Awareness Technique
LUNG BELLY ("THE SECRET")

Instructions to Clinician This is a simple exercise that encourages full, easy breathing and helps integrate mind and body.

Exercise Ask patients to pretend that you both know a secret about them that no one else knows. It is an "invisible" secret and yet it has real impact on their health.

The secret is this: The patient has an unusual anatomic anomaly. The lungs, instead of being in the usual place in the chest, are located in the belly, just behind the navel. It has apparently been this way since birth, but now you, the doctor have pointed this out, based on your examination.

This unique anatomic arrangement works just as well as the more typical or conventional one. What especially helps, though, is for the patient to check the breathing at times and make sure that the breath is reaching the "belly lungs."

Ask the patient to do this right now. "Bring your attention right now to your breathing and just check and make sure that the breath is reaching the lungs." Remind the patient that this is where it needs to go so that the oxygen can be picked up by the red blood cells and carried to all parts of the body. The patient may place one hand on the belly over the navel area to better feel the location of the lungs.

Remind the patient that it is not necessary to try and breathe deeply. Just check in with the breath and with the "belly lungs" and be sure that the breath "knows" to go there, where the "secret lungs" reside.

Encourage patients to practice this exercise when they are alone at different times during their daily routines.

Demographics

These mind-body relaxation therapies have been gaining wide acceptance, and they continue to do so. Practitioners of these therapies abound, both within and beyond the ranks of the medical establishment. They are especially widely used by clinical psychologists and other nonphysicians who, because of legal limitations on prescribing, are not tempted to use psychoactive medications for relaxation purposes.

They are useful for a wide variety of patients, including adults of all ages, men and women, and even children, who particularly enjoy the body-oriented focusing processes.

They do require a capacity to focus on specific instructions while the technique is being taught.

Indications and Reasons for Referral

These techniques are widely applicable for the stresses of everyday living. Thus, the majority of patients who make up a typical outpatient medical practice are good candidates.

In a psychiatric practice, these approaches are particularly useful for stress disorders, anxiety and panic disorders, adjustment disorders, and the treatment of addictions. For depression, the refocusing techniques are strongly recommended, but the conscious breathing and body awareness techniques may also be helpful.

In a practice of family medicine and internal medicine, these techniques are suitable for chronic illnesses of all kinds, including headache, irritable bowel syndrome, peptic ulcer disease, inflammatory bowel disease, hypertension, arrhythmias, coronary artery disease, asthma, diabetes, cancer, musculoskeletal pain, and others. Given the significance of stress in the etiology of the vast majority of illnesses and the stressful nature of illness itself, there are few conditions for which these therapies would not be suitable.

These therapies are also suitable for most hospitalized patients. They can easily be learned and taught by the nursing staff.

Office Applications

A simple ranking of conditions responsive to this form of therapy follows. As with all alternative therapies, use of relaxation therapy does not preclude the use of mainstream medical therapies in addition.

Top level: *A therapy ideally suited for these conditions*
Anxiety, headaches, and stress disorders

Second level: *One of the better therapies for these conditions*
Depression; gastritis; hypertension; irritable bowel syndrome; inflammatory bowel; musculoskeletal pain; panic disorder; and peptic ulcer disease

Practical Applications

Relaxation techniques are easy to learn by health practitioner and patient alike. As they are so widely (almost universally) useful for a range of clinical conditions, their use is highly recommended. Relaxation techniques can be taught to patients individually as part of an office visit, either by the doctor or by ancillary staff. Relaxation techniques also can be taught to patients in groups, such as "mind-body therapy" support groups or seminars.

These techniques ideally are taught in a setting with a relaxed, comfortable atmosphere. The setting itself may then set the tone for the desired effect of stress reduction and relaxation. If possible, have a special room with the designated purpose of supporting patients in becoming more relaxed and centered. Natural light, soothing music, plants, artwork and color schemes conducive to relaxation are always desirable. At minimum, the room should be quiet and free of distractions, both for practitioner and patient.

Research Base

Evidence Based

ANXIETY AND PANIC DISORDERS

Relaxation techniques are highly efficient and produce long-term benefits in the treatment of clinical anxiety.[1-4]

Drug therapy versus relaxation therapy Although much research remains to be done in this area, Lehrer and Woolfolk's review of anxiety studies comparing drug and behavioral treatments (relaxation, exposure) is worth mentioning. They concluded that both treatments have similar short-term effects, but behavioral treatments had better long-term effects than drug treatments.[5]

Generalized anxiety symptoms Different multicomponent (cognitive, relaxation, and exposure techniques) treatments for the treatment of generalized anxiety have shown significant improvements of anxiety.[6] Deffenbacher and Suinn[7] recommend teaching relaxation as a self-control procedure as part of these treatments.

HEADACHES

Relaxation techniques are useful in treating headaches in both adults[8] and children.[9,10] Relaxation or biofeedback training helps 40% to 80% of tension headache sufferers.[11]

HYPERTENSION AND HEART DISEASE

Some studies of relaxation therapy for hypertension have reported highly significant effects for relaxation therapies.[12] In 1988 the joint National Committee on Detection, Evaluation, and Treatment of High Blood Pressure recommended that relaxation be used for treatment of mild hypertension and as an adjunct to medication for treatment of more severe hypertension. There is evidence that stress management techniques can decrease the doses of antihypertensive medications needed.[13] However, where blood pressure is significantly elevated, it should not be considered safe to maintain hypertensive patients on relaxation treatment alone. Relaxation-based interventions also have a prophylactic effect against heart disease.[14-16]

IRRITABLE BOWEL SYNDROME

Studies combining relaxation and CT have shown positive results in the treatment of irritable bowel syndrome.[17,18]

INSOMNIA

PMR is an effective treatment for idiopathic insomnia (objective insomnia).[19]

PANIC SYMPTOMS

Several studies report the elimination of panic attacks via cognitive or breathing techniques in at least 80% to 90% of their patients.[20-23]

RELAXATION THERAPIES WITH CHILDREN

Children learn relaxation techniques with an equal or a better ability than adults.[24,25] Most studies show that relaxation can be beneficial in treating anxiety-related academic difficulties and pain.[26] Relaxation therapy also can be a positive addition to improving psychosomatic disorders[27] and hyperactive children's impulsivity, disruptive behavior, academic performance, and self-concept.[28]

SOCIAL PHOBIA

Relaxation appears to be effective in the treatment of social phobias. Treatment comparisons showed that either exposure, relaxation, or cognitive therapies (CT) are effective in the treatment of social phobias.[29]

SUBSTANCE ABUSE

Between 10% and 40% of alcoholics suffer panic-related anxiety disorder, and 10% to 20% of anxiety disorder patients abuse alcohol or other drugs.[30] Relaxation and self-management techniques significantly reduce anxiety and tension in alcoholics.[31,32] Relaxation seems to be highly recommended for anxious alcoholics who drink to avoid experiencing stress or in response to stress.[33]

Basic Science

THE RELAXATION RESPONSE MODEL

H. Benson, based on his observation of the relaxation effects, argued that all relaxation techniques produce a single relaxation response characterized by diminished sympathetic arousal.[34,35]

INTEGRATIVE MODEL

Schwartz, Davidson, and Goleman[36] suggests that the majority of relaxation procedures have highly specific effects, as well as more generally stress-reducing effects; therefore the specific effects of various relaxation techniques may be superimposed on a general relaxation effect. For example, autogenic training (AT) has specific effects on the autonomic functions included in the autogenic exercises, but it also produces a general decrease in physiologic arousal.

Risk and Safety

PROBLEMS ASSOCIATED WITH RELAXATION

Relaxation training is a very safe procedure. For some patients, however, the level of tension increases instead of decreases when practicing relaxation, an experience which they find to be unexpected and stressful.[37-39]

The following two adverse consequences of relaxation training have been documented:

1. Autogenic discharges: *Autogenic discharges* are emotional or physical experiences that can include pain, anxiety, palpitations, muscle twitches, and crying.[40] These AT events, which are not necessarily countertherapeutic, are sometimes experienced as unpleasant and lead the patient to abandon treatment. They may also produce effects that are medically dangerous, such as increases in blood pressure among hypertensives. Therefore patients must be carefully monitored to prevent any deleterious effect of autogenic training.
2. Relaxation-induced anxiety: *Relaxation-induced anxiety* is the heightened physiologic arousal and reactivity sometimes experienced during meditation.[41,42]

Efficacy

In the authors' experience, these therapies are highly effective (greater than 80%) in alleviating many "garden variety" symptoms of stress, such as stress headaches, anxiety, dyspepsia, diarrhea, nausea, and "bad mood" (irritability).

For more chronic conditions, there is generally some improvement in more than 75% of cases, with marked improvement in 25% to 50%.

Druglike Information

Safety

These therapies are safe to use in any circumstances in which the patient chooses to consciously cooperate with the learning process, the only exception being a borderline or psychotic patient whose reality testing may be impaired.

Warnings, Contraindications, and Precautions

These techniques are totally noninvasive and therefore carry no significant risk. The authors have found them to be counterproductive in certain schizophrenic patients and recommend using them with caution or not at all with patients who are actively psychotic.

Drug or Other Interactions

These therapies can be used safely in conjunction with all medications. However, the medication dosages should be monitored as the optimal dosage may diminish. For example, a diabetic patient's insulin needs may diminish; a hypertensive patient's dosage of antihypertensive medication may decrease; and an anxious patient may need fewer benzodiazepines.

Adverse Reactions

In depression, techniques that require inward focusing, such as conscious breathing and body awareness, can at times intensify depressed mood, so it is recommended that they be used judiciously and with attention to the patient's response as the work proceeds.

Self-Help versus Professional

For simple relaxation, these therapies are easily learned and require no special training. However, for assistance with medical or psychiatric management, training with a health professional is reasonably warranted. This suggestion is due to the complexity of selecting the appropriate method for each patient and the potential side effects of relaxation, such as relaxation-induced anxiety. There also is research evidence supporting the notion that administration of relaxation therapy by competent professionals is necessary for their success.[43] Patients may consider the following types of professionals for relaxation training: behavioral medicine specialists, physicians, psychologists, psychiatrists, school counselors, and social workers.[44] Some practitioners, especially clinical psychologists and social workers, have earned a reputation for effectiveness with this kind of approach, including some use of guided imagery.

Visiting a Professional

These techniques are often incorporated into a standard counseling session that usually occurs in the office setting of the health professional teaching these therapies.

Credentialing

No formal credentialing of relaxation therapies is currently available.

Training

Courses in relaxation therapies can be found at many professional seminars, such as National Institute for Clinical Applications of Behavioral Medicine (NICABM) and the annual conferences of the American Holistic Medical Association and the American Holistic Nurses Association. Credentialing is generally not required for practitioners who wish to teach simple relaxation techniques such as the ones described in this chapter.

What to Look for in a Provider

Providers of these therapies ideally be models of steadiness in the face of their own life challenges and capable of offering a steady, living model of relaxation and centeredness for the patient. Choose providers who exemplify, in their own being and in the manner in which they conduct their practice, that calm centeredness that you are seeking for your patient.

Barriers and Key Issues

These therapies are becoming widely accepted and are viewed as having substantial research validation.

Associations

No associations exist specifically for the dissemination and credentialing of relaxation therapies. However, the following associations are reliable sources of information.

American Holistic Medical Association
2727 Fairview Ave. East
Seattle, WA 98102
Tel: (703) 556-9245

American Holistic Nursing Association
PO Box 2130
Flagstaff, AZ 86003
Tel: (800) 278-AHNA
E-mail: AHNA-Flag@flaglink.com
http://www.ahna.org

American Holistic Health Association
PO Box 17400
Anaheim, CA 92817
Tel: (714) 779-6152
E-mail: ahha@healthy.net
http://www.ahhp.org

National Institute for the Clinical Application of Behavioral Medicine
Tel: (800) 743-2226
E-mail: nicabm@neca.com
http://www.nicabm.org

Institute of Noetic Sciences
475 Gate Five Road, Suite 300
Sausalito, CA 94965
General Inquiries: (415) 331-5650
Fax: (415) 331-5673
E-mail: webmaster@noetic.org
http://www.membership@noetic.org

Suggested Reading

1. Linden W: *Autogenics: a clinical guide*, New York, 1990, Guilford.
   This book provides a comprehensive description of the autogenic technique, with instructions for its use in clinical settings.
2. Bernstein DA, Borkovec TD: *Progressive relaxation training: a manual for the helping professions*, Champaign, Ill, 1973, Research.
   This manual offers clinicians detailed, step-by-step instructions on how to help patients learn progressive relaxation.
3. Benson H, Klipper MZ: *The relaxation response*, ed 2, New York, 1975, Avon.
   This book describes the historical roots of relaxation procedures and provides the instructions to achieve the relaxation response.
4. Davis M, Eshelman ER, McKay M: *The relaxation and stress reduction workbook*, ed 4, Oakland, Calif, 1995, New Harbinger.
   This workbook provides basic instructions and exercises to help patients learn to relax. It includes directions for progressive relaxation, autogenic training, meditation, and breathing techniques.

Bibliography

Bernstein DA, Carlson, CR: Progressive relaxation: abbreviated methods. In Lehrer PM, Woolfolk RL, editors: *Principles and practice of stress management,* ed 2, New York, 1993, Guilford.

Cooke G: Evaluation of the efficacy of the components of reciprocal inhibition psychotherapy, *J Abnorm Psychol* 73:464-467, 1968.

Lehrer PM, Woolfolk RL, Goldman N: (1986). Progressive relaxation then and now: does change always mean progress? In Davidson R, Schwartz GE, Shapiro D, editors: *Consciousness and self-regulation,* vol 4, New York, 1986, Plenum.

References

1. Borkovec TD, Sides K: Critical procedural variables related to the psychological effects of progressive relaxation: a review, *Behav Res Ther* 17:119-126, 1979.

2. Bernstein DA, Borkovec TD: *Progressive relaxation training,* Champaign, Ill, 1973, Research.

3. Clum GA, Clum GA, Surls R: A metaanalysis of treatments for panic disorder, *J Consult Clin Psychol* 61(2):317-326, 1993.

4. Rasid ZM, Parish TS: The effects of two types of relaxation training on students' levels of anxiety, *Adolescence* 33(129):99-101, 1998.

5. Lehrer PM, Woolfolk RL, editors: *Principles and practice of stress management,* ed 2, New York, 1993, Guilford.

6. Borkovec TD, Costello E: Efficacy of applied relaxation and cognitive-behavioral therapy in the treatment of generalized anxiety disorder, *J Consult Clin Psychol* 61(4):611-619, 1993.

7. Deffenbacher JL, Suinn R: Generalized anxiety syndrome. In Michelson L, Ascher M, editors: *Anxiety and stress disorders: cognitive-behavioral assessment and treatment,* New York, 1987, Guilford.

8. Primavera JP, Kaiser RS: Nonpharmacological treatment of headache: is less more? *Headache* 32(8):393-395, 1992.

9. Mehta M: Biobehavioral intervention in recurrent headaches in children, *Headache Q* 3(4):426-430, 1992.

10. Sartory G et al: A comparison of psychological and pharmacological treatment of pediatric migraine, *Behav Res Ther* 36(12):1155-1170, 1998.

11. Blanchard EB, Ahles TA, Shaw ER: Behavioral treatment of headache. In Hersen M, Eisler RM, Miller PM, editors: *Progress in behavior modification,* vol 8, New York, 1979, Academic Press.

12. Jacob RG et al: Relaxation therapy for hypertension: design effects and treatment effects, *Ann Behav Med* 13:5-17, 1991.

13. Glasgow MS, Engel BT, D'Lugoff BC: A controlled study of a standardized behavioral stepped treatment for hypertension, *Psychosom Med* 51:10-26, 1989.

14. Dath NNS et al: Behavioral approach to coronary heart disease, *J Person Clin Stud* 13(1-2):29-33, 1997.

15. Patel C, Marmot MG, Terry DJ: Controlled trial of biofeedback-aided behavioral methods in reducing mild hypertension, *Brit Med J* 282:2005-2008, 1981.

16. van Dixhoorn J: Cardiorespiratory effects of breathing and relaxation instruction in myocardical infarction patients, *Bio Psychol* 49(1-2):123-135, 1998.

17. Neff DF, Blanchard EB: A multicomponent treatment for irritable bowel syndrome, *Behav Ther* 18:70-83, 1987.

18. Blanchard EB, Schwarz SP: Two-year follow-up of behavioral treatment of irritable bowel syndrome, *Behav Ther* 19:67-73, 1988.

19. Borkovec TD: Pseudo- (experimental) insomnia and idiopathic (objective) insomnia: theoretical and therapeutic issues, *Advance Behav Res Ther* 2:27-55, 1979.

20. Barlow DH: *Anxiety and its disorders: the nature and treatment of anxiety and panic*, New York, 1988, Guilford.

21. Beck AT: Cognitive approaches to panic disorder: theory and therapy. In Rachman S, Maser JD, editors: *Panic: psychological perspectives*, Hillsdale, NJ, 1988, Erlbaum.

22. Clark DM: A cognitive approach to panic, *Behav Res Ther* 24:461-470, 1986.

23. Clark DM, Salkovskis PM, Chalkley AJ: Respiratory control as a treatment of panic attacks, *J Behav Ther Exper Psychiatry* 16:23-30, 1985.

24. Zaichkowsky LB, Zaichkowsky LD: The effects of a school-based relaxation training program on fourth-grade children, *J Clin Child Psychol* 13:81-85, 1984.

25. Hiebert B, Kirby B, Jaknovorian A: School-based relaxation: attempting primary prevention, *Can J Counsel* 23:273-287, 1989.

26. Heitkemper T et al: Brief treatment of children's dental pain and anxiety, *Percept Motor Skills* 76(1):192-194, 1993.

27. Richter NC: The efficacy of relaxation training with children, *J Abnorm Child Psychol* 12:319-344, 1984.

28. Omizo MM, Williams RE: Biofeedback-induced relaxation training as an alternative for the elementary school learning-disabled child, *Biofeedback Self-Reg* 7:139-148, 1982.

29. Heimberg RG: Cognitive and behavioral treatments for social phobia: a critical analysis, *Clin Psychol Rev* 9:107-128, 1989.

30. Cox BJ et al: Substance abuse and panic-related anxiety: a critical review, *Behav Res Ther* 28:385-393, 1990.

31. Parker JC, Gilbert G: Anxiety management in alcoholics: a study of generalized effects of relaxation techniques, *Addict Behav* 3:123-127, 1978.

32. Parker JC, Gilbert GS, Thoreson RW: Reduction of autonomic arousal in alcoholics: a comparison of relaxation and meditation techniques, *J Consult Clin Psychol* 46:879-886, 1978.

33. Kushner M, Sher K, Beitnian B: The relation between alcohol problems and the anxiety disorders, *Am J Psychiatry* 147:685-695, 1990.

34. Benson H: *The relaxation response*, ed 1, New York, 1975, Morrow.

35. Benson H: The relaxation response and norepinephrine: a new study illuminates mechanisms, *Integrat Psychiatry* 1:15-18, 1983.

36. Schwartz GE, Davidson RJ, Goleman DT: Patterning of cognitive and somatic processes in the self-regulation of anxiety: effects of meditation versus exercise, *Psychosom Med* 40:321-328, 1978.

37. Borkovec TD, Grayson JB: Consequences of increasing the functional impact of internal emotional stimuli. In Blankstein K, Pliner P, Polivy J, editors: *Assessment and modification of emotional behavior*, New York, 1980, Plenum.

38. Lazarus AA: A preliminary report in the use of directed muscular activity in counterconditioning, *Behav Res Ther* 2:301-303, 1965.

39. Ley R: Panic attacks during relaxation and relaxation-induced anxiety: a hyperventilation interpretation, *J Behav Ther Exper Psychiatry* 19:253-259, 1988.

40. Schultz JH, Luthe W: *Autogenic therapy: Vol 1. Autogenic methods*, New York, 1969, Grune & Stratton.

41. Heide FJ, Borkovec TD: Relaxation-induced anxiety: paradoxical anxiety enhancement due to relaxation training, *J Consult Clin Psychol* 51:171-182, 1983.

42. Heide FJ, Borkovec TD: Relaxation-induced anxiety: mechanisms and theoretical implications, *Behav Res Ther* 22:1-12, 1984.

43. Carey MP, Burish TG: Providing relaxation training to cancer chemotherapy patients: a comparison of three delivery techniques, *J Consult Clin Psychol* 55:732-737, 1987.

44. Miller LH, Smith AD, Rothstein L: *The stress solution: an action plan to manage the stress in your life*, New York, 1993, Pocket Books.

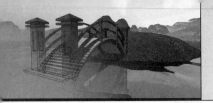

Spiritual Healing and Prayer

HAROLD G. KOENIG

Origins and History

According to a recent Gallup poll, 9 out of 10 Americans pray, and 75% pray every day.[1] To whom or what do most people pray? According to this Gallup poll, 75% pray to a supreme being such as God, 16% pray to Jesus Christ, 3% pray to the Lord, 1% pray to Jehovah, 1% pray to a transcendent or cosmic force, and 1% pray to an inner self or the God within. What do Americans pray about? The most common object of prayer is family's well-being (98%), which is followed by prayers of thanks (94%), prayers for strength or guidance in meeting a challenge (92%), and prayers asking for forgiveness (92%). Further down the list are prayers for personal health—82% of the population prays for health and healing.

In the study by Eisenberg et al, 25% of participants used prayer as an unconventional therapy, a prevalence rate that was second only to exercise (26%).[2] Prayer is indeed one of the most common unconventional therapies that complement traditional medical therapies for many illnesses.

Mechanism of Action According to Its Own Theory

There are many theories about the mechanism by which prayer and other religious and spiritual coping strategies work. According to Levin, there are four mechanisms by which prayer may have its effects: local-naturalistic, local-supernatural, nonlocal–naturalistic, and nonlocal-supernatural mechanisms. By *local-naturalistic mechanism*, Levin refers to health-related behavior, social support, stressor buffering effect, cognitive effect, and the power of belief. *Nonlocal–naturalistic mechanisms* refers to naturalistic mechanisms based on an understanding of the universe based on "new physics" that attempts to explain effects as happening outside of traditional time-space concepts (extended mind, morphic field, subtle energy, consciousness, and others). *Supernatural mechanisms* refers to phenomena occurring either locally or at a distance that are due to a force outside of nature.[3] The focus of this author and of the Center for the Study of Religion/Spirituality and Health at Duke University has been primarily on the study of local-naturalistic mechanisms.

Biologic Mechanism of Action

Prayer and related religious coping strategies likely operate through a mind-body effect. In other words, prayer has a calming effect that reduces stress and the stress-related physiological changes involving the neurologic, endocrine, immune, and cardiovascular systems. Woods et al[4] examined the association between religious beliefs and behaviors and immune functioning in 106 HIV seropositive gay men. Religious activities—prayer or meditation, religious attendance, spiritual discussions, reading religious or spiritual literature—were associated with significantly higher CD4+ counts and CD4+ percentages (T-helper-inducer cells) (controlling for self-efficacy and active coping with health situation, using regression modeling).

Forms of Therapy

People can be trained in meditation techniques, which frequently are used in relaxation therapies to help treat problems such as anxiety, chronic pain, hypertension, and other stress-related disorders. Pastoral counseling takes advantage of the religious or spiritual beliefs of the patient in the treatment of emotional disorders and adjustment problems. Some physicians pray with patients and believe that this is beneficial.[5]

Different Types of Prayer

According to Poloma and Pendleton,[6] based on a random sample of 560 persons, most types of prayer can be divided into four categories: meditative prayer; ritualistic prayer; petitionary prayer; and conversational prayer. *Meditative prayer* involves quieting the mind and focusing on a particular topic, word, sound, or phrase. Eastern types of meditative prayer involve the repetition of a sound or word that induces a deep state of relaxation and concentrated attention. Western types of meditative prayer may focus on God and attempt to create a receptive state in which one *listens* to God; alternatively, an individual may focus the mind on a phrase such as "Lord Jesus Christ, have mercy on me." Herbert Benson[7,8] studied the health consequences of such repetitive prayer and found profound physiologic changes, including reduction of blood pressure, cardiac arrhythmias, reduction of cortisol, and many other health benefits.

Ritualistic prayer involves the saying of memorized standardized prayers that have been learned as part of a religious tradition or training. *Petitionary prayer* involves praying directly to a Divine being to request something, often something very specific, such as physical healing. Petitionary prayer is the most common form of prayer in the U.S. and largely reflects the type of praying reported by the Gallup poll previously mentioned. *Conversational prayer* involves speaking on an intimate level with God, and outpouring of feelings, thoughts and needs, as if speaking to a friend.

One variant of petitionary prayer is *intercessory prayer*, which involves praying for another individual. This occurs most effectively when the subjects of the prayer know that they are being prayed for. However, the "double-blind" variety of intercessory prayer remains unproven.

Religious Coping

Prayer may often be used to help persons cope with the consequences of a stressor, such as physical illness. Religious coping frequently involves a variety of activities, such as petitionary or conversational prayer, trusting in God, turning problems over to God, and seeking support from a minister or members of a church congregation. In a study of 332 consecutively admitted medical patients aged 60 years or more to Duke Hospital, we found that more than 42% of these patients spontaneously reported religion was *the most important factor* used to help them cope.[9] More than 90% of patients indicated that they used religious or spiritual beliefs and practices in at least a moderate degree when coping with physical health problems and difficult life circumstances. In an earlier study we had found that religious coping was significantly and inversely related to depression, and we predicted lower depression scores 6 months following discharge from the hospital.[10]

Prayer often provides the sick person with a form of control over physical illness and uncontrollable life circumstances that others who do not believe in prayer do not have. For example, some individuals pray to God believing that God is all-powerful, can change the situation for the better, and responds to prayer. Thus, these individuals can now *do something* that they believe can change their situations and therefore do not feel as helpless or out of control. Such people may "put things in God's hands" and not worry about or obsess over their problems as they otherwise might. Consequently, religious cognitions play a very important role in relieving stress and helping a person cope with difficult life circumstances—circumstances that frequently involve health problems.

Demographics

The United States (particularly the southern region), India, and many of the Muslim countries are those areas of the world where prayer and religious beliefs and practices are most valued, although worldwide studies examining the prevalence of these activities are limited. Religious beliefs and activities tend to be associated with religious organizations where people who rely heavily on prayer tend to congregate, such as churches, synagogues, and mosques. Women, minority groups (African-Americans, Mexican-Americans, and others), and older adults tend to be the most religious groups in the U.S.[1]

Any health professional can administer prayer, although clergy have specific training in this regard. There is some question about whether any training is needed for prayer to be effective. The efficacy may lie in the intention behind the prayer. Locations are doctors' offices, churches, and private homes.

Indications and Reasons for Referral

Persons who may benefit most from prayer and related religious and spiritual therapies are those with adjustment problems, anxiety, depression, and almost any of the stress-related diseases. Also, persons with chronic disability and other health problems often benefit greatly from a religious or spiritual approach that gives them control over their situations and helps to infuse life with purpose, meaning, and hope.

Office Applications

Stress-related diseases can be effectively treated (as a supplemental therapy) with prayer and pastoral counseling. These diseases include generalized anxiety disorder, milder forms of depression, adjustment disorders involving medical illness, substance abuse, and some physical conditions such as hypertension, peptic ulcer disease, and possibly pain associated with rheumatoid arthritis. However, many of the physical health indications need further study given the relatively minimal research base.

Practical Applications

A clinician may decide to support the religious or spiritual beliefs of the patient. In certain circumstances the clinician may decide to pray with the patient, but only after explicit consent from the patient has been obtained. Any religious or spiritual intervention should always be patient-centered. If the clinician is uncomfortable with addressing religious or spiritual needs of patients, then the patient should be referred to a chaplain or pastoral counselor.

Research Base

Evidence Based

EPIDEMIOLOGIC STUDIES

Does prayer really work? Does prayer facilitate healing? If so, what types of prayer are we talking about? And is it only *physical healing* that we should be concerned about, or can prayer produced healing that goes far beyond the physical, to the psychologic, relational, and spiritual?

A number of studies at Duke University have shown the combination of frequent prayer and active involvement in a religious community has particularly powerful effects on health. Two of these studies are described here.

Blood pressure and religious activities were assessed in a probability sample of 3963 persons age 65 years or older who participated in the Duke site of the Establishment of Populations or Epidemiologic Studies in the Elderly (EPESE) survey.[11] Cross-sectional analyses revealed consistent differences in measured systolic and diastolic blood pressures between frequent (once per week) and infrequent (less than once per week) religious service attenders. Lower blood pressures also were observed among those who frequently prayed or studied the Bible (daily or more often). Blood pressure differences were particularly notable in Black and younger older adult patients, in whom religious activity at one wave predicted blood pressures 4 years later. Among participants who attended religious services and also prayed or studied the Bible frequently, the likelihood of having a diastolic blood pressure of 90 mmHg or higher was 40% lower than that of participants who attended religious services infrequently and prayed or studied the Bible infrequently (odds ratio 0.60; confidence intervals 95% 0.48-0.75; $p < 0.0001$).

Although most religious activity was associated with lower blood pressure, those who frequently watched religious television or listening to religious radio actually had higher blood pressures.

Prayer also may influence health behaviors. Among all health behaviors, cigarette smoking is perhaps associated with the worst health outcomes, including lung cancer, chronic obstructive pulmonary disease, hypertension, and coronary artery disease. We examined cigarette smoking and religious activities among the 3968 participants of the Duke EPESE survey.[12] Cross-sectional analyses revealed that participants who frequently attended religious services were significantly less likely to smoke. Total number of pack-years smoked also was inversely related to attendance at religious services and to private religious activities. Watching religious television or listening to religious radio, on the other hand, was unrelated to current smoking or total pack-years smoked and was related to greater rates of current smoking in certain study subsets.

In both of these studies it was the combination of frequent prayer and frequent religious community involvement that was the strongest predictor of health outcomes, much stronger than either activity alone. We have recently examined the effects of religious activity on 6-year survival of the EPESE cohort, finding that lower blood pressure, less smoking, and other consequences of devout religious or spiritual practice may significantly extend survival.[13]

INTERCESSORY PRAYER STUDIES

A number of studies have examined the effects of intercessory prayer on health outcomes. Intercessory prayer may involve praying for people who do know that they are being prayed for or praying for people who do not know that they are being prayed for. I will review prayer studies in chronologic order of their publication.

Galton[14] conducted a retrospective case-control study of petitionary and intercessory prayer, concluding that there was no statistical evidence for the objective value of prayer. In that study Galton refers to a memoir by Dr. Guy from the *Journal of the Statistical Society* in which he compares the mean age of death among males from various occupations between 1758 and 1843. Guy apparently found that clergy only lived slightly longer than persons in other professions (69.5 years, although this was the longest of 10 other groups except the gentry, with 70.2 years). Eminent clergy tended to live slightly shorter lives than either lawyers or medical professionals. Galton also reported that members of royal houses had the lowest average lifespan of all, despite traditions of praying for the sovereign. Galton also claimed that mortality rates of missionaries were not any better than others and possibly worse, a finding that is hardly surprising given the health risks of missionaries. He also looked at rates of stillbirth among members of the "praying and the nonpraying classes," again noting few survival benefits for the praying classes. This clearly was a flawed examination, however, because groups likely to be prayed for or likely to be praying are also those with the most psychosocial stressors and hardship, which are likely to shorten survival.

Parker and St. Johns studied 45 volunteers between the ages of 22 and 60, all with psychosomatic symptoms or severe emotional distress. Subjects in a directed group prayer-therapy session had greater improvement over weekly psychotherapy sessions, and both had greater improvement over personal undirected prayer alone. However, design flaws related to subject assignment and the multifaceted nature of prayer therapy made conclusions about verbal prayer impossible.[15]

Joyce and Welldon conducted the first randomized double-blind controlled trial of intercessory prayer. Subjects included 48 outpatients treated for psychologic or rheumatoid disease in London. The prayer method used was "the practice of the presence of God." Subjects in the intervention group were prayed for by 6 prayer teams; five were organized by the Guild of Health and one was organized by the Friends' Spiritual Healing Fellowship. The prayed-for group (5/16 improved) did not statistically differ from the not-prayed-for group (1/16 improved).[16]

Collipp, chairman of the Department of Pediatrics at Meadowbrook Hospital in East Meadow, New York, conducted the next randomized clinical trial of prayer. Subjects included 18 children with leukemia between the ages of 1 and 19 years. 50% of the children were prayed for daily for 15 months by an intercessory Protestant group in Washington, D.C. The health outcome was 15-month survival. Results indicated that 70% of the prayed-for children survived, versus only 25% of the not-prayed-for children. These results were not statistically significant, most likely due to the small sample size.[17]

In the most famous prayer study ever published in a medical journal, Byrd conducted a randomized clinical trial involving 393 patients randomized to intercessory prayer ($n = 192$) to a control group ($n = 201$). Neither doctors nor patients knew who was being prayed for. Intercessory petitionary prayer to the Judeo-Christian God was the intervention. The intercessory prayer group had fewer patients with congestive heart failure (8 versus 20; $p < 0.05$), needed less diuretics (5 versus 15; $p < 0.05$), experienced fewer cardiac arrests (3 versus 14; $p < 0.05$) and fewer pneumonias (3 versus 13; $p < 0.05$), were prescribed fewer antibiotics (3 versus 17; $p < 0.005$), and none of the intercessory group were intubated (versus 12 of the control group; $p < 0.05$). Controlling for other variables demonstrated that the prayer group overall required less respirator support and less medication ($p < .0001$).[18]

A number of other intercessory prayer studies have either been completed recently or are currently ongoing (Dale Matthews at Georgetown University, Jerry Kolb at Saint Luke's Hospital of Kansas City, and Herbert Benson at Harvard Medical School). No published studies have yet replicated the Byrd study.

In a more recent study,[19] predictors of depression outcome were examined in a sample of 87 hospitalized older adult patients at Duke Hospital. This study, to our knowledge, was the first to examine the effects of religiousness on the course of a major psychiatric. Significant predictors of outcome included family history of depression, low quality of life, declining physical functioning, and low social support. We also measured religious attendance, frequency of private religious activities, and intrinsic religiosity. All religious measures were associated with a faster remission of depression, although only intrinsic religiosity achieved statistical significance. We discovered that religion appears to be particularly beneficial for persons with chronic disability that is unresponsive to medical treatments.

Intrinsic religiosity is a concept developed by psychologist Gordon Allport at Harvard in the 1950s. He defined it as follows: "Persons with this orientation find their master motive in religion. Other needs, strong as they may be, are regarded as of less ultimate significance, and they are, so far as possible, brought into harmony with the religious beliefs and prescriptions. Having embraced a creed, the individual endeavors to internalize it and follow it fully. It is in this sense that he lives his religion."[20] Intrinsic religiosity is strongly correlated with prayer.[9]

Note that in the previous study, patients were asked at baseline what coping behaviors they believed were most helpful to them in coping with their physical health problems. Almost two-thirds indicated that religion (praying to God or having faith in God) was an important factor in this regard, and one-third indicated that it was the most important factor of all their coping behaviors. Thus, even before we began the follow-up, these patients reported to us that religion and prayer were important factors in coping with health problems and illness.

Basic Science

Neuroendocrine and Immunologic Changes and Prayer

Sudsuang et al[21] conducted a clinical trial to study the effects of Buddhist meditation on serum cortisol and other biologic measures. Biologic and physiologic measurements were obtained 1 hour after meditation began in the morning. Cortisol levels on follow-up were significantly reduced in meditators compared with controls ($p < 0.01$).

Koenig et al[22] conducted a prospective cohort study to evaluate the effect of religious activity on interleukin-6 and other biologic indicators of immune function in persons over age 65. The likelihood of having high IL-6 levels (>5 pg/ml) among persons attending religious services to any degree in a 1992 sample was almost 50% less than in nonattendees (odds ratio 0.51; 95% confidence intervals 0.35-0.73; $p \leq 0.001$ uncontrolled; odds ratio 0.58; 95% confidence intervals 0.40-0.84; $p < 0.005$, controlled for age, sex, race, education, chronic illness, and physical functioning).

Most recently, Woods et al[4] surveyed 106 HIV-seropositive gay men to determine whether religious activity was associated with depression or immune status in symptomatic HIV-infected gay men. Religious activities, such as prayer, religious attendance, spiritual discussions, and reading religious or spiritual literature, were associated with significantly higher CD4+ counts and CD4+ percentages. Religious coping (putting trust in God, seeking God's help, increased praying) was related to lower Beck Depression Inventory scores and lower Spielberger Trait Anxiety Inventory scores, but not with specific immune markers. However, subjects with more severe disease may have turned to prayer for comfort, canceling out a cross-sectional association between religious coping and better immune functioning.

Risk and Safety

There are few risks with regard to prayer; however, like any good thing it can be abused. Some persons may choose prayer over traditional medical care and thus delay seeking of appropriate medical treatment. This is particularly problematic when it involves children. Also, practitioners may impose their own religious beliefs on patients and encourage them to pray without being sensitive to the religious beliefs (or lack thereof) and spiritual path of the individual patient.

Efficacy

Based on the current research data, it is difficult to determine how often and to what extent prayer and other religious therapies work. The best data available is on attendance at religious services. The effect of attending services once per week or more (compared with less often) may be equivalent to 40-pack years of smoking or as long as 7 to 14 years of additional life.[23,24] Approximately 25% to 33% of older adults have had a life-changing religious experience; this is almost always a very significant event in the life of the person that is retold years after it happens. The effect sizes in prayer studies have ranged from 0% to as high as 45%.[17]

Future Research Opportunities and Priorities

Further studies are needed to examine the efficacy of hands-on prayer in the treatment of different stress-related diseases. Although such studies cannot be double-blinded, they can certainly be randomized with attention controls.

Self-Help versus Professional

Spontaneous prayer performed alone is likely to be helpful. Prayer with clergy, pastoral counselor, a clinician, or a friend may be particularly helpful (although not studied), because this combines the social support effects with the cognitive effects of prayer in facilitating healing. Often prayer groups formed within congregations can be very helpful to combat isolation and form friendships.

Visiting a Professional

A clergyperson, chaplain, or pastoral council can assist with prayer. Religious professionals are those who are specifically trained to pray with people within the context of their religious tradition.

A religious professional encourages patients to pray in a way that is comfortable to them and then agree with an "Amen," or says a brief prayer to God that is encouraging and supportive, requesting healing of a patient's physical body, mind, relationships, and spirit.

Training

There are many self-help books on prayer and meditation. Herbert Benson's *The Relaxation Response* is perhaps one of the best resources.[25] Alternatively, individuals can ask a pastor or other clergyperson to teach them ways to pray.

Credentialing

Chaplains and pastoral counselors receive extensive training to help meet both spiritual and mental health needs of patients. Physicians should feel free to refer patients to chaplains for counseling and addressing of religious or spiritual needs.

What to Look for in a Provider

A person should choose a religious professional that is nonjudgmental and has specific training in meeting emotional and spiritual needs. Such professionals include a priest, nun, pastor, rabbi, chaplain, or pastoral counselor; these often are found in churches, hospitals, and private practices. Ordinarily the religious background of the helping professional and patient should be the same.

Associations

The American Association of Pastoral Counselors provides certification for pastoral counselors and is a national organization for this group.

American Association of Pastoral Counselors
9504-A Lee Highway
Fairfax, VA 22031
Tel: (703) 385-6967
E-mail: info@aapc.org
www.aapc.org

Suggested Reading

1. Koenig HG, McConnell M: *The healing power of faith*, New York, 1999, Simon & Schuster. This book was written for the nonprofessional reader, but it integrates the existing research with powerful personal stories of people whose faith has provided healing in their lives. The book is written by an editor at *Reader's Digest* and therefore is quick, easy, and inspiring reading.

2. Koenig HG: *Is religion good for your health? The effects of religion on mental and physical health,* Binghamton, NY, 1997, Haworth.

This book is an excellent overview of the topic and a good primer for someone just learning about the relationship between religious or spiritual beliefs and practices and health. It contains references to many of the major studies.

Bibliography

Finney JR, Maloney HN: An empirical study of contemplative prayer as an adjunct to psychotherapy, *J Psychol Theol* 13:172-181, 1985.

References

1. Princeton Religion Research Group: *Religion in America, 1996 report,* Princeton, NJ, 1996, Gallup.
2. Eisenberg DM et al: Unconventional medicine in the United States, *New Engl J Med* 328:246-252, 1993.
3. Levin JS: How prayer heals: a theoretical model, *Alt Ther* 2:66-73, 1996.
4. Woods TE et al: Religiosity is associated with affective and immune status in symptomatic HIV-infected gay men, *J Psychosom Res* 46:165-176, 1999.
5. Matthews DA: *The faith factor,* New York, 1988, Viking.
6. Poloma MM, Pendleton BF: (1989). Exploring types of prayer and quality of life: a research note, *Rev Relig Res* 31:46-53, 1989.
7. Benson H: *Beyond the relaxation response,* New York, 1994, Times Books.
8. Benson H: *Timeless healing: the power and biology of belief,* New York, 1996, Scribner.
9. Koenig HG: Religious beliefs and practices of hospitalized medically ill older adults, *Int J Geriatric Psychiatry* 13:213-224, 1998.
10. Koenig HG et al: Religious coping and depression in elderly hospitalized medically ill men, *Am J Psychiatry* 149:1693-1700, 1992.
11. Koenig HG et al: The relationship between religious activities and blood pressure in older adults, *Int J Psychiatry Med* 28:189-213, 1998b.
12. Koenig HG et al: The relationship between religious activities and cigarette smoking in older adults, *J Gerontol Med Sci* 53A:M426-434, 1998c.
13. Koenig HG et al: Does religious attendance prolong survival? A six-year follow-up study of 3968 older adults, *J Gerontol Med Sci,* in press.
14. Galton FL: Statistical inquiries into the efficacy of prayer, *Fortnight Rev* 12:124-135, 1872.
15. Parker WR, St Johns E: *Prayer can change your life,* Carmel, NY, 1957, Guideposts.
16. Joyce CRB, Welldon RMC: The objective efficacy of prayer, a double-blind clinical trial, *J Chronic Disease* 18:367-377, 1965.
17. Collipp PJ: The efficacy of prayer: a triple-blind study, *Med Times* 97:201-204, 1969.
18. Byrd RC: Positive therapeutic effects of intercessory prayer in a coronary care unit population, *South Med J* 81:826-829, 1988.

19. Koenig HG, George LK, Peterson BL: Religiosity and remission from depression in medically ill older patients, *Am J Psychiatry* 155:536-542, 1998a.

20. Allport GW, Ross JML: Personal religious orientation and prejudice, *J Person Soc Psychol* 5:432-443, 1967.

21. Sudsuang R, Chentanez V, Veluvan K: Effect of Buddhist meditation on serum cortisol and total protein levels, blood pressure, pulse rate, lung volume and reaction time, *Physiol Behav* 50:543-548, 1991.

22. Koenig HG et al: Attendance at religious services, interleukin-6, and other biological indicators of immune function in older adults, *Int J Psychiatry Med* 27:233-250, 1997.

23. Strawbridge WJ et al: Frequent attendance at religious services and mortality over 28 years, *Am J Pub Health* 87:957-961, 1997.

24. Hummer R et al: Religious attendance and mortality in the U.S. adult population, *Demography* 36(2):273-285,1999.

25. Benson H: *The relaxation response*, New York, 1975, William Morrow.

Yoga

DELIA QUIGLEY

CAROLYN F.A. DEAN

Origins and History

The emergence of yoga as a therapeutic modality is just now being recognized by Western medical practice because of its treatment of the body-mind connection. As scientific research and the new field of psychoneuroimmunology points more to the integration of the whole person in healing disease, the medical community can no longer ignore the efficacy of yoga when treating illness.

Yoga is thought to have first reached American shores in the 1890s, when the young Indian, Swami Vivkananda, began lecturing about the importance of conscious control of diet, breathing, and posture to enhance meditation for spiritual practices. Over 100 years later, Western students have come to find what has been known for centuries: With consistent and earnest practice, personal transformation can take place on numerous levels. These changes can include improved health and energy, reduced stress, feelings of wellbeing, and the healing of disease in the body. What may have started as a search for increased flexibility and stress reduction slowly opens to a greater understanding of the self, emotional growth, and spiritual awakening.

The word *yoga* means "yoke" or union of the personal self with the Divine source. Dr. Andrew Weil describes it as "the joining of the mind, body, and spirit to enrich the quality of one's life and to enhance one's health."[1] It is both a profound study and pragmatic discipline.

There are a number of different systems of yoga, hatha yoga being the most familiar in the U.S. However, all systems recognize the validity of certain basic principles, including control of the body through correct posture and breathing, control of the emotions and mind, and meditation and contemplation.

A regular practice of yoga can tone the muscles that balance all parts of the body, including the internal organs, heart, lungs, glands, and nerves. It increases flexibility of the spine and therefore is good for treating chronic back problems. It is beneficial for the nervous system, promoting deep relaxation and reduction of stress. Everyone can practice yoga—children, athletes, and older adults, as well as those seeking a stronger, more supple body.

141

History of Yoga

From available records we learn that yoga began in India more than 6000 years ago. However, most researchers agree that yoga's emergence as a full-fledged tradition did not occur until 500 BCE. There are a number of ancient texts that speak of yoga, including *The Vedas*, *The Upanishads*, *The Bhagavad Gita*, and *The Yoga Sutras*. The origins of yoga can be found in *The Vedas*, the oldest written record of Indian culture. This 3000-year-old text has the earliest actual written reference to yogic activities inscribed within its hymns and rituals.

In the sixth chapter of *The Bhagavad Gita*, Sri Krishan explains the meaning of yoga:

When his mind, intellect and self are under control, freed from restless desire, so that they rest in the spirit within, a man becomes a Yukta—one in communion with God. A lamp does not flicker in a place where no winds blow; so it is with a yogi, who controls his mind, intellect and self, being absorbed in the spirit within him. When the restlessness of the mind, intellect and self is stilled through the practice of Yoga, the yogi by the grace of the Spirit within himself finds fulfillment. Then he knows the joy eternal, which is beyond the pale of the senses, which his reason cannot grasp. He abides in this reality and moves not therefrom. He has found the treasure above all others. There is nothing higher than this. He, who has achieved it, shall not be moved by the greatest sorrow. This is the real meaning of Yoga—a deliverance from contact with pain and sorrow.

Today *The Yoga Sutras* are regarded as the most coherent documentation of yoga teachings. Near 300 BCE, Patanjali described the eight limbs of yoga, known as Astanga yoga: yama (restraint); niyama (observances); asana (postures); pranayama (breath control); pratyahara (withdrawal of the senses); dharana (concentration); dhyana (meditation); and samadhi (super consciousness, or bliss).

There are four distinct paths of yoga that can be followed to achieve the goal of self-realization. It is best not to follow just one path at a time but to attempt to incorporate all four into your life.

- Bhakti yoga is the way of devotion or love. It is the surrender of the self to the Divine or supreme Spirit.
- Karma yoga aims to bring union with the supreme Spirit through right action—in other words, action that has been undertaken with unconditional selflessness and with no intention of reward.
- Jnana yoga aims to find union through knowledge and realize the truth about life, not sought through the external world of objects but rather through the realm of reality.
- Hatha yoga is the system of physical postures or *asanas*. In our Western culture it is the best known, although the growing number of styles can be confusing for the beginning student.

In 1960 Swami Vishnu-devananda wrote *The Complete Illustrated Book of Yoga*, demonstrating over 100 asanas in the Hatha yoga system. B.K.S. Iyengar followed in 1966 with the now-classic *Light on Yoga*. Included in both these volumes are teachings on pranayama breathing, meditation practice, and the importance of proper diet.

Today there are many more books written about yoga. Some follow a certain style developed by a Teacher or Guru to develop discipline and order in the student's practice, but they are all based on the traditional Hatha yoga postures.

Mechanism of Action According to Its Own Theory

There are more than 1000 asanas in Hatha yoga. This is a progressive system of learning that ranges from simple postures to more difficult ones to very challenging postures that at first seem impossible. These asanas are designed to promote a state of mental and physical well-being. This comes about because the organs begin to function efficiently, the mind becomes clear and focused, and the entire system is brought into a state of balance.

It has been said that longevity and a youthful appearance are the result of a flexible spine and a clean, efficient colon. Asanas focus on increasing the flexibility of the spine through gentle stretching, twisting, and bending movements, which work the joints, muscles, internal organs, and glands. Thus internal digestion and elimination are enhanced and there is an improvement in blood circulation to every cell of the body, carrying nutrients with a rich supply of fresh oxygen.

B.K.S. Iyengar writes in *Light On Yoga,*

> *Asana brings steadiness, health and lightness of limb. A steady and pleasant posture produces mental equilibrium and prevents fickleness of mind. Asanas are not merely gymnastic exercises; they are postures. Asanas can be done alone, as the limbs of the body provide the necessary weights and counterweights. By practicing them, one develops agility, balance, endurance and great vitality. Asanas have been evolved over the centuries so as to exercise every muscle, nerve, and gland in the body. They secure a fine physique, which is strong and elastic without being muscle-bound, and they keep the body free from disease. They reduce fatigue and soothe the nerves. But their real importance is how they train and discipline the mind.*

In the practice of Hatha yoga, the asanas are held for certain lengths of time, allowing the mind to focus and become free of disturbing and distracting thoughts. As a result concentration is increased, the mind becomes steady, and a feeling of calmness becomes an integral part of one's life. Hatha yoga was developed to prepare the body to sit for long periods of time in meditation. Patanjali in *The Yoga Sutras* stressed the practice of meditation to still and transcend the mind. In his system of Raja yoga, he prescribed three steps: concentration, meditation, and contemplation.

Meditation is a state of consciousness that can be understood only on a direct, intuitive level. Time, space, and the laws of causality limit ordinary experiences, but the meditative state transcends all boundaries. The physical benefits of meditation provide a lasting spiritual rest, which must be experienced to be understood. The individual becomes more peaceful and rested. Stress is reduced by lowering the heart rate and the consumption of oxygen. The body is able to relax at a cellular level. Meditation helps to prolong the body's period of growth and cell production and reduces the decaying process. On a mental level, new patterns of thinking begin to emerge as the individual develops a new view of the world. Negative tendencies tend to vanish, and the mind becomes filled with thoughts of peace, harmony, and happiness.

Pranayama Breathing

As one of the eight limbs of yoga, *prana* is seen as the manifestation of the vital force or energy that flows through the physical body. The word *prana* means life. B.K.S. Iyengar calls *Pranayama* "the science of breath." By learning to control the breath, the practitioner can begin to control the subtle energies within the body and finally gain full control over the mind. The benefits of pranayama breathing is a powerful vitalizing and regenerating force that can be used to heal the physical body.

Iyengar states the following:

The yogi's life is not measured by the number of his days but by the number of his breaths. Therefore he follows the proper rhythmic patterns of slow deep breathing. These rhythmic patterns strengthen the respiratory system, soothe the nervous system, and reduce cravings. As desire and cravings diminish, the mind is set free and becomes a fit vehicle for concentration. It is the oneness of the breath and mind and so also of the senses and the abandonment of all conditions of existence and thought that is designated Yoga.

Forms of Therapy

Styles

Although there are many styles of yoga, they all focus on strict alignment of the body, coordination of breath and movement, and holding the postures or flowing from one posture to another. All the styles are based in Hatha yoga, as a number of founders shared the same teacher. This was the case with Astanga, Iyengar, and Viniyoga, whose founders were all students of Krishnamacharya, a famous teacher at the Yoga Institute at the Mysore Palace in India. No style is better than another; the beginning student should explore several styles and teachers before settling on one to work with.

ANUSARA Anusara (a-nu-SAR-a) means "to step into the current of divine will," "following your heart." This is a new style developed by John Friend; it is described as heart-oriented, spiritually inspiring, yet grounded in a deep knowledge of outer and inner body alignment.

ASTANGA Astanga is also known as Power Yoga and is for those who want a serious workout. Developed by K. Pattabhi Jois, Astanga is a physically demanding practice. Students move through a series of flows, jumping from one posture to another to build strength, flexibility, and stamina.

BIKRAM Bikram is a series of 26 asanas developed by Bikram Choudhury and practiced in 105-degree temperatures. The heat warms and stretches the muscles, ligaments, and tendons and detoxifies the body through sweat.

INTEGRAL Integral was created by Swami Satchidananda and places almost as much emphasis on pranayama and meditation as on the asanas.

IYENGAR Iyengar was created by B.K.S. Iyengar, one of the most well-known yoga teachers in the world. It is noted for great attention to detail and the precise alignment of postures, as well as the use of props, such as blocks and belts.

KRIPALU Kripalu is called "the yoga of consciousness" and places the emphasis on proper breath, alignment, coordinating breath and movement, and "honoring the wisdom of the body." There are three stages to Kripalu yoga. Stage One focuses on learning the postures and exploring the body's abilities. Stage Two involves holding the postures for an extended time, focusing, and concentration. Stage Three is like a meditation in motion in which the movement between postures arises unconsciously and spontaneously.

KUNDALINI Kundalini was brought to the West in 1969 by Yogi Bhajan and focuses on the controlled release of Kundalini energy. The practice involves classic poses, breath, coordination of breath and movement, and meditation.

SIVANANDA Sivananda is one of the world's largest schools of yoga. Developed by Vishnu-devananda and named for his teacher, Sivananda, this style of yoga follows a set structure that includes pranayama, classic asanas, and relaxation.

VINIYOGA Viniyoga was created by Krishnamacharya, the teacher of B.K.S. Iyengar and K. Pattabhi Jois. It has a gentle flow with the emphasis on the breath and breath-movement coordination. Rather than work toward idealized postures, poses and flows are chosen to suit the student's abilities.

Demographics

Although there is no documented number of students practicing yoga, there are hundreds of yoga studios and centers located in small and large cities around the world. Yoga is safe to practice by people of all ages and is becoming more popular as its benefits are reported and documented.

Indications and Reasons for Referral

Dr. Andrew Weil in 8 *Weeks to Optimum Health* recommends yoga breathing techniques to regulate heart rate, blood pressure, circulation, and digestion.[1] It has been shown to be helpful in healing chronic back pain, menstrual problems, carpal tunnel syndrome, and respiratory disease.

Office Applications

A simple ranking of conditions applicable to a yoga approach follows. As with all alternative therapies, use of Yoga does not preclude the use of mainstream medical therapies in addition:

Top level: *A therapy ideally suited for these conditions*

Back pain; children's health; constipation; female health; hyperactivity; hypertension; insomnia; male health; menstrual cramps; periodic leg movement syndrome; premenstrual syndrome; respiratory conditions; rheumatoid arthritis; sleep disorders; stress

Second level: *One of the better therapies for these conditions*

Arthritis; asthma; childbirth; chronic fatigue syndrome; chronic pain; colitis and Crohn's disease; conjunctivitis; diabetes; emphysema; endometriosis; gastritis; gastrointestinal disorders; headaches; heart disease; hemorrhoids; impotence; irritable bowel syndrome; lung cancer; menopause; mental health; multiple sclerosis; obesity and weight management; osteoarthritis; osteoporosis; preconception, pregnancy and childbirth; restless leg syndrome; sinusitis; and sleep apnea

Third level: *A valuable adjunctive therapy for these conditions*

Addictions; allergies; amenorrhea; bronchitis; cancer; diverticulosis and diverticulitis; gout; hay fever; hearing disorders; macular degeneration; and postpartum care

Practical Applications

Yoga asanas are excellent for moving the circulation throughout the entire body. They provide a gentle workout and stretch, relieve stress, open the lungs, relax the heart, and clear the mind.

Research Base

Yoga can be helpful in the treatment of all illness because the practice stimulates the organs, rejuvenates the glandular system, and strengthens the physical body. It is particularly effective for chronic back problems, digestive disorders, lung and respiratory problems, and autoimmune diseases. Eric Small's Yoga Program currently is used by the Southern California MS Society with excellent results. The Yoga Institute in Bombay, India established in 1948 the beginning of therapeutic work to fulfill the request of the academic medical authorities for an evaluation of yoga's therapeutic claims along proper scientific lines. In 1960 a laboratory was organized and patients were examined by a medical practitioner who kept case records. The results were encouraging, but it was not until 1970, when another project was organized at the behest of the Indian government, that true scientific measurements revealed the effectiveness of yoga as a medical therapy. The Institute is still active today and conducts camps once per month for patients suffering from heart disease; asthma; diabetes; ear, nose and throat complaints; and gastrointestinal problems.

Evidence Based

In the early 1970s Dr. Chandra Patel, a British general practitioner, began her work in the implementation of a yoga-based stress-reduction program for hypertensive patients.[2,3] In her first controlled study, 20 hypertensive patients were matched by age and sex to a control group. The results showed a statistically significant reduction in blood pressure among the group exposed to the relaxation techniques.

Dr. Dean Ornish's research group[4] used noninvasive endpoint measures to assess the short-term effects of intervention on coronary heart disease. They reported improvement in cardiac risk factors and better functional status, including a marked reduction in the frequency and severity of angina, as well as the consumption of angina medication, improved myocardial perfusion, and improved LV function. In their 1990 study they randomly assigned 48 middle-aged female and male outpatients with angiographically documented coronary artery disease to experimental and "usual care" control groups. The patients in the experimental group were prescribed an extremely low-fat vegetarian diet and moderate aerobic exercise, given stress management training including enhancement of social support among the group members to increase compliance, and advised to stop smoking. The patients were given a 1-hour audiocassette tape in stress management, which included yoga-based stretching exercises, breathing techniques, meditation, relaxation, and visual imagery. They were asked to use it every day. The patients in the control group were not asked to make these lifestyle changes but were free to do so. As of 1995, six major cardiology centers in the U.S. and 100 hospitals have implemented the Dean Ornish program.

In his study of yoga in the control of back pain, Nespor[5,6] argues that there are more than physical benefits to yoga exercises. In his uncontrolled studies he has found that basic asanas, relaxation, and lifestyle information for patients suffering severe, painful back problems with minimal objectively verifiable somatic findings improved after this intervention. He suggests the following pathophysiologic theories for yoga's efficacy in treating back pain: increased elasticity of the shortened muscles, general and local muscle relaxation, strengthening of the relevant muscles, local relaxation by means of activating the antagonistic muscle groups, and an improved posture. There is also a greater autonomic nervous system stability because of general relaxation, decreased anxiety, and depression; increased self-awareness; easier regeneration after psychologically-induced stress and tension; a possible improved integration of unconscious forces; a deeper self-understanding; a more relaxed approach to various problems within family and social systems; and a higher energy level that enables meaningful activity and coping.

Basic Science

Raju et al,[7] in a randomized, controlled (nonplacebo) study, observed the effect of pranayama and savasana (relaxation pose) on athletes. Before the intervention, all parameters of the experimental and control group were comparable at rest and after exercise. At the end of the study, at rest there was a significant reduction of minute ventilation in both groups and blood lactate in the experimental group only. After exercise the oxygen consumption at rest was reduced significantly in both groups, but the difference was greater in the experimental group. The respiratory frequency was reduced significantly in the experimental group and increased in the control group. The researchers concluded that the oxygen consumption per unit work and resting lactate were lower in the experimental group, which indicates better oxygen delivery or use as a result of (P/L) in volunteers who practiced yoga for months, versus a control group.

Shannahoff-Khalsa and Kennedy[8] examined the effect that alternate nostril breathing had on individuals practicing Pranayama. They found that the subjects' heart rates decreased while breathing through the left nostril and the stroke volume and end diastolic volume both increased; the heart rate increased while breathing through the right nostril. They concluded that alternate nostril breathing might prove to be a useful therapeutic technique for noninvasive regulation of cardiovascular activity.

Risk and Safety

Yoga is a physical activity and can cause injury if practiced improperly or under the guidance of an inexperienced teacher.

Efficacy

With a history of more than 5000 years, yoga has been shown to change the physical, mental, and spiritual health of the practitioner for the better.

Future Research Opportunities and Priorities

With the increasing popularity of yoga in the West, studies are being called for and carried out by reputable institutions.

Druglike Information

Warnings, Contraindications, and Precautions

It is important to consider the physical health and strength of the student before prescribing a certain level of instruction. There are styles of yoga that work more slowly and gently and are recommended for those with chronic back pain or disease. Individuals in relatively good health can consider the more intense, flow types of yoga that can require more physical exertion.

Pregnancy and Lactation

Yoga is safe and recommended to practice during pregnancy, but it should be monitored by an experienced teacher. The pranayama breathing exercises can be used during labor, while certain asanas aid in the process of delivery.

Self-Help versus Professional

Although there are many excellent books and videos on the market, these materials should not replace an experienced teacher guiding the student through a practice. Some styles of yoga recommend practicing the asanas everyday for the first few months so the body can make the necessary changes. In the beginning it is advisable to take a class that meets 2 or 3 times per week for the development of a daily practice.

Visiting a Professional

A typical yoga class consists of 10 to 15 minutes of opening meditation and pranayama breath work. This is followed by mild to strenuous asanas in both standing and seated positions, which include stretching, balancing, and holding postures and a final relaxation meditation. By the end of class the student has moved all the organs, improved bodily functions, and released stored energy, leading to heightened awareness. The student should dress in loose-fitting clothes or leotards and tights. No food should be consumed between 2 and 4 hours before a session. Class is usually conducted in a bare room and mats can be used to prevent the student from slipping. The level of difficulty is determined by the experience, strength, flexibility, and overall health of each student.

The future of yoga is currently wide open here in the West, with studios opening daily and therapy programs being developed to treat conventionally diagnosed disorders. Studies are being conducted in many hospitals and universities to scientifically prove the efficacy of yoga.

Credentialing

Presently, each style of yoga or school offers a teacher training program with some form of certification. However, a number of yoga teachers from different traditions are working to develop a national standard of teacher certification, which will meet specific requirements.

Training

Each style of yoga has its own curriculum for training teachers. However, the program should include an in-depth study of the asanas, Pranayama breathing, meditation, mantras, anatomy and physiology, history and philosophy of yoga, and proper yogic diet.

What to Look for in a Provider

With the increasing popularity of yoga in the West, it is necessary to know that the training is taught and supervised by a knowledgeable practitioner. The following considerations should be used when looking for a teacher:

- The teacher should follow a personal daily yoga practice.
- Ask teachers about their training and credentials. Teacher training varies widely in depth and scope.
- Get advice on which level of class is best to take.
- Take classes in different styles until you find one that most appeals to you.
- After taking a class, ask the following questions: Did you have a rapport with the teacher? How did you feel before and after the class? Was the intensity of the class suitable?

A class should leave you feeling invigorated, calm, and satisfied, not stressed, agitated, or in physical discomfort. Once you find a method that works for you, stick with it.

Barriers and Key Issues

Yoga is a science and a practical discipline. It is not a religion and can be practiced by those of all faiths and denominations.

Associations

California Yoga Teachers Association
Attn: Judith Lasater
c/o *Yoga Journal*
2054 University Ave.
Berkeley, CA 94704
Tel: (510) 841-9200
Fax: (510) 644-3101
www.yogajournal.com

The American Yoga Association
513 S. Orange Ave.
Sarasota, FL 34236
Tel: (941) 953-5859
(800) 226-5859
E-mail: AmYogaAssn@aol.com.

3HO International Kundalini Yoga Teachers Association
Route 2, Box 4, Shady Lane
Espanola, NM 87532
Tel: (505) 753-0423

Himalayan Institute Teachers Association.
RR1, Box 400
Honesdale, PA 18431
Tel: (717) 253-5551 ext.1305
www.himalayainstitute.org

Suggested Reading

1. Iyengar BKS: *Light on yoga,* New York, 1976, Schocken.
   This classic contains hundreds of pictures demonstrating asanas and pranayama techniques. The history and philosophy of yoga is detailed, and daily practice sessions are included for all levels of student.
2. Vishnu-devananda S: *The complete illustrated book of yoga,* New York, 1988, Three Rivers Press.
   One of the first written books on the practice of yoga, it is illustrated with photographs that show each posture as well as descriptions for ways to create a complete practice.

3. Birch BB: *Power yoga*, New York, 1995, Simon & Schuster.
   Power Yoga demonstrates the Astanga yoga method, with photographs and text. This method is a choreographed sequence of postures that flow into one another, building strength, unwinding tight joints, and loosening muscles.
4. Desikachar TKV: *The heart of yoga*, Rochester, Vt, 1995, Inner Traditions International.
   This book is a distillation of Sri Tirumalai Krishnamacharya's system of yoga, now known as Viniyoga, written by his son as "basically a program for the spine at every level—physical, mental, and spiritual."

Bibliography

Birch BB: *Power Yoga*, New York, 1995, Simon & Schuster.

Dekisachar TKV: *The heart of yoga: developing a personal practice*, Rochester, Vt, 1995, Inner Traditions International.

Iyengar BKS: *Light on yoga*, New York, 1976, Schocken.

Patel C, Marmot MG, Terry DJ: Controlled trial of biofeedback-aided behavioral methods in reducing mild hypertension, *Brit Med J* 282:2005-2008, 1981.

Patel C et al: Trial of relaxation in reducing coronary risk: four year follow-up, *Brit Med J* 290:1103-1106, 1985.

Schneider C: Yogis, *Self*, July: 122, 1998.

The Yoga Institute: *Yoga therapy in asthma, diabetes, and heart disease*, www.healthlibrary.com

Vishnu-devananda S: *The complete illustrated book of yoga*, New York, 1960, Three Rivers Press.

Yoga Journal 135:56-66, 99, August 1997.

Yoga Paths: *An overview of different schools and traditions*, www.spiritweb.org

References

1. Weil A: *8 weeks to optimal health*, New York, 1996, Knopf.
2. Patel CH: Yoga and biofeedback in the management of hypertension, *Lancet* 10(2):1053-1055, 1973.
3. Patel C, North WR: Randomized controlled trial of yoga and biofeedback in management of hypertension, *Lancet* 19(2):93-95, 1975.
4. Ornish DM et al: Effects of stress management training and dietary changes in treating ischemic heart disease, *JAMA* 249(7):54-59, 1983.
5. Nespor K: Psychosomatics of back pain and the use of yoga, *Int J Psychosom* 36(1):72-78, 1989.
6. Nespor K: Pain management and yoga, *Int J Psychosom* 38 (1):76-81, 1991.
7. Raju PS, Madhavi S, Prasad KV: Comparison of effects of yoga and physical exercise, *India J Med Res* 100:81-86, 1994.
8. Sharinahoff-Khalsa DS, Kennedy D: The effects of unilateral forced nostril breathing, *Int J Neurosci* 73(1): 47-60, 1993.

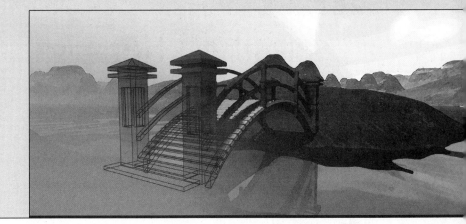

Bioelectromagnetic Applications in Medicine

Light Therapy, **154**
Magnetic Field Therapy, **164**

Light Therapy

LARRY B. WALLACE

Origins and History

Light therapy is the therapeutic application of electromagnetic energy in the visible spectrum to treat a wide range of health disorders. Phototherapies use ultraviolet, bright white, colored, monochrome, and laser light to treat health conditions. The treatment usually involves the use of instrumentation to produce specific frequencies of light energy that activate biochemical and energetic reactions. It may require shining light on a person's body, into acupuncture points, the eyes, or the body using fiberoptics to balance and restore health.

Color therapy has been part of occult sciences for thousands of years and part of oriental Eastern medicines since the earliest recorded times. Light has been associated with the transformation of consciousness and has served as a reflection of society's values since ancient times.[1] During the transcendental and spiritual movements of the nineteenth century, light and color therapy was associated with the unification of science and religion. This was the essential theme of one of the milestones in color therapy, *The Principles of White Color*, which was published in 1878 by Dr. Edwin Babbitt. Babbitt developed a specific instrumentation to provide color therapy for plants, animals, and humans. Babbitt's description of the harmonic laws in the universe, ethereal atomic philosophy, chromotherapies, and the general philosophy of fine forces preceded modern quantum physics.[2] As science became increasingly more materialistic, color therapies focused more on physical emotional factors and less on metaphysical aspects.

The work of physician Carl Loeb involved treating all health conditions as mind-body problems and attempted to treat the emotional and the physical problems simultaneously. His instrumentation, called the *mountain sun*, cast colored light onto the body using a dozen filters, with the purpose of curing a wide range of diseases and emotional problems. Loeb believed that light affected cell protoplasm and nutrition and regulated circadian rhythms.[3] Dinshah Gadiali, a healer and scientist, published a three-volume *Spectrachrome Metric Encyclopedia* based on 23 years of work evaluating color as a healing system. Gadiali found that color had a chemical potency for all the elements in a higher octave of vibration, which could affect each organ of the body and regulate metabolic activity.[4] Gadiali used 12 colored filters in different combinations to "tonate" different areas of the body and treat more than 400 diagnosed disorders.

Syntonics, a therapeutic practice that fully embraced biologic sciences, was developed by Spitler, a physician and optometrist. He began experimentation in the 1920s with animal studies and later with humans, which convinced him that the portions of the brain that control the autonomic nervous system and endocrine system are regulated by light entering the eyes. Spitler developed scientific models of light therapy documenting how light affects the physiology of cells, the nervous system, the central gray matter of the brain, bodily health, ocular functions, and emotional balance. His physiology included descriptions of electrical, potential, and action currents throughout the body, incorporating quantum physics and biology. He described the retinal hypothalamic tracks, which were later elaborated by Hollwich and Liberman (see the illustration). Spitler developed the *syntonizer,* the first instrument for ocular application of light therapy. He published his theories and findings in 1941 in *Syntonic Principle,* which became the definitive text for light therapy.[5] He founded the College of Syntonic Optometry in 1933 as a research and educational center for therapeutic application of visible light to correct vision disorders.

Psychiatrists became very interested in winter depression in relation to light and melatonin production by the pineal gland. Rosenthal did many studies for the National Institute of Mental Health that revealed that bright light therapy could treat this form of depression and biologic clock disorders. He defined *seasonal affective disorder* (SAD) as a light-related depression.[6] Reiter compared light to a potent drug because of the pineal gland's extreme sensitivity to light stimulation and the profound relation of light to health.[7]

John Ott has done a great deal to educate the general public about the necessity of full spectrum and natural sunlight for health. His research on the effects of full-spectrum light on plants, animals, and humans has described a new type of malady called *malillumination.* His treatment and research focused on the necessity of assimilating the proper light spectrum for an environment has led to the development of many lighting systems to meet this need.[8]

The development of lasers paved the way for laser therapy as a surgical tool for photodynamic therapy. Laser light is manipulated to trigger biochemical reactions and photosensitive pigments in the treatment of cancer, eye disease, psoriasis, arthritis, restonosis, and immune dysfunctions.[9]

Cold laser technologies, which use monochromatic light at an average wavelength of 610 nm, have successfully treated muscle problems, circulatory conditions, and pain management.[10] An entirely new form of color acupuncture is evolving, based on the work of Peter Mandel with Kirlian photography. This method involves placing small amounts of colored light on the various acupuncture points of the body to treat a wide range of physical and emotional disorders.[11]

Mechanism of Action According to Its Own Theory

One of the most profound ways in which white color affects human health is through its application in the eyes. It is the frequency or vibratory nature of electromagnetic energy that primarily affects health, not the color or wavelength. Light entering through the eye goes through an energetic pathway, the *retinal hypothalamic pathway,* and passes directly to the pineal and pituitary glands and hypothalamus of the brain. Frequencies can be used to balance the sensory motor systems of the eye and body by regulating the electrical output of the thalamus and hypothalamus. Certain colors or frequencies stimulate sensory responses, take information into the brain, and also can affect the motor output in a selective fashion. Because it affects the hypothalamus and its electric discharge, light can affect all kinds of autonomic functions, including temperature regulation, metabolic activity, and emotions. When light is shined into the eye, the blood supply is directly irradiated. Different frequencies of light can affect pH, immune function, and blood biochemistry when they are shined into the vascular system. Light in the eye affects ionization at the retinal level, the electric potential between the eye and the brain, the eye and the liver, and it can affect cellular function by changing electric potential.

Light in the eye can have nonlocal or general physiologic effects, but it also can have local effects to the eye physiology and therefore treat ocular pathology. It also can stimulate and inhibit our emotional centers. This occurs primarily through affecting balances between the frontal orbital cortex, limbic system, and hypothalamus of the brain. Light can adjust the baroreceptors between the brain and heart that regulate mean variability rate of the heart, and it can affect autonomic limbic circuits involved with emotional content and conditioning. Applying color through the skin and the acupuncture points creates a bioelectric current along acupuncture meridians. Bioelectric currents also give off bioelectric fields that are directly affected by color. According to the German biophysicist Fa Popp, cells within the body emit tiny biophotons or particles of light whose bioluminescence reflects the cell's state of health and also serves as a primary communication system within cells and cellular networks. The application of light can facilitate this biophotonic communication between cells.

There also is a relationship between thought patterns and this cellular bioluminescence. Specific color combinations seem to have the ability to evoke a synchronization between thought and cellular activity. Ayurvedic and oriental medicines have diagnosed on the basis of blockages of *chakras*, which are certain energy centers in the body. Traditionally, most color therapies have used specific colors to represent action on chakras and their corresponding organs. Other therapies have prescribed color not on the basis on which color may affect an organ but on the perceived cause of the energy imbalance. The cause might be either physical, genetic, psychosomatic, nuclear, emotional, or toxemic; different colors correspond to each cause.

Biologic Mechanism of Action

The biologic mechanism of action seems to be primarily through the visual system and the retinal hypothalamic pathway affecting the autonomic nervous system and endocrine function. A secondary mechanism of action is through the skin affecting acupuncture meridians or (in other perspectives) chakra centers. A more conventional use of light therapy, *photodynamic therapy*, involves irradiation of certain pigments that are injected into the cells, organs, or tissues of the body and then irradiated with certain frequencies of light. These pigments react photochemically to light stimulation, causing the destruction of tissue in the treatment of cancer or a change in the vascular system in conditions such as macular degeneration.

Forms of Therapy

The most widely used form of therapy is syntonic optometric phototherapy, in which specific frequencies of light are shined into the eyes to correct various kinds of vision problems and imbalances related to the autonomic nervous system. Another form of therapy is Irlen lens therapy, which involves the wearing of certain types of tinted lenses to treat various reading disabilities. Photodynamic therapies involve using light, primarily delivered through fiberoptic systems, to radiate cellular pigment and dyes for specific biochemic functions. Another common form of phototherapy uses brief strobic colored lights in the eyes to elicit a wide range of emotional reactions for psychotherapy. White light is also flashed in combination with certain sound patterns in order to entrain brain waves for neural feedback.

Another primary form of color therapy involves placing colored lights on acupuncture points, often with Voll machines, Vega, and kinesiology testing, as well as traditional Chinese medicine diagnosis. Another form of therapy is white light therapy to treat SAD. Light boxes or high-intensity white light is looked at or placed in the environment for 1 to 3 hours per day. Ultraviolet light therapies have been used on the skin to treat certain kinds of dermatologic problems and irradiate blood in the treatment of immune system deficiencies. Cold laser applications using LED lights, primarily in long wavelengths (660 nm), reduce pain inflammation by directly lighting strained, damaged, and inflamed tissue. Another form of color therapy involves the visualization of certain colors and meditations to apply colors to areas of the body. The visualization of colors within the body also may lead to diagnosis and treatment of physical and psychoemotional ailments. Another form of color therapy irradiates water with a specific color for drinking.

Demographics

Color therapy practitioners are most common in the field of optometry, followed by medicine. In addition, phototherapy is used in the field of psychology, homeopathy, chiropractic, osteopathy, physical and occupational therapy, acupuncture and Chinese medicine, naturopathy, massage therapy, and various body work specialties. Because light therapy is practiced by few practitioners, it has received little institutional support in terms of education and research. All types of patients may use this modality, as it cuts across all age, gender, and cultural lines.

Indications and Reasons for Referral

The most widely practiced form of light therapy is for the treatment of vision problems involving sensory motor deficiencies, such as tracking and fixation problems, accommodation or focusing problems, eye coordination deficiencies, and visual field defects. Syntonic phototherapy also concentrates on treating visually-related attention, learning, and reading problems, ocular pathology, posttrauma brain syndrome, and visually-related symptoms, such as asthenopia and ocular headaches.[12] Phototherapy is also used to treat imbalances in EKG and EEG profiles. EEG diagnosis and EEG biofeedback therapies are used to treat brain energy dysfunctions and physical disorders of the autonomic nervous system, such as addiction, depression, PMS, menopause, and brain injury.[13] Color therapy and phototherapy is also used to treat endocrine and metabolic problems because light influences the regulation of pineal function, physical growth, body temperature, kidney function, blood count, general metabolism, and thyroid, sexual, adrenal, and pituitary functions.[14] Photodynamic therapies are used in dermatology, oncology, ophthalmology, and rheumatology.[15]

For the treatment of psoriasis, a light-sensitive drug, such as psoralen, is injected and absorbed by pigments in the skin. The skin is then irradiated by ultraviolet light, preventing the reproduction of diseased cells.[16] Ultraviolet therapies have successfully treated circulatory and immune dysfunctions, infections, lupus, cancer, rheumatoid arthritis, and AIDS. Blood is drawn from the body, irradiated with ultraviolet A1 light to increase blood oxidation, and then reintroduced to the body, resulting in enhanced immune response.[17]

White light therapy is particularly successful in treating SAD or winter depression. Full-spectrum therapy has been used to provide full-spectrum lighting environments to help treat hypertension, migraine, PMS, and metabolic imbalances.[18] Wolfarth and Ott[19] have demonstrated that the installation of full-spectrum lights in the classroom results in a significantly reduced amount of clinical hyperactivity. Cold-laser applications are used in reflexology and acupuncture for allergies, sinus problems, circulation problems, ulcers, arthritis, headaches, and dental problems, as well as various emotional problems.[20]

Psychotherapists also have employed color therapy. Shealy[21] has used the lumatron to treat depression in a multidisciplinary approach to healing. Vasquez[22] also has used the lumatron to tab subliminal emotions as part of a total mind-body healing. He found that certain colors elicit archetypal responses, regardless of the individual psyche. Syntonic therapy has been used in the field of chiropractic medicine to treat autonomic imbalances and restore endocrine balance in conjunction with basic chiropractic treatment.[23] Colored light has been used on the acupuncture points to treat endocrine, neural vegetative problems, toxemia within the system, and degenerative diseases. It is used in conjunction with classical Chinese acupuncture for almost every type of physical condition.[24]

Office Applications

A simple ranking of conditions responsive to this form of therapy is as follows. As with all alternative therapies, light therapy does not preclude mainstream medical therapies.

Top level: *A therapy ideally suited for these conditions*

Attention deficit disorder; cataracts; conjunctivitis; headaches; head trauma; hyperactivity; lazy eye; macular degeneration; migraine; night blindness; poor eyesight; stroke; and vision disorders

Second level: *One of the better therapies for these conditions*

Eczema; fever; psoriasis; soft-tissue fungus; spasms and strains; addictions; allergies; anxiety; asthma; autism; bronchitis; childbirth; female health; glaucoma; insomnia; muscle spasm; premenstrual syndrome; retinal detachment; retinopathy; stress; and strep throat

Third level: *A valuable adjunctive therapy for these conditions*

Depression; epilepsy; hay fever; male health; obesity and weight management; sinusitis; sleep disorders; upper respiratory infections; back pain; candidiasis; chronic fatigue syndrome; endometriosis; gastrointestinal disorders; hypertension; menopause; menstrual cramps; multiple sclerosis; neck pain; osteoarthritis; osteoporosis; otitis media; peptic ulcer; and pneumonia

Practical Applications

Light therapy complements many other treatments. Although these generally are not allopathic therapies, syntonics may be used practically along with craniosacral therapy, osteopathy, nutrition, homeopathy, acupuncture, and ayurvedic medicine. Syntonics is also used in behavioral medicine to treat attention deficit disorder and attention deficit hyperactivity disorder. Syntonics has been highly successful in conjunction with occupational and physical therapy in the rehabilitation of stroke and head trauma. Color therapy can also be part of an environmental design. A good example is the use of color psychodynamics in Canadian school systems, developed by Dr. Harry Wolfarth, which purports to improve both psychologic and physiologic health.[4] As a practical measure, light therapy and exposure to natural light should be part of wellness programs. Like air, food, and water, sunlight is a basic form of nutrition and it also is an essential energy component of life. The elimination of full-spectrum light in our environment may be a factor in an untold number of health problems. Almost every profession could use light as a complementary form of therapy. How this will be implemented in clinical practice is unclear at present.

Research Base

Evidence Based

Numerous studies have examined the effects of color therapy.[6,7,25-34]

Risk and Safety

There have been very few studies done on the safety of these therapies. One study has shown no significant side effects of short-term 10,000-lux light therapy.[35] The wavelength bandwidth seems to present little risk in the field of color therapy, with the exception of strobic lights, which are contraindicated for individuals prone to seizure disorder. Pure color therapy per se was shown to have very few side effects or "residue," because color is not absorbed or assimilated into the system when it is not needed.

Efficacy

Just as the safety and risk factors of color therapy have not been studied in any broad sense, the efficacy also has not been studied with large population groups.

Other

Other studies that might be useful in describing this therapy certainly relate to the entire field of bioelectromagnetic therapies, which use electromagnetic energy to create a host of biologic reactions and treat a wide range of health conditions. The healing effects of electromagnetism has been examined by several researchers.[36-39] A new area of research is in the psychologic, psychoemotional, and psychospiritual realms, as well as a further elaboration of quantum physics and quantum biology to explain electromagnetic energy and its effects on biology at the atomic level.

Self-Help versus Professional

Although this therapy can be self-applied without much training or from books, it is not really practical at this point to self-treat without professional guidance. However, it is not actually dangerous to do so.

Visiting a Professional

This kind of therapy is generally a very pleasant experience. Usually a person sits in front of a colored light that shines either on the body or into the eyes. In the case of syntonics the patient sits in front of a specific instrument that uses selective frequencies or filters in front of a full-spectrum light source. The patient sits and looks into this light for 20-minute periods, typically three to four times per week for 20 sessions. In the case of color acupuncture, light is applied to acupuncture points usually for about 20 to 30 seconds; usually no more than 6 to 10 points are treated per session. In the case of white light therapy used for people with SAD, the patient sits in front of high illuminated light boxes, typically for 1 hour per day. The other applications in medicine, such as photodynamic therapy, use fiberoptics with very small exposures to light outside a person's awareness or conscious involvement. In psychotherapy a person may sit in front of a brief strobic flashing colored light for up to an hour while engaged in typical talk therapy. In this particular instance there may be a very wide range of emotions felt, sometimes even to the point of reaching an emotional catharsis and a healing crisis.

Credentialing and Training

Licensed practitioners are most common in optometry, followed by medicine. In addition, phototherapy is used in the fields of psychology, homeopathy, chiropractic, osteopathy, physical and occupation therapy, acupuncture and Chinese medicine, naturopathy, massage therapy, and various body works specialties.

Training is achieved by attending seminars and continuing education in the field. The annual Conference of Light and Vision, sponsored by the College of Syntonic Optometry, has provided basic and advanced courses with certification for 66 years. The legal status and regulations of practitioners of light therapy is nonexistent. Continuing education requirements for relicensing does not include proficiency in light therapy except in the context of general practice, such as an area of vision therapy in optometry or photodynamic therapy in medicine. Certification status is created by the College of Syntonic Optometry and conferred by fellowships. At present, no states actually license this modality.

Barriers and Key Issues

The primary issues that have kept this therapy from receiving visibility or credibility are really because light therapy falls outside the major medical model. Light therapy is generally prescribed to work with physiologic and functional disorders as opposed to pathologic disorders. The recognition of subtle energies as primary in biochemistry and human physiology will create a new appreciation and recognition of these kinds of therapies. Light therapy's low cost also will help make it more attractive.

Associations

College of Syntonic Optometry
21 E. 5th St.
Bloomsburg, PA 17815
Tel: (717) 387-0900
E-mail: cgolib@sunlink.net
www.syntonicphototherapy.com

Society for Light Treatment and Biological Rhythms
10200 W. 44th Ave. Suite 304
Wheat Ridge, CO 80033
Tel: (303) 424-3694

Environmental Health and Light Research Institute
16057 Tampa Palms Blvd. Suite 227
Tampa, FL 33647
Tel: (800) 544-4878

International Institute of Light Therapy
PO Box 2146
Longmont, CO 80502
Tel: (303) 651-3173

Schools and Other Resources

Samassati School of Holographic Healing
280 Kachina Dr.
Sedona, AZ 86336
Tel: (520) 204-9391
E-mail: samassati@sedona1.net

Light Years Ahead Productions
PO Box 174
Tiburon, CA 94420
Tel: (415) 435-1578
E-mail: bbreiling@aol.com

Universal Light Technology
PO Box 520
Carbondale, CO 81623
Tel: (970) 927-0100
www.ulight.com

Suggested Reading

1. Lieberman J: *Light medicine of the future,* book 1, Santa Fe, 1991, Bear and Co.
   This is the most current and far-ranging text on the subject of light as a therapeutic tool. It covers medical and psychologic uses of light and contains an extensive bibliography. It is a must-read for anyone interested in the subject.
2. Spitler HR: *Syntonic principle,* Bloomsburg, Pa, 1941, College of Syntonic Optometry.
   This is the thesis from which the practice of phototherapy by way of the eyes, known as syntonics, was established. It is available through the College of Syntonic Optometry.
3. Ghadiali D: *Spectrachrome metricencyclopedia,* Malaga, NY, 1933, Spectrachrome Institute.
   This three-volume treatise on the systemic application of lights on the body for healing and restorative purposes is a landmark in the application of color therapy in this century. It is available through the Dinshah Society.
4. Breiling B, editor: *Light years ahead,* Berkeley, Calif, 1996, Celestial Press.
   This is a compilation of a recent conference on the various light therapies practiced around the world in the 1990s. It is one of the best texts for an overview of the different light therapies and light technologies in current use.

References

1. Zajonc A: *Catching the light,* New York, 1993, Bantam.
2. Babbitt E: *The principles of light and color,* East Orange, NJ, 1896, self-published.
3. Loeb C: *A course in specific light therapy,* Chicago, 1939, Actino Lab.
4. Liberman J: *Light, medicine of the future,* Santa Fe, NM, 1991, Bear & Co.
5. Spitler R: *The syntonic principle,* Harrisburg, Penn, 1941, College of Syntonic Optometry.
6. Rosenthal N: Seasonal affective disorder: a description of the syndrome and preliminary findings of light therapy, *Arch Gen Psychiatry* 41:72-80, 1984.
7. Reiter R: Light as a drug, lecture 56, Annual College of Syntonic Optometry Conference, Estes Park, Co, May 1988.
8. Ott J: *Health and light,* Old Greenwich, Conn, 1973, Devon-Adair.
9. QLT Phototherapeutics: *Annual report,* Vancouver, 1995.

10. Therapeutic effects of monochromatic red light, *Asklepen of light*, Seattle, 1991.

11. Mandel P: *Esogetics and non-sense of disease and pain*, Bruschal, 1994, Energetic Verlag.

12. Gottlieb R: Research grants, *J Optom Photother* Dec 1998.

13. *Megabrain report*, vol 1-2, Sausalito, Calif 1993, Megabrain Communications.

14. Hollwich F: *The influence of ocular light perception on metabolism in man and animal*, New York, 1979, Springer-Verlag.

15. QLT Phototherapy: *Delivery results, annual report*, Vancouver, 1995.

16. Leggett K: Photochemotherapy, *Biophoton Int* 3(3):50-54, 1996.

17. Washburn P: *Alternative medicine: the definitive guide*, Boston, Burton-Goldberg Group, 1993.

18. Garland F et al: Occupational sunlight exposure and melanoma in the U.S. Navy, *Arch Environ Health* 45:161-167, 1990.

19. Ott J: *Health and light*, Old Greenwich, Conn, 1973, Devon-Adair.

20. Therapeutic effects of monochromatic red light, Seattle, 1991, Asklepen of Light.

21. Washburn P: *Alternative medicine: the definitive guide*, Boston, 1993, Burton-Goldberg Group.

22. Vasquez S: Light and psychotherapy: synthesis of the future, Presentation at 61st Annual Conference of Light and Vision, Scottsdale, Ariz, May 1993.

23. *Light years ahead*, Berkeley, Calif, 1996, Celestial Arts.

24. Pagnamental NF: *Color therapy for children*, Locarno, Switzerland, 1996, self-published.

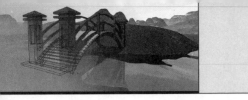

Magnetic Field Therapy

WILLIAM PAWLUK

Origins and History

The lengthy history of the use of magnets for therapy has been described elsewhere.[1] The therapy most likely dates to 200 BCE in China with an acupuncture orientation.[2] d'Arsonval first exposed a person's head to a strong electromagnetic field in a wired electric cage in 1896, demonstrating the sensitivity of neural tissues to magnetic fields. In modern times, Barker was the first to stimulate the brain with transcranial electromagnetic stimulation in 1965.[1] Eastern Europeans have used magnetic fields in various applications since the 1970s.[3] Several popular books recently have been published describing the use of magnetic fields in therapeutic applications.[4,5] Magnetic field therapy has received wide media exposure since 1996.

Before further discussing magnetic therapy, it is important to review the various types of magnetic fields that will be referenced.

Types of Magnetic Fields

Magnetic fields fall into two broad groups: static and time-varied. *Static* fields are either permanent or DC-direct current (electromagnetic). *Time-varied* fields are either pulsed or sinusoidal (radio frequency). Most therapeutic time-varied fields (either pulsed or sinusoidal) are modulated at slower "biologic" speeds or frequencies (1-100 cycles per second Hz) and can have various pulse and on/off cycle patterns. Permanent magnets only produce static fields, unless they are spun, during which they can act like sinusoidal fields. Electromagnets can be made to produce static, pulsed/sinusoidal, or radiofrequency (RF) fields, which are in megahertz or greater range. Magnetic field strength is measured in gauss or Tesla. One Tesla equals 10,000 gauss. Ten milliTesla (mT) is equal to 100 gauss.

The common bar or horseshoe magnet and the button and flat magnets commonly seen on refrigerators are *permanent*. For practical purposes, permanent and DC magnetic fields are the same, both being non-time varying. In the literature, the terms *DC*, *static*, and *permanent* are used interchangeably. In terms of magnetic materials, *ferromagnets*, which are produced from ferrous or iron materials, generally produce weaker fields. *Rare earth* magnets produce the strongest fields. Both permanent and electromagnets can be designed with an almost infinite variety of field configurations. Permanent magnet configurations may be unipole, where only one magnetic pole surface is presented to the body, or bipole designs.

Bipolar types can be designed so that both the north and the south poles are presented beside each other on the same magnet surface or in various designs using multiple repetitions of the two poles in circles, squares, triangles, or lines. In some cases the use of magnetized water has been studied.[6]

Biologic Mechanism of Action

Magnets act on the following five basic structures or processes of the body. All actions are present with every application to varying degrees.

1. **The acupuncture system:** Magnets act on acupuncture points and meridians specifically and directly.[2,7] Most trigger points are acupuncture points. Actions through acupuncture and trigger points are very rapid.[3] The tendinomuscular system of acupuncture, which is formed by the integumentary and superficial muscle and fascial systems, is an aspect of the acupuncture system.[8] As a result the placement of magnets almost anywhere on the body will activate the tendinomuscular system. These tissues readily and widely transmit electrical stimuli.[9,10] The mechanism of action of magnets is primarily mediated by the microcurrents generated through the Faraday effect.[11]

2. **The vascular and hematologic system:** Vascular effects frequently have been demonstrated with evidence of increases in tissue oxygen perfusion caused by decreased vascular resistance.[3,12,13] This in turn causes edema reduction. Clinical magnetic fields decrease thrombotic effects and platelet adhesiveness.[3] Magnets clear traumatic or surgical bruises. They also decrease the effects of reperfusion damage in vascular injuries, possibly by decreasing free radical damage.[3,4]

3. **The nervous system:** Human and animal studies have shown decreased nerve cell firing.[3,14,15] Salamanders can be put into deep surgical anesthetic sleep using electromagnets.[16] In some animal models, nerve regeneration has been produced.[17] Specially designed electromagnets[18] are also used in nerve conduction testing and brain stimulation research.

4. **Cellular effects:** Magnetic fields stimulate various cellular structures. Relatively little magnetic field energy is required to change chemical reactions in cells.[19] Changes have been observed in calcium channels, the sodium-potassium pump, RNA/DNA production, the conversion of ATP to ADP, removal of oxygen and water from the cell, and stimulation of cyclic AMP.[3,19,20] Magnetic fields permeate all body tissues without any interference. No cellular damage has been seen from even the most powerful static magnetic fields. The calcium channel in the cell wall is affected, resulting in higher intracellular calcium. Magnetic resonance imaging (MRI) is the most familiar medical application of magnetic fields. Magnetic fields affect molecular conformation.[1] Free radical production can be significantly affected by magnetic fields[3,21] at magnetic field strengths of as little as 1 to 10 mT (10 to 100 gauss).

5. **Extracellular fluid:** Extracellular fluid is very sensitive to the application of magnetic fields. The body is at least 65% fluid, which is mostly salinated electrolytic ion solu-

tion. Externally applied magnetic fields influence and charge currents and the electromagnetic field states of the body's solutions.[1]

Common physiologic responses resulting from magnetic field exposures are well-documented. These include the following actions: 1) vasodilatation; 2) analgesic action; 3) antiinflammatory action; 4) spasmolytic activity; 5) healing acceleration; and 6) antiedema activity. The probable mechanisms of these actions are reviewed extensively in Jerabek and Pawluk.[3]

Demographics

Magnetic therapy is widely used by the lay public and practitioners in Europe, Asia, and India. In these environments, most usage relates to acupuncture principles. In many countries, early use with permanent magnets has since moved mostly to time-varied fields, produced by a large variety of devices. Most usage in the U.S. is with permanent magnets introduced by Asian companies. Very few practitioners, complementary or otherwise, have enough knowledge to advise on the proper use of magnetic therapy. The clinical community has been slower than the public to understand and use it. There is no objective data to indicate the extent of its use and perceptions of effectiveness. It is primarily used for chronic pain and soft tissue injury management and general preventive health. Use among athletes seems to be especially common. Public use appears to be more among people with chronic problems and older age groups. There is little use in children. The Asian community is likely to embrace these more quickly, but all races are using them. More affluent and therapeutically open-minded people are more likely to purchase them.

Indications and Reasons for Referral

Except for nerve conduction and bone healing devices and Canadian-approved barrel-type devices for osteoarthritis, which require prescription or therapy in the clinician's office, all others devices can be recommended for use by the patient at home. Refer to "Practical Applications" for applications of specific magnet types. As with all alternative therapies, the use of magnets does not preclude the use of mainstream medical therapies.

Based on the available research and the mechanisms of action or basic effects seen with the application of magnets to the human body, and other than those noted in the corresponding table, the major indications for magnetic therapy are listed in Section Three of this book.

Practical Applications

For most problems the appropriate magnet configuration can be used locally, for example, in tendinitis the magnet is placed locally. If a systemic condition is being treated, then placement on one or more acupuncture points, spinal segments, or whole body exposure (using a mattress pad) would be considered. If local applications do not work, for example, in pain syndromes, consider nonlocal, possibly referred causes and the need for additional areas of application, including other acupuncture points. Appropriate acupuncture/ acupressure training should be undertaken if the clinician is interested in using acupuncture/acupressure principles extensively with magnetic therapy. A list of some uses for general types of magnet is as follows. The list is by no means exhaustive.

Flat pads are flexible, flat pads with various alternating bipole designs and various sizes and shapes ranging between 1 and 2 cm to 6 by 10 cm. These are useful for skin lesions, musculoskeletal problems, blisters, ulcers, dental pain, temporomandibular joint pain, sinus congestion, fibromyalgia, and superficial vascular or venous problems, among others. Larger pads are useful for back pain, dysmenorrhea, muscle tension, and spasm.

Spinning or rotating unipolar magnets are spun physically or mechanically and may simulate sinusoidal magnetic fields. Spinning magnets spun extend their magnetic field to broadcast a deeper field than stationary permanent magnets. These are useful for muscle tension, fibromyalgia, deeper hematomas, deeper sinuses, pleuritic pain, sciatic pain, deeper arthritic pain, and internal chest or abdominal problems.

Shoe inserts include several types, such as full or partially-magnetized plate design, unipole design, bipole design, magnetized metatarsal or arch bars, and pads with reflexology bumps. These are useful for all foot and ankle problems, including leg cramps and restless legs, circulation in the feet and distal lower leg, foot and leg fatigue in chronic standing, chronic hyperhidrosis of feet, plantar fasciitis, bunions, postosteotomy pain, varicose vein discomfort, general stimulation of energy, spastic neuromuscular conditions, lower extremity diabetic neuropathy, and foot ulcers.

Button or bar magnets come in various materials, shapes, sizes, and strengths. They can be free or imbedded; that is, sewn, molded, glued, or otherwise fastened into mattresses, seat cushions, pillows, back braces, joint wraps, vests, necklaces, facial masks, headbands, and other configurations designed to accommodate various anatomic areas. Uses include any for the previous configurations and types and any appropriate acupuncture applications.

If some change or relief is not experienced from magnets, it may be because of one of the following reasons: 1) the magnets were not used for a long enough time; 2) the magnets were applied in the wrong places; 3) not enough basic vitality is present, such that the person is too weak or depleted to generate a biologic response to the stimulus; or 4) the problem is severe enough to require even stronger or additional magnets. Weak vitality, from a general, prolonged or excessive, stress adaption syndrome, requires other approaches, such as nutritional adjustments, vitamin and mineral supplements, other medical therapies, et cetera, to restore these. It is important to use magnets as one of an array of approaches to consider or apply in a comprehensive therapeutic program. Numerous studies[3] have shown that magnetic therapy in combination with other accepted therapies enhances the actions of both, often allowing lower dosages of potentially toxic treatments (for example, chemotherapy).

Some other considerations include the following:

- Place magnets as close as possible to the body with no more than a layer of clothing between them.
- For acute vertebral pain syndromes, expose trigger points as well.
- Therapy is most effective if the first five exposures are performed daily or twice daily.
- If therapy does not work within 20 exposures, it will probably not be of much value, with the exception of bone healing in nonunions, where the first signs of healing occur after 30 days.
- Therapy should be applied as soon as possible after the onset of the problem.
- Exposures must be long enough and repeated. Minimum exposure time is 10 minutes and the minimum number of exposures is 10, although 15 exposures give better results. Clinical response should guide treatment.
- If possible, do not stop magnetic therapy suddenly. It is better to gradually advance the interval between exposures stepwise.

Individualization of therapy is always necessary, especially in chronic pain conditions. One other exciting new indication involves the use of repetitive transcranial magnetic stimulation. This method, which uses a rapidly pulsed magnetic field of approximately 30,000 gauss, is used by major research centers in the treatment of refractory depression. The field intensity is similar to that of an MRI session, but the location of the field is more highly focused within the cranium.[22]

Research Base

Evidence Based

The corresponding table lists the conditions that have been formally studied in humans in controlled and noncontrolled trials.[3]

Apart from the extensive studies documented from Eastern Europe,[16] significant experience is described in other research. The most widely known FDA-approved use is for nonunion bone fractures.[4] Similar benefits have been shown in Charcot joints with multiple fractures[23] and interbody spinal fusions.[24] Studies on multipole magnetic pads have been reported from Europe,[3,25] including controlled and experimental studies, case series, and even experience with 200 horses.[24] All these studies resulted in significant to moderate improvement.

Pulsed electromagnetic devices, other than those used for bone healing and nerve stimulation, are not yet available for wider clinical use in the U.S. Several devices are being readied for FDA approval, including one for the management of osteoarthritis.[26] Pulsed electromagnetic devices have received government approval in Europe for a variety of indications.[13] Randomized or controlled clinical trials in the treatment of recalcitrant venous ulcers,[27,28] diabetic neuropathy,[29] and postpolio syndrome[30] have also shown significant benefits.

Magnetic Therapy Trials in Humans by Condition

Controlled Trials in Humans		Noncontrolled Trials in Humans	
Atherosclerosis	Fibromyalgia	Amputation stumps	Legg-Perthes'
Alzheimer's disease	Fractures	Analgesia	disease
Breast fissures	Hypertension	Antiinflammatory	Neuralgia and neuritis
Burns	Infected skin wounds	Aseptic bone necrosis	Osteoarthritis
Carpal tunnel	Ischemic heart disease	Asthma	Pancreatitis
syndrome	Liver function	Atherosclerosis in	Postradiation damage
Cervicitis	Nonhealing fractures	diabetes	Retinitis pigmentosa
Chronic bronchitis	Polyneuritis	Chemotherapy	Rheumatoid arthritis
Corneal trauma	Postpolio syndrome	Enhancement	Soft tissue injuries
Diabetic neuropathy	Preoperative skin	Eczemas	Spinal cord injuries
Edema	healing	Inflammatory bowel	Thrombophlebitis
Endometriosis	Reduced clotting	disease	Vascular flow
Endometritis	Skin grafts	Intraocular pressure	Venous insufficiency

Basic Science

The basic science of the effects of magnetic fields on biologic systems is described in several texts.[3,20,31-32] Some of the practical implications of this research are summarized in this discussion.

To create biologic and thus therapeutic efficacy, the following must be considered: 1) magnetic flux density; 2) gradient; 3) field shape; 4) exposure duration; 5) volume of exposed tissue; and 6) the localization of exposure. Unipolar static magnetic fields are more likely to activate the parasympathetic system,[3] and bipolar magnets (such as multiple pole field designs) are more likely to activate the sympathetic system than the parasympathetic system.

Magnetic fields in therapeutic doses exhibit minor or no changes in healthy human volunteers. On the other hand, such doses exhibit well-established therapeutic effects in abnormal situations. This can be explained by the fact that healthy organisms are in different physiologic states than those which are diseased or ill.

Exposure duration is one of the most critical parameters. In most research exposure, durations typically varied from 10 to 60 minutes per treatment session. Static magnets may be left on for longer durations, depending on response. Generally, exposure should be for less than 24 hours per day if used daily for weeks and for any specific indication. Durations for various indications may overlap over any 24-hour period, for example, treating the low back during the day with a flat bipolar pad and sleeping on a magnetic mattress at night for stress reduction, insomnia, and general health maintenance.

Exposed volumes of tissue must be considered in designing a therapeutic program because greater volume exposure is more likely to create stronger effects. In thrombophlebitis it is recommended to expose the whole lower extremity, not only the affected area.[1] Local exposure induces less general systemic response than exposure of large areas of the body.

Simultaneous exposures of corresponding spinal segments can amplify the effect of local exposures. Examples include the thoracic spine area in ischemic heart disease, lumbar spine in lower extremity ischemia, C-spine for "tennis elbow" and "frozen shoulder," and reflex sympathetic dystrophy.

Polarity (north or south pole) is not considered critical. Much of the public literature emphasizes the importance of one pole versus the other. Except for one study on coagulation changes,[3] no firm evidence is available for its importance. However, only a few empirical observations exist regarding polarity. The north pole may exhibit higher, some, or no analgesic effect and the south pole may exhibit more vasodilating effects. The clinician may advise use based on the inclination of the patient, but the physics and basic biomedical research community does not hold to any polarity-specific effects. Any pole will do. After initial application, reassess the patient and change polarity depending on negative or nonbeneficial effects.

The question of vector orientation also is not entirely resolved. In lower extremity ischemia, perpendicular orientation of force lines to large arteries is better than parallel orientation.

MAGNETIC FIELD DOSE CONSIDERATIONS

Successful application depends on selecting the appropriate field strengths for the particular problem being treated. Optimal requirements across the spectrum of medical care will depend on more extensive research.

Magnetic field gradient (how rapidly the field drops off with distance) also is an important consideration. This varies significantly depending on the type of magnetic configuration or device used. In the case of permanent magnets (for example, permanent magnetic pads), the decay curve falls off very steeply,[3] approximately with the inverse of the distance squared. Because of this, permanent magnets are without any risk relative to exposure duration, even for hours. This means that for typical magnets with 300mT at the surface, there is almost no field strength left within 1 to 2 inches of the magnet surface.

Risk and Safety

Despite the generally recognized safety of magnet therapy, account must be taken of some possible actions that should be considered in using this therapy. Although few of these are serious, they must be anticipated and patients must be alerted to their potential. Refer to "Druglike Information."

Efficacy

The levels of benefit for magnetic therapy vary by condition. Generally with more severe problems, the later the stage of pathology, the less benefit can be expected. This also is typical of traditional, established medical therapies. For example, static magnets are ineffective in improving enzymes in acute myocardial infarction but are helpful for the pain, reducing peripheral resistance, and decreasing aldosterone, and they are mildly effective prophylactically as thrombolytics. They also are not helpful for healing gastric ulcers but they do relieve motility dyssynergia. In some cases, magnets improve problems by 20%; in others, up to 95%.[3] They have been found to accelerate wound healing time by 50% and fracture healing by a similar magnitude.

Future Research Opportunities and Priorities

Future research efforts can be directed across the spectrum of use and basic biologic processes. Research priorities have been described in the Chantilly report.[3] Some promising research results from Eastern Europe even suggest that high-strength static magnetic fields (0.5T) may create new breakthroughs in the treatment of heretofore untreatable neurologic diseases.

Druglike Information

Warnings, Contraindications, and Precautions

Absolute contraindications include the following conditions:

- Pregnancy
- Pacemakers, implanted pain modulators, insulin delivery systems, cochlear implants, and defibrillators: These may be turned off by magnets.
- Myasthenia gravis: Muscle weakness may be aggravated because of the magnets' strong action on relaxing muscle.
- Conditions with active bleeding: Because of reduced platelet aggregation (25%) and increased thrombolysis (100%), bleeding sites may not clot readily.
- Hyperthyroidism adrenal gland, hypothalamic and hypophyseal/pituitary dysfunctions

Special attention must be paid to patients with hypotension or predisposition to it, as well as patients with severe or accelerated hypertension, because sudden significant blood pressure decreases may occur, causing vertigo, fainting, et cetera. This reaction usually disappears within 30 minutes after the exposure and adaptation begins after 5 exposures.

Adverse Reactions

Some individuals report increased discomfort, usually within hours or days after starting use of magnets. This "worsening" phenomenon is seen regularly with acupuncture and massage and is thought to occur because of improving circulation in stagnated tissues or blockages of acupuncture energy flow. Magnets or acupuncture therapeutically disturb dysfunctional homeostasis (for example, in tissues hampered by chronic edema, scarring, stiffness, and atrophy) before improved or normal function can be resumed. Once the possibility for this type of reaction is explained, the increased discomfort may need to be temporarily tolerated until tissue health is restored. This reaction is normally of short duration, usually lasting a few days and rarely several weeks. If the discomfort is intolerable, the patient should stop using the magnets temporarily or reduce the number of magnets or duration of use. The magnets later can be gradually reintroduced or the frequency or duration increased again as tolerance permits.

Pregnancy and Lactation

Magnets should not be used during pregnancy.

Product Availability

Clinicians interested in magnetic therapy will have some challenges in obtaining clinically useful magnets. They are advertised in consumer catalogs and some companies have vendor representatives or distributors. Some retail outlets, such as department stores, pharmacies, health food stores, and surgical or durable medical equipment suppliers, are just beginning to make magnets available.

Electromagnets, whether static or time-varying field, are not commercially FDA-approved for therapy in the U.S. except for fracture healing, nerve conduction testing, and skin/soft tissue ulcer treatment purposes. Insurance carriers and Medicare usually approve for payment the use of electromagnetic devices for these purposes. Permanent magnets, on the other hand, have not yet been FDA-approved and are not usually approved for payment by insurance. They also are not nearly as expensive as the approved devices, ranging in price from $1.00 to $1000, with the average under $100. They do not require a prescription. Magnets made specifically for acupuncture applications are available primarily from acupuncture equipment suppliers, as are measurement devices.

Several of the books recommended for reading list some manufacturers. Many distributors of magnetic products advertise on the Internet. Search words could include biomagnetics, magnetic healing, magnetic therapy, magnet therapy, magnet(s), MRI safety and magnet manufacturers. Claims are often exaggerated and scientifically uninformed.

Self-Help versus Professional

In most cases this therapy can be self-applied with instructions for use. Once a diagnosis is made for an applicable problem, contraindications are ruled out, and precautions for use are given, the magnets may be used without any other supervision. Patients should be advised against off-label use without further assessment and guidance. Since magnetic therapy often may relieve acute pain, especially over acupuncture or trigger points or for the periodic recurrences of chronically remittent problems, such as migraines or tension headaches, patients also should be warned to consult a professional if the character of the underlying pain or problem changes before magnet application. This is similar to issues of masking potentially catastrophic acute problems with narcotics or analgesics in acute abdomen or potential intracranial bleeds.

Credentialing

Magnetic therapy is in the earliest stages of use in North America. It is still essentially an over-the-counter therapy. Any practitioner may use this therapy. There is no standardization of use. Licensing is not required for this treatment modality. New FDA-approved devices will likely only be provided through licensed professionals and may be subject to other regulations in the future. These approvals would likely also lead to insurance coverage.

Training

Formal training programs are not yet widely available and there is no officially recognized certification. The North American Academy of Magnetic Therapy, a professional organization, has been established to promote the dissemination of research knowledge on the subject, and certificate training has just been initiated.

What to Look for in a Provider

A referring practitioner should have reviewed the existing literature, understand the basic principles of magnets, and have significant experience in the clinical use of magnets. Membership in the North American Academy of Magnetic Therapy would be desirable. Belonging to a licensed health profession would be helpful.

Associations

The only clinically-related association addressing the area of magnetic therapy at present is the North American Academy of Magnetic Therapy. A web site will be available soon.

Suggested Reading

1. Polk C, Postow E, editors: *Handbook of biologic effect of electromagnetic fields*, ed 2, Boca Raton, Fla, 1996, CRC Press.
   An excellent, extensive, although technical discourse on the biologic effects seen with all types of fields.
2. Lawrence R, Rosch P, Plowden J: *Magnet therapy*, Rocklin, Calif, 1998, Prima Health.
   An easily readable, popular exposition of the why, when, what and how of magnetic therapy and is helpful for understanding some of the principles.
3. Hannemann H: *Magnet therapy: balancing your body's energy flow for self-healing*, New York, 1990, Sterling.
   Shows some of the acupuncture points and gives some treatment protocols for common conditions.
4. Jerabek J, Pawluk W: *Magnetic therapy in Eastern Europe: a review of 30 years of research*, Chicago, 1998, self-published.
   Recommended for its presentation of actual clinical research covering 30 years of experience, (primarily from human studies) and its explanation of many clinical phenomena seen.
5. Livingston JD: *Driving force: the natural magic of magnet*, Cambridge, Mass, 1997, Harvard University Press.
   A very general and readable discussion about the science of magnets. Clinical uses are not discussed.
6. Moskowitz LR: *Permanent magnet design and application handbook*, Malabar, Fla, 1986, Robert E. Krieger.
   Very technical but very useful for the more serious student because it extensively describes permanent magnets and their characteristics.

Bibliography

Barker AT, Jalinous R, Freeston AL: Noninvasive magnetic stimulation of human motor cortex, *Lancet* 1:1106-1107, 1985.

Bradley D: A new twist in the tale of nature's symmetry, *Science* 264:908, 1994.

Hanneman H: *Magnetic therapy,* New York, 1990, Sterling Publications.

Lawrence R, Rosch PJ, Plowden J: *Magnet therapy,* Rocklin, Calif, 1998, Prima Health.

MacGinitie L: Streaming and piezoelectric potentials in connective tissues. In Blank M, editor: *Electromagnetic fields: biological interactions and mechanisms,* Washington, DC, 1995, American Chemical Society.

Rubik B et al: Bioelectromagnetics applications in medicine. In Berman BM, Larson DB, editors: *Alternative medicine: expanding medical horizons, a report to the National Institutes of Health on alternative medicine systems and practices in the United States,* Washington, DC, 1992, U.S. Government Printing Office.

References

1. Malmivuo J, Plonsey R: *Bioelectromagnetism: principles and applications of bioelectric and biomagnetic fields,* New York, 1995, Oxford University Press.

2. Hsu M, Fong C: The biomagnetic effect and its application in acupuncture, *Am J Acupuncture* 6:289-296, 1978.

3. Jerabek J, Pawluk W: *Magnetic therapy in Eastern Europe: a review of 30 years of research,* Chicago, 1998, William Pawluk, MD.

4. Bassett CA: Bioelectromagnetics in the service of medicine. In Blank M, editor: *Electromagnetic fields: biological interactions and mechanisms,* Washington, DC, 1995, American Chemical Society.

5. Whitaker J, Adderly B: *The pain relief breakthrough,* Boston, 1998, Little, Brown and Company.

6. Ohno Y: The effects of magnetized mineral water on memory loss delay in Alzheimer's Disease, *Frontier Perspectives* 6:38-43, 1997.

7. Jie W: Further observations on the therapeutic effect of magnets and magnetized water against ascariasis in children—analysis of 114 cases, *J Tradition Chin Med* 9:111-112, 1989.

8. Helms J: *Acupuncture energetics: a clinical approach for physicians,* Berkeley, Calif, 1995, Medical Acupuncture Publishers.

9. Liboff AR: Bioelectromagnetic fields and acupuncture, *J Alt Complement Med* 1:77-87, 1997 (supplement).

10. Reichmanis M, Marino AA, Becker RO: Electrical correlates of acupuncture points, *IEEE Transactions on Biomedical Engineering* 22:533-535, 1975.

11. Bennett WR Jr: Health and low frequency electromagnetic fields, New Haven, Conn, 1994, Yale University Press.

12. Warnke U: Infrared radiation and oxygen partial pressure in human surfacial tissue as indicators of the therapeutic effects of pulsating magnetic fields of extremely low frequency (Report from the 2nd International Congress on Magnetomedicine), *Biophysic Med Rep* 2:1-8, 1981.

13. Weber M, editor: *Therapy with pulsating magnetic fields used in combination with other treatment methods,* Uttwil, Switzerland, 1992, Biophysics and Medicine Report.

14. McLean MJ et al: Blockade of sensory neuron action potentials by a static magnetic field in the 10mT range, *Bioelectromagnetics* 16:20-32, 1995.

15. Sullivan DR: Effect of a constant magnetic field on invertebrate neurons. In Barnothy M, editor: *Biologic effects of magnetic fields*, vol 2, New York, 1969, Plenum.

16. Becker RO: *The body electric*, ed 1, New York, 1985, Morrow.

17. Sisken BF et al: Stimulation of rat sciatic nerve regeneration with pulsed electromagnetic fields, *Brain Res* 485:309-316, 1989.

18. Chokroverty S, editor: *Magnetic stimulation in clinical neurophysiology*, ed 1, Stoneham, Mass, 1990, Butterworth.

19. Frankel RB, Liburdy RP: Biological effects of static magnetic fields. In Polk C, Postow E, editors: *Handbook of biological effects of electromagnetic fields*, ed 2, Boca Raton, Fla, 1996, CRC Press.

20. Polk C, Postow E, editors: *Handbook of biological effects of electromagnetic fields*, ed 2, Boca Raton, Fla, 1996, CRC Press.

21. Walleczek J: Magnetokinetic effects on radical pairs: a paradigm for magnetic field interactions with biologic systems at lower than thermal energy. In Blank M, editor: *Electromagnetic fields: biological interactions and mechanisms*, Washington, DC, 1995, American Chemical Society.

22. Avery DH et al: Repetitive transcranial magnetic stimulation in the treatment of medication-resistant depression: preliminary data, *J Nerv Ment Dis* 187(2):114-117, 1999.

23. Bier RR, Estersohn HS: A new treatment for Charcot joint in the diabetic foot, *J Am Pod Med Assoc* 77:63-69, 1987.

24. Mooney V: A randomized double-blind prospective study of the efficacy of pulsed electromagnetic fields for interbody lumbar fusions, *Spine* 15:708-712, 1990.

25. Latzke AW: Magnetic plaster. U.S. Patent 4,489,711, issued 12/1984.

26. Trock DH et al: A double-blind trial of the clinical effects of pulsed electromagnetic fields in osteoarthritis [see comments], *J Rheumatol* 20:456-460, 1993.

27. Ieran M et al: Effect of low frequency pulsing electromagnetic fields on skin ulcers of venous origin in humans: a double blind study, *J Orthoped Res* 8:276-282, 1990.

28. Stiller MJ et al: A portable pulsed electromagnetic field (pemf) device to enhance healing of recalcitrant venous ulcers: a double-blind, placebo-controlled clinical trial, *Br J Dermatol* 127:147-154, 1989.

29. Weintraub MI: Chronic submaximal magnetic stimulation in peripheral neuropathy: is there a beneficial therapeutic relationship? *Am J Pain Management* 8(1):12-16, 1998.

30. Vallbona C, Haywood CF, Jurida G: Response of pain to static magnetic fields in post-polio patients: a double blind pilot study, *Arch Phys Med Rehab* 78:1200-1203, 1997.

31. Barnothy M, editor: *Biological effects of magnetic fields*, vol 1, New York, 1964, Plenum.

32. Blank M, editor: *Electromagnetic fields: biological interactions and mechanisms*, Washington, DC, 1995, American Chemical Society.

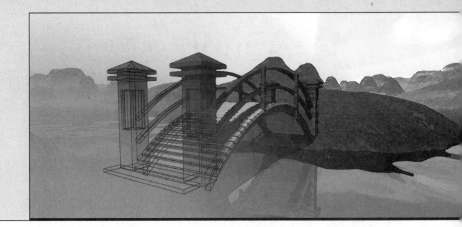

Alternative Systems of Medical Practice

Oriental Medicine Practices

Acupressure, **178**
Acupuncture, **191**
Traditional Chinese Herbal Medicine, **203**
Tai Chi, **219**
Qi Gong, **231**

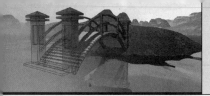

Acupressure

MICHAEL REED GACH

Origins and History

Acupressure is an ancient health care practice that uses the fingers to press key points on the surface of the skin to stimulate the body's natural self-curative abilities. Acupuncture and acupressure use the same points, but acupuncture employs needles whereas acupressure uses a gentle but firm pressure of the hands (as well as the fists, elbows, arms and feet in some techniques). Acupressure, the older of the two traditions, uses the power and sensitivity of human touch. We first will examine current research of various methods available, including massage therapy, followed by a discussion of its origins and benefits. Finally, we will cover self-care applications and the role of health education for future reform.

The origins of acupressure are as ancient as the instinct to hold your forehead or your temples when you have a headache. Everyone at one time or another has used the hands spontaneously to hold tense or painful places on the body. Since the beginning of recorded history, human beings have been instinctively drawn to hold places on the body that are blocked, ache, or hurt. People immediately hold a sprain, minor burn, or bruise to help relieve excessive pain.

> *Man's original tool is his hand, which he has instinctively used in order to alleviate pain. Whenever he is struck, strung, or seized with cramps, he involuntarily puts his hand to the painful spot in order to protect it or rub, knead, or massage it.*[1]

If you place a hand on your forehead to clear your thoughts or hold your lower back, you are actually treating yourself with acupressure. Children often instinctively demonstrate this impulse when they are hurt. This suggests that acupressure is being performed unconsciously all the time.

More than five thousand years ago the Chinese discovered that pressing certain points on the body relieved pain where it occurred and also benefited other parts of the body that were more remote from the pain and the pressure point. (Other cultures also made similar discoveries, although it did not develop into an entire medical system as it did in China.)

Chang[2] observed that in the early Chinese dynasties, when stones and arrows were the only implements of war, many soldiers wounded on the battlefield reported that symptoms of disease that had plagued them for years had suddenly vanished. Naturally, such strange occurrences baffled the physicians who could find no logical relationship between the trauma and the ensuing recovery of health. After years of meticulous observation, ancient Chinese physicians developed ways of curing certain illnesses by striking or piercing specific points on the surface of the body.

People have commonly shared their hands-on folk remedies that have proved to be effective. These shared findings have been preserved and developed through the process of objective conceptualization and reasoning. Methods of massage found to be effective for thousands of years were eventually integrated with the points and principles of acupuncture. These principles of traditional Chinese medicine were written approximately four thousand years ago in *The Yellow Emperor's Classic of Internal Medicine*. The classical references of acupuncture, as well as the conceptual teachings of traditional Chinese doctors, contributed to the development of acupressure.

Mechanism of Action According to Its Own Theory

Whether it is a sudden accident or a long-term chronic condition, illness can be the result of stressors challenging the body's homeostatic mechanisms beyond their limits. The resulting tension inhibits the body's ability to cope effectively with the disrupting condition. Acupressure enhances the body's homeostatic process by directly reducing muscular tension and stress, thus allowing the body to heal itself more effectively and obtain optimum wellness.

Muscular tension tends to concentrate around acupressure points, which in turn affects large muscle groups. Acupressure works to relax muscular tension and balance the vital life forces of the body through a system of points and meridians. The *points* are places that have a high electric conductivity on the surface of the skin where the energy forces can be manipulated and balanced. The *meridians* are the pathways along which the energy flows from point to point.

The life energy that is released in acupressure flows through the meridians, nourishing all the internal organs and systems of the body. The energy is the source of life, and its flow is the key to radiant health. It functions to regulate and balance all systems of the body, including the respiratory, digestive, endocrine, cardiovascular, lymphatic, urogenital, and nervous systems. It also functions to balance our emotions and mental state. Thus, acupressure works to effectively create a feeling of balance and well-being. When our energy is circulating properly we feel alive, happy, peaceful, and in harmony with ourselves and others. Acupressure is used in many ways. Prolonged finger pressure can be applied on the points to relieve common ailments and tensions. Acupressure also is used as a preventive health care technique to help people stay well.

An Acupressure Principle of Health

The "complementary antagonism" of positive and negative, contraction and expansion, and the balance between these forces are revealed on all levels of life. For example, the balance of positive and negative charges in atoms, ions, and molecules demonstrates yin and yang at the atomic level. In the autonomic nervous system the actions of the parasympathetic and sympathetic systems function in a *balanced antagonism*[3] that is analogous to the yin/yang principle. The constant fluctuation between both forces allows for the body to maintain homeostasis.

The principle of yin and yang also can be applied to the vital organs and tissues of the body as a whole and to an individual's social and physical environment. All aspects of life can be viewed in terms of yin and yang: Parts of the body go through periods of activity and rest; nerves fire in activity and then return to a resting state; the intestines rhythmically expand and contract to remove waste from the body. When we exercise, a yang activity, we sweat and are cooled off, a yin activity. A daily cycle of activity and sleep is also a balance of yin and yang. When we have a fever (yang), cool compresses (yin) can help relieve the heat.

Health is a result of homeostasis, the balance between these two "complementary opposites" within the human body. Acupressure works to create health in the body by balancing the extremes of yin and yang; in other words, to *harmonize the sympathetic and parasympathetic processes*. Acupressure techniques also can balance our emotions and our whole way of being in the world.

Biologic Mechanism of Action

Acupressure Pain Control

Several theories explain how acupressure effectively relieves pain. Pain perception is closely related to the amount of bodily stress, tension, and emotional anxiety present in the patient. Acupressure increases circulation, which removes lactic acid, carbon dioxide, histamines, bradykinins (mediators for pain reception), and other toxins. Circulation also brings oxygen and other nutrients to the affected areas. The patient's focus on pain is often distracted by the use of acupressure which relieves muscular tension. In these ways, acupressure provides a natural way for the patient to cope with pain.

One explanation of this phenomenon is the *pain-gateway* theory. This theory suggests that the transmission of pain impulses can be modulated by a gating mechanism in the pain signaling system. An open gate results in pain; a partially open gate results in less intense pain; and a closed gate results in no pain. This "gating" is affected in part by the activity of sensory nerves. Stimulation of these large-diameter cutaneous fibers tends to close the gate, inhibiting the transmission of pain impulses from the spinal cord to the brain.[4] Acupuncture needles and acupressure produce only a mild, fairly painless stimulation, which, as theorized, causes the gates to be closed so that painful sensations cannot pass through.[5]

Another theory is that prolonged pressure on the acupressure points releases endorphins, which have a natural analgesic effect on the body. *Endorphins* are neurotransmitters that appear to be produced by the pituitary gland.[6] It has been theorized that acupressure and acupuncture stimulate the pituitary gland to release endorphins. This analgesic effect acts at neural synaptic sites to inhibit the afferent pain receptors from connecting. Endorphins do not entirely block the sensation of pain; rather, they alter the patient's perception of the sensation in an action similar to that of administered narcotics.

Forms of Therapy

Several different styles of acupressure are currently practiced, although the same points are used in all of them. A variety of rhythms, pressures, and techniques create the different styles of acupressure. For instance, shiatsu, the most well-known style of acupressure, can be quite vigorous, with firm pressure applied to each point for only 3 to 5 seconds. The jin shin style holds at least two points at the same time for a minute or more with the fingertips. There are many different forms of both these main styles. Shiatsu for instance has several forms with its unique techiques, including zen shiatsu, barefoot shiatsu, namikoshi shiatsu, and macrobiotic shiatsu, to name a few. Similarly the jin shin style has its unique trademarked forms and point numbering systems, such as jin shin jyutsu and jin shin do.

Demographics

Practitioners and users are distributed homogeneously. The American Oriental Bodywork Therapy Association (AOBTA) publishes an annual directory of teachers and practitioners of acupressure and other styles of oriental bodywork that also stimulate these same points but in different ways. For a quarterly newsletter or a practitioner directory, contact AOBTA.

Indications and Reasons for Referral

Acupressure relieves many common complaints ranging from headaches to insomnia.[7] This author has found from 25 years of clinical experience that acupressure can be effective in helping to relieve sinus problems, shoulder and neck pain, back spasm, chronic fatigue, fibromyalgia, muscular tension, and general aches and pains. Many hundreds of this author's students, patients, and friends have been taught to use acupressure to relieve ulcer pain, menstrual cramps, lower back aches, constipation, indigestion, difficulty breathing, temporomandibular joint pain, carpal tunnel syndrome, ankle pain, sciatica, and a stiff neck. Because acupressure is so effective for releasing stress and tension, it calms and balances all the emotions including panic attacks, fears, and anxiety.

According to Dr. Serizawa, a Japanese physician who regularly uses acupressure in his medical research and practice:

The ailments from which (acupressure) can offer relief are numerous and include the following: symptoms of chilling; flushing; pain and numbness; headaches; heaviness in the head; dizziness; tinnitus; stiff shoulders arising from disorders of the autonomic nervous system; constipation; sluggishness; chills of the hands and feet; insomnia; malformations of the backbone frequent in middle age and producing pain in the shoulders, arms, and hands; pains in the back; pains in the knees experienced during standing or going up or down stairs.[8]

Office Applications

Acupressure is primary for prevention and relief of symptoms of muscle tension. Point stimulation is adjunctive for most diseases. A ranking of applicable conditions follows:

Top level: *A therapy ideally suited for these conditions*

Anxiety; carpal tunnel syndrome; chronic fatigue syndrome; menstrual cramps; neck pain; stress; wellness care; and temporomandibular joint syndrome

Second level: *One of the better therapies for these conditions*

Amenorrhea; ankle sprain; arthritis; back pain; childbirth; children's health; chronic pain; colic; female health; hiccups; insomnia; jaw problems; male health; motion sickness; nausea; periodic leg movement syndrome; postpartum care; pregnancy and childbirth; premenstrual syndrome; restless leg syndrome; sciatica; and shoulder pain

Third level: *A valuable adjunctive therapy for these conditions*

Addictions; allergies; asthma; benign prostatic hypertrophy; bronchitis; colds and flu; colitis and Crohn's disease; conjunctivitis; constipation; diabetes; diarrhea; diverticulosis and diverticulitis; ear infections; edema; emphysema; endometriosis; fever; fibrocystic breast disease; gastritis; gastrointestinal disorders; general ear pain; glaucoma; gout; hay fever; headaches; hearing disorders; hemorrhoids; hyperactivity; hypertension; immune system boosting; impotence; irritable bowel syndrome; lazy eye; menopause; mental health; multiple sclerosis; obesity and weight management; osteoarthritis; osteoporosis; poor circulation; poor eyesight; respiratory conditions; sinusitis; sleep disorders; stomach ache; strep throat; and tinnitus

Whether used to relieve pain and muscular discomfort or to prevent illness, acupressure techniques are intended to correct imbalances and work toward the regulation and harmony of all systems of the body. Because acupressure requires no special tools and many people respond to the touch of hands-on contact more than they trust needles, the growing appeal of the ancient Chinese healing arts has led to increased interest in acupressure as a means toward optimum wellness.

Practical Applications

The healing touch of acupressure reduces tension, increases circulation, and enables the body to relax deeply. A medical physician can show patients self-care applications using popular texts, such as *Acupressure's Potent Points*. Doctors also can refer their patients to professional acupressure practitioners through the AOBTA (see "Associations").

By relieving stress, acupressure strengthens resistance to disease and promotes wellness. Acupressure is very beneficial in situations of discomfort and the inability to rest or sleep. Specific points have been used traditionally to treat insomnia, anxiety, pain, general discomfort, and restlessness. All points significantly help patients relax and feel more comfortable.

Research Base

Long after acupressure was developed through instinct, the Chinese developed more technologic methods for stimulating points, first with needles and later using electricity. Thousands of scientific research projects that have been conducted around the world during the last 50 years have demonstrated that acupuncture is an effective treatment for relieving pain.

Evidence Based

Omura[9] found that acupuncture and electric stimulation not only improved the microcirculatory disturbance and relaxed spastic muscles and vasoconstrictive arteries but also reduced or eliminated the pain. Omura also found that acupuncture enhanced drug intake to the area where drugs previously could not be delivered because of existing circulatory disturbances.

In a randomized double-blind study, Garvey, Marks, and Wiesel[10] found that trigger point therapy is a useful adjunct in the treatment of lower back strain. Direct acupuncture to the trigger points gave symptomatic relief equal to that of the treatment with various types of injected medication. In animal studies, Janssens[11] found that 71% of the body's trigger points described in the literature are acupressure or acupuncture points.

ELECTRIC STIMULATION

When these points are stimulated with electricity (for instance, using TENS units) the treatment is referred to as *transcutaneous nerve stimulation*. The following two research studies dealing with dysmenorrhea and chemotherapy use this form of noninvasive stimulation of the points.

Jackson and Varner[12] studied the effects of transcutaneous electrical nerve stimulation in the relief of primary dysmenorrhea. Results revealed that at least 50% of the subjects experienced immediate posttreatment relief, indicating that acupuncture-like TENS may be useful for dysmenorrheic pain.

Dundee, Yang, and McMillan[13] studied the beneficial effects of transcutaneous electrical stimulation of the P6 antiemetic point as an adjunct to standard antiemetics. P6, known as *Neiquan* in Chinese, is an acupoint approximately the width of two fingers up the inside of the arm from the transverse crease of the wrist, located between the two tendons. It traditionally is considered an excellent point for nausea of most types, especially motion sickness. P6 was used in over 100 patients in whom chemotherapy-induced sickness was not adequately controlled by pharmaceutic antiemetics alone. Although the results were not quite as effective as with invasive acupuncture, more than 75% of the patients achieved considerable benefit from this nontoxic procedure.

Basic Science

PROVING THE EXISTENCE OF ACUPOINTS

Omura[14] attempted to track meridians and points using the "bidigital o-ring test imaging technique," with remarkable results that corroborated ancient teachings. Omura accurately localized meridians and points that correspond to specific internal organs and found that with the exception of some variables and inaccuracies, the paths of the meridians described in the literature of ancient Chinese medicine are more or less correct.

Each meridian of a specific internal organ was found to be connected to that organ's representation area in the cerebral cortex. Omura also found a high concentration of neurotransmitters and hormones within most points and meridian lines.

Another study that gave physiologic validation to the points was performed by Omura et al.[15] This study imaged the stomach and localized the stomach meridian and its acupuncture points in a human cadaver. They found more dense connective tissue network between the skin layer and the fascia on the muscle tissue at the ST36 point compared with the surrounding area.

Risk and Safety

Foremost among the advantages of acupressure's healing touch is that it is safe to do on yourself and others—even if never attempted before—as long as you follows the instructions and pay attention to the cautions. There are no side effects from drugs because there are no drugs. The only equipment needed is your hands. Patients thus can practice acupressure safely anytime, anywhere.

Efficacy

Most of the research on acupressure has used the P6 point for treating nausea. For instance, previous work by Dundee and Yang[16] (1990) has shown that P6 can be effective for 8 hours to substitute for conventional antiemetic therapy. Dundee and Yang also showed that the application of an elasticized wrist band with a stud placed over the P6 point and pressed regularly every two hours will prolong its antiemetic action for 24 hours. This proved to be more effective in hospital patients (20/20) than in outpatients (15/20), presumably because of the constant encouragement given to regularly press the stud. Although nausea and vomiting remain problems with cancer in chemotherapy, acupressure on the P6 point had an antiemetic action when using the "Sea Band," a commercially available elasticized band with a plastic stud.

The effect of using P6 on postoperative vomiting in children was studied by Lewis et al.[17] Sixty-six patients ages 3 to 12 years who were undergoing outpatient surgery to correct strabismus were allocated randomly to receive either bilateral P6 acupressure or a placebo during the postperioperative period. Acupressure on P6 did not reduce the incidence of postoperative children undergoing strabismus surgery.

Another acupressure research study on postoperative nausea was performed by Barsoum, Perry, and Fraser.[18] A total of 162 general surgical patients were randomized for one of the following three treatments for postoperative nausea and vomiting: (1) acupressure using elastic bands containing a plastic button to apply sustained pressure at the P6 point above the wrist; (2) control dummy bands without the pressure button; and (3) antiemetic injections of prochiorperazine with each opiate given as required. The incidence of postoperative vomiting and the need for unplanned antiemetic injections also were reduced by acupressure, but this was not statistically significant. Therefore the author concluded that acupressure can work and should be investigated in other clinical situations.

Self-Help Research

The following studies illustrate four different self-help approaches. The first study used a combination of exercise and relaxation for premenstrual syndromes. The second study tested self-acupressure as a treatment for menstrual distress. The third study used diaphragmatic breathing to treat asthmatics. The fourth study validated the benefits of Qi Gong, an ancient Chinese health care practice that involves conscious, deep breathing with various movements.

Pullon, Reinken, and Sparrow[19] surveyed 1826 women for the self-treatment of premenstrual syndromes. Of these women, 85% noted premenstrual syndromes of some kind. Overall there was a marked placebo response, but exercise, rest, and keeping a written diary of the symptoms were all helpful in over 80% of those who had tried them.

Fraley[20] studied 143 subjects who were randomly assigned to self-acupressure, placebo, and control groups for the treatment of menstrual distress. Results verified a significant decrease in menstrual pain among the self-acupressure group compared to the control group. Subjects in the acupressure and placebo groups took less medication than subjects in the control group. Subjects in the acupressure group were more likely both to continue and recommend acupressure treatment than subjects in the placebo group.

Girodo[21] studied 67 asthmatic adults, randomly assigned to either deep diaphragmatic breathing training, physical exercise training, or a waiting list control group, that participated in a 16-week program. Deep diaphragmatic training resulted in specific reductions in medication use, as well as decreased intensity of asthmatic symptoms. Another important result of deep, diaphragmatic breathing was that most patients tripled their time spent in physical activities.

Omura[14] found unique physical changes in patients who practiced the Qi Gong treatment. Beneficial effects of Qi Gong resulted in improvement in the circulation and lowering of high blood pressure, as well as relaxation of spastic muscles, relief of pain, and enhanced general well-being.

Druglike Information

Safety

Acupressure uses the anatomic specificity of the acupuncture points with the power and sensitivity of touch. The greatest advantages of using hands versus needles are safety, the noninvasive healing nature of touch, and the self-care applications that can be practiced anywhere.

Warnings, Contraindications, and Precautions

Patients with life-threatening diseases and serious medical problems always should consult their doctor before using acupressure or other alternative therapies. It is important for the novice to use caution in any medical emergency situation, such as a stroke or heart attack, or for any serious medical condition, such as arteriosclerosis or an illness caused by bacteria. Acupressure is not an appropriate sole treatment for cancer, contagious skin diseases, or sexually transmitted diseases. In conjunction with proper medical attention, however, gentle acupressure (safely away from the diseased area and the internal organs) can help soothe and relieve a patient's distress and pain.

Apply finger pressure in a slow, rhythmic manner to enable the layers of tissue and the internal organs to respond. Never press any area in an abrupt, forceful, or jarring way.

Use the abdominal points cautiously, especially if you are ill. Avoid the abdominal area entirely if you have a life-threatening disease, especially intestinal cancer, tuberculosis, serious cardiac conditions, and leukemia.

Lymph areas, such as the groin, the area of the throat just below the ears, and the breast near the armpits, are very sensitive. These areas should be touched only lightly and not pressed.

Do not work directly on a serious burn, an ulcerous condition, or an infection; for these conditions, medical care alone is indicated.

Do not work directly on a recently formed scar. During the first month after an injury or operation, do not apply pressure directly on the affected site. However, gentle continuous holding a few inches away from the periphery of the injury will stimulate the area and help it heal.

After an acupressure session, body heat is lowered; thus resistance to cold is also lower. Because the tensions have been released the body's vital energies are concentrating inward to maximize healing. The body will be more vulnerable, so be sure to wear extra clothing and keep warm when you finish an acupressure routine.

Pregnancy and Lactation

Avoid the abdominal area during pregnancy. Special care should be taken during pregnancy. Please refer to chapters 29 and 36 in *Acupressure's Potent Points* for the points to avoid during pregnancy and for relieving discomforts due to pregnancy, labor pain, postpartum recovery, and nursing, as well as further guidance.

Trade Products

The *Hands-On Health Care Catalog*, a free patient-wellness mail order resource, presents a wide variety of recommended books on acupressure and other alternative therapies, acupressure and reflexology charts, instructional videotapes, and self-care stress reduction tools. Free catalog copies are available through the Acupressure Institute.*

The Acupressure Institute
1533 Shattuck Ave.
Berkeley, CA 94709
Tel: (800) 442-2232
www.acupressure.com

---

*This company is owned by the author of this chapter

Self-Help versus Professional

Acupressure self-care techniques can empower patients to take some responsibility for stress relief and wellness. Self-care education increases self-reliance and boosts morale and thus enhances overall quality of life.

An additional advantage of acupressure is that it can be used on a self-help basis. People can learn to help themselves for everything from insomnia to migraine headaches and nausea. Many acupressure point combinations are well within a person's reach and take a minimal amount of time to teach their proper location and pressure.

There is a dualistic benefit derived from self-acupressure. First and most obvious is that people are able to relieve particular pains and discomforts. This ability to assume responsibility for self-treatment then boosts a person's self-confidence and trust. People can take this self-treatment knowledge home with them out of the hospital setting. Health professionals also can use acupressure on themselves for stress reduction, which can help them cope with their demanding duties.

Credentialing

The hands-on nature of acupressure has put acupressure under the auspices of massage therapy. The National Committee Certification for Acupuncture and Traditional Oriental Medicine recently created national examination and credentialing standards for oriental bodywork and acupressure. Among the many requirements are a minimum of 500 hours of training including at least 100 hours of anatomy. Although the industry standard is 500 hours of training, each state has different requirements for licensure.

Training

The Acupressure Institute in Berkeley, California, one of the foremost educational centers, offers three levels of training totaling 1000 hours. The Institute's acupressure therapy health education program provides clinical experience and teacher training and covers many of the following specialized applications: pain management, women's health, emotional balancing, stress management, sports acupressure, traditional Oriental therapy, and acupressure for older adults.

What to Look for in a Provider

A good acupressurist is knowledgeable about point therapeutics, able to apply traditional theory in a practical context, skilled in oriental bodywork techniques, and uses the art of hands-on massage with sensitivity, confidence, and compassion. To choose a quality provider of acupressure therapy, examine the practitioners' training, rapport, personal presence and alertness. Follow up on their references. In a one-on-one interview, require the practitioner to give you a 20-minute shoulder and neck release to experience the quality of touch. The way the practitioner approaches you, both verbally and hands-on, should be your deciding factor.

Associations

American Oriental Bodywork Therapy Association (AOBTA)
Laurel Oak Corporate Center
1010 Haddonfield-Berlin Rd., Suite 408
Voorhees, NJ 08043
Tel: (609) 782-1616
Fax: (609) 782-1653
E-mail: AOBTA@prodigy.net

Suggested Reading

1. Gach MR: *Acupressure's potent points*, New York, 1990, Bantam.
   A point reference book and self-treatment guide for relieving common complaints from A to Z. Forty different ailments are covered with over 500 illustrations and photographs of the most important acupressure points and a step-by-step routine for relieving each health problem. This self-care book offers quick relief from everyday aches, pains, and ailments and is an authoritative guide to self-acupressure. The last chapter provides vital guidelines for wellness, followed by five comprehensive charts of the points, a glossary, and an index.
2. Serizawa K: *Tsubo: vital points for oriental therapy*, Tokyo, 1976, Japan Publications.
   A practical fully illustrated acupressure point reference book with 256 pages.
3. Eisenberg D: *Encounters with qi*, New York, 1987, Penguin.
   A classical account by a Western physician of the extraordinary ways that the life force is used in various Asian healing and martial arts.
4. Gach MR: *Arthritis relief at your fingertips*, New York, 1989, Warner.
   Presents a key to drug-free therapy to relieve the pain, stiffness, and inflammation of chronic joint disease. Using a combination of invigorating massage, gentle stretching, and pressure point stimulation, this self-care program uses 12 antiinflammatory points for relieving specific areas of arthritic pain. Both self-care methods and techniques for helping others are described and illustrated in step-by-step detail. With a forward by rheumatologist Murray C. Sokoloff, MD, assistant clinical professor of medicine at Stanford University.
5. Gach MR: *Acu-yoga*, Tokyo, 1981, Japan Publications.
   Illustrates the ways that body postures stimulate specific acupressure points for self-treatment. After an introduction to the therapeutic components of acupressure and yoga, the book provides four complete exercise sets. The last half of *Acu-Yoga* addresses colds, constipation, cramps, headaches, insomnia, menstrual tension, nervous disorders, potency, shoulder tension, and spinal disorders. Each of these sections present step-by-step self-care instructions, illustrating the acupressure points stimulated in specific yoga postures.

Bibliography

Doehring KM: Relieving pain through touch, *Adv Clin Care* 4(5):32-33, 1989.

Gach MR: *Acu-yoga: self-help techniques to relieve tension*, Tokyo, 1981, Japan Publications.

Gach MR: *The bum back book: self-help back care*, Berkeley, Calif, 1983, Celestial Arts.

Gach MR: *Greater energy at your fingertips*, Berkeley, Calif, 1986, Celestial Arts.

Gach MR: *Arthritis relief at your fingertips*, New York, 1989, Warner.

Gach MR: *Acupressure's potent points: a guide to self-care for common ailments*, New York, 1990, Bantam.

Goats GC, Keir KA: Connective tissue massage, *Brit J Sports Med* 25(3):131-133, 1991.

McCaffery M: Nursing approaches to nonpharmacological pain control, *Int J Nurs Stud* 27(1):1-5, 1990.

Serizawa K: *Tsubo: vital points for oriental therapy*, Tokyo, 1976, Japan Publications.

Reed BV, Held JM: The effects of connective tissue massage in the autonomic nervous system, *Phys Ther* 68(8):1231-1234, 1988.

References

1. Palos S: *The Chinese art of healing*, New York, 1972, Bantam.

2. Chang ST: *The complete book of acupuncture*, Berkeley, Calif, 1976, Celestial Arts.

3. Bergenson B: *Pharmacology in nursing*, ed 13, St Louis, 1976, Mosby.

4. Brunner L, Suddarth D: *Textbook of medical-surgical nursing*, ed 3, Philadelphia, 1975, Lippincott Colk.

5. Tan LT, Tan MYC, Veith I: *Acupuncture therapy—current Chinese practice*, Philadelphia, 1973, Temple University Press.

6. Pomeranz B: Brian's opiates as they work in acupuncture, *New Science* January 6, 1977.

7. Gach MR: *Acupressure's potent points*, New York, 1990, Bantam.

8. Serizawa K: *Tsubo: vital points for oriental therapy*, Tokyo, 1976, Japan Publications.

9. Omura Y: Storing of qi energy in various materials and drugs (qi gongization): its clinical application for treatment of pain, circulatory disturbances, bacterial or viral infections, heavy metal deposits, and related intractable medical problems by selectively enhancing circulation and drug uptake, *Acupunct Electrother Res* 15(2):137-157, 1990.

10. Garvey TA, Marks MR, Wiesel SW: Trigger point injection therapy for low-back pain, *Spine* 14(9):962-964, 1989.

11. Janssens LA: Trigger point therapy, *Probl Veteran Med* 4(1):117-124. 1992.

12. Jackson JR, Varner RE: Transcutaneous electrical nerve stimulation for dysmenorrhea, *Phys Ther* 69(1):3-9, 1989.

13. Dundee JW, Yang J, McMillan C: An antiemetic point in cancer chemotherapy, *J R Soc Med* 84(4):210-212, 1991.

14. Omura Y: Connections found between each meridian (heart, stomach, triple burner, etc.) and organ representation area of corresponding internal organs in each side of the cerebral cortex; release of common neurotransmitters and hormones unique to each meridian and correspond-

ing acupuncture point and internal organ after acupuncture, electrical stimulation, mechanical stimulation (including shiatsu), soft laser stimulation, or Qi Gong, *Acupunct Electrother Res* 14(2):155-186, 1989.

15. Omura Y et al: Imaging of the stomach and localization of the stomach meridian and its acupuncture points in a human cadaver by the use of the indirect "bidigital o-ring test imaging technique," *Acupunct Electrother Res* 13(4):153-164, 1988.

16. Dundee JW, Yang J: Acupressure in cancer chemotherapy, *J R Soc Med* 83(6):360-362, 1990.

17. Lewis IH et al: Acupressure's effect on postoperative vomiting in children, *Br J Anaesth* 67(1):73-78, 1991.

18. Barsoum G, Perry EP, Fraser IA: Postoperative nausea relieved by acupressure, *J R Soc Med* 83(2):86-89, 1990.

19. Pullon SR, Reinken JA, Sparrow MJ: Treatment of premenstrual symptoms, *N Z Med J* 10(862):72-74, 1989.

20. Fraley LE: Acupressure for the treatment of menstrual distress, School Public Health, University of California-Berkeley, 1983.

21. Girodo M: *Phys Med Rehab* 73(8):717-720, 1992.

Acupuncture

CAROLYN F.A. DEAN

MARGARET MULLINS

JEFFREY YUEN

Origins and History

Acupuncture is part of a larger system of health care called *oriental medicine*, which includes diet therapy, herbal medicine, medical massage (Tui Na), exercise (Tai Chi and Qi Gong), and meditation. Diet Therapy is said to be the most important Chinese medical specialty.

Acupuncture originated in China approximately 4000 to 5000 years ago with written records from 200 BCE. The term is derived from *acus* (needle) and *punctura* (puncture) and involves puncturing the skin with needles that go into the underlying tissue or even the bone.

A more medical approach to acupuncture (separate from sorcery) is documented by Bian Que (407-310 BCE). During his time, many fundamental Chinese medicine texts were written that are being used and commented on to this day. The basic twelve meridians, which are road maps to life as well as treatment, were also delineated during this time. By the mid 200s up to the early 300s CE, information on disease pathology and its treatment by Chinese medicine were being traded along the Arab route towards the West. Surgery was also performed using cannabis paste for anesthesia.

By the Tang Dynasty (618-907 CE) subspecialties in medicine were established, including internal medicine, gynecology, obstetrics, pediatrics, dermatology, ENT, and surgery. Many famous texts also were written at this time. The trademark of classical acupuncture originated here: "The superior physician is one who can successfully prevent diseases before they develop." Acupuncture, herbs, diet, and hygiene were amalgamated. Before this time they existed as separate specialties.

During the Jin-Yuan Dynasty (1115-1368 CE) there were many foreign invasions. The turmoil led to new traditions and four new schools of healing emerged. These schools form the basis for many strategies of treatment used today. Chronic disease pathology and treatment became more defined.

The Western medicine influence arrived mainly through the Jesuits in the eighteenth century. They shared anatomy, blood letting, and some other western techniques. Much of Western medicine's influence occurred in the 1920s when Chinese medicine itself was banned in China. It was difficult to maintain the ban and it was subsequently lifted.

Even though Osler commented on the use of acupuncture for back pain in his "Principles and Practice of Medicine" of 1892, there was very little acupuncture performed in the U.S outside of Chinese immigrant communities until the 1970s, with the U.S. government's recognition of the People's Republic of China. The media was dazzled by the use of acupuncture anesthesia for a journalist's appendectomy pain and this immediately catapulted acupuncture into the spotlight. There was a flurry of visits to China and a tremendous amount of research, but acupuncture remained an experimental treatment for over 20 years.

The first major breakthrough was in 1994 when the National Institutes of Health (NIH) petitioned the Food and Drug Administration (FDA) at the conclusion of a technology assessment workshop on the safety of acupuncture needles, which included the scientific literature. The FDA reclassified needles from an experimental device to a standard medical device to be used by a qualified practitioner.

Then the debate culminated at the National Institutes of Health (NIH) Consensus Development Conference on Acupuncture held in Bethesda, Maryland on November 3-5, 1997. Although the struggle to fit this modality into a scientific model still exists, researchers feel that enough evidence is already here or forthcoming to embrace acupuncture into our medical model.

> *Promising results have emerged, showing efficacy of acupuncture in adult postoperative and chemotherapy nausea and vomiting and in postoperative dental pain. There are other situations such as addiction, stroke rehabilitation, headache, menstrual cramps, tennis elbow, fibromyalgia, myofascial pain, osteoarthritis, low back pain, carpal tunnel syndrome, and asthma, in which acupuncture may be useful as an adjunct treatment or an acceptable alternative or be included in a comprehensive management program. Further research is likely to uncover additional areas where acupuncture interventions will be useful.*

The practice of classical Chinese medicine continued throughout. The current Traditional Chinese Medicine (TCM) training in American and Chinese schools implies a long-standing institution. However, TCM began during the Communist era at a time when religion, superstition, and psychology were all suppressed. The committees that developed TCM excluded these topics and summarized a lot of traditions. That is why so many people think Chinese medicine does not deal with the mind.

There is a tremendous amount of information that is still buried in the more than 23,000 untranslated Chinese medicine texts. In China, official government policy now calls for all hospitals to incorporate both Western and Eastern modalities. Hopefully we are not going to be too far behind.

Mechanism of Action According to Its Own Theory

Chinese medicine has developed theories and approaches to treat all conditions, whether physical, mental, emotional, or spiritual. Most of the attention in the West regarding acupuncture has been on pain control and analgesia.

Acupuncture is performed at specific points that are palpable indentations on the surface of the skin that, according to most modern texts on acupuncture, display electrophysiologic and anatomic differences from surrounding areas. Acupuncture points lie along lines called *meridians* that are thought to carry a stream of life force or energy called *Qi* (pronounced *chi*) cyclically through the body, connecting with channels and organs deep inside the body. The fact that we do not yet have instruments sensitive enough to measure this energy is not a sufficient reason to deny its existence.

Meridians seem to lie along the planes of fascia between the muscles. There are many meridian systems that are used in acupuncture to create different effects, the most commonly identified ones being the 14 principal meridians. The *8-extraordinary* (curious), *Tendinomuscular, Divergent,* and *Luo* meridians comprise further systems of channels at a "postgraduate" level of acupuncture theory. There are 361 basic acupuncture points represented on the surface of the body that have specific names and functions and also many more "extra" points—trigger points, *Ah shi-pain* points, and microsystem points on the feet, hands, and ears. In fact, the total number of points can be upwards of 1500 and the number of channels over 70.

A brief oriental view of pain is that it results primarily from "stagnant" or blocked *Qi* (life force), and needling the point opens up the "dam" in the flow of energy through a meridian. When one needles a point on the body the patient often feels a sensation in some distant part of the body not directly connected to the point by the nervous system. See Dr. Bruce Pomeranz's work for further discussion.

Chinese medicine has elegant, simple, but very effective treatments which have been developed using the various energetic layers described in the classical texts to strengthen the host and to defend against the "guest" (pathologic) factors.

However, if the host cannot be adequately strengthened to expel the "guest" the "pathogenic factor" is redirected to a more superficial layer, which is usually the joints and musculoskeletal system, and maintained there, which keeps it from affecting the vital organs. Fibromyalgia is a modern example of this fascinating process.[1]

Biologic Mechanism of Action

In *Acupuncture: Textbook and Atlas*, Bruce Pomeranz reviews 228 modern scientific studies on acupuncture and focuses on acupuncture analgesia.[2]

> We conclude that acupuncture activates small myelinated nerve fibers in the muscle, which send impulses to the spinal cord, and then activates three centers (spinal cord, midbrain, and pituitary-hypothalamus) to cause analgesia. The spinal cord center uses enkephalin and dynorphin to block incoming painful information. The midbrain center uses enkephalin to activate the raphe descending system, which inhibits spinal cord pain transmission using the monoamines (serotonin and norepinephrine). The third center is the hypothalamus-pituitary, which releases beta endorphin into the blood and cerebrospinal fluid to cause analgesia at a distance.

There is speculation that as we find out more about the various neurotransmitters, we will find correspondences between their action and that of acupuncture. Recent MRI and SPECT scan results also elucidate the effects of acupuncture on the brain.

An article, "The Scientific Mechanisms of Acupuncture" in *Integrative Medicine Consult* (January 15, 1999) concluded with evidence that acupuncture involves five different methods of transmission of its effects: electric; neurologic; humoral; lymphatic (as a medium for the electroionic flow along fascial planes); and wave propagation.

Forms of Therapy

Systems

Numerous systems of acupuncture have evolved in different cultures with their own unique characteristics. This is apart from the different schools of traditional Chinese medicine. These systems include the following:

1. **Traditional Chinese Medicine** (TCM), as previously mentioned.
2. **French energetics acupuncture,** a derivative of TCM acupuncture, is practiced mostly by medical doctors who are trained either in France or through the Medical Acupuncture program at UCLA. (See "Training.")
3. **Neuroanatomic acupuncture,** which has a Western slant, is very useful for pain problems. Many of these systems may use electric stimulation of points (*electroacupuncture*) to enhance the therapeutic effects of needling. This medically-oriented form is mostly practiced by western doctors.
4. **Five-element acupuncture** is one component of Chinese medicine that originated in the *Nan Jing* writings and is derived from the Taoist philosophy of a human being's interconnectedness with the universe.
5. **Auricular acupuncture** is considered to be a microsystem of acupuncture. It originated in China but was developed in Europe after World War II by Dr. Paul Nogier of Lyon, France, who confirmed that treatment of specific points on the external ear alleviated specific problems in other parts of the body. He proposed and proved that a somatotopic relationship exists between different anatomic areas of the body and specific points on the ear. He then began mapping auricular points based on an embryologic model and found somatic correlations with mesodermal, ectodermal, and endodermal auricular structures. Treatment is with needles, pellets, seeds, or magnets, some of which can be left in place in the ear to continue the treatment.[3]
6. **EAV** (the Medical System Diagnosis Electroacupuncture according to Voll) is defined as a whole-body system of electrophysical measurements at specific anatomic points on the skin where the current state and the regulation dynamics of systems and subsystems of the human body are recorded and any malfunction and blocking of independent regulation mechanism are determined. The specifically required remedy is then selected through the resonance phenomena during the measurement.
7. **Japanese herbal medicine** uses the Chinese text *Shang Han Lun* as its foundation. Chinese monks traveled to Japan in the fifth century to spread Buddhism and by the sixth century the Japanese learned of the Chinese culture from envoys. The Japanese acupuncture variations are being translated into English by Manaka, Matsumoto, and Birch.

8. **Vietnamese traditions,** which were developed from the French when they occupied Vietnam, have more recently become available in the U.S. and are being incorporated into some of the U.S. schools.

9. An **American** style of acupuncture has been described and is beginning to evolve, but it is far from a fixed body of information that has withstood the test of time.

10. **Classical acupuncture** consists of practitioners and researchers who translate from the original texts and possess a medical and often a religious background. Philosophy cannot be separated from oriental medicine, which is applied philosophy.

11. **Korean hand acupuncture** is another microsystem of acupuncture used in the U.S. in which the hand is a said to be a representation of the whole body. For an experienced practitioner this can be used as a primary treatment modality or an adjunct. It can be taught to patients for use at home with either massage or moxa.[4]

Methods of Stimulation: Needle, Moxa, Electric, and Laser

Acupuncture needles range from 24 to 40-gauge and are between 0.5 and 2.0 inches in length. The longer ones have to be inserted through a plastic tube to keep them from bending. Historically the needles were gold, silver, and later stainless steel. Now they are essentially stainless steel and disposable. They are generally gas-sterilized and individually wrapped.

In some traditions, acupuncture is incomplete without the concurrent use of moxabustion and it is heavily used in the U.S. Moxa is the powdered leaves of *Artemisia vulgaris* or mugwort, which are burned near or on an acupuncture point. It is formed into a tiny cone that can be as small as a rice grain or as large as a small upright triangle (0.5 cm). It also can be burned on the handle of an acupuncture needle. It also can be used at a short distance from the body using a moxa pole, which resembles a long cigar. Patients can take these home with them. There also is a Japanese moxa that comes with a sticky base and a small tube of moxa that is placed over a point and burned. Moxa is generally used to warm the body where cold is a significant part of the pathology.

Silver, gold, and stainless steel pellets are also used for stimulating points mostly in the ear but also on the body. In the West they have been substituted for rice or grain kernels.

Electric stimuli also are used. A simple method that uses the body's own electricity is called *ion pumping cords,* in which copper cords are attached to needles between two points with no outside electric stimulation. The TENS unit has taught us that the best "electric window" for chronic pain (C fibers) is in the 2 to 4 Hz range, and the acute pain (A fibers) respond to the 150 to 200 Hz range. Fatiguing or habituation occurs when the same stimulus is used over and over, which at least is a partial explanation of why the TENS units have limited success. Attaching electrodes to the handles of acupuncture needles can deliver a fixed current to an acupuncture point and give greater stimulation. It is used in China as well as the West, but not all forms of Chinese medicine use this modality. It may be used more often for analgesia, paralysis, and addiction.

Laser (cold or not cutting) is also used. It is still considered experimental in the U.S. but is widely used in Canada and Europe, especially for scars and wound healing. It affects the most superficial layers of tissue and is painless. The frequencies most responsive to the various parts of the body have been analyzed and chosen for use. These lasers use helium, neon, galium, arsenic, and aluminum as laser diodes. Treatments are between 0.5 and 10.0 joules per treatment point. Ultrasound uses about 100 times the amount of energy per laser treatment. Because the diode is monochromatic (white) it is usually outside the visible spectrum of a human.[5]

Demographics

A recent *Discover* magazine article on acupuncture announced that between 9 million and 12 million acupuncture treatments are given each year in the U.S.

The National Certification Commission for Acupuncture and Oriental Certification Medicine (NCCAOM) has a database of over 8500 active acupuncturists with members in every state. Certification for each acupuncturist requires 500 patient visits per year and more than 100 patients, which gives a conservative estimate of 850,000 patients seeking acupuncture.

The American Academy of Medical Acupuncture (AAMA) has 1000 members and the postgraduate Medical Acupuncture program at UCLA has taught over 2000 doctors.

There are numerous other organizations and thousands of Chinese acupuncturists but no general census to determine the actual number of practitioners.

Indications and Reasons for Referral

The World Health Organization of the United Nations has identified more than 40 medical conditions effectively treated with acupuncture. A quote from the American Academy of Medical Acupuncture (AAMA)'s website gives an overview of the conditions treated by medical acupuncturists.

> *Acupuncture is highly effective in treating both acute and chronic pain. Studies have shown that 85% of patients with chronic pain respond positively to acupuncture with improvement or resolution of their symptoms. These conditions include sports injuries; sprains and strains; pain and "whiplash" injuries due to motor-vehicle accidents; myofascial pain syndrome; fibromyalgia; arthritis; headaches (posttraumatic, muscle-tension, migraines, cluster); low back, thoracic, and neck pain; sciatica; nerve pain due to compression on nerves; carpal tunnel syndrome; overuse syndromes; reflex sympathetic dystrophy; phantom limb pain; postsurgical pain; pain resulting from spinal cord injuries; and cancer.*
>
> *Common conditions effectively treated by acupuncture primarily or adjunctively may include sinusitis, allergies, tinnitus, sore throats, high blood pressure, asthma, gastroesophageal reflux, hyperacidity, and peptic ulcer disease, constipation, diarrhea, spastic colon, urinary incontinence, bladder and kidney infections, PMS, infertility, painful and/or abnormal menstruation, endometriosis, memory problems, insomnia, recovery from strokes (i.e. movement disorders/spasticity), multiple sclerosis, sensory disturbances, depression, anxiety and other psychological disorders.*

Acupuncture also has an extremely important role in preventing illness and may even be utilized to facilitate personal transformational and spiritual growth processes.

The list goes far beyond the NIH consensus report but is still focused largely on analgesia and pain control. As with all alternative therapies, the use of acupuncture does not preclude the use of mainstream medical therapies.

Research Base

The Chinese have chosen to use hundreds of years of observation and patient experience as their gold standard rather than the double-blind studies that are done for a relatively short time with relatively few patients. While clinical outcome studies are more amenable to evaluate acupuncture, certainly double-blind studies have been and should be done when they make sense in both Eastern and Western thinking.

Evidence Based

A comprehensive acupuncture bibliography was prepared in support of the NIH Consensus Development Conference by staff at the National Institute on Drug Abuse (NIDA) and the National Library of Medicine (NLM). The literature search spanned from January 1970 through October 1997 and identified 2302 citations in various categories including a wide range of systems.

These categories include addictions and psychiatric disorders; cardiovascular system; dermatology; face, sinuses, mouth, and throat; gastroenterology; general pain; genitourinary, pelvic, and reproductive systems; headache; low back, sciatica; lower extremities; miscellaneous; nausea, vomiting, and postoperative problems; neck and shoulders; nervous system and special senses; upper extremities and breast; and veterinary medicine.

Birch and Hammerschlag's *Acupuncture Efficacy: A Compendium of Controlled Clinical Studies* gives a more detailed appraisal of the literature.[6]

Pomeranz's groundbreaking work is also very important to review.[7] A metaanalysis by Patel et al reviews randomized controlled trials to determine efficacy of acupuncture for pain. They felt that the trial sizes were usually small and difficult to determine efficacy but when pooled the outcome was in favor of acupuncture.

Another study on postoperative nausea, vomiting, and pain by Dundee et al[8] demonstrated the efficacy of acupuncture on over 500 patients.

Future Research Opportunities and Priorities

The Office of Alternative Medicine, now the National Center for Complementary and Alternative Medicine (NCCAM), is an independent body within the NIH. With an initial budget of $50 million it has several acupuncture research projects underway.[9] We would like to see a long-term clinical outcome study that encompasses acupuncture, Chinese herbal medicine, dietary therapy, and exercise regimens for two of our most chronic diseases: fibromyalgia and chronic fatigue. Control and comparison groups could include combinations of two of these modalities and a group that makes no changes and takes no therapy.

Druglike Information

Safety

Risk of infection is negligible when sterile, disposable stainless steel needles are used and clean needle technique is applied.

Actions and Pharmacokinetics

A patient is more sensitive to alcohol on the day of treatment. Drugs can change the signs and symptoms. Beta blockers are not a contraindication for acupuncture but they slow the pulse and pulse-taking results have to be adjusted. This is one of the reasons why it is *critical* for acupuncturists to be very familiar with drugs and their actions and for all practitioners to know what medications, herbs, or therapies their patients are taking.

Warnings, Contraindications, and Precautions

As in any medical encounter where needles are used, the risk of vasovagal faint is always a possibility. For this reason, acupuncture is usually administered with the patient in the reclining position.

Drug Interactions

Some homeopaths prefer patients not to receive acupuncture concurrently with treatment.

Adverse Reactions

Acupuncture is not innocuous; pneumothorax has occurred with overzealous needling of chest points. Bruising by hitting capillaries and veins does occur. Fainting occurs either from fear of needles or vasovagal reactions. Fainting is treated with moxa at two particular acupuncture sites. Skin infection can occur around the needle site. There can also be a transient increase in symptoms, which the Chinese refer to as "chasing the dragon." The occurrence of any of these reactions is rare. Patients are encouraged to call their practitioners with any concerns. One author has had only four after-hours calls in 18 years.

Pregnancy and Lactation

Pregnancy is a contraindication. An experienced practitioner who already knows the patient before pregnancy will treat if the need arises, avoiding points that can adversely affect pregnancy. Acupuncture can facilitate lactation and has been used for many years for this purpose.

Trade Products, Administration, and Dosage

Various types of needles (mostly sterile and disposable) are on the market and reliable companies can be recommended by acupuncture organizations.

Self-Help versus Professional

Acupuncture is a skill requiring both education and experience. Only a trained professional should administer acupuncture.

Visiting a Professional

A typical first visit starts with an extensive medical and acupuncture-oriented history. Acupuncture questions might seem quite unusual: "In what season or climate do you feel better or worse?" "What colors, tastes, temperatures, food, and drink do you prefer?"

The physical exam consists of confirming the medical findings, then Chinese pulses are taken. The wrist is held for several minutes and minute changes in the radial artery are noted at different points. The tongue is examined and then trigger points are palpated. Particular note is made of skin changes, scarring, and temperature differences on the skin and the abdomen is palpated for areas of tenderness.

Usually at the same time, some explanation is given to the patient, if it is appropriate, about the pattern of pathology and a first treatment is performed. The first time needles are inserted the patient is lying down, not sitting up. This makes it less likely that the patient will faint. The needles are usually left in for 15 minutes. Sometimes they are manipulated, but often they are just left in place. The patient is usually left alone in a room with subdued lighting and has a bell to ring if they want the practitioner. (If they feel faint with the insertion of needles the practitioner takes them out and briskly rubs certain points to bring back the circulation.)

Before the needles are removed, patients are usually asked for anything they may have noticed during the time of treatment. Then with the removal of the needles, patients are reminded that they may feel better, either suddenly or (more likely) gradually, almost imperceptibly, or that sometimes symptoms may be aggravated before improving.

Follow-up visits include a much shorter history of what has happened in the interval and other pieces of history may be expanded or clarified. Then a second treatment is performed. There should be an agreement between the patient and practitioner regarding improvement or movement in the condition within a certain number of treatments.

Costs can be quite varied. The first treatment could be from $75 to $125 and follow-up visits could be from $40 to $80. However, there are insurance companies that are beginning to cover acupuncture.

Credentialing

The National Certification Commission for Acupuncture and Oriental Certification Medicine (NCCAOM) is a nonprofit organization established by the profession to create nationally recognized standards of competence and safety in acupuncture and oriental medicine. NCCAOM certification is accepted by a majority of the states requiring licensing. Acupuncture licensure is now available in 36 states and the District of Columbia. The NCCAOM is a member of the National Organization for Competency Assurance (NOCA) and is accredited by the National Commission for Certifying Agencies (NCCA).

NCCAOM certification in acupuncture offers a diploma in acupuncture (Dipl. Ac. NCCAOM). The NCCAOM examination in acupuncture includes acupuncture, clean needle technique, and point location skills.

There are several levels of criteria for the acupuncture examination, including the following:

1. Completion of an acupuncture program with a minimum of 3 years after a 2-year undergraduate program and 1350 hours of entry-level acupuncture education, including at least 500 clinical hours
2. Apprenticeship
3. Professional practice (see "Resources")

The American Academy of Medicine Acupuncture (AAMA) offers a certification exam for medical doctors. However, most states do not restrict the practice of acupuncture for doctors. Some states do require a minimum of 200 hours of formal training and certification. In reality most physicians spend 10 hours for every classroom hour totaling approximately 2000 hours of study to incorporate acupuncture into their practices.

Training

The Accreditation Commission for Acupuncture and Oriental Medicine (ACAOM) sets standards for a master's degrees in either acupuncture or oriental medicine. There are more than 50 schools of acupuncture in the country, and practitioners function in every state; however, not all may be accredited by ACAOM.

Medical Acupuncture for Physicians identifies itself as the most convenient and reliable training program for busy physicians to obtain the clinical skills needed to incorporate acupuncture into their practices. The program has been taught since 1983 through the Office of Continuing Medicine Education at the UCLA School of Medicine. The founder, Dr. Joseph Helms, trained in France, where acupuncture has been practiced for more than several hundred years.

What to Look for in a Provider

See "Credentialing." A good reputation in the community is an essential component of a good referral.

Associations

There are possibly hundreds of smaller or younger organizations in the country that operate on a more local level. The American Association of Oriental Medicine (AAOM) is the oldest organization representing individual practitioners of Acupuncture and Oriental Medicine in the United States. The American Academy of Medicine Acupuncture (AAMA) was founded in 1987 and is the only national professional society of North American physicians who have incorporated acupuncture into their medical practices. Often more than 1000 requests are fulfilled each month for their patient referral service.

NCCAOM
11 Canal Center Plaza, Suite 300
Alexandria, VA 22314
Tel: (703) 548-9004
Fax: (703) 548-9079
www.nccaom.org

The American Association of Oriental Medicine
Tel (patient referrals): (888) 500-7999
www.aaom.org

AAMA
5820 Wilshire Blvd., Suite 500
Los Angeles, CA 90036
Tel (patient referrals): (800) 521-2262
www.aama-ntl.org/index

Suggested Reading

1. Stux G, Pomeranz B: *Basics of acupuncture*, ed 3. Translations from Chinese by Sahm KA. Berlin, 1995, Springer-Verlag.
   This is an introductory book combining Western medicine and traditional Chinese concepts. Pomeranz is noted for his discovery of the endorphin effect of acupuncture.
2. Schneideman J: *Medical acupuncture*, Hong Kong, 1988, Mayfield Medical.
   A textbook of modern acupuncture. The author shares his teaching and the lessons learned from years of experience in medical acupuncture in the context of holistic medicine. The presentations venture into important areas, such as nutrition and other holistic concepts, but are adapted to the Western setting.
3. Ellis A et al: *Fundamentals of Chinese acupuncture*, Brookline, Mass, 1994, Paradigm.
   This book is compiled from both modern TCM and classical Chinese texts, creating a clinical text that reflects both. It also addresses the most common learning problems identified by acupuncture students and clinicians.
4. Kaptchuk T: *The web that has no weaver: understanding Chinese medicine*, New York, 1983, Congdon & Weed.
   This book is the easiest source for someone trying to understand the modern application of ancient Chinese medicine from the practitioner's point of view.
5. Deadman P et al: *A manual of acupuncture*, Nove, England, 1998, Journal of Chinese Medicine Publications.
   An excellent book researched over many years. For each point there is a dedicated drawing followed by regional body drawings. The high quality of the 500 drawings also is conveyed in the "Acupuncture Point Cards," a companion card set.

Book Sources

Redwing Book Company
Tel: (800) 873-3946
www.redwingbooks.com

Blue Poppy Press
Tel: (303) 447-8372
www.healthy.net/bluepoppy/

M.E.D. Servi Systems Canada Ltd.
Tel: (800) 267-6868
www.medserv.ca

Bibliography

Dold C: Needles and nerves, *Discover* 19:9, 1998.

Ergil KV: Acupuncture: history, theory, and practice, *Integrat Med Consult* 1:20-23, 1999.

Helms J: *Acupuncture energetics: a clinical approach for physicians*, Berkeley, Calif, 1995, Medical Acupuncture Publishers.

Klein LJ, Trachtenberg AI, compilers: *Acupuncture bibliography online*, Bethesda, Md, Oct. 1997, National Library of Medicine. Citations from Jan. 1970 through Oct. 1997. Available from www.nlm.nih.gov/pubs/resources or in print from the NIH.

Manaka Y: The layman's guide to acupuncture, New York, 1984, Weatherhill.

Matsumoto K, Birch S: *Five elements and ten stems*, Brookline, Mass, 1983, Paradigm Publications.

Patel M et al: A metaanalysis of acupuncture for chronic pain, *Internal J Epidemiol* 18(4):900-906, 1989.

References

1. Yuen JC: *Chinese medicine history and quotes from class transcriptions by Dr. C. Dean, 1997-1999.* Presented by GAIA Inc. at the Swedish Massage Institute, November 22-23, 1997, New York.

2. Stux G, Pomeranx B: *Acupuncture: textbook and atlas*, Berlin, 1987, Springer-Verlag.

3. Oelson T: *Auricular acupuncture*, Brookline, Mass, 1991, Paradigm Publications.

4. Yoo TW, Eum YMJ, Koryho SC: *Korean hand acupuncture*, Seoul, 1988.

5. Kert J, Rose L: *Clinical laser therapy, low level laser therapy*, Scandinavian Medica Laser Technology, 1989.

6. Birch S, Hammerschlag, R: *Acupuncture efficacy: a compendium of controlled clinical studies*, National Academy of Acupuncture and Oriental Medicine, 1996.

7. Stux G, Pomeranz B: *Basics of acupuncture*, Berlin, 1995, Springer-Verlag.

8. Dundee JW et al: Effect of stimulation of the P-6 antiemetic point on postoperative nausea and vomiting, *Branch J Anaesth* 63(5):612-618, 1989.

9. *Alt Ther* 5(1):24-26, 1999.

Traditional Chinese Herbal Medicine

MARGO JORDAN PARKER

Origins and History

Traditional Chinese medicine (also known as oriental medicine, TCM, or acupuncture and oriental medicine [AOM]) is a completely articulated system of natural medicine, which looks at the entire body, mind, and spirit as an integrated whole. Central to Chinese medicine is the concept of *Qi* (chi), which is described as the body's "vital life force" that connects the body, mind, and spirit. Our Qi also connects us with the outer world. Our relative health is dependent on the balance of all the internal and external factors. The promotion of balance, the maintenance of health and well-being, and the prevention of disease are the main aims of Chinese medicine, but it often excels as a natural first line of defense. TCM includes acupuncture, Chinese herbs, moxabustion, massage (Tui Na), movement and breathing exercises (Tai Chi and Qi Gong), as well as food therapy (Chinese nutrition), and lifestyle modification. This discussion addresses Chinese herbal medicine.

Chinese herbology has a rich tradition in medical literature which, according to scholars Joseph Needham and Lu Gwei-Djen of the East Asian History of Science Library at Cambridge, began with the *Shen Nong Ben Cao Jing* (Pharmacopeia of the Heavenly Husbandman) in the second century BCE. Much later in CE 659 came the imperially commissioned *Hsin Hsiu Pen Ts'as* (Newly Reorganized Pharmacopoeia), a world-reknowned history of natural pharmaceutics. It was not until CE 1600 that the *Pharmacopoeia Londiniensis*, the first official pharmacopoeia of the Western world, was compiled.

Mechanisms of Action According to Its Own Theory

Chinese herbs are most effective when used in accordance with the traditional indications whereby each patient's constitution and collective symptoms are taken into account in a holistic way according to their pattern of disharmony. This is the point where TCM differs significantly from modern medicine. In TCM not all patients suffering from a specific disease would be given the same medication. A central tenant to TCM is an elaborate philosophy and diagnostic technique that places greater emphasis on the whole person, which we will review briefly.

The Chinese model is very different from the anatomy, physiology and disease theory in allopathic medicine. TCM considers the body/mind as a dynamic system that reflects the cycles of change and its environment. The system has been completely articulated over thousands of years and views the components along with that of structure. The emphasis is on supporting what Weil referred to as the body's healing system.[1] Chinese medicine articulated how that works thousands of years ago in its own language, and it has been transmitted to us for use in these modern times.

The basic substances, which range from the material to the immaterial, are Qi, Jing, Blood, Body Fluids, and Shen.[2]

Qi (Chi)

Qi has variously been translated as "energy," "life force," and "bioelectroenergy." It also has been compared to the concept of *prana* (the breath of life) in ayurvedic medicine; perhaps it is similar to ATP. Similar to electricity, we cannot see it; but we know its potential and applications. The flow and quality of Qi in the body is intimately connected to health and disease.

Jing

Jing is usually translated as "essence" and may be considered the underpinning of all aspects of organic life. Qi is responsible for the ongoing, day-to-day movements in the body, whereas Jing can be considered an individual's constitutional makeup and is associated with slow developmental change that characterizes the organism's growth from a fetus through life and ultimately to old age and death.

Blood

Blood in Chinese medicine is not the same substance that is recognized as blood in Western medicine. Chinese medicine sees Blood as a very material and fluid manifestation of Qi.

Body Fluids

Body fluids (Jin Ye) are considered to be the organic liquids that moisten and lubricate the body in addition to Blood, which is considered separately because of its importance to Chinese medicine.

Shen

The last basic substance that we will briefly discuss is the Shen, which can be translated as the mind or psyche of the individual. Jing, Qi and Shen are referred to collectively in Chinese medicine as the "Three Treasures" and are believed to be the essential components of life. The Three Treasures, along with Blood and Body Fluids, comprise the basic substances in the body, according to Chinese medicine. When the basic substances are in harmony the individual will be radiant with life, physically fit, mentally sharp and alert, and free of disease.

The Organ Systems

In Chinese medicine, although organ systems are translated with our common Western names, they are actually considered complete networks rather than just individual structures, with meridians that traverse the body and specific functions on energetic as well as physical levels. Illness is seen as a process, which is referred to as a pattern of disharmony of the fundamental substances of the organism. The therapeutic goal is to balance these substances and bring the healing system back to homeostasis. The functions of the organ systems in this medical theory are outlined in the table below. Understanding these functions aids in applying the appropriate herb to obtain the therapeutic result of returning the body to a state of health.

The Causes of Disharmony

Chinese medicine thinks of disease as arising from influences that have disturbed the harmony and balance of the whole energy system, including the physical body and emotions.

The Functions of the Organs in Chinese Medicine

Organ	Function
Heart	Governs the blood, controls the blood vessels, houses the shen, manifests in the complexion, opens into the tongue, controls sweat, and maintains joy.
Pericardium	Protects the heart and guides joy and pleasures.
Triple energizer	Coordinates transformation and transportation of fluids in the body and regulates the warming function of the body.
Small intestine	Separates the pure from the impure.
Spleen	Governs transportation and transformation of food and fluids, contains the blood, dominates the muscles and the limbs, opens into the mouth and manifests itself in the lips, controls the raising of the qi, and houses thought.
Stomach	Receives and stores food; stomach qi should descend.
Kidneys	Stores jing, dominates reproduction, growth, and development, produces marrow, fills the brain, dominates the bones, manufactures blood, and maintain the gate of vitality or adrenal glands. Governs water in the body, controls the reception of qi from the lungs, opens into the sense organ of the ear, manifests in the health of the hair, houses the will, and controls fear.
Bladder	Stores urine and controls excretion.
Lungs	Govern qi flow and respiration, control dispersion and descending of breath, energy, and fluids, regulate the water passage of the body, control the skin and hair, open into the nose, and connect to the world.
Large intestine	Absorbs the pure and excretes the impure.
Liver	Stores blood, controls the smooth flow of qi, controls the tendons, manifests in the nails, opens into the eyes, and exercises control.
Gallbladder	Stores bile and dominates decision making.

These terms may be equated to modern biomedical conditions, but looking at the conditions within the paradigm of the theory of TCM provides a more balanced, integrated perspective.

EXTERNAL CAUSES

In Chinese medicine there are considered to be six external causes of disharmony that relate to climate conditions. These include wind, cold, damp, fire and heat, dryness, and summer heat wind. Wind causes movement, sudden change, and shaking and swaying.

INTERNAL CAUSES

The major internal causes of disharmony are considered physiologic in nature and are termed the seven emotions. These seven emotions are anger, joy, sadness, grief, pensiveness, fear, and fright. Clearly the experience of emotion is intrinsic to the human experience, and in Chinese medicine these emotions are as important for maintaining health as they are for creating potential ill health. It is always seen as a matter of degree. If there is an excess or a lack of emotional expression in any area, then this will likely lead to disharmony. The seven emotions are considered neither "good" nor "bad"; it is how they balance out in an individual's life that is considered important. The seven emotions are central to the concept of how disharmonies occur in Chinese medicine, and an observation of the emotions may lead to a disharmony of the organ system involved, as in the following examples:

> Evidence of anxiety may suggest a Heart pattern and disturbed Shen.
> Evidence of depression may suggest Lung or Heart disharmony.
> Evidence of anger or frustration may suggest a Liver disharmony.
> Evidence of poor concentration may suggest a Spleen disharmony.
> Evidence of undue fear may suggest a Kidney disharmony.

Miscellaneous causes of disharmony in Chinese medicine consist of constitutional factors, lifestyle factors, work, exercise, sexual activity, and diet.

Whether they are emotions or external pernicious influences, these all may lead to a disharmony that may be treated by Chinese medicine. Chinese medicine recognizes the manner in which a whole variety of influences may create patterns of disharmony in the individual.

Diagnostic Approaches

In Chinese medicine the diagnostic process is considered in the four examinations. These four areas include looking, hearing and smelling, questioning, and palpation. *Looking* details the physical exam and observation of the skin, hair, posture, and affect (or Shen in Chinese medicine). The tongue diagnosis is critical and is elaborated in the following section. *Hearing and smelling* observes the patient's body odors and the sound of the voice. *Questioning* asks basic questions to determine the pattern of disharmony. *Palpation* may involve an abdominal exam that often is used for diagnostic purposes in Japan by palpating for tender areas along the meridians or traditional pulse diagnosis. (See "Acupuncture" for more details.)

Observation of the tongue is a reliable and accurate diagnostic tool that is helpful in any clinical practice to determine what internal imbalance is occurring. The "geography" of the tongue is considered important. Various areas relate to the condition of specific internal organs, as shown in the figure below. By observing the tongue condition in each of the areas, information is gathered regarding the condition of the organ system corresponding to that area and the general characteristics of the tongue itself. The important tongue characteristics are provided in the box on page 208.[3]

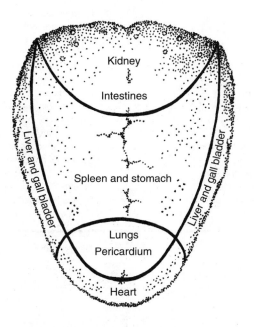

Tongue diagnosis in Chinese Medicine. Representation of the condition of internal organ systems at different parts of the tongue.

Principles of Treatment

The following guidelines are basic to Chinese herbal formulation. If a deficiency exists, or to prevent deficiency, the system must be tonified by ingesting tonic herbs. If an excess exists, it must be reduced by dispersing herbs. If the excess is hot, it must be cooled with cooling herbs; if the excess is cold, it must be warmed with warming herbs. If there is excess damp or phlegm, this must be resolved using herbs that specifically balance each condition. If there is stagnation of Qi or Blood, these should be unblocked with stronger herbs for a brief course of treatment, and then tonifying herbs should be used to "support the root" (Fu Zheng) and restore health. The herbs have been classified according to their characteristics of temperature, action, meridian influence, and therapeutic properties. This classification of the herbs was developed and perfected over many centuries and are classical formulas applicable today.

Tongue Characteristics	
Characteristics	**Significance**
Thin white coating	Normal
Thick coat	Presence of pathogenic influence
No coat or peeled	Yin deficiency present (false heat)
White coat	Cold present (normal when thin)
Yellow coat	Heat present
Slightly moist	Normal
Wet tongue	Internal damp present
Sticky tongue	Phlegm present
Dry tongue	Heat present
Pale red tone	Normal
Pale tone	Deficient condition
Red tongue	Presence of internal heat
Purple tongue	Stagnation of blood
Blue or black tongue	Internal cold present
Thin tongue	Deficient condition
Swollen tongue	Internal damp present
Stiff or deviated tongue	Internal wind present
Quivering tongue	Spleen Qi deficiency
Short horizontal cracks	Spleen Qi deficiency
Toothmarks at side	Spleen Qi deficiency
Shallow midline crack (not at tip)	Stomach deficiency
Long deep midline crack (to tip)	Heart condition present

Biologic Mechanisms of Action

Bensky et al state in their introduction to *The Chinese Materia Medica* (revised edition) that "herbs of all types, including those from China, are composed of a multitude of ingredients and their interactions with the body are exceedingly complex. A high level of sophistication of research methodology is necessary to describe the interaction between the human body and substances as complex as those contained in the *Materia Medica*. Only recently has such a rigorous methodology begun to develop. For example, the herb *Herba hedyotitis diffusae* has been shown to be clinically effective in the prevention and treatment of a variety of infectious diseases. However, it has not demonstrated a significant inhibitory effect in vitro against any major pathogen. Only as techniques became available to test the immunological system did it become apparent that at least part of this herb's effect was due to its enhancement of the body's immune response."[4]

Forms of Therapy

Chinese herbal medicine may be prescribed in an office setting by a practitioner trained and licensed in acupuncture and oriental medicine. Patent formulas from China, which have been in question as to their efficacy, labeling, and occasional presence of contaminants or adulterants, are available over the counter in Chinatowns and Asian markets. There are many traditional Chinese herbal pharmacies where handwritten prescriptions for raw herbs are filled and the herbs are then brewed at home by the patient. This practice is most common in the Asian community as the American consumer does not comply with the typically bitter flavor of Chinese herbal medicinals.

The superior and middle class herbs that are tonics are pleasant-tasting and may be used for long periods of time to fortify the system. These herbs, which include ginseng, lycii berries, jujube dates, ginger, and shiitake mushrooms, are very well tolerated and many Westerners seek them out in their raw form for inclusion in the diet for health maintenence. The newest trend is in concentrated formulas manufactured by a reputable source using modern facilities either in the West or Asia. These formulations are based on the time-tested formulas from the ancient Chinese texts or newer revised versions. These formulations are marketed to physicians or lay persons for specific conditions or imbalances, along with information on their application, in a manner similar to the way pharmaceuticals are marketed to physicians. Practitioners who are educated in the formulation of traditional Chinese herbal medicine may also use the refined herbs to build a formula specific to an individual patient's needs. Some manufacturers also provide this service to their physicians.[5]

Demographics

Practitioners who are licensed to prescribe traditional Chinese herbs or formulas are most heavily populated in the western part of the U.S. This form of therapy is extremely popular in California, Oregon, Washington, Florida, New Mexico, and in the Tri-State area (New York, New Jersey, and Connecticut) on the East Coast. There are more than two dozen schools that have 2 to 4 year academic and clinical programs, which qualify graduates for licensing exams in 32 states and the District of Columbia. There are now more than 15,000 licensed providers of acupuncture and oriental medicine (AOM) nationally.

The use of Chinese herbal medicine has spread beyond the Chinese community and the patent formulas available in Chinatowns across the country. Chinese medicine has caught the attention of Westerners interested in health and disease prevention. At this time, Chinese herbal medicine is most popular on the West and East coasts, but it is catching on across the country as did the acceptance of acupuncture.

Indications and Reasons for Referral

Classical ailments and conditions for referring to Chinese herbal medicine stem from the functional disorders that have not responded well to Western medicine. These include the following conditions: chronic or acute pain; allergies; menopausal issues; arthritis; symptoms of stress; fatigue; and digestive disorders. Patients who are seeking optimal well-being and prevention of disease are also interested in herbal medicine to strengthen their resistance and immune system. Similarly, in trained hands, it is commonly used in preconception, pregnancy, and postpartum care. Chinese herbal medicine is now being used extensively in Japan, where it is known as *Kampo*. The Kampo formulations are recommended by the Japanese Ministry of Health.[6] Chinese herbal prescriptions are available on the national medical benefits plan because of their cost-effectiveness in Japanese health care. The Japanese have found that Kampo shows the best results with chronic illnesses, such as chronic arthritis, chronic kidney conditions, hepatitis, diabetes, and women's conditions such as PMS, dysmennorhea (painful periods), and menopausal symptoms. Traditional remedies also have had marked success with the common cold. Some of the best of these remedies can be traced back to the Chinese medical classic, the *Shang Han Lun (The Treatise on Cold and Febrile Disease)*, which is probably about 1800 years old.

Office Applications

Chinese herbal medicine is used for allergies, PMS, stress, and postpartum care (care is taken with lactating mothers). It also is used for arthritis, back pain, pulmonary, gynecologic, and ENT concerns such as asthma, pneumonia, pharyngitis, sinusitis, and tinnitus, cystitis, amenorrhea, uterine fibroids, prostate disease, and various infections.

A simple ranking of conditions responsive to Chinese herbal treatments is as follows. As with all alternative therapies, use of Chinese herbal medicines does not preclude the use of mainstream medical therapies in addition.

Top level: *A therapy ideally suited for these conditions*
Allergies; postpartum care; premenstrual syndrome; and stress

Second level: *One of the better therapies for these conditions*
Addictions; amenorrhea; restless leg syndrome; arthritis; asthma; back pain; benign prostatic hypertrophy; bladder infection; bronchitis; candidiasis; pneumonia; pregnancy and childbirth; prostatic cancer; prostatitis; respiratory conditions; rheumatoid arthritis; sinusitis; sleep disorders; stomachache; strep throat; tinnitus; ulcers; uterine fibroids; vaginal infection; and viral and bacterial infections

Third level: *A valuable adjunctive therapy for these conditions*
AIDS; cancer; cataracts; cervical cancer; periodic leg movement syndrome; pinworms; retinopathy; sexually transmitted disease; sleep apnea; syphilis; trichomosis; and vision disorders

Practical Applications

Because of the complexity of Chinese herbal medicine, formal diagnosis and treatment is best referred to an experienced provider. Common conditions and preventive health care may be addressed by modern patent medicines and formulary notes. Few forms of nontraditional medicine are as complex as Chinese herbal medicine, and proper study takes years. In addition the proper use of Chinese herbal medicine requires availability from a manufacturer that complies with the manufacturing industry standards (good manufacturing practice or GMP) to insure correct dispensing of herbal preparations and avoid the possibility of products containing contaminants or adulterants.

Research Base

Evidence Based

Many studies confirm the effectiveness of this modality. Medline lists many positive studies reported in just the past 2 years and research has been reported in the English language since the late 1970s. Because of the number of studies available the reader is referred to standard journal references sources, such as Medline.

Risk and Safety

In Hong Kong, where the use of Chinese herbs is both widespread and unregulated, it has been shown that only 0.2% of the general medical admissions to the Prince of Wales Hospital were due to adverse reactions to Chinese medicine, as compared to 4.4% of admissions caused by Western pharmaceutics.[7] Hu[8] has recently developed an outline of the toxicity of Chinese herbal medicine. He identifies the three classes of Chinese herbs, their characteristics, and toxicity levels. Treatment of a disease entity is more of a last resort in Chinese medicine and the use of herbs that support the body's healing system and are closer to high-nutrient foods are preferred over the lower class herbs, which are toxic to treat disease.

> Upper class herbs: Nontoxic, possess rejuvenating properties. Examples: *Radix ginseng, Ganoderma, Fructus schizandrae,* and others
>
> Middle class herbs: Most are nontoxic and help to maintain health. Examples: *Radix angelicae sinensis* (tang-kuei), *Rhizoma zingerberis siccatum* (ginger), and others
>
> Lower class herbs: Toxic and used to treat various diseases. Examples: *Tuberaconiti, Radix et Rhizoma Rhei*

Safety is a primary interest of consumers, practitioners, and regulatory agencies. To insure a maximum degree of safety, Hu proposes that the coalition of manufacturers work cooperatively in developing adequate use and safety guidelines for every herb in trade, both through health professionals and the commercial market. Safety may be addressed in the following ways:

1. Identify those herbs that should be dispensed only by experts in their use.
2. Provide manufacturers with labeling guidelines that outline proper use of botanicals available in the open market, including dose limitations, contraindications, and restrictions.
3. Develop a "pharmaco-vigilance" program that can monitor adverse side-effects.
4. Develop botanic monographs outlining proper use and manufacturing parameters.
5. Adhere to appropriate GMP for the manufacture of herbal supplements.

Efficacy

The efficacy of Chinese herbal medicine is dependent on the following conditions: 1) the quality of the herbal formula; 2) patient compliance with the form of delivery, which may be raw unprepared herbs, capsules, tablets, tinctures, or granules; and 3) correct diagnosis and indication for the herb or formula.

Future Research Opportunities and Priorities

Future research opportunities abound that will help to integrate TCM and Western medicine. A study designed to explore the benefit of Fu Zheng therapy ("support the root") in conduction with modern cancer treatments would be very exciting.

Druglike Information

Safety

See "Research."

Actions and Pharmokinetics

The pharmokinetics and actions obviously vary depending on the herb. The pharmocologically active constituents of ginseng, for example, are identified as dammarane-type triterpenoidal glycosides. Japanese studies have reported 15 separate glycosides of this type, which were named *ginsenosides*. Shibita et al gave them the code R (Ra, Rb, Rc, and so on). All of them have been isolated and their structures are completely known. They fall into two groups of compounds, each group consisting of different sugars combined with the same core triterpene and are called *protopanaxadiol* and *protopanaxatriol*. This is just for one type of ginseng; other types have shown completely different types of saponins.[9] Although the active constituents of the herbs may now be isolated, there is a strong argument against simply using the isolated active constituents in order for the pharmacology or the future to evolve beyond pathology into preventive medicine.[10]

Warnings, Contraindications, and Precautions

Some problems have occurred when single herbs in the medicinal categories are used apart from their traditional combinations because the formulas use herbs to counterbalance any side effects. Side effects have also been noted when the active component of a single herb is used rather than the complete herb or traditional formula.[11]

Drug or Other Interactions

Drug interactions, patient sensitivity, and untreated or undiagnosed medical conditions are the key points for awareness. There are certain Chinese herbs that are incompatible with each other. There are Chinese herbal formulas that should not be used with basic constitutional types; this information would be known by the practitioner prescribing the formulas. And there are specific herbs that should not be used together and with other substances.*, 12

Adverse Reactions

Usually, Chinese herbs are mixed with other herbs to make up a formula to minimize side effects. The traditional prescribing method uses herbs that work synergistically together to be maximally effective. This is because of the highly evolved system of classification that has been empirically tested since ancient times on billions of people in the vast Chinese population. The more ancient formulas have fewer ingredients and the more modern formulas may include many herbs, each of which perform a specific function in the formula. The Chinese herbs have been studied and classified for thousands of years.

Pregnancy and Lactation

Given the wide range of toxicities of Chinese herbs, their use should be avoided in pregnancy and lactation unless under the direction of an experienced practitioner. As Chinese herbal therapy is an integral part of women's health care in China, a number of preparations have been given with an acceptable empiric safety record.

Trade Products, Administration, and Dosage

Chinese herbs are available as encapsulations, tablets, tinctures, and granules. The following is only a representative selection of suppliers.

Herbal Fortress
4750 West Red Wolf Dr.
Tucson, AZ 85742
Tel: (520) 579-3267
Toll Free: (888) 454-3267
www.herbalfortress.com

---

*The classics list eighteen incompatibilities and nineteen antagonisms. The eighteen incompatibilities are as follows Rx. Glycyrrhizae Uralensis (gan cao) is incompatible with the following prescriptions: Rx. Euphorbia Kansui (gan sui), Rx. Euphorbia seu Knoxiae (da ji), Flos Daphnes Genkwa (yuan hua), and Herba Sargasii (hai zao). Rx. Aconiti (wu tou) is incompatible with Bulbus Fritillariae (gua lou), Fr. Pinelliae Ternatae (ba xia), Fr. Trichosanthis (gua lou), Rz. Pinelliae Ternatae (ban xia), Rx. Ampelopsis (bai lian), and Rz. Bletillae Striatae (bai ji). Rhizoma et Radix Veratri (li lu) is incompatible with Rx. Ginseng (ren shen), Rx Adenophorae seu Glenhniae (sha shen), Rx. Salviae Miltiorrhizae (dan shen), Rx Sophorae Flavenscentis (ku shen), Herba cum Radice Asarii (xi xin), and Rx Paeoniae Lactiflorae (bai shao). The "nineteen antagonisms" are as follows: Cortex Cinnamomi Cassiae (rou gui) antagonizes Halloysitum Rubrum (chi shi zhi); Sulpher (liu huang) antagonizes Sal Glauberis (po xiao); Hydargyrum (shui yin) antagonizes Arsenicum (pi shuang); Rx. Euphorbiae Fischerianae (lang du) antagonizes Lithargyrum (mi tuo seng); Sm. Croton Tiglii (ba dou) antagonizes Sm. Pharbitidis (gian niu zi); Nitrum (ya xiao) antagonizes Rz. Sparganii (san leng); Flos Caryophylli (ding xiang) antagonizes Tuber Curcumae (yu jin); Rx. Aconiti (wu tou) (two varieties) Cornu Rhinoceri (xi jiao); and Rx. Ginseng (ren shen) antagonizes Ex. Trogopterori seu Pteromi (wu ling zhi).

Brion/Sunten Herb Corporation
9200 Jeronimo Rd.
Irvine, CA 92618
Tel: (949) 587-1238
Toll-Free: (800) 333-HERB
Fax: (949) 587-1260

Crane Herb Company
435 Falmouth Rd.
Mashipee, MA 02649
Tel: (800) 227-4118
Fax: (508) 539-2369

Zand-McZand Herbal Products
PO Box 5312
Santa Monica, CA 90409
Tel: (800) 800-0405

Self-Help versus Professional

The complexities of Chinese herbal therapy preclude self-diagnosis and treatment for serious or chronic conditions. However, in Asian families, basic knowledge is often passed down from parents to children in terms of treatment for simple conditions. As with mainstream medicine, more complex diagnosis and treatment requires a visit to an experienced practitioner.

Visiting a Professional

A professional TCM provider may have a very relaxing office atmosphere. Providers meet with the patient. They ask pertinent questions in the TCM framework and ask to observe the tongue and note its appearance. They may palpate to locate tender points on the channels or on the abdomen to diagnose obstruction in the related organs; this is called *Hara diagnosis* from the Japanese. A highly skilled TCM practitioner employs observation of the pulses as well. It is said that it takes many years to become truly skilled in Chinese pulse diagnosis, and 40 years to master the art. In TCM the radial pulse is divided into three positions on each wrist, with two organ systems in each position. There are over 30 qualities attributed to the pulses. Providers trained in the Japanese style may rely more on other forms of diagnosis than the pulse, such as point tenderness and Hara. After diagnosing the patient, providers determine the combination of acupoints or herbal treatment plan to prescribe. This is where intense training comes into play. They may treat the patient with acupuncture, moxabustion or cupping, or perhaps they may massage specific points or the abdomen—whatever treatment providers feel in their experience will alleviate the patient's existing discomfort or enhance the patient's healing system to restore balance. The provider then may prescribe an herb or herbal formula for the patient. Provider might have in their own office a pharmacy of raw herbs, modern encapsulations, or tinctures or rely on a local dispensing pharmacy. Someone who specializes exclusively in Chinese herbal medicine may not provide any physical treatment and recommend an herb or formula based on the four diagnosis, questions, or palpation.

Credentialing

The Accreditation Commission for Acupuncture and Oriental Medicine (ACAOM), formerly known as the National Accreditation Commission for Schools and Colleges of Acupuncture and Oriental Medicine (NACSCAOM), is a federal accreditation commission for schools and colleges of acupuncture and oriental medicine. The student must graduate from an accredited school before sitting for the state board exam or national certification commission Exam (NCCAOM). The manner in which states use the NCCAOM process varies. In some jurisdictions, NCCAOM certification is the only educational, training, or examination criteria for licensure. Other jurisdictions have set additional eligibility criteria. A small number of states have additional jurisprudence or practical examination requirements. Texas was the first state to pass legislation on licensure for Chinese herbology.

Training

Training in Chinese herbal medicine is part of the total training in acupuncture and oriental medicine. The programs range in length from 2 to 4 years depending on the state requirements and degree level. There is an accrediting body of schools called National Accreditation Commission for Schools and Colleges of Acupuncture and Oriental Medicine (NACSCAOM) and the American Association For Teachers in Oriental Medicine (AATOM). Some schools are accredited by their state; some also are federally accredited by ACAOM. The accreditation status listed on the schools list reflects the federal accreditation. Federal accreditation means that the school has raised its standards to the minimum requirements set forth by the federal government. It also means that federally guaranteed student loans are available for tuition and living expenses while studying at these schools.

Each state has different requirements for licensure and the lengths and qualities of the programs at these schools vary greatly. California schools are among the more challenging in that they require 3 years minimum training, although most students study for 4 years. Most California schools require 60 semester units to enter their program. Their programs are about one-third acupuncture and theory, one-third herbology, and one-third Western science.

A list of accredited schools and colleges is available from the following organization:

The National Acupuncture Foundation
1718 M St., Suite 195
Washington, D.C. 20036
Tel: (202) 332-5794
www.acupuncture.com

What to Look for in a Provider

Practitioners should be licensed in accordance with the laws of your state or country. A list of practitioners worldwide is available at www.acupuncture.com. or by contacting the NCCAOM, AAAOM, or ITM for herbalists who have been practicing for many years. (See "Associations.") This ensures that the provider has received more than a superficial education of Chinese herbal medicine. The patient should feel comfortable with the provider and the provider should be able to demonstrate competence and education. The provider should be aware of the latest research and issues related to the manufacture of Chinese herbal formulation and provide products that comply with GMP established by the industry.

Barriers and Key Issues

The National Institutes of Health (NIH), the Office of Alternative Medicine (OAM), and the Food and Drug Administration (FDA) are currently wrestling with the best way to regulate Chinese herbal remedies without disregarding the basics of traditional Chinese medicine.

Associations

The National Commission for the Certification of Acupuncture and Oriental Medicine
1421 16th St. N.W. Suite 501
Washington, D.C. 20036
Tel: (202) 232-1404
www.nccaom.org

The National Acupuncture and Oriental Medicine Alliance
14637 Starr Rd. SE
Olalla, WA 98359
Tel: (253) 851-6896
Fax: (253) 851-6883

Institute of Traditional Medicine
2017 SE Hawthorne Blvd.
Portland, OR 97214
www.itm.com

American Association of Acupuncture and Oriental Medicine
433 Front St.
Catasauqua, PA 18031
Tel: (610) 433-2448

Suggested Reading

1. Bensky D, Gamble A, Kaptchuck T: *Chinese herbal medicine materia medica*, Seattle, 1993, East-land.

    Lists the major known ingredients, as well as the pharmacologic and clinical research, with a subsection on toxicity and contraindications for each substance. Contains summaries of abstracts regarding modern pharmacologic and clinical research.

2. Fulder S: *The tao of medicine: ginseng, oriental remedies, and the pharmacology of harmony*, New York, 1982, Destiny Books.

    A well-written and thought-provoking book about research on traditional Chinese herbs. Makes a plea the development of a new class of "harmony drugs" based on the ancient Chinese view of healing, using certain vitalizing and harmonizing substances that repair and tune the body.

3. Ni M: *The yellow emperor's classic of medicine: a new translation of the NeiJing Suwen with commentary*, Boston, 1995, Shambala.

    A clear and concise modern translation of one of the important classics on traditional Chinese medicine with the translators' comments to help clarify the meaning of the text. A highly readable narrative that explains the underlying principles of Chinese medicine.

4. Teeguarden R: Radiant health: the ancient wisdom of the Chinese tonic herbs, New York, 1998, Warner.

    A comprehensive study of the superior class or tonic herbs used for prevention, mental energy, fertility, and longevity. Lists and describes more than 70 tonic herbs and formulas for their preparation. Cites scientific research studies to explain the efficacy of the herbs.

5. *International Journal of Oriental Medicine*

    The Journal of Traditional Chinese Medicine (English version)

    Bulletin of the Oriental Healing Arts Institute of the U.S.A.

    Bulletin of The Chinese Medicinal Material Research Centre, Chinese University of Hong Kong

    These journals and bulletins all contain research reports from Asia and the U.S.

Other Resources

HerbalGram
American Botanical Council
PO Box 201660
Austin, TX 78720
Tel: (512) 331-8868
Toll-Free: (800) 272-7105
Fax: (512) 331-1924

The quarterly magazine of the American Botanical Council and the Herb Research Foundation. Contains information on the medical and scientific updates on herbs, feature articles, reviews on medicinal plants, review of media coverage, updates on legal and regulatory matters, conferences, and book reviews.

Blue Poppy Seminars
3450 Penrose Place, Suite 10
Boulder, Colorado 80301
Tel: (800) 448-8372
Fax: (303) 444-3633
www.bluepoppyseminars.com
www.acupuncture.com

An excellent noncommercial website that reports on all aspects of TCM including Chinese
herbal medicine. With links to Medline and other informational sites. Lists licensing requirements for acupuncture and oriental medicine in the U.S. and worldwide. Contains
book reviews, frequently asked questions, research articles, and much more.

References

1. Weil A: *Spontaneous healing*, New York, 1995, Faucett Columbine.
2. Beijing College of Traditional Chinese Medicine et al: *The essentials of Chinese acupuncture*, Beijing, 1980, Foreign Languages Press.
3. Ma CC, Yang CY, Pao TP: Methods of tongue diagnosis, *Bull Orient Healing Arts Inst* 6(1):1-43, 1981.
4. Bensky D, Gamble A, Kaptchuck T: *Chinese herbal medicine materia medica*, revised edition, Seattle, 1993, Eastland Press.
5. Brion/Sun Ten will prepare a custom formula for a physician or patient. Address and phone are listed in the Reference section.
6. Borchers A et al: Complementary medicine: a review of immunomodulatory effects of Chinese herbal medicines, *Am J Clin Nutr* 66:1303-1312, 1997.
7. Chan TYK et al: Hospital admissions due to adverse reactions to Chinese herbal medicines, *J Trop Med Hygiene* 95:296, 1992.
8. Hu QF: unpublished paper on safety for the herbal manufacturing industry, 1/28/99.
9. Shibita S et al: Tetrahedron letter, *Chem Pharm Bull* 11:959-961, 1963. Cited in Fulder S: *The tao of medicine*, New York, 1980, Destiny Books.
10. Fulder S: *The tao of medicine*, New York, 1980, Destiny Books.
11. Blackwell R: Adverse events involving certain Chinese herbal medicines and the response of the profession, *J Chinese Med* Jan 1990 (reprint). (Available electronically at www.acupuncture.com)
12. Hsu HY: An outline of oriental materia medica, *Bull Orient Healing Arts Inst* 9(4), 1984.

Tai Chi

(Taiji, Taijiquan)

YUZENG LIU

THERESA M. MORGAN

Origins and History

Tai Chi is referred to by many names, including Taiji and Taijiquan. For consistency, Tai Chi is used throughout this discussion. Tai Chi originated in what is now the People's Republic of China. According to legend, Zhang Sanfeng (ca. 1550-1600 CE), a hermit living in the Wudang mountains, created the 13 basic postures. Wang Zongyue wrote down these postures in *Treatise on Taijiquan*. The postures are based on a combination of the four directions and the four corners—south (ward off), north (roll back), west (press), east (push), southeast (elbow), northwest (shoulder), southwest (pull down), northeast (split)—and five elements: metal (entering), wood (leaving), water (look left), fire (look right), and earth (centering). Each element also contains the element of earth (centering).

Many forms and styles of Tai Chi have developed from the original 13 postures. Forms differ in their application of principles and in the practice of movements. There are traditional forms such as Wudang Tai Chi and modern forms such as the 24-step short form. Traditional family forms include Chen, Yang, Wu, Sun, Wuhao, Ching, and others. Elements from the four family styles of Chen, Yang, Wu, and Sun make up the 42-step combined form that is compulsory at international Wushu competitions. Each system and style has unique characteristics and methods for practice. Style variations can be attributed to differences in teaching methods, teachers, and interpretations of the classical principles.

Mechanism of Action According to Its Own Theory

All Tai Chi systems share certain foundation principles, such as open and close, full and empty, yielding, entering, leaving, continuous and connected movement, to name a few, which clearly distinguish yin and yang. The foundations of Tai Chi are derived from the principle of yin and yang. Yin is the feminine, female, receptive, dark, negative, closed, ·

empty principle. Yang is the masculine, male, creative, bright, positive, open, full principle. Without both, there is potential but not substance. Wang Zongyue wrote in his "Treatise on Taijiquan," "Yang is not separate from yin; yin is not separate from yang" (available online at www.wudang.com). In movement, the smooth alternation between full and empty creates harmony and balance. Correct Tai Chi practice develops connections, unity, and harmony inside and outside, between the movement and the breathing, the body and the *qi,* the *qi* and the mind, the *qi* and the energy, the energy and the spirit.

Moreover, correct Tai Chi practice especially requires that the heart must be quiet, the attention must be concentrated, and one must understand and pay attention to "using mind, not physical strength." Tai Chi movements require "integrated *qi.*" The spirit shines from the eyes and extends through the upper limbs, torso, and lower limbs. The upper and lower body are connected; there should not be the slightest confusion or disorder. Advance and retreat are consistent. The movements of Tai Chi unfold with elegance and composure and are continuous and unbroken. This encourages every part of the body to be relaxed and alert. Tai Chi movements require coordinated and timed breathing, which encourages natural respiration and can strengthen the respiratory system.

People who regularly practice Tai Chi report that their entire bodies feel comfortable and their spirits are "glowing" and that when two people practice *push hands,* their bodies feel lively and agile. This heightened feeling gives the body's physiologic mechanisms an invigorated sensation, which clearly can strengthen and enhance the efficacy and results of many treatments.

Biologic Mechanism of Action

The physiologic effects of Tai Chi have been clinically studied in many countries with a great deal of research in China. This contributor has conducted several group studies in China, with results that verify the positive effects of Tai Chi practice on respiratory, cardiovascular, and cerebral functions in both children and older adults. In the United States, a primary focus group for Tai Chi research has been older adults, with significant results. Research shows that regular Tai Chi practice can reduce the incidence of falls in older people by 47%.[1] Tai Chi practice requires consistent movement, round motion, and alignment of the joints throughout the body. During Tai Chi practice, the individual should keep the spinal column upright, sink the chest, relax the elbows, and raise the back. The shape and alignment of the spinal column are important because of the principal roles of the waist and back during movement.

In addition to its ability to increase outer body mass strength, Tai Chi can assist in the treatment of high blood pressure, heart disease, pulmonary tuberculosis, dyspepsia, and ulcers.[2] It is especially beneficial in the treatment of the liver, kidneys, spleen, and stomach. The relaxed and gentle movements of Tai Chi strengthen the body in normal physiologic patterns and encourage regular functioning of the internal organs. Tai Chi has a positive influence on central nervous system functions. It strengthens the heart, blood vessels, and respiratory functions, improves digestive and metabolic processes, and can decrease static blood in the body.[3]

During Tai Chi practice, the contraction-expansion cycle of the musculoskeletal system can strengthen and calm arterial blood circulation. Respiratory movement also can accelerate the returning flow of blood in the veins. Tai Chi increases chest volume during inhalation and raises internal negative pressure, which consequently reduces venous pressure in the upper and lower cavities and accelerates the return flow in the veins.

The expansion and contraction of the diaphragm and abdominal muscles during Tai Chi practice cause the continuous change in abdominal pressure, which has a beneficial effect on blood circulation. The massaging action of this movement on the liver helps to eliminate static blood and strengthen the liver's function. Respiratory movement also stimulates the stomach and intestinal tract mechanisms and can improve blood circulation in the digestive system. Consequently, it can accelerate digestive functions and prevent constipation, which is a very important consideration for older adults.

Good control and balance are required in Tai Chi, owing to the relative complexity of some movements. The cerebrum is required to be intensely active and complete, thus increasing activity in the central nervous system and strengthening the cerebrum's regulating functions.

Forms of Therapy

There are many styles of Tai Chi and many variations within each system. All have the same foundation principles but style practices differ according to the basis for movement and the theory of the individual form. Wudang Tai Chi uses spiraling circular patterns that vary in size and direction. The movements of the form are dynamic and changing and use a wide range of movements. Yang Tai Chi uses lateral circular patterns that maintain a similar size and direction throughout the form. The movements of the form are regular and elegant, with a quiet strength and hidden potential. Wu Tai Chi uses small intricate circles and smooth flowing motions that require fine muscle control. The movements of the form are deceptive and close and use vertical patterns. Chen Tai Chi uses a spiral pattern that sometimes is combined with an explosive release of energy. The movements of the form employ a characteristic *silk-reeling* pattern. Wuhao Tai Chi is similar in dynamic to Chen Tai Chi but uses compact, close circles performed with a characteristic "start-connect-open-close" pattern. Sun Tai Chi has small circles that open and close. The movements have a distinct rolling motion and subtle changes in direction.

Demographics

The majority of those who practice and teach Tai Chi in the United States are adults. Although there are some children who practice, they are a very small minority. People who practiced other martial arts as teenagers and young adults often later adopt Tai Chi. In China, older adults (age 50 to 80 years) make up a large proportion of those practicing; in the U.S., the majority of those practicing are between 30 and 60 years of age. A greater number of Tai Chi practitioners and teachers are located in larger cities. As more people have demonstrated the health benefits of Tai Chi practice, many hospital wellness clinics and seniors groups have begun Tai Chi programs.

Indications and Reasons for Referral

Tai Chi practice can help decrease the side effects of arthritis, osteoporosis, balance disorders, arteriosclerosis, heart disease, high and low blood pressure, gastrointestinal problems, stress-related disorders, depression, and other disorders of the nervous system. By increasing the body's resistance to disease, Tai Chi practice can preserve health. As a preventive therapy, Tai Chi can help reduce susceptibility to infectious disease by strengthening the body's natural homeostatic mechanisms, which benefits individuals with AIDS or a weakened immune system.

Tai Chi practice strengthens the sense of equilibrium and musculoskeletal system functioning, thereby reducing the incidence of falls and broken bones in older adults. For underweight individuals, Tai Chi practice can help stimulate the appetite and increase muscle mass. For overweight individuals, Tai Chi can help increase the sense of well-being during exercise and reduce the postpractice intake of superfluous calories because of anxiety or punishment/reward syndromes, as well as burn fat and improve muscle tone. Because Tai Chi requires quiet, continuous, circular, complete, and connected movements, it may be practiced by individuals that require some physical activity but cannot engage in strenuous exercises.

Regular Tai Chi practice helps regulate the respiratory organs, increases lung capacity, and calms the respiratory patterns, making it an effective therapy for asthma, chronic respiratory distress, anxiety, and shortness of breath. It could be an effective therapy for individuals who wish to quit smoking. The continuous motion and diaphragmatic breathing can provide an internal massage for the stomach, kidneys, liver, spleen, small and large intestines, and the cardiopulmonary organs. Tai Chi improves and helps maintain functioning by stimulating blood flow to these organs. Tai Chi practice helps regulate and enhance the central nervous system functions, which in turn regulate and govern stress response, mental health, cardiovascular functions, and other vital physiologic functions.

Office Applications

Tai Chi practice can preserve the natural alignment of the spinal column and flexibility in all joints, which makes it an effective adjunctive treatment for rheumatoid arthritis, gout, back pain, and osteoporosis.

During Tai Chi practice the body must be straight and erect and the *qi* must sink down. This is known as "sinking the *qi* to the *dan tian*" and is one type of diaphragm breathing. The expansion and contraction of the diaphragm and abdominal muscles cause the abdominal pressure to continually change and provide a massaging action for the internal organs, thus stimulating their functions. This can alleviate constipation, gastrointestinal disorders, gastritis, and irritable bowel syndrome, and can aid in postpartum care.

Regular Tai Chi practice can keep the heart and coronary arteries' blood supply in the best condition, maintain the strength of the heart systole, and strengthen blood movement and the cardiovascular processes. It is an excellent therapy for heart disease, hypertension, menstrual cramps, menorrhagia, and impotence.

Tai Chi exercises can strengthen the functions of the central nervous system. Because the heart must be quiet, the attention must be concentrated, and one must understand and pay attention to "using mind, not using physical strength," the cerebrum is required to be intensely active and complete, thus increasing central nervous system activity and strengthening the cerebrum's regulating functions. This makes Tai Chi an excellent therapy for stress, mental health, chronic fatigue syndrome, obesity and weight management, sleep apnea, and chronic pain.

Tai Chi's well-distributed respiration, abdominal muscle, and diaphragm activity can regulate and control abdominal pressure, increasing the rate of blood flow and lung tissue functioning, thereby preserving lung elasticity and preventing weak bones and ossification. This makes it an excellent therapy for bronchitis, emphysema, and sinusitis. It can also be effective in the treatment of asthma, hay fever, lung cancer, and respiratory infections.

The following list presents a simple ranking of conditions responsive to Tai Chi treatments. As with all alternative therapies, Tai Chi does not preclude the additional use of mainstream medicine in addition.

Top level: *A therapy ideally suited for these conditions*
Back pain; bronchitis; chronic pain; constipation; emphysema; female health; gastrointestinal disorders; gout; heart disease; hypertension; male health; mental health; postpartum care; rheumatoid arthritis; sleep apnea; and sinusitis

Second level: *One of the better therapies for these conditions*
Asthma; arthritis; gastritis; headaches; impotence; irritable bowel syndrome; menstrual cramps; osteoporosis; pneumonia; sleep disorders; stomachache; and ulcers

Third level: *A valuable adjunctive therapy for these conditions*
Colds and flu syndromes and diarrhea

Practical Applications

The benefits of Tai Chi are derived from the correct practice of a linked set of movements. The person first must learn the correct movements, then apply this knowledge in practice. A physician may become familiar with reputable teachers in the area for referral. The physician could learn Tai Chi and then select elements of the forms for use in a physical therapy session. For example, the practice exercise *Wave Hands Like Clouds* works the entire body and helps to align the spinal column, open the hip joints, free the waist, provide flexibility in the upper back, and open the shoulders. Its rhythmic patterns adhere to basic Tai Chi principles, so there is also an excellent massage and stimulation for the internal organs. It can be performed in a limited space as it only requires room for standing. The rudiments of the exercise can be learned in 1 hour but require years for refinement. The foundation principles of Tai Chi can be applied to relationships and situations in our lives and promote balance and harmony. The inner peacefulness that is part of Tai Chi training—the idea of calm and tranquility—can be applied with positive therapeutic effects.

Research Base

Evidence Based

Studies have been conducted on the effectiveness of Tai Chi as a treatment for ailments which commonly affect older adults and as a preventive practice to reduce the rate of deterioration.[4] Evidence shows that Tai Chi is an effective treatment for many cardiovascular ailments, including heart disease, arteriosclerosis, skeletal deterioration, and fractures due to falls.[4,5] Tai Chi is also effective in improving intellectual functions in children.[6] In addition to its physiologic effectiveness, individuals that practice Tai Chi report an increased sense of well-being and a willingness to continue with an exercise program.[7]

Basic Science

A 12-month study evaluated cardiopulmonary function, strength, flexibility, and body fat percentage.[2] The Tai Chi group had an average increase of 18.7% in VO2max ($P < 0.01$), an increase of 9.9% in thoracic/lumbar flexibility ($P < 0.05$), and an increase of 19.2% in muscle strength of the knee extensor. The control group showed no significant change in these variables.

A group of 34 older adults that regularly practiced Tai Chi were compared with a group of 56 older adults that did not practice Tai Chi.[3] The occurrence of spinal deformities in the Tai Chi group was only 25.8%, compared to 47.2% in the control group. Those who regularly practiced Tai Chi also had a better range of movement in the spinal column. In the Tai Chi group, 77.4% could bend forward at the waist and touch the floor with their hands, compared to 16.6% in the control group. The incidence of bone density loss was lower (36.6% compared with 63.8% in the control group). In the Tai Chi group, average blood pressure was 134.1/80.8, compared to 154.5/82.7 in the control group. The arteriosclerosis rate in the Tai Chi group was 39.5%, compared to 46.4% in the control group.

In another study, 45 primary school children with an average age of 11.5 years, practiced Tai Chi for 30 minutes twice a day for 4 months.[7] They were compared with a group of 30 children with an average age of 11.9 years. The children in the Tai Chi group showed marked improvements in memory, calculation skill, and concentration, reflected in improved scores on standard tests.

Risk and Safety

Tai Chi is safe for everyone. Because Tai Chi works in harmony with the body, anyone can practice it. The range of movement applied depends on the person, not on any external requirement. Injuries among solo Tai Chi practitioners are quite rare but are more common among *push hands* practitioners. This is natural. Studies have focused on the benefits of Tai Chi practice because, unlike pharmacologically active agents or other therapies, Tai Chi practitioners have not reported adverse effects. Some beginners report a slight burning sensation in the knee area that disappears with the increase in muscle strength. Tai Chi can be compared to many movement arts. The relative risk and safety depend on the extent of the movement, the strength with which it is performed, and whether the person has prepared the body for the movement.

Efficacy

China's Exercise Medicine Research Institute studied 100 people between the ages of 50 and 90 years.[3] Thirty-four people practiced Tai Chi regularly and 56 did not. According to the evidence observed, the cardiovascular system functions, metabolism, and skeletal matter of the Tai Chi group, regardless of their individual physique, were better than that of the control group.

Steven L. Wolf and colleagues at Emory University School of Medicine found that older adults enrolled in a 15-week Tai Chi program reduced their risk of falling by 47.5 percent.[1] Another study by Leslie Wolfson and colleagues at the University of Connecticut studied the effectiveness of several interventions to improve balance and strength among older adults. These improvements, particularly in strength, were preserved over a 6-month period in Tai Chi exercise.[8]

Future Research Opportunities and Priorities

Many published studies focus on one or two particular aspects of practice. Although this is a generally accepted practice and yields good results, it would be quite useful to have a comprehensive study that would include a Tai Chi group, a group practicing another type of exercise, and a sedentary control group. Both physiologic and psychologic factors should be included, as well as participant logs. Another useful focus would be in the area of cardiovascular health, specifically circulatory problems, heart disease, and hypertension brought on by stress-related conditions. An interesting investigation would be to compare Tai Chi and a standard aerobic routine for respiratory and cardiac functions, overall muscle tone, and flexibility.

Druglike Information

Safety

Tai Chi can be practiced by anyone, regardless of age. As with any movement therapy, safe practice relies on common sense. Correct body alignment is essential, not only in performing Tai Chi movements correctly, but also in preventing injuries. For example, Tai Chi movements require bending the knees. Correct toe alignment is critical to the prevention of knee injuries. If an individual is too full or too hungry, too sad or too happy, too anxious or too angry, too tired or too upset, it is not a good time to practice the full movements. The individual should practice more slowly, which can help balance the condition.

Actions and Pharmacokinetics

Tai Chi movements provide a gentle massaging action for the internal organs, stimulate the cerebrum and central nervous system, and help regulate both the cardiovascular and respiratory systems. The overall practice works to stimulate and enhance natural homeostatic functions and can aid in the elimination of toxic substances from the body.

Warnings, Contraindications, and Precautions

Most contraindications for Tai Chi relate to the way exercises are practiced, not to the practice itself. This has to do with the extent of movement, the relative strength applied, and the ability of the practitioner to sustain movements over time. Common sense should prevail. People who are recovering from an illness should practice slowly and rest after 2 or 3 minutes. Individuals with lower back problems should practice higher stances to open the hips and release the spine.

Drug Interactions

Tai Chi may enhance the effects of medications due to its stimulating effects on the body's systems, but it has no other interactions. The results of Tai Chi practice can be diminished by drugs that inhibit cerebral, central nervous system, or muscle functions.

Adverse Reactions

Muscle strain can occur because of overexertion, excessive force, or misalignment of the body during practice. Complaints of knee strain are common until the person learns to use and strengthens the correct muscles in the legs. Complaints of lower back discomfort also are common because Tai Chi requires use of the legs. This discomfort usually occurs from incorrect spine-hip alignment, locked hips, uneven weight distribution through the legs, and failure to use the abdominal muscles to support the torso.

Pregnancy and Lactation

Tai Chi can be safely practiced during pregnancy although the extent of some movements may be limited by term. Its relaxed, gentle, flowing motion and internal massaging action can have the same calming and stimulating effect on the fetus as it has on the mother's internal organs. After delivery, Tai Chi can help stimulate and increase lactation by calming the mother's central nervous system.

Trade Products, Administration, and Dosage

All Tai Chi systems have beneficial effects; the best Tai Chi is that which is correctly practiced. The choice of system or style may depend on the available teacher or personal preference, according to the type of movement and the knowledge level of the teacher.

Traditionally, the best time to practice Tai Chi is early in the morning, when yang energy is rising. As a general rule, one should not practice between the hours of 11:00 and 1:00, whether morning or night. During these times, yang and yin energies are at their strongest and practice can create an imbalance in the body's natural yang and yin energies. However, certain imbalance conditions can be treated by practice during these times.

Practice duration can be as short as 5 minutes or as long as several hours, depending on the person's circumstances. A short Tai Chi form can be completed once in approximately 3 to 5 minutes; a long form may take 15 to 30 minutes or more, depending on the rate of speed of the movements. Regular practice is essential to achieve the benefits of Tai Chi.

Daily practice is highly encouraged, but it is fine to set a regular schedule of 2 or 3 days per week.

Self-Help versus Professional

Some people try to learn Tai Chi from a videotape or book. A major problem with either of these methods is that neither a video nor a book can tell the person whether a movement is being practiced correctly. Videotapes and books have a very limited ability to communicate the timing, character, and quality of a movement. Although some movements may be learned from these sources, essential aspects of the practice are not addressed. It is not usually dangerous to learn in this way, but it is definitely incomplete.

Visiting a Professional

Typically a person joins a Tai Chi class. If the class emphasizes the physical aspects, the mood of the class should be upbeat with a high level of concentration. If the emphasis is on the internal aspects, the mood should be quiet and intense. Outside disturbances should not distract the participants. Some instructors use music to help students with timing and to enhance the character of the movements. Everyone in the class should be moving at the same speed at the same time with the same quality of movement. The whole room is focused on one thing and one time: the present. Everyone is concentrating on the small nuances of each movement and connecting the whole with the parts. Everyone moves together as one body, just as the parts should all move together within each person. A harmonious spirit and energy fills the room. There is a sense of mindfulness and presence about each movement, yet each movement seems effortless and natural. After practice, the feeling of rhythm and harmony remains; a soft but strong quality radiates from the body. The eyes are bright and the breathing is deep and regular. The whole body is comfortable and refreshed.

Credentialing

There is no national agency for licensing or credentialing in the U.S. In general, peer review and recognition determine whether a given practitioner is competent.

Training

Training is a lifelong endeavor. Individual schools and international organizations may issue training completion or teaching authorization certificates. The President's Council on Fitness offers a participation award for sports activities, including Tai Chi, based on regular participation. However, there are no nationally recognized agencies that issue credentials or certificates for training in Tai Chi.

A person's level of competence is measured subjectively by demonstration and observation. The training evaluations are the same as for individual progress. Evaluations are generally performed by the teacher, although various seminars and competitive events offer an opportunity to obtain evaluations from other recognized experts.

What to Look for in a Provider

A provider should offer referral services or should be a teacher available for study. A teacher should have a sufficient understanding of Tai Chi practice and philosophy as well as some knowledge of general movement theory and basic human anatomy. As a general rule of thumb, a qualified teacher should have had at least 3 to 5 years of previous or current study with a master before teaching independently. The provider should have a sufficient understanding of form theory to explain key principles, be able to explain the differing requirements at each level of practice, and be able to demonstrate correct, coordinated (inside and outside), and full Tai Chi movements. The types of internal practice vary, but the ability to combine at will movement with internal energies is essential in all Tai Chi systems. The provider should have at least a basic understanding of Tai Chi history and a clear knowledge of the lineage of the style or system being taught.

Barriers and Key Issues

Language and the differences in Western and Eastern conceptualizations of physiologic mechanisms are the two greatest barriers to the widespread acceptance of Tai Chi in the U.S. The problems of conceptualization are compounded by the variations in translation of Chinese characters (*taijiquan* or *t'ai chi ch'uan*; *qigong* or *chi kung*). Despite these difficulties, there has been a great deal of clinical evidence collected on the benefits of Tai Chi practice. The increased availability of clinical information in English would help foster an understanding of Tai Chi in terms of physiologic mechanisms that would in turn increase its acceptance as an effective therapy. The cultural and language difficulties are exacerbated by the promotion of misconceptions in various media, incomplete knowledge on the part of some instructors, and misunderstanding of basic Tai Chi principles. Since there are no regulatory or licensing agencies, it is difficult to determine whether a provider is qualified. Reference and background checks can help determine qualification.

Associations

Tai Chi associations are as varied as the styles and systems. There is no governing body for all Tai Chi practitioners, nor is there any regulation of associations in the U.S. Although there are national associations in the Chinese martial arts that include Tai Chi members, most Tai Chi associations are governed by the head of a particular style, system, or school.

Suggested Reading

1. Jou TH: *The tao of t'ai chi ch'uan: way to rejuvenation*, Rutland, Vt, 1980, Charles E. Tuttle.
   This comprehensive book on Tai Chi includes history, drawings, translations, and commentaries from the classics. The genealogic tables are excellent as well as the complete, step-by-step illustrations of three forms (Yang, Chen, Wu). The discussions are complex and introduce classic concepts.

2. Kaptchuk T: *The web that has no weaver: understanding Chinese medicine*, Chicago, 1983, Congdon and Weed.
   The author's purpose is to bridge the cultural gaps between Chinese and Western medicine. As a Western-trained physician, he presents Chinese medicine from the Western point of view and provides both insight and connection.

3. Veith I, trans: *The yellow emperor's classic of internal medicine (Huangdi Neijing Shuwen)*, Berkely, 1949, University of California Press.
   This book is an excellent translation of one of the earliest (ca. 2697-2597 BCE) and most important texts on Chinese medicine, theories, and practices. It details the foundation principles that have guided many centuries of practice and research in traditional Chinese medicine. Background material is provided by the translator.

4. Wile D: *Lost tai chi classics of the late Ching dynasty*, Albany, 1996, State University of New York Press.
   This book provides the four major classic works with translations, extensive notes, and charts, as well as background material and the original Chinese texts. The author also provided an excellent translation in *T'ai Chi Touchstones: Yang Family Secret Transmissions* (Brooklyn, Sweet Chi Press, 1983).

Internet Links

There are a vast number of resources on the Internet that pertain to Tai Chi. The following are some of the better websites and should allow the reader to browse a variety of interest areas.

www.chebucto.ns.ca/Philosophy/Taichi/other
www.nih.gov/nia/new/press/taichi
www.mtsu.edu/~jpurcell/taichi/tc-links
www.wudang.com
www.sunflower.singnet.com.sg/~limttk/index

Magazines

1. *Tai Chi* www.tai-chi.com/magazine
   Tai Chi is a very good print resource with a catalog of tapes and directory of providers.

2. *Journal of Asian Martial Arts*
   The *Journal of Asian Martial Arts* is much more scholarly than the others. It is published quarterly and frequently has articles on Tai Chi and Qigong, as well as a directory of providers.

3. *Qigong and Kung Fu*

   Qigong and Kung Fu covers the U.S. and international tournament circuits and has many good articles by national instructors. It is a good contact point as it includes lists of providers, seminars, workshops, and other resources.

4. *Shaolin and Taiji* (in Chinese)

   Qi Journal also carries articles on Tai Chi but focuses more on Qigong. It also provides a directory of providers. It is only available in the Chinese language.

Bibliography

Jin P: Efficacy of Tai Chi, brisk walking, meditation, and reading in reducing mental and emotional stress, *J Psychosom Res*, 36(4):361-370, 1992.

References

1. Wolf S: *Tai Chi for older people reduces falls, may help maintain strength (Atlanta, Ga)*, National Institutes of Health (U.S.) Public Information Office, May 2, 1996.
2. Lan C et al: 12-month tai chi training in the elderly: its effect on health fitness, *Med Sci Sports Exer* 30(3):345-351, 1998.
3. Liu Y: Comparison study of 100 people, 50-90 years old, China Sports Medical Research Institute, 1994.
4. Lai JS et al: Two-year trends in cardiorespiratory function among older tai chi chuan practitioners and sedentary subjects, *J Am Geriatr Soc* 43(11):1222-1227, 1995.
5. Kessenich CR: Tai chi as a method of fall prevention in the elderly, *Orthoped Nurs* 17(4):27-29, 1998.
6. Kuthner NG et al: Self-report benefits of tai chi practice by older adults, *J Gerontol Behav Psychol Sci Soc Sci* 52(5):242-246, 1997.
7. Liu Y: The influence of taijiquan on intellectual functions in children, Wudang Research Association, study conducted between 12/15/1997 and 5/5/1998.
8. Wolfson L: Tai chi for older people reduces falls, may help maintain strength (Farmington, Conn), National Institute of Health (U.S.), Public Information Office, May 2, 1996.

Qi Gong

DONALD LONDORF

MICHAEL WINN

Origins and History

Qi Gong (pronounced "chee kung") is an ancient healing art that uses various forms of meditation, movement exercises, self-massage, and special healing techniques to regulate internal functions of the human body. Qi Gong is part of the four branches of Traditional Chinese Medicine (TCM), along with acupuncture and moxibustion, herbology, and *tuina* (massage). Through the integration of mind, body, and breathing, a person can learn to promote, preserve, circulate, balance and store *Qi* (vital energy) within the body to achieve health and longevity.

Archeologic finds in China trace back the origins of Qi Gong at least 3000 years. Many relics and texts have survived the rise and fall of Chinese dynasties to attest to the importance of Qi Gong in the development and practice of TCM. In fact, Qi Gong may have played a significant role in the development of some of the basic theories of TCM, namely those of Qi, yin and yang, and the meridians.[1,2] (Examples: *ki* is the Japanese word for Qi, *do* is the word for Tao: Ai-ki-do, Rei-ki, and Jin Shin-do are all derivative schools.)

The major schools of Qi Gong are Taoist, Buddhist, and Confucian. The three major types are martial, medical, and spiritual, with Taoism being famous for its medical styles. Although there are literally hundreds, if not thousands, of different styles of Qi Gong in existence today,[3] most have the common purposes of relaxing and strengthening the body, improving mental capacity, nurturing innate potential, promoting longevity, and preventing and treating disease. Millions of people around the world today practice Qi Gong on a daily basis for these benefits.

Mechanism of Action According to Its Own Theory

Qi Gong shares the same philosophic foundation as TCM. This includes the use of the theories of Qi and Blood, yin/yang, meridians and collaterals, Zang-Fu organs, the Five Elements, and the pathogenesis of disease. However, the therapeutic tools of Qi Gong differ from those of acupuncture, herbology, and tuina.

According to TCM theory, all things in the universe, including the human body, are believed to be composed of Qi. This energy flows in the body along channels called *meridians* and *collaterals,* which connect all the organ systems and tissues. In this philosophy, all phenomena occur as a result of changes and movements in the flow of Qi.

When Qi is abundant, flowing freely, and in balance, a person usually enjoys good health and longevity. However, when Qi becomes deficient or excessive, stagnant or blocked in different parts of the body, or unable to ward off pathogenic factors, a pattern of imbalance is set up that can lead to physical, mental, or emotional problems. Imbalances in Qi can occur as a result of improper diet, over strain, stress, lack of physical exercise, traumatic injury, toxins, the six exogenous or environmental factors (wind, cold, summer heat, dampness, dryness, and fire), or the seven emotional factors (anger, worry, sadness, grief, fear, fright, and joy). When the body's natural ability to cope with change and challenges is overcome by any of these factors, its equilibrium is lost and disease can occur.

Qi Gong meditation or exercises aim to promote good circulation of energy in the body. These techniques can be learned and practiced by people with various problems to maintain general health and wellness or for specific purposes or conditions. For instance, some schools may teach specific techniques for people who have asthma or arthritis. The application of awareness, intent, and consciousness toward the body's energy results in the physiologic changes that foster healing.

In contrast, Qi Gong therapy or Qi healing requires specially trained individuals who are capable of sensing and emitting Qi at will and detecting and correcting imbalances in the flow of Qi in another person. In addition to individual therapy sessions, daily Qi Gong meditation or exercises are often prescribed for patients according to their body type, specific condition, and situation.

The theory of yin/yang helps us understand how someone can effect a physiologic change in another person's body without necessarily coming in contact with that person. Simply stated, yin and yang are the dual aspects of all things: night and day, inside and outside, front and back, stillness and motion, and so on. Yin and yang oppose and control each other. They also depend on each other: without yin there is no yang; without yang there is no yin. These two aspects coexist within the same space in a state of constant, dynamic equilibrium. A change in one necessarily results in a change in the other.

By correcting imbalances in the circulation of Qi outside of the body (yang aspect), a corresponding change is set forth in the Qi inside the body (yin aspect). The same is true for the reverse, as in treating a person with herbs or medications from the inside. The belief that the outside world is a reflection of the inside world and vice versa is a central component of this theory.

Qi healing and Qi Gong involve consciousness and intent applied to the body to trigger its innate healing ability. They are applied according to the theories of TCM and always according to the condition of the person and the relevant situation.

Biologic Mechanism of Action

The physiologic effects of Qi Gong have been extensively scientifically studied in the past 20 years. The computerized Qi Gong database (Qi Gong Institute) has more than 1300 studies. Qi Gong has been shown to decrease blood pressure,[4,5] decrease oxygen consumption, increase respiratory efficiency,[6] alter and integrate brain wave patterns,[7-12] decrease stress hormone levels,[13,14] and improve cellular and humoral immunity.[15,16] These changes are characteristic of effects on central and autonomic nervous systems, hormones, and neurotransmitters. The overall relaxation response is believed to play a significant role in the mitigation of the devastating effects of stress and the prevention and treatment of illness.

As for the study of the mechanisms of emitted Qi on biologic systems, no other field has the potential to unsettle the foundation of established, modern science and thinking as much as this area of research. It is important to understand that Qi Gong does not appear to behave entirely according to the laws of linear physics. Instead, it may have more to do with the advanced concepts brought forward in quantum and chaos theories.

In a series of preliminary experiments on the physiologic effects of externally emitted qi from Qi Gong Masters on various biologic substrates and chemical compounds, emitted Qi was found to affect DNA synthesis and structure,[17,18] protein synthesis,[17] artificial cell membranes,[19] chemical reactions,[20-22] and polarized light beams.[23]

In similar preliminary experiments involving long-distance Qi emission and its effects on molecular structures, evidence was found to suggest the existence of such a phenomenon.[24,25] If the phenomena just described can be reproduced with other Qi Gong Masters under different conditions, it could help explain some of the specific properties of Qi, as well as the physiologic effects of emitted Qi on the body. Research into Qi Gong and emitted Qi is still in its infancy, but it is rapidly expanding our knowledge of human biomagnetic energy.

Forms of Therapy

Internal (self-practice) and external (Qi emission) Qi Gong are the two broad divisions. Internal Qi Gong consists of meditation and movement exercises that are self-practiced by individuals to regulate their own Qi. The patient is taught ways to do Qi Gong movements and meditations that will benefit their particular condition. Some are specifically designed for different illnesses (for example, asthma, a special anti-cancer walk, or joint disease), and others are meant to balance the Qi of summer, winter, or the heart or lung meridian, and so on. All are easily performed even by older adults or people in a weak condition. The patient usually feels improvement immediately and a general sense of well-being.

The powerful Qi meditation methods known as *neigong* create "internal Qi movements" using the mind to flow Qi in the meridians. Most famous is the *microcosmic orbit,* which circulates Qi up the spine and down the front of the body. Others might use subvocal sound frequencies focused on the vital organs (the "six healing sounds") or by evoking postive feeling states (the "inner smile"). There is even a sexual Qi Gong for redirecting sexual Qi to alleviate impotence and premenstrual syndrome and stimulate the production of hormonal precursors in the bone marrow.

The self-practice approach requires self-discipline on the part of the patient, but because patients are taught to take responsibility for their own healing it generally produces the most effective and lasting results. Once patients learn to generate "Qi" within themselves the results are not limited to self-healing. Patients may continue to practice the Qi Gong to achieve ever higher levels of wellness and spiritual awareness. Qi Gong is so simple yet powerful that many healers use Qi Gong to repair themselves from "healer burnout."

External Qi Gong is performed by a trained Qi Gong practitioner to detect and correct imbalances in the circulation of Qi in another person. The Qi Gong healer may tap into either personal or universal energy, which is then focused and radiated into the patient's body lying on a table or while sitting. This alters the energetic matrix of the patient's meridians and causes the physical body to be regenerated. The patient may feel a gentle warmth or tingling begin to flow in different parts of the body. Depending on the skill of the healer, it can be used with great success on anything from mild headache to broken bones to sexual dysfunction, as well as chronic illnesses such as cancer and AIDS. Some healers can work at a distance and even hundreds of miles away.

Demographics

Qi Gong exercises and meditations are practiced on a daily basis by an estimated 100 million people in China and in growing numbers throughout the world. The profile of those using Qi healing outside of China is not well known. In the authors' experience, the typical profile of a patient seeking Qi healing is female, professional, with higher education, and between the ages of 30 and 50.

Qi Gong teachers and self-practitioners are now relatively easy to find in North America, especially in large cities and communities with strong Asian roots. Practitioners can be found through contacts with local or national Qi Gong associations, Qi Gong or TCM schools, Chinese associations, herbal pharmacies, health food stores, martial arts stores and schools, alternative/complementary medicine publications, and occasionally in the Yellow Pages under holistic listings. Traditional Masters tend to be very discreet and operate mostly by word of mouth referral.

Indications and Reasons for Referral

Most older children and adults can learn to practice simple Qi Gong meditation or exercises. This can be done to increase their sense of well-being, decrease stress, improve health, prevent illness, and treat different conditions.

It is important to realize that Qi Gong is a valuable adjunct to Western medicine in that it supports a proactive, preventative approach to health. People do not need to be sick in order to practice Qi Gong. For those patients in search of something to do to maximize their state of wellness, Qi Gong has much to offer.

When prevention fails and a patient is faced with treating an illness, Qi Gong can also be used as a therapeutic option. Qi Gong therapy alone is not appropriate for the treatment of acute or emergency situations, although it can be used as an adjunct to Western medicine if the practitioner is highly skilled and experienced. Qi Gong is a gentle and honoring tool for the management of many chronic illnesses.

Common reasons for referring someone to Qi Gong instruction or therapy include the following:

- Management of chronic illness
- Wellness promotion or preventive medicine

- Stress management
- Inability of Western medicine to clearly diagnose an illness or condition, such as strange or bizarre symptoms that do not conform to any known Western pattern of disease
- Patient requests "holistic or natural" treatment options
- Unacceptable risk (to patient or physician) of proposed medical interventions
- Terminal illness: palliative or therapeutic stages

Office Applications

Qi Gong can infuse Qi into everything that acupuncture needles can reach, and it can reach even deeper into the mind-body relationship. This makes it a premier treatment choice for most chronic conditions, including the following:

Hypertension: Benefits include improved blood pressure control (systolic and diastolic), decreased medication use, decreased mortality, decreased incidence and mortality of stroke, offset of the progression of cardiovascular lesions, and retinopathy.[4,5]

Asthma: Disorders that are affected by emotional components or stress are very amenable to Qi Gong, which improves respiratory efficiency.[6]

Allergies: Studies show Qi Gong can affect the immune system and stabilize the effects of stress and emotions.

Stress and stress-related disorders: (for example, fatigue, tension headaches, poor concentration, difficulty sleeping, problems with appetite, vague aches and pains, and others) Sitting and moving Qi Gong are excellent tools to mitigate the devastating effects of stress on the mind, body and spirit.[13,14]

Cancer: Because of experimental data about the effects of Qi on DNA,[17,18] protein synthesis,[17] chemical reactions,[20-22] cell growth,[17] the immune system,[15,16] emotional well-being, and improved quality of life,[28] Qi Gong should be an integral part of all programs dealing with cancer. Many studies have been presented at scientific meetings about the beneficial effects of Qi Gong on cancer cells and tumors. No peer-reviewed, English language references can be found.

AIDS: Same reasons as for cancer.

Gastrointestinal: (such as irritable bowel, peptic ulcer disease, poor appetite, constipation, hemorrhoids, and others) The effects of Qi Gong on the functional aspects of digestion are well-recognized by practitioners of Qi Gong. Some of these effects have been documented by research.[28]

Chronic fatigue and fibromyalgia: These syndromes can be frustrating to treat with Western medicine. Qi Gong can help these patients rebuild their stores of Qi and balance their energy circulation.

Diabetes: There is evidence that Qi Gong can alter hormonal levels in the body. Specific Qi Gong techniques exist for diabetes mellitus.

Arthritis: Qi Gong is often used for arthritis. It appears to benefit rheumatoid as well as osteoarthritis. The exercises are gentle and generally easy to learn.

Musculoskeletal pains and sports injuries (acute or chronic): Best used under the guidance of a trained practitioner to avoid further injury.

Low energy states: If Western medical investigations reveal no clear cause for fatigue or low energy states, it is likely due to Qi deficiency.

Hepatitis: Anecdotal reports of benefits. Some schools have specific Qi Gong techniques for hepatitis and liver problems.

A simple ranking of conditions responsive to this therapy follows. As with all alternative therapies, Qi Gong does not preclude the use of mainstream medical therapies in addition.

Top level: *A therapy ideally suited for these conditions*

Chronic fatigue syndrome; colds and flu; female health (wellness); tension headaches; male health (wellness); stress; and tinnitus[1]

Second level: *One of the better therapies for these conditions*

AIDS; allergies; asthma; bronchitis; cancer; cervical cancer; emphysema; gastritis; gastrointestinal disorders; hay fever; hypertension; migraine headache; hemorrhoids; impotence; infertility; irritable bowel syndrome; lung cancer; Meniere's disease; depression and anxiety; multiple sclerosis; ovarian cancer; ovarian cysts; preconception; prostatic cancer; respiratory conditions; sinusitis; stomach ache; and peptic ulcers

Third level: *A valuable adjunctive therapy for these conditions*

Arthritis; chronic pain; constipation; diabetes; diarrhea; ear infections; general ear pain; gout; hearing disorders; hearing loss; heart disease; osteoarthritis; otitis media; pneumonia; rheumatoid arthritis; uterine fibroids; and viral and bacterial infections

Practical Applications

Most Qi Gong schools or instructors in the United States teach Qi Gong self-practice, which includes meditation or gentle movement exercises. For patients who practice methods to promote well-being, deal with stress, "recharge their batteries," balance their mind-body-spirit, or handle functional complaints or disorders, Qi Gong is a great tool.

As for Qi Gong therapy (external Qi emission), most physician initiated-referrals (in the author's personal practice) tend to be for conditions that do not respond to standard medical treatment, strange symptoms that do not fit into the Western model, or requests from patients for more "natural or holistic" approaches. A Qi Gong practitioner should be used as any other consultant when a physician needs a fresh look from a different theoretic healing model and the patient is open to it.

Research Base

Most of the research on Qi Gong in the past 30 years are in abstracts in proceedings from international scientific meetings[27] or published in Chinese. Many are now available through the Qi Gong Institute research database.

Evidence Based

Several studies support the findings that the practice of Qi Gong can reduce both systolic and diastolic high blood pressure and decrease the amount of medication required to stabilize hypertension. Kuang et al found a significant decrease in 18-hydroxy-11-deoxycorticosterone and blood pressure in hypertensive patients practicing internal Qi Gong twice a day. This suggests that Qi Gong may reduce excessive responses to stress and improve the function of the hypothalamic-pituitary-adrenal axis.[14]

In an impressive 22-year controlled study of 244 hypertensive patients, Qi Gong practice was shown to decrease overall mortality (19.3% Qi Gong versus 41.7% control), decrease the incidence (18% Qi Gong versus 41% control) and mortality for stroke (13.9% Qi Gong versus 24.7% control), improve control of systolic and diastolic blood pressure, and help reduce antihypertensive medication dosages (47.7% Qi Gong versus an increased dosage requirement in 30.85% control). Qi Gong also helps offset cardiovascular lesions, such as progressive retinopathy and abnormal ECG findings.[4,5]

Studies suggest that Qi Gong affects hormonal balance by decreasing estradiol levels in hypertensive men and increasing estradiol and testosterone levels in postmenopausal women. It also improves left ventricular function, increases cardiac output, and decreases peripheral vascular resistance in patients with essential hypertension and coronary heart disease.[5]

Hemodialysis patients reported subjective improvements in appetite, increased frequency of bowel movements, increase in general well-being and physical strength, improved sexual activity, and sleep quality. In the Qi Gong group, 42% reduced their antihypertensive drug use compared with only 8% in the control group.[28]

Basic Science

The existence and measurement of Qi has been the object of several studies. Seto et al measured an extraordinarily large magnetic field (10^{-3} gauss) emanating from the palms of three individuals emitting Qi. This is 1000 times stronger than the known, naturally occurring human biomagnetic field (10^{-6} gauss). This can not be explained by our present knowledge of the human body. The frequency of this unusual magnetic wave was 4 to 10 Hz.[29]

Chien et al documented the effects of emitted Qi on human fibroblast cell growth, DNA synthesis, protein synthesis, and boar sperm respiration.

Studies suggest several possible mechanisms for the physiologic effects of Qi Gong. Emitted Qi is able to affect RNA and DNA UV absorption,[18] change artificial phospholipid membranes,[19] and alter molecular compositions of nonliving substances similar to those found in the body.[30] Similar results at long distances defy our current understanding of physical laws.[24,25]

The effects of Qi Gong on the nervous system have been well studied. The Qi Gong state is different from the waking state, resting with eyes closed, drowsiness, sleep, or any state in between.[7,8,12] EEG studies show slowing of alpha peak frequency and increase in alpha-1 (8 to 10 Hz) components in the anterior-frontal regions.[7,12] This suggests internal inhibitory changes in the cerebral cortex of practitioners of this type of meditation.

Qi Gong meditation with active abdominal breathing is a method common to many schools. In one study this was found to improve ventilatory efficiency for oxygen and carbon dioxide by about 20%.[6]

Risk and Safety

Qi Gong enjoys an enviable and remarkable safety profile but is not without possible side effects. Side effects are infrequent and usually are not due to the techniques themselves but rather to incorrect practice. Patients with acute infections should avoid vigorous types of Qi Gong that may circulate the infected blood. Some White Crane styles with rapid fluttering of limbs have been reported to overstimulate frail individuals, causing nervous breakdown.

Qi Gong "deviation syndrome" (dizziness, headache, nausea, palpitation, feeling hot or cold, and dissociative feeling) is easily corrected by the practitioner with relaxation and correct mindset, body posture, or breathing. Qi Gong-induced psychosis has been described in rare cases with auditory hallucinations and delusions.[33] This is usually self-limited and resolves soon after stopping Qi Gong. When this fails an experienced Qi Gong practitioner or Master can help.

In one series, self-taught, unguided exercises accounted for 67.8% of cases seen.[34] Some of the possible psychologic symptoms include anxiety, depression, agitation, neurosis, excitement, behavior disturbance, and delusions usually limited to Qi Gong topics. The psychologic symptoms are classically less severe than in primary affective or psychotic disorders and tend to have a short course with no recurrence.[34]

The diagnosis of Qi Gong deviation syndrome meets the following criteria: normal behavior prior to doing Qi Gong; psychologic or physical reactions during or following Qi Gong practice; and failure to meet *Diagnostic and Statistical Manual IV* (DSM-IV) criteria for schizophrenia, affective disorder, or neuroses. It is unclear how often the psychologic deviations occur outside of the Chinese cultural setting, as it is believed by some to be related to cultural background.[35]

Efficacy

The percentage of patients who respond to Qi Gong vary according to the level of experience and skill of the practitioner. Common estimates of benefits run from 80% to 90%. With greater length of practice and experience, the benefits appear to increase.

Efficacy is enhanced if people fully commit to practice on a daily basis. In a study of hypertensive patients, the overall mortality rate of people who practiced more than three-fourths of the time was 11.2%, compared with 29.3% in the inconsistent group.[4]

Future Research Opportunities and Priorities

Further research likely will be directed toward demonstrating effectiveness rather than understanding why and how Qi Gong works.

Druglike Information

Qi Gong works very well with Western medicine and does not interfere with medications. Numerous studies in China show patients on chemotherapy and radiation recover faster and survive longer when Qi Gong is practiced.

Self-Help versus Professional

Basic Qi Gong meditation or movement exercises can be learned through books or videos. However, it is preferable to learn from a trained instructor with experience, if this is available. Because proper body posture, breathing, and mindset are essential for the correct and safe performance of a technique, quality instruction is of great value. It also prevents patients from attempting a technique that is inappropriate for their level of training or physical and mental condition. External Qi Gong or Qi healing requires a trained practitioner with experience.

Visiting a Professional

The setting for learning internal Qi Gong can vary greatly, from a private session to a group lesson, depending on the instructor, school, tradition, and particular needs of the person. Lessons may be given in an office, school, home, or even in a park. Prospective students should find out what the class format is like, which exercise or meditation is being taught, whether it will suit their specific needs, how long it usually takes to learn the technique with this format, and how frequently they should attend. It is easier to learn a technique in a private session because of the individual attention but the group classes can be a lot of fun and are great for motivation.

Some Qi Gong movements use the walking, sitting, or lying positions, but most are performed standing. All share the same underlying principles. The visible physical movements of the arms and waist are usually very gentle and circular in nature and are often accompanied by rhythmic breathing methods and subtle shifts in body weight between the left and right foot or between the toe and heel.

There probably is no such a thing as a typical setting for Qi Gong therapy or healing. Some practitioners have home offices and others work out of a more conventional office or clinic setting. The decor depends on the individual practitioner, the style of practice, and the Qi Gong roots. An oriental theme is common. Offices tend to be calm and soothing in keeping with the ultimate goal of balance.

The style of practice pretty much dictates the interactions. Practitioners will ask patients some questions to determine what is going on and then go on to their form of assessment and treatment. This varies significantly from tradition to tradition. Patients remain clothed during the session and may be sitting or lying down. The assessment is usually based on an individual's appearance and demeanor, as well as the interpretation of imbalances in the flow of Qi. This is done through sight, light touch of different parts of the body, or commonly through *Qi scanning*. Scanning for energy imbalances is done with the palms, without contact, at a distance of 3 to 12 inches from the body.

External Qi Gong healing methods also vary widely. They may consist of guided meditations or exercises, specific or flowing movements over the patient's body, emitting Qi with the palms or fingers, physical contact on acupoints, or light contacts on the body with the palms. Some healers may utter certain sounds to vibrate the internal organs or expel the "sick" or "perverse" Qi that is causing the illness or psychosomatic symptoms. Some may stamp their foot to activate earth chi or move their hands over the patient's body to stimulate or sedate the flow of Qi. Most patients report a wonderful sense of relaxation, warmth, and lightness after the session.

Follow-up frequency depends on the particular situation and severity of symptoms. At the beginning, weekly follow-up visits are common for most problems. More frequent sessions may be scheduled to work on difficult issues. The interval between visits is usually lengthened as Qi imbalances improve and the system remains balanced. Some patients like to schedule a wellness session once per month for prevention. Conditions that have been present for a long time or that are severe or life-threatening require more work. Patients with these significant challenges on average feel some kind of shift in their symptoms or improvement in their quality of life within 12 to 16 visits. People who are sensitive to this work may experience changes after one session. Others may take months or years to heal. It may depend on whether they practice at home or make lifestyle changes to support their Qi cultivation process.

As with any other healing modality, Qi Gong may not work all the time. It is not meant as a "quick fix." However, it can lead to long-term healing, greater insight, self-discovery, and improvement in quality of life.

Credentialing and Training

Currently there is no official credentialing or licensing of Qi Gong instructors in the U.S. or guideline for what is required to be called a Master or Qi Gong therapist. There is a National Qi Gong (Chi Kung) Association working to establish recommended minimum curriculum, hours of training, and ethical guidelines for both general Qi Gong and medical Qi Gong therapy.

Setting a uniform curriculum is difficult because schools have different roots and the mastery of Qi Gong is a lifetime process. Currently each school has its own internal regulations and credentials. Some people train in Qi Gong schools in China and receive official credentials. So it is not always easy to determine the quality, level, and experience of a Qi Gong practitioner.

Many Qi Gong teachers in the West are only skilled in martial arts and not as Qi therapists. They often use Qi Gong as warmups for Tai Chi, and many of the same health benefits will accrue. But if Qi training is done mostly with the intention to fight the health results may not be the same if the Qi is tied up in anger or defensive boundary setting.

In the U.S., standards of practice or code of ethics are not in place yet. Not all Qi Gong practitioners are conversant with principles of TCM or can do external Qi Gong healing. Many practitioners practice and teach only internal Qi Gong.

Everyone who has read a book, watched a video, and learned a Qi Gong form can call themselves an instructor or teacher, but this does not necessarily make them qualified to teach.

One of the difficulties of credentialing Qi Gong is the fact that for many schools there is a very strong spiritual aspect to the personal practice and learning of Qi Gong. Many practitioners have to go through long apprenticeship periods with Masters to learn advanced techniques, which are often well-guarded secrets. The degree of spiritual development of a student or practitioner is difficult to measure using written and laboratory-like practical tests. To retain only the intellectual and so-called medical aspects of Qi Gong would be to separate mind, body, and spirit, which would miss the essence of this art.

What to Look for in a Provider

Look for practitioners who practice and teach Qi Gong on a full-time basis. Ask about the length of their training, their experience with specific issues or conditions, and the name of their Master(s) or teacher(s). Ask for references and check them. Contact the schools where the practitioners studied and ask about their training and abilities. Beware of those who make exaggerated claims such as vast experience and incredible abilities (even though they have taken only a few classes and have been practicing for a few years), ability to cure everything, being the only person to hold the true knowledge of a lineage, and so on. You can check with the National Qi Gong Association (U.S.) regarding the issue of lineage.

The moral character and energy of a Qi Gong teacher or practitioner are important factors. Look for someone with a strong moral character who appears calm, caring, warm, and compassionate. This person should inspire trust and reflect the qualities of gentleness, humility, health, and balance. Healing Qi Gong is practiced from the heart for the benefit of all beings. After all this, your patient will still have to feel comfortable with the practitioner, the modality, and the setting.

Barriers and Key Issues

Several issues stand in the way of the widespread acceptance of this healing art by the medical community. One is the difference between the theoretical healing models of TCM and Western medicine. The apparently contradicting paradigms are in fact the strength of the merging of TCM and Western medicine. Some problems are best addressed with Western medicine, some with Chinese medicine, and others with both. In China, many hospitals have Qi Gong departments working with Western-trained doctors.

The concept of Qi appears to be a large stumbling block. Energy medicine incorporates the concepts of mind, body, and spirit into a whole that is inseparable from the universe we live in. It incorporates the meaning of life and death, and champions quality of life through natural connectedness. Its healing power is experiential rather than purely intellectual or mechanic. To overcome this barrier we need to accept the importance of personal experience in our daily lives. This requires openness, suspension of judgment, and expansion of our field of vision to include different systems of science. Qi Gong must be first experienced before it can be understood.

To further scientific and mainstream acceptance, the meticulousness of the experimental designs and statistical analyses must increase. Future research will have to be clearer about which Qi Gong techniques and styles are used in studies and the level of experience and training of the Master or practitioner. It is easy to discount the results of experiments that defy conventional theories, especially when we do not understand or believe a phenomenon. Science must remain objective and examine all phenomena, believable or not.

Associations

Healing Tao International
PO Box 20028
New York, NY 10014
Tel: (800) 497-1017
www.healing-tao.com

National Qi Gong (Chi Kung) Association USA
PO Box 20218
Boulder, CO 80308
Tel: (888) 218-7788
Fax: (415) 389-9465
www.nqa.org

Qi Gong Institute
561 Berkeley Ave.
Menlo Park, CA 94025
www.healthy.net/QiGonginstitute

World Academic Society of Medical Qi Gong
No. 11, Bei San Huan Dong Lu
Beijing, 100029, China
Fax: 0086 10 6421 1591

Suggested Reading

1. Cohen KS: *The way of Qi Gong: the art and science of Chinese energy healing,* New York, 1997, Ballatine Books.

    This is a well-written, scholarly, yet readable book on Qi Gong. It presents a great overview of the subject and introduces the reader to basic theories, meditations, and exercises.

2. Shih TK: *Qi Gong therapy: the Chinese art of healing with energy*, Barrytown, NY, 1994, Station Hill Press.

This is a short introduction to Qi Gong concepts and some of the principles of Chinese medicine and Qi Gong therapy.

3. Wang S, Liu JL: *Qi Gong for health and longevity: the ancient Chinese art of relaxation/meditation/physical fitness*, Tustin, Calif, 1995, The East Health Development Group.

This is an easy-to-read overview of Qi Gong with historical notes and guidelines for training.

References

1. Ding L: *Acupuncture, meridian theory, and acupuncture points*, San Francisco, 1992, China Books and Periodicals.

2. Shih TK: *Qi Gong therapy: the Chinese art of healing with energy*, Barrytown, NY, 1994, Station Hill Press.

3. Cohen KS: *The way of Qi Gong: the art and science of Chinese energy healing*, New York, 1997, Ballatine Books.

4. Kuang A et al: Long-term observation on Qi Gong in prevention of stroke: follow-up of 244 hypertensive patients for 18-22 years, *J Trad Chinese Med* 6(4):235-238, 1986.

5. Kuang A et al: Research on "anti-aging" effect of Qi Gong, *J Trad Chinese Med* 11(2):153-158, 1991.

6. Lim YA et al: Effects of Qi Gong on cardiorespiratory changes: a preliminary study, *Am J Chinese Med* 21(1):1-6, 1993.

7. He Q, Zhang J, Li J: The effects of long-term Qi Gong exercise on brain function as manifested by computer analysis, *J Trad Chinese Med* 8(3):177-182, 1988.

8. Liu GL, Cui RQ, Li GZ: Neural mechanisms of Qi Gong state: an experimental study by the method of auditory evoked responses, *J Trad Chinese Med* 7(2):123-126, 1987.

9. Liu GL et al: Changes in brainstem and cortical auditory potentials during Qi-Gong meditation, *Am J Chinese Med* 18(3-4):95-103, 1990.

10. Pan W, Zhang L, Xia Y: The difference in EEG theta waves between concentrative and non-concentrative Qi Gong states: a power spectrum and topographic mapping study, *J Trad Chinese Med* 14(3):212-218, 1994.

11. Zhang W et al: An observation on flash evoked cortical potentials and Qi Gong meditation, *Am J Chinese Med* 21(3-4):243-249, 1993.

12. Zhang JZ, Li JZ, He QN: Statistical brain topographic mapping analysis for EEGs recorded during Qi Gong state, *Int J Neurosci* 38:415-425, 1988.

13. Ryu H et al: Acute effect of Qi Gong training on stress hormonal levels in man, *Am J Chinese Med* 24(2):193-198, 1996.

14. Kuang A et al: Effect of Qi Gong therapy on plasma 18-OH-DOC level in hypertensives, *J Trad Chinese Med* 7(3):169-170, 1987.

15. Ryu H et al: Effect of Qi Gong training on proportions of T-lymphocyte subsets in human peripheral blood, *Am J Chinese Med* 23 (1):27-36, 1995.

16. Ryu H et al: Delayed cutaneous hypersensitivity reactions in Qi Gong (Chun Do Sun Bup) trainees by multitest cell mediated immunity, *Am J Chinese Med* 23(2):139-144, 1995.

17. Chien CH et al: Effects of emitted bioenergy on biochemical functions of cells, *Am J Chinese Med* 19(3-4):285-292, 1991.

18. Yan X et al: Observations of the effects of external Qi of Qi Gong on the ultraviolet absorption of nucleic acids [translated], originally published in *Ziran Zazhi (Nature Journal)* [Chinese] 11:647-649, 1988. Available electronically at www.interlog.com/~yuan/yanuv.

19. Yan X et al: The effect of external Qi of Qi Gong on the liposome phase behavior. [translated], originally published in *Ziran Zazhi (Nature Journal)* [Chinese] 11:572-573, 1988. Available electronically at www.interlog.com/~yuan/yanlip.

20. Yan X et al: Observations of the bromination reaction in n-hexane and bromine system under the influence of the external Qi of Qi Gong. [translated], originally published in *Ziran Zazhi (Nature Journal)* [Chinese] 11:653-655, 1988. Available electronically at www.interlog.com/~yuan/yanbro.

21. Yan X et al: The influence of the external Qi of Qi Gong on the radioactive decay rate of 241 Am. [translated], originally published in *Ziran Zazhi (Nature Journal)* [Chinese] 11:809-812, 1988. Available electronically at www.interlog.com/~yuan/yan241.

22. Yan X et al: The observation of effect of the external Qi of Qi Gong on synthetic gas system [translated], originally published in *Ziran Zazhi (Nature Journal)* [Chinese] 11:650-652, 1988. Available electronically at www.interlog.com/~yuan/yanbro.

23. Yan X et al: Measurement of the effects of the external Qi on the polarization plane of a linearly polarized laser beam [translated], originally published in *Ziran Zazhi (Nature Journal)* [Chinese] 11:653-655, 1988. Available electronically at www.interlog.com/~yuan/yanbro.

24. Li S et al: An experimental study on ultra-long distance (2000 km) effects of the external Qi of Qi Gong on the molecular structure of matter [translated], originally published in *Ziran Zazhi (Nature Journal)* [Chinese] 11:770-775, 1988. Available electronically at www.interlog.com/~yuan/yanmol.

25. Lu Z et al: The external Qi experiments from the United States to Beijing, China [translated], originally published in *Zhongguo Qi Gong (China Qi Gong)* [Chinese] 1:4-6, 1993. Available electronically at www.interlog.com/~yuan/yanus.

26. Pearl WS, Leo P, Tsang WO: Use of Chinese therapies among Chinese patients seeking emergency department care, *Annu Emerg Med* 26(6):735-738, 1995.

27. Sancier KM: Medical applications of Qi Gong, *Alt Ther* 2(1):40-46, 1996.

28. Tsai TJ et al: Breathing-coordinated exercise improves the quality of life in hemodialysis patients, *J Am Soc Nephrology* 6(5):1392-1400, 1995.

29. Seto A et al: Detection of extraordinary large biomagnetic field strength from human hand during external Qi emission, *Acupunct Electrother Res Int J* 17:75-94, 1992.

30. Yan X et al: Laser raman observation on tap water, saline, glucose and medemycine solutions under the influence of the external Qi of Qi Gong [translated], originally published in *Ziran Zazhi (Nature Journal)* [Chinese] 11:567-571, 1988. Available electronically at www.interlog.com/~yuan/yanwat.

31. Takeshige C, Sato M: Comparison of pain relief mechanisms between needling to the muscle, static magnetic field, external Qi Gong and needling to the acupuncture point, *Acupunct Electrother Res Int J* 21:119-131, 1996.

32. Housheng L, Peiyu L: *300 questions on Qi Gong exercises*, Guangzhou, China, 1994, Guangdong Science and Technology Press.

33. Lim R, Lin KM: Cultural formulation of psychiatric diagnosis: case no.3, psychosis following Qi-Gong in a Chinese immigrant, *Cult Med Psychiatry* 20:369-378, 1996.

34. Shan HH et al: Clinical phenomenology of mental disorders caused by Qi Gong exercise, *Chinese Med J* 102(6):445-448, 1989.

35. Xu SH: Psychophysiological reactions associated with Qi Gong therapy, *Chinese Med J* 107(3):230-233, 1994.

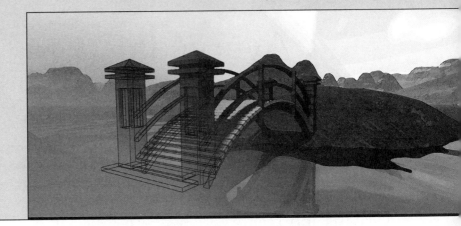

Professionalized Health Care Systems

Ayurveda, **246**
Homeopathy, **258**
Naturopathic Medicine, **274**

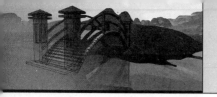

Ayurveda

MARC HALPERN

Origins and History

Ayurveda, which literally translated means "the science or knowledge of life," is the traditional medical system of India. Its origin dates back an estimated 5000 to 10,000 years, and it is considered to be the oldest form of health care in the world's history. The knowledge of Ayurveda has its written origins in *The Vedas,* which are the sacred texts of India.

Current knowledge of Ayurveda originates from relatively later writings, primarily the *Caraka Samhita* (written approximately 1500 BCE), the *Ashtang Hrdyam* (written approximately CE 500), and the *Sushrut Samhita* (written approximately CE 300 to 400). These three classics describe the basic principles and theories from which Ayurveda has evolved. Later writings and research expand on this early clinical information presented in these three classics.

Mechanism of Action According to Its Own Theory

Ayurveda is based on the premise that disease is the natural end result of living out of harmony with our environment. *Natural* is an important word because Ayurveda understands that symptoms of disease are the body's normal way of communicating disharmony. With this understanding of disease, Ayurveda's approach to healing becomes obvious: To reestablish harmony between the self and the environment. Once this is reestablished the need for the body to communicate disharmony diminishes, symptoms dissipate, and healing has occurred.

Ayurveda understands that each person and the disease the person is manifesting is a unique entity. Therefore Ayurveda does not approach the cure of a disease as much as it approaches the cure of a person. Where allopathic medicine looks for a drug that will cure a statistically significant number of people for a specific condition, ayurvedic medicine looks for a treatment that will cure an individual of the unique presentation of the disease. Because no disease affects two people in exactly the same way, no two cures are exactly the same.

Principles

For the Ayurvedic practitioner it is necessary to understand the nature of the patient, the nature of the disease, and the nature of the remedy. The qualities of Nature are said to be either heavy or light, cold or hot, stable or mobile, sharp or dull, moist or dry, subtle or gross, dense or flowing, soft or hard, smooth or rough, and cloudy or clear. A person, a disease, or a remedy is understood to have a unique combination of these qualities. It is the goal of Ayurvedic practitioners to understand as many of the qualities as they can about their patient and their patient's condition.

A person may be heavy or light, move quickly or slowly, feel more warm or cool, have a sharp or dull mind, and have moist or dry skin. These are examples of understanding the nature of a person. Similarly, a disease like arthritis may be defined as producing sharp or dull pain, migrating (mobile) or localized to one or more joints (stable), and producing vasodilatation around the joint (warm), or vascular constriction (cool). By understanding the presentation of a disease through its qualities, the uniqueness of a disease is understood.

Remedies, whether herbs, diet, colors, aromas, or sounds, are also understood in terms of their qualities. The fundamental principle of treatment in Ayurveda is to treat the disease with the qualities opposite to its nature. Cold diseases are treated with warm remedies, heavy diseases are treated with light remedies, and so on. Ayurveda describes the human being as composed of five elements, three *doshas* (biologic energies), seven *dhatus* (tissues), and numerous *srotas* (channels). The five elements are ether, air, fire, water, and earth. These five elements, which make up all of Nature, are not meant to be taken literally. They are ideas described as elements. These are the ideas of space, motion, heat, flow, and solidity, respectively.

DOSHAS

Vata dosha is a biologic force that governs all motion in the body. Composed of ether and air, it is light, dry, mobile, hard, and cool. People with a predominance of this energy in their bodies tend to exhibit these characteristics. They tend to be thin, have dry skin, feel cold easily, and move and speak quickly. They also tend to have a greater amount of cold emotion, such as anxiety and fear. Vata imbalance can cause physiologic disturbance in any system of the body and cause an increase in those qualities. For instance, the respiratory system becomes dry as seen in nonproductive coughs. An increase in the motile quality of vata in the nervous system is understood to cause tremors. The cold nature of vata can become severely disturbed and cause Raynaud's syndrome. Wasting conditions are viewed as an increase in the light quality of vata.

Pitta dosha is a force that governs all digestion in the body. Composed primarily of fire, it is hot, light, exhibits flow, and is sharp. It contains a little water and thus it is neither very moist or dry. People with a predominance of pitta in their bodies exhibit these qualities. They feel warm, have a rosy complexion, are moderate and steady in their weight, have a mesomorphic body build, and can have a sharp and intense personality. This personality tends to be challenged by a greater amount of heated emotion such as anger, resentment, and jealousy. As pitta governs digestion, the digestive system tends to be strong. Bowel movements occur frequently, two or three times per day. When pitta imbalance affects a system, heat builds up at that location. Hepatitis, hyperacidity, acne, and conjunctivitis and infection are examples of heated pitta conditions.

Kapha dosha is a biologic force that governs growth in the body. Composed of water and earth, it is heavy, moist, stable, soft, and dull. People with a predominance of kapha in their bodies tend to carry more weight, have thicker, denser bones and skin, and have a more traditional endomorphic body build. They also tend to have moist supple skin and full, thick hair. This person's personality tends toward being quiet and relaxed. They talk and move slowly. They can be challenged by heavy feelings, such as lethargy. When kapha increases in the body, there is a greater production of mucous. There may also be swelling and weight gain. Conditions such as obesity, chronic bronchitis, and fluid retention syndromes have a kapha disturbance as a component of their pathophysiology.

While the doshas are seen as the causative agents of disease, *dhatus, upadhatus,* and *srotas* are understood to be the site of the disease. Dhatus are tissues; upadhatus are secondary tissues; and srotas are channel systems.

There are the following seven tissues or dhatus in the body: plasma, blood, muscle, fat, bone, marrow, and reproductive tissue. Unlike Western medicine, which understands each tissue to be separate, Ayurveda understands each to be dependent on the tissues preceding it for its nourishment and health. Therefore if the preceding tissues are not healthy, the health of the proximate tissues will eventually suffer and the disease becomes systemic.

During the formation of the dhatus, additional secondary tissues are formed. These tissues are called upadhatus. For example, in the formation of plasma (*rasa*) the breast milk and menstrual fluids are formed. These also may become the site of doshic disturbance. In addition, during the formation of each tissue, a waste product (*mala*) is formed. These are examined and give clues to the pathology.

A srota is a channel. The channel systems of the body are numerous. Some channels are gross while others are so subtle they are imperceptible. Channels supply tissues with nourishment and remove waste. Gross channels include the digestive tract, urinary tract, respiratory system, reproductive channels, and the sebaceous channels. Subtler channels are those channels that carry thought and nourish the dhatus and the energetic channels called *nadi.* (A nadi is a channel that carries the energy of the subtle body).

Pathology in Ayurveda can be partially understood in terms of which dosha is affecting which tissue or organ system.

When vata enters a dhatu or srota, that tissue becomes lighter, drier, and hypermobile. When pitta enters, it becomes heated; when kapha enters, it becomes heavier, moister, and more stable. In a muscle, vata disturbance causes wasting, pitta disturbance causes infection, and kapha disturbance causes hypertrophy.

All physical disease is understood to affect the digestive system. It is this system that Ayurveda understands to be the root of most disease. Here doshas accumulate, become aggravated, overflow into the blood stream, and then relocate to other weakened areas of the body where they manifest and diversify into specific conditions.

CONSTITUTION AND IMBALANCE

According to Ayurveda, each person has a constitution that was determined at conception. This constitution is the inherent balance of these three doshas. The constitution determines a person's basic body type and personality. Although other factors influence the formation of both the body and personality, the constitution provides the predisposition in much the same way as a person's genetics. There are infinite combinations and permutations of these three basic energies in each person. Therefore we see that each person is understood to be unique. The ayurvedic practitioner's first objective is to understand the nature or constitution of the patient. Next the practitioner attempts to understand the disease or the nature of the imbalance and the overall strength (ojas) of the body. Ojas is a substance that gives the body the ability to endure stress.

Methods of evaluation include a detailed case history, abdominal palpation, and examination of the pulse, tongue, and physical features.

Although pathology is important to understanding the nature of the disease, etiology is equally important. Etiology is understood according to how the patient's lifestyle, habits, and environment caused the doshas to become disturbed. A lifestyle that emphasizes a fast pace and dry, light foods, such as a raw foods or a vegetarian diet, is likely to cause an aggravation to vata dosha. A lifestyle that is intense, competitive, and emphasizes spicy hot foods will aggravate pitta. Kapha is aggravated by a sedentary lifestyle and a diet of heavy, moist foods, such as yogurt and meat.

Biologic Mechanism of Action

Ayurveda is health care science, which approaches the understanding of a person physically, emotionally, and spiritually. The physical model is based on establishing optimal physiology of the patient's unique body. Disease progresses as a result of a breakdown of the body's normal homeostatic mechanisms. This is understood to occur because the body's normal immune and homeostatic mechanisms can no longer function appropriately due to a lifestyle of stress that weakens these systems. Ayurvedic lifestyle counseling uses a behavioral approach toward correcting the etiology of disease.

The psychologic model of disease is based on the spirit-mind-body connection. A disturbed and distracted mind cannot be at peace. A peaceful mind is a prerequisite for a healthy body. Thus, Ayurveda employs the principles of its sister science, yoga, toward this end. Stress reduction through proper lifestyle and meditation play an integral role.

The spiritual side of Ayurveda is most important as disease is understood to begin when individuals forget their true nature as spirit. This forgetfulness results in the perception of the self as a physical being only who is dominated by the senses and the pursuit of pleasure. This perception leads to overindulgence, which weakens the body and upsets the doshas. Ayurveda employs spiritual counseling and meditation to lead a person toward greater faith in a higher power, compassion for all people, and nonattachment (a greater reliance on internal fulfillment than external actions or events).

Forms of Therapy

Ayurvedic treatment programs use what is commonly called *five sense therapies* as their foundation, along with specialized treatments for purification and rejuvenation called *Pancha karma*. Using the sense of taste the practitioner is able to prescribe diet and herbs consisting of the opposite qualities of the disease or imbalance. This diet is very specific and describes the exact foods in each category a patient may consume (see the table "Representative Examples of Foods and Herbs for Each Dosha"). This includes specific meats, dairy, nuts, vegetables, and others. Herbs also exert a strong effect on specific organs and symptoms.

Representative Examples of Foods and Herbs for Each Dosha

Dosha	Increase	Decrease
Vata	**FOODS** Raw vegetables and bitter greens Dry grains such as cornmeal Excessive fruit Dry nuts such as peanuts Bitter, astringent, and pungent food in general	**FOODS** Vegetables cooked with sesame oil Heavy grains such wheat and oats Oily nuts such as almonds Meat Milk taken warm Sweet, sour, and salty foods in general
	HERBS Bitter alteratives such as dandelion, kutki, and neem	**HERBS** Sweet herbs such as licorice, ashwaganda and slippery elm; warm herbs such as cinnamon and garlic
Pitta	**FOODS** Cooked vegetables Warming grains such as buckwheat Most fruit Sour, salty and astringent foods in general	**FOODS** Raw vegetables and bitter greens Cool heavy grains such as wheat and oats Dry sunflower seeds Milk and dairy products Bitter, astringent and sweet foods in general
	HERBS Pungents such as cayenne pepper, hot mustard, or dry ginger	**HERBS** Sweet herbs such as licorice, slippery elm, and shatavari Bitters such as kutki and neem
Kapha	**FOODS** Heavy grains such as wheat Sour foods such as pickles Oily nuts such as almonds Milk and dairy Sweet, sour, and salty foods in general	**FOODS** Most cooked or raw vegetables and bitter greens Dry, light, or warm grains such as buckwheat and cornmeal Pungent, bitter, and astringent foods in general
	HERBS Sweet herbs such as licorice, slippery elm, and shatavari	**HERBS** Bitters such as kutki and neem Pungents such as cayenne pepper, hot mustard, or dry ginger

Color therapies are used with the sense of vision. Colors possess the same qualities as all of Nature and are prescribed according to the opposite qualities of the disease (see the table "Colors, Their Qualities, and Their Effects on the Doshas"). Colors can also have strong special effects on specific diseases.

The ears provide a vehicle for treatment using sound therapies. Ayurveda has traditionally used sound energies called *mantras* for healing. These sound energies are understood to stimulate specific organs and endocrine glands, possibly affecting hormonal production.

Aromatherapy provides treatment through the sense of smell. The qualities of a smell have different effects upon the doshas. For example, sweet-smelling fragrances increase kapha but bring balance to vata and pitta.

Treatment through the skin involves the application of specific medicated oils and massage. Different strokes and pressures affect the doshas in different ways. Patients may be told to massage themselves, or massage may be applied by the practitioner.

Colors, Their Qualities, and Their Effects on the Doshas*

Color	Qualities	Actions on the Doshas
White	Cool, moist	P − V − K+
Red	Hot, dry	K − V + P+
Orange	Warm, dry	K − V − P+
Yellow	Warm	K − V − P+
Green	Cool, moist	P − V − K+
Blue	Cool, dry	P − K − V+
Brown	Cool, stable, moist	P − V − K+
Black	Cool, dry	V + P + K+

*A minus (−) sign after the doshic designation indicates that the color decreases the dosha; a plus (+) sign indicates that the color increases the dosha.

For the treatment of the mind, Ayurveda merges with its sister science, yoga. By using yoga and meditation the patient is encouraged to adopt a lifestyle emphasizing peace of mind and connection to God. The resulting stress reduction is an understood component of the healing process.

Ayurveda also emphasizes the importance of keeping the body clean and pure. Toxins, both external and intrinsic to the body, interfere with the flow of waste material out of the cells, resulting in impaired function. To remove these toxins, Ayurveda employs a technique known as pancha karma, meaning "the five actions." This is a program performed for 7 to 28 days at a specialized center that uses a restricted diet, herbs, massage therapies, additional medicated oil therapies, medicated steam therapies, and elimination therapies, such as enemas, purgation, and nasal or sinus cleansing. In addition to these physical modalities the patient retreats from the world and enjoys time for meditation and reflection. While each therapy is understood to be important, Ayurveda emphasizes lifestyle analysis and change as the most significant aspect of the healing process.

After evaluating the patient, the Ayurvedic practitioner designs a program using the therapies previously noted. These therapies may be instituted over a period of 6 to 12 months.

Demographics

There are no formal studies on how many patients use ayurvedic medicine and principles in their lives. Since Ayurveda is a relatively new science in the West the percentage is low. Worldwide, the traditional medicine of Ayurveda is still used primarily by the poor in India who are unable to afford Western medicine.

Indications and Reasons for Referral

Ayurveda is a complete medical science that should be considered whenever allopathic medicine is unable to produce the desired results.

As Ayurveda includes protocols for the care of every system of the body, it can play a role in the management of any case. It is being used most effectively in the U.S. on patients with chronic and subacute disease. It is not generally recommended for acute diseases where heroic measures are required. Ayurvedic lifestyle therapies may also be effectively used to enhance wellness and prevent disease.

Indications for Referral

The following is a partial list of indications for Ayurvedic referral, presented alphabetically:

Allergies; amennorrhea; anxiety; arthritis; asthma; attention deficit disorder; back pain; benign prostatic hypertrophy; bladder infections (chronic); candidiasis; childbirth preparation; chronic fatigue syndrome; chronic pain and fibromyalgia; colic; conjunctivitis; depression; diabetes Type II; endometriosis; fibrocystic breast disease; gastritis; hay fever; headaches; hemorrhoids; hypertension; insomnia; irritable bowel syndrome; menopause; menstrual cramps; multiple sclerosis; multiple chemical sensitivity syndrome; obesity and weight management; otitis media (chronic); ovarian cysts; parasitic infections; pinworms; pneumonia (chronic); postpartum care, postpartum depression, and diminished milk supply; preconception; premenstrual syndrome; sinusitis; stress; ulcers; ulcerative colitis (chronic); urinary tract infections (chronic); uterine fibroids; vulvadynia; and yeast infections

Practical Applications

Ayurveda is typically used as a complement or alternative to Western allopathy. Although the lifestyle and sense therapies easily compliment any treatment, herbs and metal oxides may be effective as an alternative to pharmaceutic drugs. The medical practitioner untrained in Ayurveda may choose to employ a Clinical Ayurvedic Specialist in the practice to address chronic and difficult cases or to work on lifestyle as a complement to traditional therapy.

Research Base

Research on the effectiveness and Indian herbs is abundant in the literature. Nadkarni's *Indian Materia Medica* summarizes the vast research and historic usage of the multitude of herbs used in Ayurveda. The classical texts of Ayurveda contain vast references to using literally hundreds if not thousands of herbs for different disease conditions described in Ayurveda

Although research in Ayurveda has focused primarily on the pharmacologic use of Indian herbs, a paper published in 1995 presented a possible theoretic explanation for the success of the broader Ayurvedic model of healing. The January 1995 issue of the *Indian Journal of Physiology and Pharmacology* published a paper presented by Walton and Pugh outlining the relationship between stress and disease in both Ayurveda and the West.[1] The paper explores the relationship between the Ayurvedic concept of ojas, which is believed to be responsible for maintaining the physiologic equilibrium of the body, and what is known about the functions of steroids in the body's reactions to stress.

Recent herbal research from the Southern Illinois University School of Medicine has confirmed the effectiveness of the Indian herb *Mucuna pruriens*, which has been used historically for the treatment of neurologic disease and specifically for paralysis and tremors called *Kampavata* in Ayurveda. In 1990 Manyam published his findings in *The Journal of Movement Disorders*. He found that *Mucuna pruriens* contains Levodopa, which is effective in treating Parkinson's disease.[2] Then in 1995 *The Journal of Alternative and Complimentary Medicine* published research performed in The Netherlands at the Department of Biology of the University of Groningen. A controlled clinical trial using HP-200 derived from *Mucuna pruriens* was performed. The study followed 60 patients with a mean age of 59 years for 12 weeks. The study concluded that HP 200 was an effective treatment for patients with Parkinson's disease.[3]

In 1995 *The Journal of Ethnopharmacology* published additional research performed in The Netherlands at the Department of Biology of the University of Groningen. The research revealed that alcohol extracts of the Indian herbs *Caltropis procera* and *Semecarpus anacardium* displayed strong cytotoxic activity when tested on COLO 320 tumor cells.[4]

Risk and Safety

No studies have been performed to assess risks involved with ayurvedic therapies. Ayurvedic herbal and metal oxide remedies pose the greatest potential risks as they are ingested internally and through enemas. Ayurvedic practitioners believe that special methods of preparation applied to the metals renders them nontoxic when taken in the appropriate dosage.

Efficacy

In the author's experience the success of ayurvedic therapies depends on patient compliance, as much of the therapy is lifestyle-based. Compliance varies in accordance with the counseling skills of the practitioner and the relationship developed with the patient. When compliance is good, ayurvedic care is successful in greater than 80% of chronic disease cases. Success diminishes as compliance diminishes.

Future Research Opportunities and Priorities

Research opportunities are vast and interesting. In addition to continued pharmacologic research into the vast compendium of ayurvedic herbs and metal oxides, research on the effects of dosha-specific ayurvedic lifestyle, sense therapies, and diet would either prove or disprove the ayurvedic model of constitutional individuality.

Druglike Information

The actions of most herbs and the cross-reactions of herbs and drugs have not been studied in great detail. History suggests few harmful interactions, and most herbs are safe in the hands of a qualified practitioner. Practitioners are educated regarding which herbs and procedures are to be avoided by pregnant and lactating woman. For more information, see "Risk and Safety."

Sampling of 5 Common Indian Herbs According to Ayurvedic Principles*

Latin Name	Common Name	Doshic Effect	Actions	Pharmacology	Indications
Termin alia arjuna	Arjuna	VPK−	Cardiac Tonic and lithotropic	Contains large amounts of calcium and salts	Angina, cardiac valve abnormalities
Saraca iIndica	Ashok	P− VK(neutral)	Hemostat, analgesic, uterine sedative	Contains a fair amount of tannin, catachin and iron	Menstrual bleeding disorders, fibroids, uterine cramping
Withani a somnifera	Ashwagan da	VK− P+	Rejuvenative and nervine sedative	Contains alkaloid somniferin	Multiple sclerosis, oligospermia, general debility
Phyllan thus niruri	Bhumyama alaki	PK− V+	Alterative, diuretic	Contains phyllanthin, a bitter neutral substance	Hepatitis C, hyperacidity, diabetes, hyperacidity
Cucurma longa	Turmeric	KV− P+	Alterative, antibacterial, carminative, anticoagulant	Contains the alcohol turmerol and an alkaloid curcumin	Prevention of thrombus and embolus, Raynaud's disease, and other circulatory diseases

*A minus (−) sign after the doshic designation indicates that the color decreases the dosha; a plus (+) sign indicates that the color increases the dosha

Drug or Other Interactions

See "Risk and Safety" and "Druglike Information."

Adverse Reactions

See "Risk and Safety" and "Druglike Information."

Trade Products, Administration, and Dosage

There is a growing market for ayurvedic products in the health food stores. These products are herbal in nature, and they are designed according to allopathic usage and are condition-specific. Proper use according to ayurvedic principles requires a patient evaluation for the specific nature of the condition. Failure to use the products according to the nature of the constitution and imbalance is not the practice of Ayurveda, but rather, it is the pratice of allopathic herbalism.

Self-Help versus Professional

Ayurvedic lifestyle and dietary treatment may be applied by the general public on a cursory level after a proper evaluation to determine the constitution of the individual and the nature of the imbalance. Five sense therapies, with the exception of herbalism, may be self-applied with no significant risk and patients report that they enjoy being involved in their own healing. The use of herbs and ayurvedic purification and rejuvenation programs require greater training and patients should visit with a clinical ayurvedic specialist.

Visiting a Professional

A patient who visits an ayurvedic practitioner should expect to receive an evaluation consisting of a minimum of a history of the chief complaint, past medical history, a review of systems, and a review of any medications, herbs, and vitamins the patient may be taking.

Examination of body structure and the tongue and the taking of the pulse and vital signs completes the evaluation. A report of finding follows the physical examination to educate the patient. Follow-up visits are scheduled to support patients as they make progress and confront challenges. If necessary, additional therapies are integrated into the program slowly.

Training

Currently the only place in the U.S. where practitioners receive complete clinical training including internship is the California College of Ayurveda located in Grass Valley, California. Additional training programs in the basic principles of Ayurveda are available in Massachusetts at the New England Institute of Ayurveda, in New Mexico at the Ayurvedic Institute, in New York at the Ayurveda Holistic Center, and in Florida at the Florida Vedic College. Programs vary from 1 to 2 years in duration and often include part-time classroom education and independent study. In California, graduates of the California College of Ayurveda receive certification as a "Clinical Ayurvedic Specialist" and use the initials C.A.S. There are also home-study programs offered through the American Institute of Vedic Studies.

Credentialing

At this time there is no licensing available for the practice of Ayurveda in any of the 50 states. Credentials are issued by schools, which create their own standards to insure competency. State associations are forming to correct this situation. In California, graduates of the California College of Ayurveda receive a certificate upon completing the program and practice as a clinical ayurvedic specialist. Graduates may educate their patients, council them on lifestyle changes, and use the five sense therapies but may not diagnose or treat disease except under the direction of a licensed health care provider.

What to Look for in a Provider

When looking to refer a patient to a practitioner of Ayurveda, check to see if the practitioner is a graduate of one of the programs noted above. Always try to meet with practitioners and discuss the cases they have managed and their results. The California College of Ayurveda maintains a list of graduate practitioners throughout the U.S.

Barriers and Key Issues

The ayurvedic practitioner's thought processes and perceptions of the patient vary significantly from the allopathic physician and this is reflected in the de-emphasis of therapeutic drugs and herbs in the overall treatment approach. Emphasis on the psychospiritual nature of the mind-body connection reflects the holistic and spiritual nature of their approach. In addition, Ayurveda introduces a new vocabulary into the healing community that expresses these different ideas. These fundamental differences may make it difficult for the mainstream community to immediately understand and embrace Ayurveda.

Associations

The California Association of Ayurvedic Medicine
PO Box 2272
Loomis, CA 95650

Suggested Reading

1. Chopra D: *Perfect health*, New York, 1991, Harmony Books.
   A popular classic that introduced the principles of Ayurveda to the Western masses.
2. Frawley, Lad V: *The yoga of herbs*, Twin Lakes, Wis, 1986, Lotus Press.
   A classic in the field of Ayurvedic herbalism.
3. Frawley D: *Ayurveda and the mind*, Twin Lakes, Wis, 1997, Lotus Press.
   The best book that approaches the subject of Ayurvedic psychology.

4. Frawley D: *Ayurvedic healing,* Salt Lake City, 1989, Passage Press.
   The first book approaching the Ayurvedic management of disease in the West.
5. Svoboda R: *Prakruti,* Wilmont, Wis, 1989, Lotus Light Press.
   A poetic discussion of the basic principles of Ayurveda.

Bibliography

Murthy S: *Ashtang samgraha,* Varanasi, India, 1995, Chaukaumba Orientalia.

Dash B, Sharma RK: *Caraka samhita,* Varanasi, India, 1995, Chaukaumba Orientalia.

Dash B, Junius R: *Handbook of Ayurveda,* New Delhi, 1983, Concept Publishing.

Nadkarni AK: *Indian materia medica,* Bombay, 1982, Popular Prakashan.

Bishagratna KL: *Sushrut samhita,* Varanasi, India, 1998, Chaukaumba Orientalia.

Frawley D, Lad V: *Yoga of herbs,* Twin Lakes, Wis, 1986, Lotus Press.

References

1. Walton KG, Pugh ND: Stress, steroids, and ojas: neuroendocrine mechanisms and current promise of ancient approaches to disease prevention, *Indian J Physiol Pharmacol* 39(1):3-36, 1995.
2. Manyam BV: Paralysis agitans and levodopa in Ayurveda: ancient Indian medical treatise, *Mov Disord* 5(1):47-48, 1990.
3. An alternative medicine treatment for Parkinson's disease: results of a multicenter clinical trial. HP-200 in Parkinson's Disease Study Group, *J Altern Complement Med* 1(3):249-255, 1995.
4. Smit HF et al: Ayurvedic herbal drugs with possible cytostatic activity, *J Ethnopharmacol* 47(2):75-84, 1995.

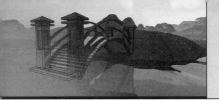

Homeopathy

EDWARD V. KONDROT

EILEEN NAUMAN

TODD ROWE

Origins and History

Classical homeopathy is an empiric system of medicine established by Samuel Hahnemann, MD, who was born in Dresden, Germany in 1755. The word *homeopathy* is derived from the Greek word *homoios* (similar) and *pathos* (suffering or disease).

While translating *A Treatise on Materia Medica* by Dr. William Cullen, Hahnemann came across a passage describing the use of cinchona bark in the treatment of malaria. Cullen stated that cinchona was a valuable drug because of its astringent qualities. Hahnemann decided to take the cinchona and observe in detail his own symptoms. To his surprise he developed a symptom complex very similar to the malaria. This supported the law of healing described by Hippocrates called the *Law of Similars*. Drugs that produce symptoms in a healthy person will treat those symptoms in a disease state. Hahnemann then proceeded to test or "prove" many other compounds, including aconite, belladonna, and calcarea carbonica.

The symptoms were carefully recorded and were published in the *Materia Medica Pura* and *Chronic Diseases*. Hahnemann, using his skills of critical observation, developed this system of homeopathy over many years. Additional provings based on experiments led to a system of healing.*

Other experiments were conducted, and these provings became the basis for inclusion in the *Homeopathic Pharmacopoeia*. The current (ninth) edition describes how more than 1000 substances are prepared for homeopathic use. These provings became the foundation for homeopathic prescribing. Hahnemann further developed this system of homeopathy over a course of many years and performed many additional proofs. Hahnemann's

---

* A *proving* is a method of experimentation using a highly diluted homeopathic substance that is administered to healthy volunteers to create symptoms. These symptoms are then carefully recorded. From this compilation of substance-induced symptoms, the homeopathic repertory is created.

very critical observation transformed itself into a system of healing based on the following laws:

The law of similars: The symptoms of the patient must be matched to the proving symptoms of the remedy for the drug to act homeopathically. This is the basic and most important law in homeopathy. In selecting a remedy, not only the physical particular symptoms of the disease but also mental, emotional, and general symptoms must match the remedy. The physical particulars need to be defined as accurately as possible, including precise location, extension (symptoms that extend into other parts of the body), and modalities (circumstances that will cause an aggravation or amelioration of the symptoms). In addition, concomitants are also important. They are unrelated symptoms that may not be explained by the commonly understood pathophysiologic process of the disease. An example of a concomitant would be a headache that occurs during diarrhea. Homeopathic remedies that are used have been tested by provings of a single remedy. Combination remedies are untested and their proving symptoms are not known. It is impossible to then match symptoms of the patient with these theoretic combinations. Hahnemann in his writings emphasized the importance of only using one remedy at a time. He felt that the combination of remedies was dangerous and this combination would produce a different set of symptoms that may not match those of the person. It is important to understand the action of one remedy and the response of the person to that remedy. If a person has a positive response or negative response when using combination remedies, it would not be known what remedy was responsible for the action. This would interfere with future treatment when repetition or changing of the dose is required.

Single dose: One dose will stimulate the body and create a change. It is important to let this action continue and not be disturbed by repeating the remedy. If the remedy is repeated too soon its action will interfere with the action of the first dose, resulting in an aggravation or a neutralization of its action.

Minimum dose: This is another one of the basic tenets of homeopathy. The lowest possible dose should be used to stimulate the natural healing action of the body. The homeopathic remedy is similar to an enzyme or a hormone in its action. A small amount is all that is needed to effect a change. Hahnemann taught that additional doses of medicine would cease to be therapeutic.

The law of dilution and succussion: Hahnemann was concerned about the side effects of many of the medications that were commonly used. Through a serious of carefully controlled experiments, Hahnemann discovered that medications could be diluted and still maintain medicinal properties. It was also noted that the dilute medications produced fewer side effects. Hahnemann also discovered that by succussing (striking or shaking the medicated solution), an apparent activation of the substance developed, which increased its healing power. The more the medication is diluted and succussed, the stronger are the medicinal effects. These are the most difficult concepts of homeopathy to understand. How can these extremely dilute substances have any effect? How can succussion activate the medication? Is it nothing more than a placebo response? There have been several experiments conducted in water physics to demonstrate that water crystals develop that can act much like an enzyme substrate reaction to transfer the characteristics of the material substance. (See "Basic Science.")

Laws of cure: The homeopath Constantine Herring observed this phenomena. It is not enough to rid the body of symptoms of disease; the goal is cure. Disease moves in a specific direction during cure. It moves from vital organs to less vital organs, from within to without, from above to below, and in the reverse order of appearance. The background that led up to the formation and refinement of this modality as it is exists in its present form. Classical homeopaths practice according to the *Organon* written by Samuel Hahnemann 250 years ago.

Mechanism of Action According to Its Own Theory

The belief in homeopathy is that each individual has a self-healing capacity or a healer within. Homeopathy works by activating the self-healing capacity of the individual organism. What is curable in homeopathy is what individuals can heal within themselves. This self-healing brings individuals into balance wherever they are out of balance, and it then restores homeostasis. The mechanism of action is dynamic rather than material. Throughout history there have been two dominant approaches to healing. These two approaches are the rationalistic and empiric schools. Allopathic medicine is an example of the rationalistic school. This type of healing focuses on a bimolecular understanding of life, and it attempts to find the root or fundamental cause of the disease. Homeopathy is an example of the empiric form of healing. Here the focus is on energy and attempting to see the whole person and to understand that individual on all levels of being. Homeopathic remedies act by affecting what is termed the *vital force* or the energetic or dynamic level of an organism. According to Hahnemann, the remedies create a stronger dynamic disease, one that is capable of eclipsing the weaker dynamic disease within the organism, and thereby producing cure. Remedies each have their own resonant frequency. The goal of the homeopathy practitioner is to choose a medicine that resonates with the frequency of the disease. In essence, homeopathic remedies are thought to act more on a bioenergetic level, rather than a bimolecular level.

Hormesis is the name of a fairly new and popular scientific field that studies the effects of extremely small doses of otherwise toxic substances to promote growth or healing processes. This field in part is an outgrowth of the Ardnt Schultz Law, which states the following: that for every substance, small doses stimulate, moderate doses inhibit, and large doses kill.

Another theory about the mechanism of action of homeopathic remedies is the idea of "smart water." The understanding here is that the solvent (usually water) can carry information that is formed as a vibratory imprint of its solute. Every substance leaves a different vibratory imprint and as this imprint gets stronger and clearer, the remedy is more potentized. This theory has been experimentally substantiated by the work of Dr. Shui-Yin Lo with ice crystals (see "Research Base").

Biologic Mechanism of Action

It remains unknown as to how homeopathy really works on the cellular structure. More research needs to be done. The Arndt-Schultz Law with reference to biologic activity provides justification for the use of minute doses. This law states that small doses of drugs encourage life activity, large material doses of drugs impede life activity, and very large doses destroy life activity. To put it another way, the function of the dose of the drug is inversely proportional to the effect of the drug.

The posologic concept of the infinitesimally small dose is the second basic principle of homeopathy. Apart from their therapeutic effectiveness, minute homeopathic dosages render even the most toxic substances used in their preparation safe and free from unwanted side effects.

Forms of Therapy

The method of homeopathy described in this chapter is based on classical principles described by Samuel Hahnemann. Nonclassical methods include combination remedies, disease-oriented prescribing, formula prescribing, electronic testing, and Radionics. Combination remedies are one or more remedies formulated to treat common diseases, but they do not represent classical homeopathic treatment and healing. Homeopathy is not herbal medicine.

Electronic testing and Radionics also are methods used to select a homeopathic remedy in a nonclassical manner.

Demographics

Homeopaths are found throughout the U.S. and the world. Many types of persons, regardless of gender and age, use homeopathy.

To locate a homeopathic practitioner, contact The National Center of Homeopathy (NCH), listed in "Associations."

Indications and Reasons for Referral

Homeopathy can address nearly any condition. It cannot cure everything, but even in incurable cases it can stop or limit progression of the disease. There are many conditions where homeopathy can work curatively, even though there is no effective standard medical treatment. If a person is not improving with conventional medicine for the chronic symptoms, homeopathy may be sought as an alternative for cure. A person who is sensitive to conventional drugs, suffers from adverse reactions or side effects, refuses conventional drug treatment could look to homeopathy for help and support.

In disease prevention, homeopathy can be used prophylactically for acute epidemics. For example, people who refuse flu shots can use homeopathy instead.

In pregnancy the gentle efficacy of homeopathy can be instituted when drug therapy is not an option to the pregnant woman.

Many chronic conditions, such as asthma, arthritis, and migraine headaches, can be effectively addressed. The goal here is not just to manage the chronic symptoms but to cure the underlying disease.

Acute conditions that are too numerous to name here but include injuries, colds, and flu can be addressed directly by homeopathy. What are the classic reasons for referring to this type of therapy?

Reasons include wanting a "safer" medicine, disliking conventional drugs, preferring a less expensive alternative, seeking a more holistic approach to healing, and wanting a stronger relationship with the doctor.

See "Office Applications" as a partial list of conditions treated by homeopathy. Homeopathy can effectively treat nearly all problems and diseases. A few conditions may not be curable with homeopathy, including AIDS, insulin-dependent diabetes mellitus, cancer, surgical conditions, and schizophrenia. However, although the remedies are not curative in these cases, they still can substantially alleviate symptoms and suffering. The remedies only can heal what the body itself can heal. They work curatively if the following criteria are met: (1) the person's vital force is sufficiently strong; and (2) the person is not engaged in treatment that antidotes the homeopathic remedy. Factors that influence the strength of the vital force include age, severity of physical pathology, family history, and history of suppression of symptoms with conventional medications.

Office Applications

Because of the extent of the conditions that can be applied to homeopathic evaluation and treatment, please refer to the following list of conditions. A simple ranking of conditions responsive to this form of therapy is as follows. As with all alternative therapies, use of homeopathy does not preclude the use of mainstream medical therapies in addition.

Top level: *A therapy ideally suited for these conditions*

Abscess; acne; acute diseases; agoraphobia; allergies; amenorrhea; anger; uncontrolled anxiety; arthritis (rheumatoid or osteoarthritis); asthma; attention deficit disorder; belching; benign prostatic hypertrophy; bites and stings (animal, insect, reptiles); bladder infection; blepharitis; boils; bone ailments; botulism; breast feeding; bronchitis; bruises; bruxism; bursitis; carpal tunnel syndrome; cerebral concussion; chancre sores, chickenpox; childbirth; childhood parasites; children's health; cholecystitis; chronic fatigue syndrome; chronic obstructive pulmonary disease; chronic pain, circulation disorders; cold sores; colds; colic; colitis; compulsive disorder; confusion; conjunctivitis; compulsive disorders; conjunctivitis; connective tissue disorders; constipation; convulsions; coughs; cramps; crohn's disease; croup; cuts; cystitis; cysts; dacryocystitis; delirium; delusions; depression; dermatitis; diarrhea; digestive problems; diverticulitis; diverticulosis; dry eyes; dysphasia; ear infections; ear injuries; earaches; eczema; edema; emotional disorders; encopresis; endometriosis; enuresis; epilepsy; esophageal spasm; esophagitis; exhibitionism;

eyestrain; fears; febrile convulsion; female health; fever; fibromyalgia; fibrocystic breast disease; fibrosis; flatulence; floaters; food poisoning; foot injuries; fractures, frost bite; gallbladder disease; gallstones; gastritis; gastroenteritis; gastrointestinal disorders; general ear pain; genital warts; german measles (rubella); gout; growing pains (in children); hay fever; head injury; headaches; headaches (migraine); headaches (tension); heartburn; hemorrhoids; herpes simplex and zoster; high altitude sickness; hives; hoarseness; hypertension; indigestion; influenza; insomnia; intestinal disorders; irritable bowel syndrome; knee disorders; knee injuries; laryngospasm; laryngysmus; laryngitis; lung disorders; Lyme disease; lymph gland disorders; lymph gland swelling; measles; memory disorders; men's health problems; Meniere's disease; menopause; menstrual cramps; mental health; migraines; mononucleosis; motion sickness; mouth disorders; multiple sclerosis; mumps; muscle injuries; narcolepsy; nausea; necrosis; neuralgia; nerve disorders; night blindness; nose disorders; nose injuries; otitis media; pain of any kind; panic attack; paranoid; periodic leg movement syndrome; pelvic disorders; peptic ulcers; phantom limb pain; pharyngitis; phobias; photosensitivity; pleurisy; pneumonia; poison ivy/oak; postpartum care; posttraumatic stress disorder; pregnancy and childbirth; premenstrual syndrome; prostatitis; psoriasis; pulmonary disease; puncture wounds; Reynaud's syndrome; rectum disorders; renal disorders; respiratory disorders; restless leg syndrome; rheumatoid arthritis; rheumatism; Rocky Mountain spotted fever; salmonella; sea sickness; shingles; shortness of breath (dyspnea); sinus disorders (acute and chronic); sinusitis (acute and chronic); skin diseases; sleep apnea; sleep disorders; soft tissue injuries; sore throat; spastic colon; spider bites; spleen injury; sports injuries; sprains; stings (all kinds); stomach disorders; strains; strep throat; stress; styes; surgical (presurgical and postsurgical); teething; tinnitus; tonsillitis; toothache; ulcers; ulcerative colitis; uterine fibroids; urethritis; vaginal infections; vertigo; viral and bacterial infections; vision disorders; warts; whiplash; women's health; yeast infections; vaccination alternative; vaccination reactions; and vomiting

Second level: *One of the better therapies for these conditions*

Accidents of any kind; acid reflux; anaphylactic reaction; anesthesia reaction; angina pectoris; arrhythmia; backache; back pain; bad breath; blood clots; breathing disorders; candidiasis; cardiovascular disease; central nervous system diseases; cerebral hematoma; coma; congestive heart failure; dehydration; dislocation; drug overdose; electrical trauma; emphysema; epidural hematoma; exposures to environmental poisons; gangrene; glaucoma; gonorrhea; hallucinations; hearing loss; heart attack; heart disease; heat cramps; heat exhaustion; heat stroke; hip disease; hypoglycemia; hypothermia, hypoxia; incontinence; infection; internal injuries; kidney stone; lightning strike injury; liver disease; locomotor ataxia; lower back disorders; lower back injury; manic behavior; manic depressive illness; narcotic overdose; obsessive compulsive disorder; osteoarthritis; osteoporosis; ovarian cysts; Parkinson's disease; pedal foot edema; pertussis; phlebitis; poisoning (any type); psychologic problems; psychotic behavior; pulmonary edema; renal colic; retinitis; retinal degeneration; rheumatic fever; schizophrenia; sciatica; scoliosis; sepsis; sexual dysfunction (male and female); sexually transmitted diseases; snakebite; speech difficulty; speech disorders; spinal injury; spleen disorders; stammering; stroke; syphilis; TMJ; tick bite; and violent behavior

Third level: *A valuable adjunctive therapy for these conditions*

Abdominal injury; addictions; allergic reaction; Alzheimer's disease; appendicitis; autism; bleeding (control of); cardiovascular accident; carbon monoxide poisoning; cardiac arrest; cataracts; chemical poisoning; cornea disorders; detached retina; diabetes; double vision; eclampsia; embolism; eye diseases; head lice; hearing disorders; hemoptysis; hemorrhage; hip dislocation; hyphema; iritis; macular degeneration; myasthenia gravis; myocardial infarction; neck injuries; paralysis; parasitic infections; shock (treatment of); and shoulder dislocation

Practical Applications

Homeopathy has a value in almost all clinical situations. The homeopath must match as closely as possible the symptoms of a patient with the symptoms of a homeopathic remedy. Two types of books that are indispensable in this process are the repertory and the materia medica.

Research Base

Evidence Based

Reilly, Taylor, and Beattie[1] successfully reproduced evidence from two previous double-blinded trials, all of which used the same model of homeopathic immunotherapy in inhalant allergy. In this third study, 9 of 11 patients on homeopathic treatment improved, compared to only 5 of 13 patients on placebo. The researchers concluded that either homeopathic medicines work or controlled studies do not work. Their work has been recently replicated again and is submitted for publication.[2]

Jacobs, Jimenez, and Margarita[3] demonstrated the value of homeopathy in acute childhood diarrhea. Reilly[1,2] also has presented compelling evidence on the effectiveness of homeopathy.

Basic Science

Lo[4] proposes a theoretic framework to explain some unique physical properties of very dilute water solutions of common chemical compounds. These solutions are prepared in a manner similar to potentized remedies. Lo's principal claim is that at least some substances dissolved in water can lead to the formation of tiny ice-like crystals, which can then exist and grow independently of the original substance that induced their formation.

This theory supports homeopathic succussion: That in successively diluted or shaken solutions there is then a very physical presence, which is due to but does not require any concentration of the original solute. Lo estimates that these crystals incorporate up to a few percent of the water in a solution. This is an anomalous state of ice, which can be induced to form under the action of ions in very dilute solutions. These stable structures change the UV transmission characteristic of water. Different structures formed from different ions are shown to have similar UV transmission characteristics.

These structures can be filtered, concentrated, and photographed using a transmission electron microscope. A dipole-dipole interaction model is constructed to suggest an explanation of the elongated shape of these structures. There are considerable experiments in the field of biology, biochemistry, and pharmacology indicating that ultra low doses have significant effects on living organisms. The experiments here show that ultra small amounts of acid, base, or salt can induce stable rigid ice crystal (IE) structures in water itself. These IE structures have different UV transmission characteristics from pure water. Transmission electron microscope pictures are consistent with the idea that these IE structures are made up of electric dipoles.

Studies by Benveniste[5-8] demonstrate the effect of ultra high dilutions on specific biologic processes.

Risk and Safety

Because of their extreme dilution, homeopathic remedies are generally quite safe. It is rare to have an adverse reaction except the proving symptoms that already have been noted. However, no formal studies exist evaluating the safety of this therapy.

Efficacy

Most experienced homeopathy practitioners have success rates between 75% and 90% in the treatment of chronic disease.

Future Research Opportunities and Priorities

There are three studies currently listed with the National Institutes of Health examining the effectiveness of homeopathy. Clearly, the highest priority is to prove that the homeopathic medical model works to the satisfaction of the conventional medical and science world.

Druglike Information

Safety

Homeopathic medicines are safe when used by a professional homeopath. Because of the extremely dilute substance used, homeopathic remedies are virtually nontoxic. Homeopathic remedies are extremely dilute, and potencies above 12 C contain no physical substance.

Warnings, Contraindications, and Precautions

There are few warnings or contraindications in the homeopathic literature due to the safety of this form of healing. One of the warnings relates to the remedies containing either phosphorus or silica, which can be dangerous if misapplied. In addition, taking a specified homeopathic remedy after the symptoms have disappeared can cause problems.

Drug or Other Interactions

Steroids, chemotherapeutic agents, and antibiotics are major contraindications in the use of homeopathic medications. Acupuncture frequently interferes with the action of the homeopathic remedy.

There are many things that can antidote (neutralize) a homeopathic remedy. The following is a partial listing of these substances and treatments:

1. Coffee (including decaffeinated)
2. Camphor, menthol, and strong herbal oil products
3. Dental work (High speed drills can sometimes approximate the "frequency" of the remedy and antidote it.)
4. Certain herbs
5. Certain allopathic medications
6. Energy treatments
7. Recreational drugs

In addition, certain foods, chemicals, or substances can antidote if the patient is quite sensitive. Consistent use of electric blankets and exposure to strong overpowering odors may also antidote a remedy.

Adverse Reactions

Aggravation of presenting symptoms sometimes occur with the use of homeopathic medications. Often called a *healing crisis*, the aggravation is generally brief, lasting several hours to several weeks.

Pregnancy and Lactation

No contraindications exist.

Trade Products, Administration, and Dosage

There are three categories of homeopathic potencies: decimal potencies (diluted 1 part per 10), centesimal potencies (diluted one part per 100), and M potencies. These are described as X, C, and M dilutions. An easy way to calculate dilution is to consider the scale logarithmically. A 6X dilution therefore translates as 10^{-6}. A 200C dilution translates as 10^{-400}, and a 1M dilution equals 1000C, which translates as 10^{-2000}.

Classically the remedy is given either as a dilution (fluid), pellet (sucrose) or tablet (lactose), mother tincture, or ointment.

Homeopathy, unlike many other alternative medicines, is well-regulated and approved by the FDA. For remedies to be sold in the U.S., they must first be *proven* and listed in *Homeopathic Pharmacopoeia of the United States* (HPUS). Most health food stores carry some of the remedies but very rarely do they carry all of them.

The following is only a partial listing of recommended sources for homeopathic products:

Dolisos
Tel: (800) 365-4767
Fax: (702) 871-9670

Hahnemann Pharmacy
Tel: (888) 427-6422

Standard Homeopathic Co.
Tel: (800) 624-9659
Fax: (310) 516-8579

Boericke & Tafel
Tel: (800) 876-9505
(707) 571-8202, extension 105
Fax: (707) 571-8237

Boiron
Telephone orders: (800) 258-8823
Consumer information: (800) 264-7661
Fax: (800) 999-4373

Washington Homeopathic Products
Telephone orders: (800) 336-1696
(301) 656-1695
Fax: (301) 656-1847

Luyties
Tel: (800) 466-3672
Fax: (314) 535-9600

Self-Help versus Professional

In acute cases, many people will purchase an introductory how-to book on homeopathy. In chronic cases, a person should never try to self-treat.

Visiting a Professional

The constitutional case-taking is a prolonged interview, which may take anywhere between 1 and 2 hours. After the evaluation is completed, a homeopathic remedy is usually provided. At the 4 or 6-week check-in, progress is reevaluated and, if necessary, the entire case is retaken.

Credentialing

The Council for Homeopathic Certification (CHC) is the only certification board that certifies competency in homeopathy regardless of professional training. The designation is CCH. Homeopathy is currently licensed in only three states. Their governing bodies are the Arizona Board of Homeopathic Medical Examiners; Connecticut Department of Health Homeopathic Licensure; and Nevada State Board of Homeopathic Medical Examiners.

In most other states, homeopathic medicine is considered a process of diagnosis and treatment. For this reason it is included in the license of *physician*, which definition varies from state to state. Lay homeopaths also practice but in an unlicensed capacity except for the states previously listed.

Certification

The Council on Homeopathic Certification (CHC)
1199 Sanchez
San Francisco, CA 94114
www.homeopathy-council.org

There is a movement by many homeopaths to get all homeopathic practitioners certified by the CHC. Currently, many good homeopathic practitioners still are not certified.

Training

Numerous schools and training programs exist. The following list is only a representative sample:

WEST COAST:
National College of Naturopathic Medicine
Tel: (530) 255-4860

Bastyr University
Tel: (206) 823-1300

Southwest College of Naturopathic Medicine
Tel: (602) 858-9100

Hahnemann Medical Clinic
Tel: (510) 232-2079

SOUTHWEST:
Desert Institute of Classical Homeopathy
Tel: (602) 347-7950
Fax: (602) 864-2949

MIDWEST:
Robin Murphy, ND, offers training programs. She can be contacted at (303) 264-2460

EAST COAST:
The Teleosis School of Homeopathy
Tel: (518) 392-7975

SPECIALIZED TRAINING:
Dental Seminars
PO Box 123
Marengo, IL 60152

Training in Veterinary Homeopathy
Tel: (503) 342-7665

CORRESPONDENCE COURSES:
The British Institute
Tel: (800) 498-6323
Fax: (800) 495-8277

The School of Homeopathy
Tel/Fax: (203) 624-8783

The Desert Institute of Classical Homeopathy
Tel: (602) 864-1776

What to Look for in a Provider

Because there is no one organization leading homeopathy in the U.S. today, the person
looking for homeopathic treatment must do some self-educating before setting out to look
for a practitioner. There is a movement by many homeopaths to get all homeopathic practitioners certified by the Council for Homeopathic Certification (CHC). Currently, many
good homeopathic practitioners are still not certified. Until this is accomplished, the following list of questions should be asked:

1. How long has the practitioner been in practice? Typically, the more time they have
   practiced, the better they are at their skills. Ideally, five years of practice as a homeopath is a good guideline.
2. What is the quality of their education? There are many homeopathic schools available of varying quality. The Council for Homeopathic Education (CHE) is in the
   process of accrediting homeopathic schools throughout the country. This is one good
   standard to determine the quality of the school. We would suggest that a good quality

program has a minimum of 500 hours of didactic instruction. Clinical training is also an important component to homeopathic education, yet many schools still lack this in their curriculum.

3. Is the homeopath a classically trained homeopath? *Classical* means that the practitioner gives a single dose of a single remedy at a time and then wait for the remedy to act. This is the form of homeopathy that is most practiced in the world today, as set forth by Samuel Hahnemann.

4. Does the practitioner have adequate medical training? It is imperative that the homeopath have adequate background medical knowledge. The homeopath must be able to discern a medical emergency and when it is important to refer to a more experienced medical practitioner. This question is especially important if the practitioner does not have a medical license (such as MD, DO, ND, DC, LAC, and others). However, the practice of homeopathy requires much more than medical training.

5. Does the homeopathic practitioner regularly attend seminars or workshops on classical homeopathy? Homeopathy is enjoying a powerful resurgence worldwide with much new information on provings and cured cases. It is imperative that a homeopath keep up with new developments in the homeopathic field.

Barriers and Key Issues

There is a strong need for greater funding of research studies into the mechanism of action and efficacy of homeopathy.

Like most forms of nontraditional therapy, the greatest barrier to acceptance in mainstream medicine is the lack of literacy among physicians and other practitioners regarding homeopathy. This could be effectively addressed by the following:

1. Introductory classes in homeopathy within medical school and residency training programs
2. Introductory workshops on homeopathy at hospitals within the integrative medicine departments
3. Introductory talks at standard medical conferences
4. Reading from the book list provided in "Suggested Reading"
5. The creation of greater public awareness of homeopathy
6. Promoting good quality homeopathic research through the National Institutes of Health (NIH)

Associations

NOTE: There are many international organizations, but space limitations prevent listing them here.

United States Organizations

The National Center of Homeopathy (NCH)
801 North Fairfax St., Suite 306
Alexandria, VA 22314
Tel: (703) 548-7790
Fax: (703) 548-7792
E-mail: nchinfo@igc.org
www.homeopathic.org

State Associations for Licensed Professionals

Please visit www.healthy.net/nch for information. States that have homeopathic associations include Arizona, California, Connecticut, Illinois, Michigan, Nevada, New York, Ohio, Pennsylvania, Virginia, and Texas.

Internet Resources

This is not a complete list.

HOMEOPATHIC WEBSITES

www.alchemilla.com
www.gn.apc.org/ecch.icch
www.homeopathic.com
www.homeopathy.ch(Switzerland)
www.medicinegarden.com
www.simillibus.com

HOMEOPATHIC EDUCATION INFORMATION

E-mail: jkreisberg@igc.apc.org

REPERTOIRES ONLINE

Kent Repertory online: www.homeoint.org
Complete Repertory online: www.irhis.nl

HOW TO MAKE A HOMEOPATHIC REMEDY

www.medicinegarden.com/Homeopathy/How_to_make_a_remedy_1

HOMEOPATHIC MAGAZINE ONLINE

Homeopathy Online: A Journal of Homeopathic Medicine: www.lyghtforce.com

HOMEOPATHIC LISTS

http://www.dungeon.com/~cam/homfaq.html
www.medicinegarden.com/Athena

HOMEOPATHIC DIRECTORIES IN THE U.S.

www.healthy.net/nch

HOMEOPATHIC BOOKSTORES ONLINE

www.homeopathic.com
www.minimum.com

Homeopathic Computer Software

CARA Pro
Tel: (905) 886-1060
Fax: (905) 886-1418
E-mail: basilziv@web.net

Kent Homeopathic Associates
Tel: (415) 457-0678
Fax: (415) 457-0688
E-mail: kha@igc.org

RADAR Canada
Tel: (800) 668-7543

Suggested Reading

1. Vithoulkas G: *The science of homeopathy*, New York, 1980, Grove Press.
   Vithoulkas is considered one of our most brilliant, forward-thinking homeopaths in the world. His book brings homeopathy from the 1800s into more modern language and parallels of the twentieth century.
2. O'Reilly WB: *Organon of the medical art by Dr. Samuel Hahnemann*, Redmond, Wash, 1996, Birdcage Books.
   This book elaborates in plain English the *Organon of Medical Art* by the founder of homeopathy, Samuel Hahnemann.
3. Bellavite P, Signorini A: *Homeopathy: a frontier in medical science*, Berkeley, Calif, 1995, North Atlantic.
   This book puts homeopathy into a better understood context for traditional medicine and Western science.
4. Kent JT: *Repertory of the homeopathic materia medica*, New Delhi, 1981, B. Jain.
   This repertory is the one most commonly used in the world today.
5. Clarke JH: *A dictionary of practical materia medica*, vol 3, New Delhi, 1984, B. Jain.
   This repertory is one of our best *Materia Medicas*.
6. Rowe T: *Homeopathic repertory, case-taking, and case analysis methodology*, Berkeley, Calif, 1998, North Atlantic Books.
   This is an introduction to repertory, case-taking, and case analysis.

7. Schiff M: *The memory of water: homeopathy and the battle of ideas in the new science*, London, 1998, Thorsons Publishing.

   Jacques Benveniste's ground-breaking work in France shows that water has memory and therefore adds growing proof of how homeopathy works.

8. Nauman E, Derin-Kellogg G: *Homeopathy 911*, New York, 1999, Kensington.

   This book provides bridgework showing the ways homeopathy can help during medical emergencies.

Bibliography

Clarke JH: *A dictionary of practical materia medica*, vol 3, New Delhi, 1984, B. Jain.

Farrington H: Homeopathy and homeopathic prescribing, New Delhi, 1993, B. Jain.

Kent TK: *Lectures on homeopathic materia medica*, New Delhi, 1986, B. Jain.

Kent TK: *Lectures on homeopathic philosophy*, Richmond, Calif, 1979, North Atlantic Books.

Kunzli J, Naude A, Pendelton P: *Organon of medicine of Samuel Hahnemann*, translation from German, ed 6, Los Angeles, 1982, J.P. Tarcher.

Nauman E, Derin-Kellogg G: *Homeopathy 911*, New York, 1999, Kensington.

Nauman E: *Poisons that heal*, Sedona, Ariz, 1995, Light Technology.

Rowe T: *Homeopathic methodology: repertory, case-taking, and case analysis*, Berkeley, Calif, 1998, North Atlantic Books.

Simon B: Communications, April 1998.

Vithoulkas G: *The science of homeopathy*, New York, 1980, Grove Press.

References

1. Reilly D et al: Is evidence for homeopathy reproducible? *Lancet* 10(344):1601-1606, 1994.

2. Jacobs J et al: Treatment of acute childhood diarrhea with homeopathic medicine: a randomized clinical trial in Nicaragua, *Pediatrics* 93(4):719-725, 1994.

3. Reilly D et al: Is homeopathy a placebo response? Controlled trial of homeopathic potency, with pollen in hayfever as model, *Lancet* 18:881-886, 1986.

4. Lo SY: Anomalous state of ice. Excerpt from *Modern Physics Letters B* 10(19):909-916, 1996.

5. Benviste J: Further biological effects induced by ultra high dilutions: inhibition by a magnetic field. In Endler PC, Schulte J, editors: *Ultra High Dilution*, Dordrecht, 1994, Kluwer Academic.

6. Benviste J, Arnoux B, Hadji L: Highly dilute antigen increases coronary flow of isolated hart from immunized guinea pigs, Abstract 1610, *FASEB J* 6, 1992.

7. Benviste J et al: L'agitation de solutions hautement diluees n'induit pas d'activite biologique specifique, *C R Acad Sci Paris* 312:461, 1991.

8. Benviste J: Human basophil degranulation triggered by very dilute antiserum against IgE, *Nature* 333:816-818, 1988.

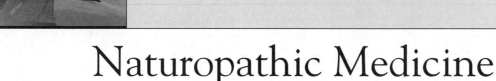

Naturopathic Medicine

CATHERINE DOWNEY*

Origins and History

Naturopathic medicine is a distinctively natural approach to health and healing that recognizes the integration of the whole person. Naturopathic medicine is heir to the vitalistic tradition of medicine in the Western world, emphasizing the treatment of disease through the stimulation, enhancement, and support of the inherent healing capacity of the person. Methods of treatment are chosen to work with the patient's life force, respecting the natural healing process.

The philosophy of naturopathic medicine traces its roots to Hippocrates with the concepts of *tolle causam,* supporting the *vis medicatrix naturae* and *primum no nocere.* From a therapeutic standpoint, naturopathic medicine relies on the oldest known remedies: food, herbs, baths (hydrotherapy), and massage or manipulation.

The practice of naturopathic medicine actually emerges from six principles of healing. These principles are based on the objective observation of the nature of health and disease and are examined continually in the light of scientific analysis. These principles distinguish the profession from other medical approaches.

The Healing Power of Nature *(Vis medicatix naturae):* The body has the inherent ability to establish, maintain, and restore health. The healing process is ordered and intelligent: Nature heals through the response of the life force. The physician's role is to facilitate and augment this process, act to identify and remove obstacles to health and recovery, and support the creation of a healthy internal and external environment.

Treat the Whole Person *(The multifactorial nature of health and disease):* Health and disease are conditions of the whole organism, involving a complex interaction of physical, spiritual, mental, emotional, genetic, environmental, and social factors. The physician must treat the whole person by taking all of these factors into account. The harmonious functioning of all aspects of the individual is essential to

*The author wishes to thank the staff of the National College of Naturopathic Medicine for its participation in the writing of this chapter.

recovery from and prevention of disease and requires a personalized and comprehensive approach to diagnosis and treatment.

First Do No Harm (*Primum no nocere*): Illness is a purposeful process of the organism. The process of healing includes the generation of symptoms, which in fact are an expression of the life force attempting to heal itself. Therapeutic actions should be complementary to and synergistic with this healing process. The physician's actions can support or antagonize the actions of the *vis mediatrix naturae*; therefore methods designed to suppress symptoms without removing underlying causes are considered harmful and are avoided or minimized. Therapeutic actions are applied in an ordered fashion congruent with the internal order of the organism.

Identify and Treat the Cause (*Tolle causam*): Illness does not occur without cause. Underlying causes of disease must be discovered and removed or treated before a person can recover completely from illness. Symptoms are expressions of the body's attempt to heal but are not the cause of disease; therefore naturopathic medicine addresses itself promptly to the underlying causes of disease rather than symptoms. Causes may occur on many levels, including physical, mental-emotional, and spiritual. The physician must evaluate fundamental underlying causes on all levels, directing treatment at root cause rather than at symptomatic expression.

Prevention (*Prevention is the best "cure"*): The ultimate goal of naturopathic medicine is prevention. This is accomplished through education and promotion of lifestyle habits that create good health. The physician assesses risk factors and hereditary susceptibility to disease and makes appropriate interventions to avoid further harm and risk to the patient. The emphasis is on building health rather than fighting disease. Because it is difficult to be healthy in an unhealthy world, it is the responsibility of both the physician and patient to create a healthier environment in which to live.

The Physician as Teacher (*Docere*): Beyond an accurate diagnosis and appropriate prescription the physician must work to create a health-sensitive interpersonal relationship with the patient. A cooperative doctor-patient relationship has inherent therapeutic value. The physician's major role is to educate and encourage the patient to take responsibility for health. The physician is a catalyst for healthful change, empowering and motivating the patient to assume responsibility. It is the patient, not the doctor, who ultimately creates or accomplishes healing. The physician must strive to inspire hope as well as understanding. Physicians also must make a commitment to their personal and spiritual development in order to be good teachers.

A History of Naturopathic Medicine

The 1800s saw a rough-and-tumble free-market approach to medicine in the US, with states first licensing then revoking licensing laws. Education was spotty, many practitioners were self-taught, and there were many styles of practice. By the late nineteenth century, patients could choose between eclectics, homeopaths, osteopaths, and chiropractors, as well as lay practitioners of various drugless therapies.

As a distinct American health care profession, naturopathic medicine is almost 100 years old, tracing its origins to Dr. Benedict Lust and Dr. Robert Foster. In this century, "naturopathy" came together in the U.S. as an eclectic group of drugless healers sought consolidation and recognition around 1900, spurred by an influx of European "nature cure" doctors. There were dozens of colleges of naturopathy, ranging from 2 to 4 years, and often in conjunction with chiropractic colleges. Throughout the first quarter of this century, there were tens of thousands of naturopathic healers, numerous journals, annual conventions, and professional associations, complete with dissension about what constitutes "real" naturopathic medicine. To this day there is a dissenting group (ineligible for state licensure) that professes naturopathy and naturopathic medicine are two different and contradictory practices, although they claim the same history and tradition.

While allopathic medicine was consolidating its political power, the Flexner report came out in 1910, which examined various medical colleges. Fueled by politics, technology, pharmaceuticals, and immunization, allopathic medicine eclipsed the drugless healers by midcentury. States allowed their naturopathic licensing laws to lapse. A few attempts at naturopathic colleges came and went, but one, the National College of Naturopathic Medicine, has endured since 1956 and others have grown from it, including Bastyr University, Southwest College of Naturopathic Medicine and Health Sciences, and The Naturopathic College at Bridgeport University.

The basic philosophy and practice that naturopathic medicine has espoused have gone in and out of fashion. During the rise of scientific medicine, naturopathic medicine was "out." Now it is back "in." Research is proving daily that what we eat *does* matter, that the patient's symptoms cannot be treated in isolation, and that practitioners in various disciplines can work together for the good of the patient.

Mechanism of Action According to Its Own Theory

Naturopathic medicine is based on a philosophy rather than simply a system of "this is what we do for that disease." It is not based on any particular modality as are most other health care systems, and there are a large variety of therapies that are used. In this manner, naturopathic doctors remain open to new ideas and concepts of healing. The practice of this philosophy might be summarized in the following sentence: Whenever possible, naturopathic doctors use medicines and techniques that are the least invasive and most curative.

Forms of Therapy

In practice, naturopathic physicians (NDs) use standard diagnostic procedures such as radiographs, physical examinations, laboratory testing, gynecologic exams, and metabolic analysis, although such practices vary from state to state. In addition, NDs are the only licensed primary care physicians who are clinically trained to use a variety of natural therapeutics. They tailor their treatments to meet the individual needs of each patient.

NDs are trained in clinical nutrition, botanic medicine, homeopathy, physical medicine (such as massage, manipulation, applications of hot and cold water, electrical stimulation, and others), body-mind connection, and minor or superficial surgery (such as warts, moles, skin tags, and others). Often practitioners will gravitate to those methods for which they feel they possess a particular gift. In naturopathic medicine the issue is the philosophy within which these methods are applied, as much as with the natural, gentle, noninvasive methods themselves.

Forms of Therapy

Clinical Nutrition

A cornerstone of naturopathic practice is that food is the best medicine. Many medical conditions can be treated more effectively with dietary changes, nutritional supplements, and with fewer complications and side effects than they can by other means. NDs use dietetics, natural hygiene, metabolic cleansing, and nutritional supplementation in practice.

Botanic Medicine

Many plant substances are powerful medicines with some advantages over conventional drugs. They are effective and safe when used properly, in the right dose, and in proper combination with other herbs and treatments. Their organic nature makes botanicals compatible with the body's own chemistry; they can be gentle and effective with few toxic side effects. A resurgence of scientific research in Europe and Asia demonstrates that some plant substances are superior to synthetic drugs in clinical situations.

Homeopathic Medicine

In contrast to drugs, homeopathic medicine is based on the principle of "like cures like." This powerful system of medicine is more than 200 years old and is widely accepted in other countries. Homeopathic medicine acts to strengthen the body's innate immune responses and seldom has side effects. Some conditions that have not responded to conventional medicine will respond well to homeopathy.

Hydrotherapy

The use of water is an ancient form of healing that comes to us from Hippocrates. Naturopathic doctors are trained to know the physiologic principles underlying the therapeutic use of water, heat, and cold.

Physical Medicine

A variety of treatments are used to help stimulate the healing process of muscle tissue and the immune system. This may include a gentle form of manipulation, the specific application of heat and cold, the use of ultrasound, massage, and exercise therapy. All of these treatments are designed to be noninvasive and gentle.

Minor Surgery

NDs are trained and licensed to perform minor surgery in an outpatient setting. This includes the removal of moles, warts, and hemorrhoids and the suturing of cuts and lacerations.

Natural Childbirth and Midwifery

Naturopathic physicians provide natural childbirth care in a nonhospital setting. They offer prenatal and postnatal care using the most modern diagnostic techniques and are sensitive to the power of the birthing process. The naturopathic approach strengthens the mother so that complications associated with pregnancy may be prevented. As family practitioners of natural medicine, NDs treat the whole family throughout the cycles of life.

This is just a sampling of the therapies used by naturopathic physicians. Anyone can read a book and decide what herb would be good for a disease, but it is the biochemical individuality that is addressed when seeing an ND. Too often we think of natural medicine as just substituting a herb or vitamin for a drug. It is so much more than that. It is the ability to find the root or the cause of the problem underlying the symptoms and addressing the patient's individual health needs. One person's rash might be an allergic reaction while another person's rash could be an underlying weakness of liver function, and yet another person's rash could be a digestive tract that is in need of rejuvenating.

Demographics

Licensed NDs are found in many states of the U.S. as well as Canadian provinces. For a listing of NDs that are members of the American Association of Naturopathic Physicians please visit www.naturopathic.org. Their referral line is (206) 298-0125. The largest concentration of NDs is in the Pacific Northwest of both Canada and the U.S. Naturopathic colleges as well as professional organizations receive dozens of calls daily for referrals to NDs from everywhere in North America. Consumers cross racial as well as socioeconomic boundaries.

Indications and Reasons for Referral

Naturopathic medicine is a primary care form of practice that is applicable to acute as well as chronic disease. It is this author's opinion that the first physician a patient should see is a naturopathic doctor. Drugs and surgery would then become the "alternative" medicine.

All too frequently, people come to naturopathic medicine as a last resort. They are hoping for a way to avoid surgery or they have exhausted all that allopathic medicine has to offer them and are told to seek the aid of a psychiatrist. They still do not believe it is all in their heads if no disease can be named. Often people with cancer are seeking ways to ease the side effects of chemotherapy, or those who are HIV-positive want help strengthening their immune system. Patients seek out NDs when they are tired all the time or have insomnia. They want natural therapies to treat their children's chronic otitis media, asthma, or allergies. Patients want alternatives to antibiotics or cortisone. Women find that plant-based hormones, vitamins, minerals, and herbs address their menopause symptoms more effectively than prescription synthetic estrogen and progesterone preparations. Young mothers want advice on nutrition for their children and older men are helped with benign prostate hypertrophy without drugs and surgery. Arthritis responds well to our natural therapies as do migraines and other types of chronic pain. As with all alternative therapies, use of naturopathic medicine does not preclude the use of mainstream medical therapies in addition.

Naturopathic doctors do not perform heroic medicine. They do not compete with medical physicians in the emergency room or in major surgery. Sometimes surgery is best for the patient and NDs refer to their colleagues in the hospital.

Office Applications

Patients who seek naturopathic doctors are the same as those who see any physician. NDs treat all types of diseases and conditions, much the same as an allopathic general practitioner. Students from the accredited colleges are trained as general practitioners with a specialty in natural medicine and its applications.

Research Base

Open any newspaper or magazine these days and you are likely to find an article on the latest contemporary medical research supporting the use of clinical nutrition, herbal medicine, or mind-body healing, the types of therapeutics that exemplify the premises of naturopathic medicine.

At colleges of naturopathic medicine, faculty and alumni are making their contributions to this new knowledge with research on detoxification, dysglycemia, asthma, women's health, and cancer.

Self-Help versus Professional

Much has been made in the popular and professional literature about the fact that just because remedies are "natural" does not mean they are totally safe under any conditions. In fact, NDs themselves are generating literature about drug-nutrient interaction and nutrient-nutrient interaction.

As with allopathic medicine, some over-the-counter remedies may be safe if "used as directed," such as aspirin, but we are well aware of the danger of abuse and ignorance. Similarly, there are nutritional, herbal, and physical therapies that may be applied safely within certain guidelines, although from an ND standpoint it takes a well-trained professional to address the whole picture and prescribe therapies to ensure their effectiveness as well as to avoid harm.

Just as we fear negative consequences of self-dosage, so should we be concerned about ineffectual use of potentially helpful remedies.

Visiting a Professional

The typical first visit to an ND lasts for 1 hour. The ND takes a detailed history of the patient's past medical history and lifestyle history, as well as a review of symptoms. The ND asks detailed questions regarding diet, mental/emotional components, and how these symptoms are related to each other. An ND will work with the patient to find the root cause of illness.

Credentialing

Naturopathic physicians who are eligible for state licensure are those who have graduated from an accredited, 4-year postgraduate naturopathic college of medicine. Accreditation means under the auspices of the Council on Naturopathic Medical Education (CNME), which is recognized by the U.S. Department of Education as a special accrediting body for this purpose.

States that license naturopathic medicine include Alaska, Arizona, Connecticut, Hawaii, Maine, Montana, New Hampshire, Oregon, Utah, and Washington, as well as several Canadian provinces. In addition, Florida has some naturopaths practicing under a sunsetted licensure law.

States with licensure have a board of naturopathic medical examiners to which patients can appeal, and physicians must take a test in order to practice there in addition to the academic degree they have earned. Scope of practice may vary according to state licensure.

Training

State licensure requires graduation from an accredited 4-year college of naturopathic medicine. Two years of basic medical sciences, such as anatomy, physiology, biochemistry, pharmacology, pathology, and microbiology/immunology (total 1025 hours) are meshed with 2 years of naturopathic philosophy and therapeutics, plus 869 hours of clinical education and 1500 hours of clinical training.

There are four accredited or accreditation-candidate naturopathic medical colleges in the U.S. These are 4-year, in-residence graduate schools that offer a doctoral level degree.

National College of Naturopathic Medicine (founded 1956)
Clyde B. Jensen, PhD, President
49 SW Porter
Portland, OR 97201
Tel: (503) 499-4343
www.ncnm.edu

Bastyr University (founded 1978)
Joe Pizzorno, ND, President
14500 Juanita Dr. NE
Bothell, WA 98011
Tel: (425) 602-3322
www.bastyr.edu

Southwest College of Naturopathic Medicine & Health Sciences
David Marchese, Interim President
2140 E. Broadway Rd.
Tempe, AZ 85282
Tel: (602) 858-9100
www.scnm.edu

Canadian College of Naturopathic Medicine
60 Berl Ave.
Toronto, ONT M8Y 3C7
Tel: (416) 498-1255
Fax: (416) 498-1576

What to Look for in a Provider

The best way for patients and practitioners alike to gauge the quality of a consulting ND is to check whether the ND has graduated from an accredited 4-year college of naturopathic medicine (see "Training") and whether the person is licensed to practice (where applicable, as not all state legislatures have passed licensure laws).

Barriers and Key Issues

Naturopathic medicine has been hampered by an extremely small population; even with explosive growth in the past five years, there are fewer than 2000 NDs eligible for state licensure. However, more colleges are forming and existing colleges are growing to increase the supply.

Education also is the key to more complementary and multidisciplinary practices. As medical doctors become more aware of the training and education of licensed NDs, they become more comfortable in working together for patient care.

Detractors say there is no proof that the methods used according to naturopathic philosophy work. In fact, there is abundant proof in peer-reviewed journals on such methods as clinical nutrition and botanic medicine. Generally these elements are studied in isolation, such as a single active ingredient in gingko biloba.

One stumbling block may be the intentional lack of standardized treatment protocols, which is the "gold standard" of allopathic medicine. Standardized protocol is anathema to the ND, who believes that each patient is to be treated individually.

If we were to take a disease state as an example of how a naturopathic doctor treats a patient, we might consider benign prostatic hypertrophy (BPH). Nutritionally, NDs would emphasize a vegan diet, decreased use of simple carbohydrates, and decreased sodium and alcohol use. They might ask the patient to increase the use of omega oils and high fiber foods and encourage them to eat pumpkin seeds as a snack food. The patient would be encouraged to eat foods rich in zinc as well as estrogenic foods. On the other hand the patient would be asked to stay away from saturated fats, dairy products, caffeine, and pesticides found in nonorganic foods. The supplements would include vitamins C and E, mineral zinc picolinate, amino acids glycine, glutamic acid, and alanine. Quercetine and selenium might also be added.

Certain exercises as well as hot and cold sitz baths might be recommended for this patient. There are over 18 different botanicals that are used in formulas for BPH, with *Serenoa repens* (saw palmetto) leading the pack. Another physician might prescribe a constitutional homeopathic remedy that fits the patient's symptom picture. For many BPH patients, naturopathic doctors recommend cleansing programs and detoxification protocols.

From this we can see that treatments used by NDs are numerous and varied. One of the blessings of being an ND is the wide range of modalities and treatment possibilities that can be tailored to fit each individual.

Associations

American Association of Naturopathic Physicians (AANP)
601 Valley St. Suite 105
Seattle, WA 98109
Tel: (206) 298-0126
Referral Line: (206) 298-0125
Fax: (206) 298-0129
E-mail: GartleyME@compuserve.com
www.aanp.net

Each state has a Naturopathic Association that can be found listed with the AANP.

Suggested Reading

1. Boice J: *Pocket guide to naturopathic medicine*, Freedom, Calif, 1996, The Crossing Press.
2. Murray M, Pizzorno J: *Encyclopedia of natural medicine*, Rocklin, Calif, 1998, Prima Health.
3. Marz RB: *Medical nutrition from Marz*, Portland, Ore, 1994, Omni-Press.
4. Kirchfeld F, Boyle W: *Nature doctors, pioneers in naturopathic medicine*, East Palestine, Ohio, 1994 Medicina Biologica.

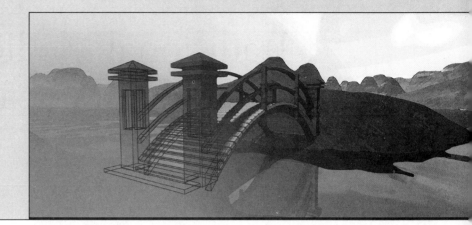

Community-Based Health Care Practices

Traditional Medicine in Latin America, **284**
Native American Medicine, **293**
Shamanism, **301**

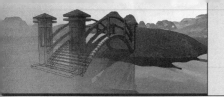

Traditional Medicine in Latin America

JAMIE L. FELDMAN

Origins and History

Latin America is home to a variety of people, cultures, and healing practices. Although there is no standardized medical system equivalent to traditional Chinese medicine, Latin American-based practices often share elements derived from humoral medicine, spiritism, Catholicism, and herbalism. The precise nature of Latin American healing interventions varies, depending on the culture of the practitioner, the cultural and geographic location of the patients, and the illness.

Historically, colonization of Latin America by the Spanish in the sixteenth century brought humoral medicine (also known as *Galenic* or *Hispano-Arabic medicine*) and Catholicism into contact with indigenous systems.[1] Among both cultures, spiritual beliefs played a large role in healing. Colonial suppression of native religions led to increasingly syncretic healing rituals, with Catholic symbols and saints alongside of or instead of indigenous ones. The rise of biomedicine introduced yet another set of beliefs and practices into Hispanic culture, ultimately leading to the present ethnomedical system. Known in Mexico as *curanderismo*, the ethnomedical system is representative of many healing practices throughout Latin America.

This chapter will review the theory and basic practices of curanderismo, the demographics of its patients and practitioners, and its clinical applications. In addition, two folk illnesses common to Hispanics—*susto* and *empacho*—will be discussed, along with interaction of Hispanic health beliefs regarding the biomedical diseases of diabetes and HIV infection. Healers are known as *curanderas* or *curanderos,* and the masculine and feminine designations will be used interchangeably in this chapter.

Mechanism of Action According to Its Own Theory

As noted earlier, curanderismo combines a variety of theoretical elements into a holistic approach to illness. The etiology of illness is often framed in terms of imbalance, between the hot and cold in the body, between parts of the body, between patients and the social environment, or between patients and the spiritual realm.[2] Finally, illness can have either a natural or supernatural cause, each potentially having identical symptoms. Although both curanderismo and biomedicine can treat naturally caused illness, only the *curandero* can treat supernatural ailments.[3]

Historically, humoral medicine is based on the ancient Greek concept of four bodily humors, which in turn combine the fundamental qualities of hot, cold, wet, and dry. Illness is caused by an overabundance or deficit in a given quality or qualities and is cured by supplying the opposing quality. For example, a hot remedy treats a cold illness, be it a food, activity, or medication. In present day Latin America, the wet and dry qualities have dropped out, and illness is often ascribed to an invasion of the body by heat or cold.[4] Although the hot and cold theory is present in popular culture throughout the region, which illnesses, medications, and foods are specifically defined as hot or cold varies. In some regions, this model plays a minimal role.[3]

Illness may also be caused by a displacement of parts of the body that need to be restored through a manipulation, herbs, or rituals. Examples include susto (soul loss, discussed on p. 287), *caida de la mollera* (fallen fontanelle, most common in infants), and *caida de la matriz* (fallen womb). Caida de la mollera, for example, is often treated by pushing on the palate. These illnesses are often treated at home, with severe cases requiring a visit to the *curandera*.[3]

In curanderismo, however, illness ultimately arises from disordered social or spiritual relationships and unlike biomedicine, there is little distinction between medical, emotional, and social problems; healers are asked to handle both infidelity and diabetes. Envy by another, conscious or unconscious, may precipitate illness. A hex cast by a witch, or *bruja*, can cause prolonged misfortune or even natural diseases such as cancer. Treatment often involves reestablishing accepted social roles or reconciliation between patients and others, such as family, friends, and neighbors, through the use of rituals or other actions prescribed by the healer.[3]

Illness arising from spiritual offense is treated similarly. Among many Hispanic people, health is perceived as a gift from God, and disease serves as punishment for sins. Cure is accomplished only through God's mediation.[5] The curandero helps to relieve patients of their sins, and through these rituals enables patients to bring their lives in line with divine will.[2] Sufferers may undertake pilgrimages, either to saints' shrines or shrines of famous folk healers.[4] In one study, non-Mexican Hispanics sought out Catholic priests more often than curanderas,[5] and personal faith may be used more often than either.[6] Spirits also bring suffering and may need to be exorcised or appeased.[3] In a study of elderly Mexican-Americans, however, belief in the existence of spirits was common, but belief in their etiologic role in chronic disease was limited.[6]

Latin Americans use herbs to treat both natural and supernatural illness. Home remedies involving herbs are often the first line of treatment, rather than a trip to the curandera or biomedical doctor.[6] The type of herbs used by patients and curanderos varies considerably with locale. *Yerba buena*, for example, can refer variously to mint, savory or other species.[7,8] Herbs may be chosen for their symbolism (for example, plants in the shape of a cross or the affected organ), their hot and cold properties, or simply tradition of use. Of note, nonherbal ingestions are also common and may rarely include laxatives, lead compounds, mercury, or laundry bluing.[8]

Demographics

Curanderos or curanderas are loosely defined as folk healers recognized by the community to treat physical, mental, and spiritual ailments.[3] Other folk practitioners include herbalists (*yeberos*), bone and muscle healers (*heuseros, sobadores*), midwives (*parteras*), and spiritualists (*espiritualistas*). There is, however, great overlap in beliefs and practices among these categories, and curanderas will generally use multiple healing modalities. Curanderos are perceived as having a divine gift and they may be "called" (sometimes involuntarily) through an illness experience of their own.[4] There is no standardized training; rather individuals are apprenticed to an older, experienced healer. In some cases, the curandera is divinely guided rather than specifically trained. In either case, the healer's reputation for cure, easing suffering, and affordability builds a following.[4] Curanderos may make a full-time living seeing patients.

It is difficult to estimate the number and distribution of curanderos in North and Latin America, due in part to the difficulty of distinguishing them from other folk healers. More importantly, their existence is kept secret from outsiders.[6] In the United States, their patients include illegal immigrants and migrant workers; two groups less likely to speak with government representatives. It is likely, however, that U.S. curanderos can be found wherever there is a large Hispanic (and primarily Mexican) population, such as border states, cities with significant Hispanic communities, and regions reliant on migrant farm workers.

Likewise, it is difficult to estimate the number of people who use curanderas. The 1982-1984 Hispanic Health and Nutrition Examination Survey (HHANES) sampled 3,623 adult Mexican Americans from the Southwestern United States. Only 4.2% reported consulting a folk healer of any kind in the previous year. Users of curanderos were more likely to be male, less well-educated, and foreign-born. Being interviewed in Spanish was highly predictive of use, and acculturation, martial status, community size, age, or insurance statuses were not related. Those people who sought folk healers were more likely to rate their health status as fair or poor and to believe that they had little personal control over their health. However, they also consulted physicians in addition to folk healers.[9]

Its focus on Mexican-Americans in the Southwest and use, limit this study only over the previous year. Data from a 1996 study of Mexican-American women attending migrant health clinics in Washington State revealed that 21.4% had used curanderos within the last 5 years.[10] The use of folk healers may be also higher for culturally defined illnesses[11] although Trotter and Chavira suggest these ailments compose a small fraction of a healer's practice.[3] If one expands the use of folk healing to include home remedies, then evidence suggests that use of herbs, cleansing rituals, and other interventions may be as high as 50% to 80%.[5,6,12]

Forms of Therapy

Latin American healing methods include herbal therapies, hot and cold adjustments to diet and activities (outlined previously), religious interventions such as prayer and pilgrimage, massage or other body manipulation, and ritual activities. There is considerable overlap among these categories. For example, herbs can be used for their recognized physiologic properties (purgative, laxative, and so on), their hot and cold properties, or their spiritual properties. Most herbal therapies consist of common household materials such as olive oil, oregano, anise, fruits, and spices.[3] Manipulation of the body may also have both physical and spiritual elements. Caida de mollera is treated by pressing on the infant's palate, and massaging the head with oils gives mental strength during other healing rituals.

Most healing, however, is accomplished through a ritual combining multiple therapies acting on multiple levels—material, spiritual, and mental. Not all healers are proficient in all techniques; spiritual and mental healers are less common. In most cases, the curandera diagnoses patients through one of a variety of methods, such as card-reading, "sweeping" patients with an egg, consulting the spirits, or assessing the patients' aura. The basic therapeutic ritual is known as a *barrida*, or spiritual cleansing. The purpose is to eliminate negative vibrations affecting patients by transferring them to another object. While concentrating on God (or other benevolent spirits) patients are swept from head to toe using an appropriate object, often an egg. If the suffering is in a particular body area, that place is given greater attention. While sweeping patients, the curandero recites prayers petitioning help from God, saints, or other spirits.[3]

The *sahumerio*, or incensing, is a ritual designed to purify the living environment of disruptive problems, such as bad luck, marital problems, or business rivalry. A *sortilegio* ritual uses material objects to bind up negative influences, particularly personal shortcomings, on patients.[3] Other objects used in healing rituals include candles, magically prepared water, perfumes, incense, crucifixes, and religious pictures.

The curandera shares a common worldview with their patients and understands their beliefs and lifestyles. They involve the family in healing rituals and any aftercare instructions. Finally, the curandera manipulates culturally recognizable symbols to relieve the biological, social, emotional, and spiritual suffering of their patients.

Indications and Reasons for Referral

Patients are likely to self-diagnose and self-refer to a folk healer before the ailment comes to the attention of a physician. This appears more likely in the case of ethnomedical (culturally defined) illnesses. Sometimes called *culture bound* syndromes, these disorders cross geographic and ethnic boundaries and may be psychiatric and/or somatic in nature.[13] Ethnomedical illnesses do not usually correspond to a particular biomedical disease, despite attempts at direct correlation.[13-15] Three ethnomedical disorders common to Latin America are described in the following section and include susto, or soul-loss, empacho, or "blocked digestion," and *mal de ojo*, or "evil eye."

Susto is a condition in which a frightening event is believed to cause the soul to become dislodged from the body, resulting inevitably in illness. The inciting event can be either emotional or physical trauma, sometimes occurring years prior to the onset of symptoms. The severity of the event does not correlate with severity of symptoms.[13] Susto affects individuals of all genders, ages (including infants), and socioeconomic and acculturation levels. Symptoms are variable, usually consisting of decreased energy, diminished appetite, lack of initiative, diarrhea, and insomnia. Studies show that *asustados* experience significant morbidity and mortality, having both a higher burden of disease and higher likelihood of death than matched controls.[14] Often diagnosed by physicians as depression, these patients scored no differently than matched controls on psychiatric testing. Those suffering from susto tend to live on the margins, with small and impoverished social networks. Although no single biomedical pathology underlies susto, it strongly correlates with perceived failure in the patient's social role.[13] Left untreated, susto becomes a chronic, life-threatening illness. Treatments include herbal teas, barrida or ritual cleansing (described earlier), marking the sign of the cross, and prayer.

Empacho is a gastrointestinal disorder believed to be caused by blockage in the stomach or intestines. Symptoms include bloating, constipation, lethargy, vomiting, and diarrhea. Infants are at greatest risk, followed by children, teenagers, and postpartum women,[8] although anyone may get it. Improper dietary habits are considered the primary cause, such as too much food, poorly cooked food, or the wrong types of food. Swallowing of saliva (as in teething) or chewing gum are other factors. A study by Weller et al[15] demonstrates a high degree of consistency in descriptions of empacho by Guatemalan, Mexican, Mexican-American (Texas), and Puerto Rican (Connecticut) informants. Empacho can worsen if left untreated, and treatments include stomach massage, "popping" the skin on the back to free the blockage, rolling an egg on the stomach, or ingesting olive oil or herbal teas.[8,15]

Mal de ojo is a condition primarily affecting children and is characterized by fever, irritability, headache, and weeping. Related to the Mediterranean concept of "evil eye," mal de ojo is caused by the envious gaze of another, either conscious or unconscious. Classically, a nonfamily member will admire a child, and the child later develops symptoms. The illness can be prevented by having a family member touch the child being admired. Once a person develops mal de ojo, it can progress if left untreated. Physicians are thought not to diagnose or treat this problem correctly, and therefore a female relative (or a curandera in severe cases) usually does treatment. An egg is rolled over the child's body, then cracked into a glass of water, and placed under the child's bed. The egg and water solution is discarded the next day, along with the affliction.[3,14]

Although the symptoms of susto, empacho, and mal de ojo can be aided by biomedicine, the underlying cause can not. Similarly, diabetes is often perceived as the result of God's will. A study of non-Mexican-American Hispanics demonstrated a high degree of fatalism in regards to both having diabetes and developing complications. Overwhelmingly, participants agreed that "Only God can control my diabetes,"[5] although self-care, family, and priests were also helpful. Only a small percentage used herbs or spiritualists in their diabetes care. A 1998 study of diabetic Mexican-Americans described participants combining biomedical causal explanations with provoking factors from their individual behavior or life events.[14] Finally, biomedical therapies such as insulin can be seen as harmful or signifying a terminal stage in the illness.[15] Home remedies, prayer, and faith appear more common approaches to chronic diseases of aging than use of curanderas, although use may increase when biomedicine has no more to offer.[6]

AIDS, like diabetes, has no medical cure, which readily lends itself to alternative explanatory models and treatments. A 1996 study of inner-city Hispanics indicated that most responders believed in spirits and that half of those believed that spirits played a role caus-ing AIDS. Two-thirds engaged in folk healing for AIDS, desiring spiritual and physical re-lief and protection from evil.[16] Latino women, in a qualitative study, demonstrated a mix of biomedical, popular, and traditional explanatory models of AIDS. Contact with impu-rities such as perspiration, imbalances in the body, and sin or curses were all seen as causal factors. As with diabetes, herbs and religious interventions were considered appropriate treatments, along with antibiotics and injectable vitamins. U.S.-born Latinos were less likely to offer traditional interpretations of AIDS.[17]

As seen in the previous examples, Hispanic explanatory models encompass several com-mon elements for all illnesses. First, illness may have a natural or supernatural cause. Ill-ness and its relief are due ultimately to the will of God, and faith is thus a powerful heal-ing technique. Home remedies, or in more severe cases, biomedical physicians can be used to treat natural illness. Curanderismo also offers relief from suffering, particularly when bio-medicine has no more to offer. Curanderos or knowledgeable family and community mem-bers best treat supernatural and ethnomedical ailments through herbs, manipulation, and specific rituals.

Practical Applications

Few physicians would be equipped to practice Hispanic healing techniques in the office setting. Rather, physicians can use this knowledge to better understand their patients' ap-proach to health and illness, to recognize ethnomedical conditions, and to work in part-nership with their patients regarding complementary treatments. Patients may not openly admit to using home remedies or curanderos due to fear of rejection by the physician, de-sire to be seen as "American," or the secrecy involved in coping with supernatural forces such as spirits and curses. Biomedical practitioners may need to inquire after the patients' explanatory model with open-ended questions, following up with more culturally specific inquiry. For example, the practitioner may ask, "Some people believe that certain herbs can help this problem. Are you taking any herbal medicines?" Physicians should recognize that there are many acculturated Hispanic patients with little knowledge or interest in folk healing, and referral to a curandera would be inappropriate. It is important to elicit use of herbal, topical, or other ingested remedies, remembering that most healing is done at home. Finally, physicians should also ask but not pressure patients regarding the use of comple-mentary healers.

Adjunct therapy with traditional methods can be helpful for diseases with few effective biomedical treatments (such as Alzheimer's dementia), for chronic conditions (such as arthritis, chronic fatigue), and psychosocial issues (grief, marital stress). If the physician or patients suspect a culturally defined ailment, referral to a folk healer is appropriate. Mild, self-limiting illnesses are likely to be self-treated by patients and generally do not precipi-tate referral. Due to the deeply spiritual basis of many Hispanic health beliefs, physicians may wish to acknowledge faith-based interventions in addition to biomedical ones. Finally, physicians working with a large Hispanic community can work with local healers to help patients access both realms of care.

Druglike Information

Safety

There are few studies on the overall safety of Latin American healing practices. For serious diseases such as diabetes, the use of curanderismo to the exclusion of biomedicine can be dangerous. However, most patients use complementary systems simultaneously.[3] Herbal remedies can have interactions with medications or may have dangerous side effects of their own. As most Hispanic herbal medicines involve household foods and spices, however, serious reactions are uncommon. As noted previously, toxic nonherbal ingestions, although rare, do occur, resulting in acute or chronic poisoning.

Self-Help versus Professional

Patients of all ethnicity tend to self-treat prior to consulting any healer. As the primary care physician refers to a specialist in severe or recalcitrant cases, Hispanic patients will turn to the curandera (or physician) when home remedies fail. The best recourse is to ask patients whether a professional healer is needed.

Visiting a Professional

A visit to the curandero can vary widely in location, procedure, type of therapy, and payment. Some healers visit patients at their home, and other healers maintain busy practices at their own home. Full-time healers may have a separate room set aside for their practice. Most curanderas do not have scheduled appointments. Patients are usually seen on a first-come, first-served basis. If patients do not know the healer, they are usually accompanied by someone who does. In any case, patients often bring a family member or friend. The curandero's workroom generally has chairs or benches, along with an altar filled with objects used in healing, such as crucifixes, saint's images, candles, and oils. The healer will invite patients into the room and start a conversation. The initial contact is social and aimed at developing rapport. Patients will then present their symptoms, and the curandero will make a diagnosis through a variety of procedures (see "Indications and Reasons for Referral"). Depending on the ailment and the specialty of the healer, a therapeutic intervention will be performed, such as herbal remedy, barrida, or another ritual. The healer then recommends any self-care and follow-up visits that are needed. Many curanderas see themselves as doing the work of God, with an obligation to help those in need. However, as the healers themselves may make a living at their work, payment for services is usually expected.[3]

Barriers and Key Issues

The existence and number of curanderos and other Hispanic healers is not widely known. The use of traditional healing methods has historically been suppressed for a variety of reasons, such as misperception of curanderismo as witchcraft, uncivilized, dangerous, or ineffective. The use of healers as a symbol of being "foreign" or "backwards" is another stereotype. As a result, those outside the Hispanic communities do not know about this healing system, nor do patients readily admit using it. Some patients, such as migrant workers and the uninsured, cannot easily access biomedical care, relying on home remedies and non-biomedical healers.

A wider dialogue between physicians, patients, the biomedical community, and Hispanic communities would alleviate this problem. Community-oriented clinics can develop partnerships with local healers to better serve patients' health needs.

Suggested Reading

1. Trotter R, Chavira JA: *Curanderismo: Mexican-American folk healing,* ed 2, Athens, Ga, 1997, University of Georgia Press.
    A seminal and comprehensive study based on ethnography in the Lower Rio Grande Valley.
2. Rubel AJ, O'Nell C, Collado-Ardon R: *Susto: a folk illness,* Berkeley, 1984, University of California Press.
    The predominent work on susto.
3. Foster G, Anderson BG: *Medical anthropology,* New York, 1978, John Wiley and Sons.
    A basic medical anthropology text with multiple references to Hispanic healing.

References

1. Kidwell C: Aztec and European medicine in the New World, 1521-1600. In Romananucci-Ross L et al, editors: *The anthropology of medicine,* S Hadley, Mass, 1983, Bergin and Garvey.
2. Ruiz P: Cultural barriers to effective medical care among Hispanic-American patients, *Annu Rev Med* 36:63-71, 1985.
3. Trotter R, Chavira JA: *Curanderismo: Mexican-American folk healing,* ed 2, Athens, Ga, 1997, University of Georgia Press, p 42.
4. Foster G, Anderson BG: *Medical anthropology,* New York, 1978, John Wiley and Sons, pp 57-60.
5. Zaldivar A, Smolowitz J: Perceptions of the importance placed on religion and folk medicine by non-Mexican-American Hispanic adults with diabetes, *Diabetes Ed* 20 (4):303-361, 1994.
6. Applewhite S: Curanderismo: demystifying the health beliefs and practices of elderly Mexican-Americans, *Health Soc Work* 20 (4):247-254, 1995.
7. Lewis W, Elvin-Lewis M: *Medical botany,* New York, 1977, John Wiley and Sons.
8. Trotter R: Folk medicine in the Southwest: myth and medical facts, *Postgraduate Medicine* 78 (8):167-179, 1985.
9. Higginbotham J et al: Utilization of curanderos by Mexican-Americans: prevalence and predictors from HHANES 1982-84, *Am J Public Health* 80:32-35, 1990.
10. Skaer TL et al: Utlization of curanderos among foreign born Mexican-American women attending migrant health clinics, *J Cult Divers* 3 (2):29-34, 1996.

11. Risser AL, Mazur LJ: Use of folk remedies in a Hispanic population, *Arch Pediatr Adolesc Med* 149 (9):978-981, 1995.

12. Mikhail BI: Hispanic mothers' beliefs and practices regarding selected children's health problems, *West J Nurs Res* 16 (6):623-638, 1994.

13. Logan M: New lines of inquiry on the illness of susto, *Med Anthropol* 15:189-200, 1993.

14. Baer R, Bustillo M: Susto and mal de ojo among Florida farmworkers: emic and etic perspectives, *Med Anthropol Q* 7 (1):90-100, 1993.

15. Weller S et al: Empacho in four Latino groups: a study of intra- and inter-cultural variation in beliefs, *Med Anthropol* 15:109-136, 1993.

16. Hunt LM et al: Porque me toco a mi? Mexican-American diabetes patients' causal stories and their relationship to treatment behaviors, *Soc Sci Med* 46 (8):959-969, 1998.

17. Hunt LM et al: NIDDM patients' fears and hopes about insulin therapy, *Diabetes Care* 20 (3):292-298, 1997.

18. Suarez M et al: Use of folk healing practices by HIV-infected Hispanics living in the United States, *AIDS Care* 8 (6):683-690, 1996.

19. Flaskerud J, Calvillo ER: Beliefs about AIDS, health and illness among low-income Latina Women, *Res Nurs Health* 14:431-438, 1991.

Native American Medicine

EILEEN NAUMAN

Origins and History

The practice of medicine means a *skill* or *talent*. A Native American medicine man or woman has a skill in healing. Among Native Americans, there are different types of medicine people, depending upon their Nation. Herbs, ceremony, shamanism, songs, feathers, dancing, and engaging the spirits of Nature are all a part of medicine. Usually, if people are trained in herbal medicine, they are not a shaman; although they can be both. There are uniquely different ceremonies for healing for each Nation. Underlying this, there is a commonality of themes that emerge, despite the labels placed upon them. To practice Native American medicine means to acknowledge that all of us are related to animals, plants, minerals, and human beings. Spirit inhabits all things; not just humans. Energy is a real and living element and is recognized as an essential underpinning to healing. Medicine people realize that they are catalysts to the healing process and are also intercessors to the spirit world—they can engage and talk to the spirit of the plant, animal, or mineral, and pray for help from it, in the name of their patients.

Native American culture includes an earth-based religion and belief system. They acknowledge and pay tribute and prayers to Mother Earth. They see Her as everyone's Mother and they see themselves as simply a small part of the greater whole of cycles and seasons that are a part of Her. All of Nature plays a part in medicine. Life does not consist of pieces; rather, it is interconnected and related. Disease is not looked at as being imposed upon the person. Instead, all causes of disease must be considered, such as the person's deeds, their words, their state of mind and emotions, if they have strayed from their spiritual path, or if they have inadvertently angered a spirit or spirits, and so on. To the medicine person, everything is related spiritually and energetically and is intertwined with what is causing the sickness in this individual.

Special attention is paid to the person's spirit. It is either *well* or *out of harmony* or *imbalanced*. When the spirit is imbalanced, one gets ill. In Native American medicine, it is recognized that sickness or health has to do directly with a person's spirit. Medicine people engage the spirit of plants, trees, rocks, winged ones, or four-legged ones to help a people get back into harmony with themselves. Spiritual considerations, such as a dead person or animal coming back to harm the patient, are also a common motif. They can "talk" to the spirits directly, telepathically, through feeling and sensing, through prayer, or through song and ceremony.

Mechanism of Action According to Its Own Theory

Native American medicine is the opposite of science. It is, for lack of better terminology, the *heart of spirit*. Medicine people acknowledge that the spirit, mind, and emotions all have interplay with the environment. One's connection to Nature, Mother Earth, and communion with the spirit world is either in harmony or out of harmony. They acknowledge the unique energies of the eight directions, or the medicine wheel. The sky, Sun, Moon, and the Earth, all play an integral part in Native American cosmology. Faith is a vehicle for cure. Prayer is the vehicle to get in touch with the spirits. Humility and asking for help when sick is part of this cosmology.

People contract illness because they are out of harmony or balance with their spirit. All the symptoms are seen as connected with spirit. Energy, then, must be used as a catalyst to help patients come back into harmony. It is the medicine person's job to create a ceremonial environment in which patients can call back their spirit, or make peace within or outside of themselves, to bring them back into harmony, spiritually speaking.

Native American medicine interacts more on a bioenergetic level (energy medicine) than a bimolecular level. By working with *energy* with different "tools" as outlined in "Forms of Therapy" the medicine person is able to make changes in sick peoples' spirit, mind, emotions, and physical body in order to reintroduce harmony or balance to their life.

The body's mechanisms are stimulated to heal itself from the spirit, downward, into the mind, the emotions, and physical form. All healing comes from the *Great Spirit*. The energy that is all around us connects with and through us. When medicine people, who are our intercessors, ask and engage this energy on patients' behalf, it heals them.

Demographics

Every reservation in the United States has a medicine man or woman; usually many, depending upon the size of the reservation. In some Nations, such as the Navajo Nation, they have what is known as the *Medicine Man Society*. If people wanted to get a hold of such a person, they would simply call the chief of the Nation and ask for that society.

Native Americans use their medicine people all of the time. Some will go to "whiteman's" medicine but will inevitably go back to the medicine man or woman for treatment afterward. Most Native Americans do not like the drugs dispensed by modern medicine and eventually will stop taking it and seek out more "natural" medicine through their medicine people. When there is no recourse, they will, however, use mainstream medicine, particularly if diabetes is diagnosed.

Forms of Therapy

The following forms of therapy are used, often in combination, and include the following:

1. In a sweat lodge ceremony, "medicine" sweats are used to heal.
2. The sacred pipe is used and prayed with for the patient. Or the smoke may be blown on the sick person.

3. Sacred sage, sweet grass, and cedar, among other dried herbs that is wafted over the patient with the use of a feather are used. These herbs are considered healing to the energy and spirit of the person who is sick.

4. A specific ceremony that is hundreds or thousands of years old is performed on behalf of the sick person. It may last less than an hour or up to 10 or 12 days, depending upon the Nation involved. Ceremony usually includes sacred songs, the use of the drum, singing, herbs, feather or feathers, gemstones (quartz crystal), a rattle, or other things from Nature that the medicine person may use from their repertoire and that of the ceremony.

5. Feathers are said to be from Spirit. They are used to remove "blocks" of energy from the aura or energy around the sick person. It is also used to "unruffle" the energy field around a person and remove "debris" from it, which is making the person ill.

6. Herbs are often used. They can be drank as a tea, eaten, used in a bath for the person, or used in a sweat lodge ceremony. They may also be burned, and the smoke is inhaled.

7. Rattles are used to break up blocks of dead or jammed energy in the aura or energy field of the sick person.

8. Drums are used to align the person's spirit with the heartbeat of Mother Earth. Once this is done, harmony can, once again, begin to be established.

9. Sacred songs are sung. There are sounds, names, and words that are sung in a certain way and cadence that dramatically affect the aura or energy field of the sick person. Songs are also used to beseech spirits to come and help cure the sick person.

10. Shamanic intervention is used to bring back the missing pieces from the sick person that may have been taken by someone else.

11. Possession can occur by another person, dead or alive, or by another earth-based spirit (animal, plant, bird, and so on). The medicine person then uses his or her spirit guides to remove the possession from the ill person.

12. Mud is used to *cleanse* the sick person.

13. Sacred stone is used and rubbed in the area where the person is ailing. The stone is said to absorb or soak up the *bad* energy so that the person can get well.

14. Laying on of hands is done to remove something either from the person's body (they usually suck it out with their mouth) or pluck the energy or spirit out of the person's aura or energy field.

15. Vision quest is done to put people in direct touch with the spirits so they can ask for and hopefully receive a vision that will guide them like a symbol.

16. Dreams are very important, and medicine people use them to understand the *disease* and *disharmony* of the person. They may also use them as an indicator of how to get the person well once again.

Indications and Reasons for Referral

Native American medicine is often used to address acute and chronic conditions by the individuals who seek out this form of therapy. All diseases have been treated with Native

American medicine, from cancer to colds. As with all alternative therapies, use of Native American medicine does not preclude the use of additional mainstream medical therapies.

If people have a belief system that is Earth-based, then they may resonate well with a more spiritually based medicine. Or if people have a strong belief or need of Native American healing being performed, they should be supported in this direction. People can rarely do this type of healing for themselves.

Practical Applications

Native Americans, because of their belief in spirit with all things, with connection, will often move toward a more "natural" medicine rather than standard pharmaceutical drugs. They want something with "spirit" in it; not removed and not synthetic and certainly not "man-made." They will use medicine and ceremony because they come from this background and belief system. Mainstream medicine does not generally believe in *spirit*, nor does it include spirit as part of its care of people. This is very strange to Native Americans because of the belief that people cannot get well unless their spirit is considered in all healing attempts. The medicine people acknowledge spirit as most important in the process of healing patients. They recognize that ceremony is important to be a catalyst for people giving themselves permission to heal.

Research Base

Formal research is nonexistent for this form of therapy. True medicine people do not write down their sacred ways or ceremonies for fear they will be misused or abused by those who do not have the proper mind, perspective, training, or education to use the energies with which they work.

Efficacy

The author observes a roughly 75% rate of responsiveness. Its effectiveness comes in part from the patients' belief in this system of medicine, of spirit and connection to all things that will help them get well. There is a placebo effect in about 25% of the people, where the disease symptoms will disappear for weeks or months but return eventually to their original intensity.

Future Research Opportunities and Priorities

Native American medicine does not lend itself to studies. Rather, personal experiencing of it is the best teacher. Actions speak louder than words, and this is the case with this model of medicine. Readers who could arrange to attend a sweat lodge session would find the experience an excellent introduction to this form of therapy.

Druglike Information

The Native American medicine people know from information that is handed down through generations of practice what a certain herb will do, and they know how to use it and apply it.

Safety

Native American medicine is a safe medical modality when a medicine person is asked to participate. If people try it for themselves, there may be many risks incurred because they do not have the education or training needed for this modality. The medicine person is an essential part of the overall strategy to help patients return to a state of harmony. When a medicine person works with the spirit as well as the body, the two work in concert with each other. A medicine person knows when to stop engaging the energy and spirit or spirits. The objective of Native American medicine persons is to catalyze patients back into harmony. Once they see that this is being done, they do no more.

Warnings, Contraindications, and Precautions

This form of therapy is safe for the majority of people. However, during a sweat lodge session, patients' blood pressure may elevate significantly, and people with hypertension should monitor themselves throughout the ceremony. People with asthma may have a problem when sage or cedar smoke is wafted around a sweat lodge as this might provoke an asthma episode. People who are claustrophobic may find the close, dark, hot confines of a sweat lodge overwhelming.

Drug or Other Interactions

Spirit medicine and energy medicine, as used by medicine people, do not counteract any type of therapy. It is supportive.

Adverse Reactions

Depending upon the herb used, there can be some nausea, vomiting, or diarrhea. All this is seen as good. "Better out than in" is acknowledged. Purging and cleansing the *physical vehicle* is considered healing. In other words, Native Americans, this therapy's most prominent users, seldom consider these as adverse reactions.

Conversely, this same population is often averse to mainstream prescription medications. If side effects are experienced from them, patients are more likely to stop taking them and find a medicine person instead to help cure them.

Pregnancy and Lactation

Medicine people work with pregnant women without problems.

Self-Help versus Professional

Native American ways of healing involves not only the medicine person but also the sick person's family. Many times neighbors are also involved in healing. The strength of family and friends is recognized and an important key to the healing process. All this energy and heart-felt prayers are brought to the sick person to help them get well. This is not a modality that one can do alone.

Visiting a Professional

Depending upon the Nation involved, medicine people are paid with money or goods. What the price is depends upon the Nation and the individual and how sick the person is. The more sick the person, the more ceremony and time is involved. The services are usually more expensive. The therapy is usually applied through ceremony, song, herbs, drumming, paintings (desert), and use of the sacred pipe, among many instruments from Nature that are used. Patients are not taught the ceremony. Patients *experience* the ceremony. This therapy embodies spirit medicine, energy, and the engaging of spirit energy from around the person, bringing it into the healing for them. Native American medicine is interactive between the individual and the medicine person at all times.

Credentialing

Nearly every Nation has a medicine family or clan that is self-taught, generation to generation. One's credentials are in proving that one can heal a person of their ailment or ailments. In some Nations, such as the Navajo, they have a formal society of medicine men, but many nations do not.

Training

If people want to be trained in Native American medicine, they must approach the medicine person with gifts, a sincere heart, and with humility. They often may need to ask two or three times before the medicine person gives them the answer. Medicine people are very good about perceiving those who would come to "steal" what they know and then irresponsibly give it out to those who are not trained to handle it properly. Most medicine people are not trained until they are at least 40 years old. Training usually takes 10 to 20 years as an apprentice. In the Apache Nation, a woman cannot become a medicine woman until she goes through menopause. Each Nation is different.

Native American medicine has been passed down by word-of-mouth for hundreds or thousands of years. There is usually one clan or one family who passes on this knowledge from one generation to another. Nothing is ever written down. There are many secrets to the ceremonies that are used in the healing of an individual and they will never be divulged to the public. The ceremonies are kept and passed down generationally.

Medicine people do not sell what they know. These are family and generational secrets that are considered sacred. Only an assistant to the medicine man or woman is taught this knowledge so it can be carried forward to the next generation.

What to Look for in a Provider

To locate a medicine person, contact the reservation and talk to the chief. He or she will be able to direct you to the medicine people. Every Native American reservation has their medicine people. Very few practice off the reservation. Talk to people who have gone to the medicine man or woman. They make their name by being effective at what they do. Good feedback from patients is the only way to know about the healer. This is a word-of-mouth "referral" system.

Generally, if a non-Indian seeks out such a service, they must go to the reservation, bring gifts of food, blankets, and so on and give them to the medicine person. The medicine person will then decide whether or not to heal them. And if the medicine person refuses, the gifts remain with the medicine person and then they are distributed among the poor and the elderly.

When you find such a medicine person, there should be a connection of trust that automatically establishes itself between one another. The medicine person is a listener and a counselor. Often, they listen without ever saying much of anything. Most medicine people are not counselors of the variety that most of us expect. They are keen listeners. They perceive deeply into our disharmony. They say little, and let their actions (the ceremony) speak for them.

Associations

No formal associations exist to the knowledge of this author. One educational location is the following:

The Psychocultural Institute
School of Soul Retrieval & Extraction
45A Simpson Ave.
Toronto, Ontario
Canada M4K 1A1
Tel: (416) 469-5155
Fax: (416) 469-4605
E-mail: hep@interlog.com
www.interlog.com/~hep

Barriers and Key Issues

Individuals without an Earth-based belief system, or a religious perspective that embraces that all things have a spirit and have energy, will keep a person from using this modality.

People who do not believe in ceremony will also have difficulty in finding this therapy a useful tool.

A bridge could be built more quickly between mainstream medicine and Native American medicine if the following could occur:

1. Having qualified medicine people from the different Native American Nations speak to medical personnel about their healing techniques.

2. Having mainstream medical personnel attend a sweat lodge ceremony. This is considered the fastest introduction into Native American healing procedures.

3. Working with a medicine person and observing what they do.

4. Understanding how medicine people use herbs and compiling information on them and their medical applications.

Suggested Reading

1. McGaa EE: *Mother earth spirituality*, San Francisco, Calif, 1990, Harper Collins.
    Gives an excellent example of Native American thinking and belief system of the Lakota Nation.
2. Waya, AG: *Soul recovery and extraction*, ed 3, Cottonwood, Ariz, 1997, Blue Turtle.
    Information on what is shamanism, signs of soul loss, and case histories from a Native American perspective.
3. Waya, AG: *Path of the mystic*, Sedona, Ariz, 1997, Light Technology.
    Stories based upon Native American belief system.
4. Wolf, FA: *The eagle's quest*, New York, 1992, Touchstone Book.
    Theoretical physicist looks at shamanism and explains it in scientific terms.

Shamanism

JANNEKE KOOLE

Origins and History

This chapter discusses shamanic healing, the *twisted hairs blessed beauty way*. The path of shamanic healing described in this chapter is only *one* lineage of the Twisted Hairs Way, and the Twisted Hairs is only *one* line of shamanic healing. The author acknowledges that this is a very small section of the very large field of shamanism and shamanic healing.

Within the general collective of the modern Western world there is, of recent, a growing interest in shamanism. Especially as modern diseases and treatments elude the expertise of modern Western medicine, people are again demanding help from a "higher power." Very simply put, shamanic healing allows access to that "higher power" for personal healing, transformation, and regeneration.

It is generally accepted that shamanism originated simultaneously in North Asia and North America. Shamans were men and women who could access worlds beyond the ordinary to affect the natural world of human existence. Using basic alchemic ritual and ceremonial practices with specific healing tools, shamans created magic, healed the sick, and indicated the probabilities of the future. Shamanism is therefore the use of spiritual energies to affect the physical world.

Any study of tribal peoples and ancient civilizations will reveal that each tribe had their shaman, medicine women and men, or spiritual healers of the people. Sometimes they were revered; sometimes they were feared. Always they were respected for the power they were able to wield.

In "Turtle Island" (that is, North America, South America, Central America, New Zealand, and Australia) there have always been those men and women who were driven to find knowledge that worked to heal their people. Not satisfied with only their tribal ways, they wandered from tribe to tribe searching out this knowledge. As they wove the different strands of knowledge into one braid, they became known as "Twisted Hairs." The Twisted Hairs Elders gathered together in council. They preserved the ancient knowledge over time—taking it into hiding, into secret societies, through those times in American history when the shamanic practices of the indigenous people were threatened by those who came to conquer the land and control the people. They waited for the day when that which was held in secret could again be released to all that were dedicated to the healing of the planet and of humanity.

In 1974, the Twisted Hairs Council of Elders of Turtle Island voted to begin releasing the knowledge back to those individuals who were seeking to once again find the ways of beauty, blessing, and balance. Harley Swift Deer Reagan was charged with the task of translating into English the Wheels and Keys given to him in the ancient language. As Swift Deer began to share this knowledge, students began to learn and practice the ancient healing ways. Thus the Twisted Hairs Blessed Beauty Way of Shamanic Healing became available once again.

Mechanism of Action According to Its Own Theory

The belief system of shamanism encompasses the following:

> Out of the void, the great womb of creation, air, fire, water, and earth gave birth to all forms of life, as we know them. There is nothing which exists that does not have these four (or rather five) elements. Within humans these are known as the emotional (water), mental (wind), physical (earth), and spiritual (fire) aspects. The void is the soul force energy, the chi (or ki) that pulses through our body, most undeniably felt within the intensive experiences of sexuality. We are created in such a way that these elements or aspects are balanced, in harmony, with one another. When something happens that puts them out of balance or creates disharmony within our essential nature, we get sick, diseased, or ill. Sickness, disease, and illness are nothing more than indicators (a constellation of symptoms) that an imbalance is present.

Practitioners of the Twisted Hairs Blessed Beauty Way of Shamanic Healing are first of all scouts. They hunt for the *cause* of the sickness, illness, or disease. Through an intricate application of the Wheels and Keys of the healing paradigm and based on a thorough case history, the symptoms are examined in all five aspects. A clear pattern of choice for the sickness, disease, and illness will be seen. An alchemical ceremony is then designed specifically to address this pattern in patients.

Healing is not done to or for patients. Patients have chosen the illness; patients must choose to be whole again. Healing is rarely done by "the shaman" on an individual basis. The ceremonies within the Twisted Hairs Blessed Beauty Way of Shamanic Healing take place within a circle of people who form a sacred space for patients to do their healing. The powers of the universe are called into this space through ancient evocation, invocation, and conjuring anchored in the four elements. This establishes a clear matrix of interconnection, interreliability, and interdependence (all forms of one thing are linked to all forms of all other things within this space). The patient comes into the center of this circle and is surrounded by the presence of spiritual power. This power enters the psyche of the soul and establishes contact with the higher self. Through this contact with a "higher power," patients have the greatest potential to see the cause for their choice, learn the lesson of that choice, and give away the symptom or symptoms, including all affects and effects associated with them. The shamanic practitioners assist patients to make their changes through the use of crystal doctoring, sandpainting, body painting, and other shamanic healing tools.

There are no such things as miracles; there is only the correct application of knowledge that works and the spiritual determination of patients to heal.

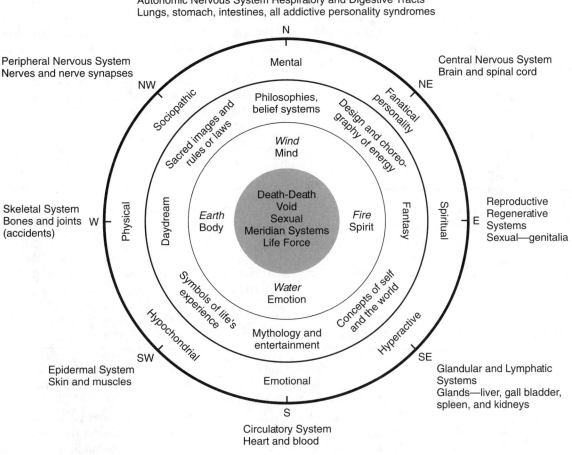

Autonomic Nervous System Respiratory and Digestive Tracts
Lungs, stomach, intestines, all addictive personality syndromes

Peripheral Nervous System
Nerves and nerve synapses

Central Nervous System
Brain and spinal cord

Skeletal System
Bones and joints
(accidents)

Reproductive
Regenerative
Systems
Sexual—genitalia

Epidermal System
Skin and muscles

Glandular and Lymphatic
Systems
Glands—liver, gall bladder,
spleen, and kidneys

Circulatory System
Heart and blood

Courtesy DTMMS/Doorways, 1998.

The illustration shows the key driver wheel (a cognitive map) for the Twisted Hairs Blessed Beauty Way of Shamanic Healing. All medical diagnoses have a place on the wheel of life. This is the instrument that is used to place those medical diagnoses within a context of care for all five aspects of the human.

Forms of Therapy

There are many kinds of therapy within the Twisted Hairs Blessed Beauty Way of Shamanic Healing. They fall into five different kinds (connected to the five elements). In the South are all forms of shamanic counseling, including one-to-one therapy and ceremonies known as "Balancing the Shields, Walk Talk Circles." The therapies and ceremonies of the North address concepts and belief systems that have created patterns of dysfunction or disease and are known as the "Crystal Circle Sound Sings." The ceremonies of the West occur primarily in a purification lodge—either a sweat lodge or an underground kiva. In the East are all ceremonies that include the use of shamanic dreaming techniques and body and sandpaintings to enter altered states of consciousness. In the center of the wheel are those ceremonies and shamanic techniques that address the life force of patients directly. The most notable of these is the process of recapitulated shamanic dearmoring.

Demographics

There are currently only a handful of shamanic practitioners who are qualified in the Twisted Hairs Blessed Beauty Way of Shamanic Healing. They are scattered throughout the United States, Canada, and Europe.

Those who come to this form of therapy for healing, range in age from infancy through into the eighties. There is no limitation of culture, religion, or creed because belief in these therapies is not necessary in order to use the alchemical ways.

Indications and Reasons for Referral

Most of the patients who seek this form of therapy have exhausted the resources of Western medicine and even many of the alternatives available. Shamanic healing is often a last resort when all else has failed to bring healing.

There are two requirements for patients to achieve success in the ways of shamanic healing. First, people must be willing to take responsibility for the creation of the disease and therefore be able to assume authority for their desire to be whole. Secondly, people must be open to the nonphysical realities of life and be willing to engage with their inner spirit and their higher selves.

Office Applications

As with all alternative therapies, use of shamanic healing does not preclude the use of mainstream medical therapies in addition. Shamanic healing is considered highly effective for the following ailments:

All forms of sexual dysfunctions and diseases in the reproductive systems
Chronic fatigue syndrome
Confrontation with death and loss
Mental health concerns, including schizophrenia
Most forms of cancer

Obesity and other eating disorders

Respiratory conditions such as bronchitis, pneumonia, asthma, emphysema, and so on

The illnesses that are rarely addressed in shamanic healing include the following:

Bacterial and viral infections

Childhood illnesses such as chicken pox, and so on

Routine eye problems

The common cold or flu

Practical Applications

Without specific training in shamanic healing, the reader is unlikely to apply this form of therapy in practice. However, there are certain key concepts that can be easily integrated into other forms of healing to increase their effectiveness.

The first is the concept that patients are in charge of their own body and therefore their state of health. Whether or not they ever step into an alchemical, shamanic healing circle, patients are given an opportunity to stand in the center of their own inner circle and claim their own power to change and heal.

The second concept is the holistic model of the wheel of life. Patients do not exist in isolation; symptoms do not exist without affecting the whole of their health. All health practitioners will enhance their care when the treatment they offer is placed within the context of a greater picture of the patients.

The third concept is that of our interconnection with all forms of life. Send patients out into nature and encourage them to walk and talk with the natural worlds. Spirit will greet them there and they will open to the natural healing powers within themselves.

With some basic continuing education in the paradigm and cognitive maps of the Twisted Hairs Blessed Beauty Way of Shamanic Healing, health practitioners can enrich their practice with simple tools in diagnosis and treatment.

Research Base

At this stage in the development of the Twisted Hairs Blessed Beauty Way of Shamanic Healing, research is only at the beginning stages. Thorough records of ceremonial healings are maintained and the data is being compiled. It is anticipated that documented research will become available over the next few years.

Self-Help versus Professional

Once a person has been initiated into the Twisted Hairs Blessed Beauty Way of Shamanic Healing, there are certain practices that can easily be done, and in fact are recommended to be done, as a measure of self-help. However, it is irresponsible and can be dangerous for someone who is not trained in the intricate alchemy to administer shamanic healing on another. Shamanic healing enters the realm of the soul and thus demands a high level of spiritual accountability in its practitioners.

Visiting a Professional

When patients visit a professional shamanic counselor or healer, they can expect to step into a very safe space of deep acceptance and caring. At the same time, they may feel exposed because the intake questionnaire they will be asked to fill in is very comprehensive in all five aspects. As well, the cognitive maps used to analyze that information and design the appropriate therapy, treatment, or ceremony allows the shamanic counselor to enter inside their matrix and "see" them. The shaman is able to see through the physical world and into the spiritual world; to analyze the past, project into the future, and be fully present all at the same time. This can be slightly disconcerting for new patients. They are entering into a great unknown, and some fear and apprehension usually accompanies that.

Once the initial assessment is complete, treatment sessions vary depending on the modality that is chosen. One-to-one therapy is one option. Intense shamanic de-armoring of pain tapes in the body is a second option. An evening of ceremony is the third option. Regardless of which option is selected, each person is given full preparation and offered a choice to fully participate or not.

Credentialing

Those who are fully qualified practitioners of the Twisted Hairs Blessed Beauty Way of Shamanic Healing are all accountable to our Standards of Excellence Committee. A Review Board may request a full review and demand that necessary adjustment, re-training, or refinement be completed within a designated period.

Training

The training to become a fully qualified practitioner of the Twisted Hairs Blessed Beauty Way of Shamanic Healing takes several years. Although each training program is totally individualized, the training for the basic qualifications is rarely completed in less than 5 years.

The training incorporates analytical study, practical experience, personal transformation or self-development, and the disciplined application of spiritual practices. Students of this way of healing become apprentices on a spiritual path with heart. When a measure of unity of mind, body, and heart are achieved, spirit begins to work through the apprentice. It is only as a wounded healer that the apprentice can be of service to others. This is not an easy training. It requires an unbending will and a fearless heart to enter into the unknown and confront death (change) each step of the way. It requires one to be a spiritual warrior.

The Deer Tribe Metis Medicine Society (DTMMS)
PO Box 12397
Scottsdale, AZ 85267
Tel: (602) 443-3851
Fax: (602) 998-2569
E-mail: dtmms@amug.org
www.amug.org/~dtmms/

What to Look for in a Provider

It is highly recommended that you request to see documentation of the qualifications of the practitioner chosen. Qualified practitioners should have a certificate and diploma and a "scroll." The latter is the diploma of old. Painted on an animal hide, it depicts each of the thirty steps taken to accomplish the basic training in ceremonial alchemy. You can also call DTMMS/Doorways to ask for a list of qualified practitioners.

Barriers and Key Issues

The main factor that keeps shamanic healing from receiving visibility or credibility is a lack of internal readiness to meet the mainstream medical community. Although on the one hand this form of healing is ancient, on the other hand it is relatively new in its modern phase. In its presence as a viable alternative medicine within our modern world, it is young and vulnerable. There are a growing number who claim to be working as shamanic counselors, teachers, healers, and so on. These individuals and varying approaches have not yet gathered into an association that would give them visibility and allow them to develop credibility.

Associations

No formalized national associations exist yet for shamanic healing.

Suggested Reading

1. Reagan, HS: *Shamanic wheels and keys: the teachings of the twisted hairs elders of turtle island,* vol 1, Scottsdale, Ariz, 1994, The Deer Tribe Metis Medicine Society.
   This is a volume of the basic knowledge and the cognitive maps, which are the foundation for the entire healing paradigm. It is a critical study for anyone who desires to apply shamanic healing techniques within their own practice.
2. Storm H: *The song of heyoehkah,* San Francisco, Calif, 1981, HarperCollins.
   This is a book for inspiration and delight. It holds stories of the ancient mystery ways . . . and messages for modern day application.

3. Bear S, Wind W, Mulligan C: *Dancing with the wheel: the medicine wheel workbook,* 1980, New Leaf Distributors.

4. Bear S, Wind W: *The medicine wheel: earth astrology,* 1992, New Leaf Distributors.
Sun Bear held a vision of the gathering together of peoples from all paths, all ways. The gathering together would be in the form of a medicine wheel. Each has its own place; each cannot thrive without the other also thriving. In simple language, it gives the reader something to play and work with immediately.

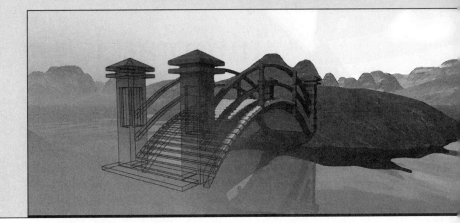

Manual Healing Methods

Chiropractic, **310**
Osteopathic Medicine, **325**
Massage Therapy, **338**

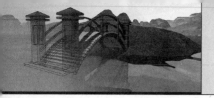

Chiropractic

DANIEL T. HANSEN

JOHN J. TRIANO

Origins and History

At the turn of the century, health care seemed more a craft than a science. In this early time before the integration of science and treatment method and the assumption of cultural authority over health care by allopathic medicine, chiropractic emerged in the midst of magnetic healers, herbal healers, bonesetters, and homeopaths. Historical accounts place the origin of chiropractic to an event that occurred on September 18, 1895 when Daniel David Palmer placed his hands upon an irregular protrusion of the spine of a janitor, and with a forceful thrust reduced the irregularity. As a result, Palmer's patient claimed to "hear wagons on the street," something he could not do before the treatment.

From its earliest origin, opposition grew between chiropractic and allopathic medicine. The practices were separate. Emphasizing their differences, the chiropractic community developed different lexicon and clinical rationale and opposed the use of medicines and surgery. Chiropractic was conceived as a more natural approach to healing, basing its philosophy on facilitating the body's own recuperative powers.

Through most of its history, the chiropractic profession has been criticized by medicine for lack of scientific underpinning. With its relative isolation from public research funding, critical investigation of chiropractic methods largely remained intramural. Access to federal grants and formal appropriateness research has occurred recently. Scientific study has focused primarily on the effectiveness of chiropractic methods for common back and neck complaints. The results of these studies have found their way into recognized refereed literature and has affected changes in health policy. In recent years the interprofessional controversies have narrowed and we are witnessing growing collaboration between chiropractors and the greater scientific and medical communities. Cooperation is occurring in basic and applied research, clinical practice and policy development. Research has demonstrated that manipulation, the primary mode of care for the doctor of chiropractic, offers benefits for acute and chronic low back pain patients. It has been recognized as such in federal guidelines for treatment of adult acute low back pain. While the number of studies remain small, similar results appear to be emerging for the treatment of neck pain and headaches. For these recognized applications for which chiropractors are most often involved, the label of chiropractic as an unscientific cult has difficulty sticking.[1]

Mechanism of Action According to Its Own Theory

Chiropractic beliefs were born out of the principles of vitalism. Early chiropractors rationalized a system of thinking about the body's self-healing capacity. Even now, some chiropractors espouse this perspective. Historical efforts attempted to evaluate the role of body structure in the healing process. Early chiropractic literature can be found that intertwines self-healing vitalism with reasonable discussions of physiology and anatomy.

The simplest explanation of what a chiropractic practitioner does can be reduced into elements of structure and function. Chiropractors work primarily with patients that have musculoskeletal complaints. Initially, the patient is evaluated to diagnose the problem and determine an appropriate treatment plan that may include conservative management with chiropractic care, patient education, self-care recommendations, rehabilitation, and medical consultation or referral where necessary. The objective of chiropractic care is to restore and preserve musculoskeletal function and alleviate symptoms. The lesions that are treated are commonly termed *subluxations*. Although the scientific details remain unknown, the response to treatment has been demonstrated. The subluxation in its simplest form is a local, uncontrolled mechanic response to spine environment loads that manifest clinically as a set of symptoms. They are known to initiate or aggravate inflammatory or degenerative conditions and are amenable to manipulation. The chiropractic *adjustment*, a form of manipulation, is achieved by applying controlled and directed forces and moments to the effected joint to alter its function. The effect of treatment is dependent on the tissue that has been stressed (for example, muscle, joint, ligament, or nerve) and any coexisting pathology.

Modern chiropractic practices emphasize a patient-centered, hands-on approach intent on influencing function through structure. And currently chiropractors embrace practice attitudes that strive toward early intervention emphasizing timely diagnosis and treatment of functional, reversible conditions. In more severe cases, medical intervention coordinated with chiropractic care can be complementary, solving problems that neither have been able to solve alone.

Biologic Mechanism of Action

The initial insult associated with spinal complaints is generally considered mechanic in nature.[2] Tissue injury may take the form of deformation by trauma, degeneration, or stenosis, generating local concentration of compressive, tensile, or shearing forces. The function of the spinal joint is altered by virtue of static misalignment, or reduction of motion (for example, hypomobility). Associated mechanisms of segmental derangement include entrapment of the facet joint meniscoid; entrapment of a fragment of posterior annular material of the intervertebral disc; stiffness induced by adhesions, scar tissue and degenerative changes; and excessive activity (spasm, hypertonicity) of the deep intrinsic spinal musculature. Through nerve irritation or release of chemical byproducts of tissue damage, pain production may arise either with or without local inflammation. Prolonged painful stimulation may cause an increased reactivity of the spinal cord perceived as hypersensitivity and pain from normal activities and stresses.

These biochemic and physiologic complications of mechanical injury explain persistent symptoms even when the acute phase of injury has passed. Chiropractic care attempts to alter the local tissue stresses and reduce the mechanic stimulation, allowing the body to recover. When biochemic mechanisms become too severe or self-perpetuating, an integrated treatment program that combines medical antiinflammatory interventions with manipulation and rehabilitation may be necessary.

Many aspects of these theories remain speculative, supported by indirect evidence. Basic science investigations continue, including human studies. Models of biomechanic and physiologic effects of manipulation with consideration to complications and natural events are now emerging in the literature.[3,4]

Forms of Therapy

Chiropractic treatments, as well as diagnostic practices, vary by geographic region largely because of differences in state laws governing the scope of practice. The therapeutic procedure most closely associated with chiropractic is spinal manipulation, traditionally termed an adjustment. However, chiropractic patient management also includes lifestyle counseling, nutritional management, rehabilitation, various physiotherapeutic modalities, and a variety of other interventions.

There are at least 100 distinct chiropractic, osteopathic, and medical manipulation techniques, a large array of highly specialized adjusting tables and equipment, and a great deal of variation in the specific techniques used by individual practitioners. Although there is biomechanical evidence for differing mechanisms for individual procedures, there has been no formal study comparing the clinical effectiveness between techniques. There have been significant studies comparing spinal manipulation against physical therapy, medications, bed rest, use of corsets, and no treatment for low back pain, neck pain, and headache. Most studies show comparative benefit of manipulation, other studies show no difference, and some have shown enhanced benefit of manipulation when coupled with medical management (such as nonsteroidal antiinflammatory medications).

The term *spinal manipulative therapy* is often used to encompass all types of manual technique systems used by chiropractors and other manual therapists. *Mobilization* is a slow, passive oscillating motion of a joint within its physiologic range of motion. Manipulation, on the other hand, is a mechanic procedure that is most often carried out by hand. Forces and moments are administered to the patient along specific intended lines of action and within an intended range of peak amplitudes and displacements. Cavitation of the joint can occur which typically produces an audible "pop" in a synovial joint. Both manipulation and mobilization are used to facilitate joint motion.[8]

Demographics

Chiropractic represents the third largest health profession after medicine and dentistry. In 1994 there were approximately 50,000 chiropractors licensed in the U.S., roughly one chiropractor for every 5000 U.S. residents. It is estimated that 82% of the chiropractors are in full-time practice, and the majority are in solo practices. Over the course of the 1980s and 1990s an increasing number of doctors are in group or multidisciplinary practices. In 1995 there were 14,040 students enrolled in the 16 accredited chiropractic colleges in North America, 2864 of whom graduated in that year.

Data from the Federation of Chiropractic Licensing Boards (1995) reveals that distribution of chiropractors tends to be proportionate to state and regional populations. States with more than 3000 chiropractors include California, New York, Florida, Pennsylvania, and Texas. Twenty-two states have more than 1000 chiropractors. About 60% of chiropractors work in urban or suburban communities, 35% work in small towns, and 5% work in rural areas.[5] The proportion of the U.S. population that uses chiropractors and the number of chiropractic visits per capita have nearly doubled in the past 15 to 20 years.[6]

The cross-section of people that use chiropractic services favors 18 to 55 year-olds, females slightly more than males, and typically people with at least a high school education. The use of chiropractors tends to be higher in the western states and lowest in the northeastern United States. Geriatric populations also tend to use chiropractors, as chiropractic manipulation is a covered service under Medicare. Although many chiropractors espouse the benefits of care to children, the use of chiropractic services by the pediatric population is minimal.

More than 80% of American workers in conventional insurance plans, preferred provider organizations (PPOs), and point-of-service plans now have health insurance that cover at least part of the costs of care. It is only in health maintenance organizations (HMOs) that a majority of enrollees still lack chiropractic coverage; however, public demand and evidence of cost-effectiveness from appropriate use are increasing the availability of benefits. All workers' compensation systems—state and federal, personal injury protection insurance, and Medicare—cover chiropractic services.[7]

Indications and Reasons for Referral

Conservative management of acute low back pain, subacute and chronic neck pain, and certain kinds of nonmigraine headaches with spinal manipulation now is considered more a part of mainstream rather than alternative medicine. Results of formal randomized studies have demonstrated the effectiveness of manipulation as performed by chiropractors. Considering the evidence and clinical experience, multidisciplinary consensus panels have clearly identified those circumstances where chiropractic manipulation is considered appropriate (and inappropriate) for low back and neck problems. These results have found their way into health policy, setting insurance benefits as well as quality management protocols. Low back, leg pain and related conditions make up 68% of patient visits to chiropractors. Most of the remaining 32% of visits are for headaches and pain or injury to the neck, middle back, arm, or legs. Approximately 5% of the visits to chiropractors represent consultation for other organic disorders (for example, asthma, menstrual disorders, upper respiratory conditions, and others). These reasons are truly the "alternative" complaints for which people seek chiropractic care.[8,9]

Chiropractic Management: Indications and Contraindications
Consensus-based protocols

What Leads a Patient to a Chiropractor		**Services the Chiropractor Provides**	
Circumstances, patient complaints, or patient symptoms that lead to seeking chiropractic consultation or appointment:		Administrative, clinical, and consultative procedures and services provided by chiropractic providers:	

ACCESS / TRIAGE DECISIONS

☐ Direct referral from MD/DO/DC	☐ **No Red Flags** (B) **and:**	☐ 1st physician-available triage	☐ Physical examination
☐ Direct referral from PT/OT/LMT	• Headache	☐ Conservative care consultation	☐ Ortho or neuro examination
☐ Physician requests DC or manip.	• Neck pain	☐ Pre or postsurgic consultation	☐ Noninvasive imaging
☐ Patient requests DC or manip/adj	• Midback (thoracic) pain	☐ MVA or work injury work-up	☐ Biomechanic assessment
☐ Patient request no surg or meds	• Low back or pelvis pain	☐ Impairment rating	☐ Scoliosis evaluation
☐ Noncritical trauma (A)	• Extremity symptoms		
☐ Favorable response to prev. manip			

ASSESSMENT DECISIONS

☐ Painful spine motion	☐ Painful incr stiffness in local jnt	☐ Biomechanical assessment	☐ Physical examination
☐ Focal tenderness over joint	☐ Normal or stable motor function	☐ Scoliosis evaluation	☐ Ortho or neuro examination
☐ Focal muscle hypertonicity	☐ Normal or stable sensory function	☐ Health risk assessment	☐ Noninvasive imaging
☐ Focal muscle tenderness		☐ Ergonomic assessment	

MANAGEMENT DECISIONS

☐ Acute LBP w/in 1st month of sympts	☐ Cumulative trauma disorders	☐ Tolerance to manual methods	■ Manipulation, postinjection
☐ Acute soft tissue injury	☐ Uncomplicated DJD or DDD	☐ Passive care: manipulation	■ Postsurgical mgmt (mechanical)
☐ Subacute neck pain - manip	☐ Referred UE/LE spine rel sympt	☐ Passive care: cont. passive mob	■ Failed surgery management
☐ Pain or spasm assoc w/acute radic	☐ Extremity pain or dysfunction	☐ Passive care: muscle or trig point	■ Chronic pain management
☐ Recurrent back or neck pain	☐ Nonprogr spondylo (w&w/o slip)	☐ Active care: therapeutic stretch	■ Chronic pain behav/emotional overlay
☐ Chronic neck pain	■ Patient refusal of surgery	☐ Active care: therapeutic exercise	■ Pain management (w/ meds)
☐ Chr back pain w/ or w/o leg pain	■ Complicated multijoint disorders	☐ Pt education: biomechanics	■ Supportive care, disability syndr
☐ Chronically limited ROM	■ Suspected or known instability	☐ Scoliosis management or bracing	■ Supportive care, compl rehab
☐ Tension, other nonmigraine HA	■ Consult: nonsurgical options		

CONTRAINDICATIONS TO MANIPULATIVE THERAPIES

■ Undiagnosed neuro deficits	■ Suspected or known acute fx (C)	■ Area w/ malignancy	■ Clin evidence or vert-basilar synd
■ Congen or acquired deformities	■ Region w/ acute episode of RA	■ Area w/ bone or joint infection	■ Advanced osteoporosis
■ Hx circ. (CVA or TIA) deficits (C)	■ Acute myelopathy or cauda equina	■ Progressive neuro deficits	
■ Benign bone tumors	■ Spondy w/ progressive slippage		

Relative contraindication: team manage; absolute contraindication; (A) Noncritical spinal trauma: lack of any spinal fracture or hard neurologic signs; (B) Red flags: history or findings indicative of infection, fracture, cancer, or progressive neurologic deficits; (C) Contraindicated until complication or risk of complication has been ruled out by appropriate diagnostic testing. (Courtesy Texas Back Institute, Plano, TX.)

The figure "Chiropractic Management: Indications and Contraindications" is a physician job aid developed in a large, multidisciplinary spine care center. It concisely describes appropriate reasons for chiropractic referral.[10] It vertically catalogues reasons that a patient might need a chiropractor on the left. On the right, the services that might meet the patient needs are listed. Horizontal stratification divides the reasons into stages of patient encounter.

Office Applications

A simple ranking of conditions responsive to this form of therapy is as follows. As with all alternative therapies, the use of chiropractic does not preclude the use of mainstream medical therapies in addition.

Top level: *A therapy ideally suited for these conditions*
Back pain and headaches

Second level: *One of the better therapies for these conditions*
Arthritis; childbirth; chronic pain; menstrual cramps; osteoarthritis; and pregnancy

Third level: *A valuable adjunctive therapy for these conditions*
Chronic fatigue syndrome; colic; female health; hypertension; male health; menopause; otitis media; periodic leg movement syndrome; postpartum care; premenstrual syndrome; rheumatoid arthritis; and tinnitus

Practical Applications

In 1993 the National Board of Chiropractic Examiners released a report from their survey of chiropractic practice in the U.S. They used this data to better perform a job analysis for chiropractors in practice for the purposes of testing for appropriate competencies. Recalling from previous descriptions, the chiropractic practice involves more than just manipulation or adjustment of spine and other articulations. Chiropractors frequently engage in rehabilitation efforts, application of physical modalities, and counseling on diet, nutrition, exercise, fitness, and stress management. The diagnostic and treatments procedures used and the ancillary processes employed will likely vary from provider to provider based on specialization and practice philosophy. The following is the hierarchy of presenting and concurrent patient conditions seen by chiropractors, based on frequency:[25]

Routinely seen: Spinal sublaxation and joint dysfunction; low back pain; neck pain; headaches; and thoracic pain

Often seen: Muscular strain and tear; extremity sublaxation and joint dysfunction; osteoarthritis and degenerative joint disease; hyperlordosis of cervical or lumbar spine; peripheral neuritis or neuralgia; scoliosis; tendonitis and tenosynovitis; bursitis or synovitis; radiculitis or radiculopathy; high or low blood pressure; vertebral facet syndrome; allergies; intervertebral disc syndrome; obesity; and sprain or dislocation of any joint

Sometimes seen: Kyphosis of thoracic spine; respiratory, viral, or bacterial infection; osteoporosis or osteomalacia; acne, dermatitis, or psoriasis; carpal or tarsal tunnel syndrome; loss of equilibrium; skeletal congenital or developmental anomaly; diabetes; articular joint anomaly; psychologic disorders; TMJ syndrome; eating disorders; thoracic outlet syndrome; ear or hearing disorders; systemic rheumatoid arthritis or gout; eye or vision disorders; occupational or environmental disorder; hiatus or inguinal hernia; muscular atrophy; gastrointestinal bacteria or viral infection; nutritional disorders; infection of kidney or urinary tract; menstrual disorders; colitis or diverticulitis; asthma, emphysema, or obstructive lung disease; thyroid or parathyroid disorder; upper respiratory or ear infection; hemorrhoids; and pregnancy

This list represents the complaints for which patients typically seek help from a chiropractor. It is not known how effective chiropractors are in managing some of the conditions, especially those that are "sometimes seen." Most competent chiropractors would assess a patient for any of these conditions, evaluate for the appropriateness of any care provided in the office, and determine the appropriate provider in the community for referral or a co-management relationship. Certainly, there is concern by many in the allopathic community that there is potential for delay or failure for timely referral on patients that may have disorders with grave prognoses or high potential for complications. Most commonly, however, patients may present with conditions or complaints such as "sometimes seen," and be managed appropriately for collateral joint dysfunction problems that may affect the patient's quality of life. Patients that are treated by chiropractors are typically those having musculoskeletal problems as cited earlier. Clearly 95% of patients treated by chiropractors have a primary diagnosis of back pain, neck pain, arm or leg pain, or headache.

Research Base

Evidence Based

There are more randomized clinical trials of manipulation for spine related disorders from various sources than exist for any other single approach. In addition to these direct tests of chiropractic effectiveness, formal and independent consensus processes have been sponsored through the U.S. Agency for Health Care Policy and Research (AHCPR),[11] the RAND corporation,[12] as well as related formal efforts in Great Britain and New Zealand. For review, these authoritative sources can be grouped according to the topic matter into evidence for treatment of low back and leg pain, headaches, and neck and arm pain.

For lower back and leg pain, both acute and chronic, there is strong evidence that chiropractic manipulation should be a first line of management provided that there is no sign of progressive neurologic deficit.[13,14] Patients with back pain can expect up to a 17% greater rate of recovery and those with leg pain can expect an 8% greater rate of recovery.[15]

Unfortunately, the evidence for headache and neck pain is not as plentiful. Evidence from the few studies and consensus panels that have addressed neck and arm pain consider a trial of manipulation to be an appropriate approach to these complaints[16] and more effective than mobilization.[17]

Basic Science

Basic science studies of manipulation have focused on the biomechanic and physiologic effects. Most of the pertinent and critical literature has been reviewed and summarized.[4] For the most common system of manipulation, there are more than 45 procedures for the lumbar spine, 25 procedures for the neck, and 17 procedures for the thoracic spine. The administration of the procedures is complex, simultaneously accounting for the nature of the manipulatable lesion, patient pathology, and stature. The loads applied are significant and rapid, taking place in less than 0.25 second, requiring the doctor to be skilled and practiced in their application. As emphasized by Spitzer et al,[18] a patient should submit to these procedures only when performed by a doctor with adequate training. Manipulation is a mechanic procedure that is most often carried out by hand. Forces and moments are administered to the patient along specific intended lines of action and within an intended range of peak amplitudes and displacements. Investigators have quantified the loads required to achieve selected biologic effects. To determine systematic differences as a consequence of load amplitudes, it is necessary that the operators be able to manually generate graded increments in forces and moments. Recent evidence suggests that proficiency is not transferable between procedures even for the same spinal region but requires persistent practice for adequate administration. The skill levels of the provider can be assessed by both biomechanic and skill-rating systems.

Physiologic studies have been carried out to examine a few of the effects of manipulation on muscle activity, range of motion, and circulating serum components. The results of these works demonstrate that manipulation may have both local and remote effects.[19] Locally, range of motion is increased and muscle activity is altered. At remote locations, muscle activity mediated by nerves from the level of the spine being treated may be relaxed. Clinical studies also demonstrate reduction in pain levels immediately following manipulation, a response that persists without apparent accommodation with time. Such effects have obvious corollaries to clinical evidence of treatment efficacy. Enhanced respiratory burst of white blood cells and associated biochemic activity for substance P and tumor necrosis factor have been described over short intervals and are examples of purely physiologic studies in progress. The clinical importance of the temporary phenomenon is unknown.[20]

Risk and Safety

A wide variety of procedures are available and the doctor must be familiar with a number of options for each clinical circumstance, particularly when there is comorbidity in functional and structural pathologies. The evidence shows that when administered by a competent, skillful, and knowledgeable practitioner, manipulation is extraordinarily safe.[21] Complications do occur. Self-limiting, mild symptoms of new local pain account for the majority and occur in as many as 12.5% of patients. The rate of other minor complications requiring appropriate diagnosis management is 3%, comparable to the risk rate of many surgical and medical procedures. Severe complications have been reported including stroke and damage to the spinal cord. Although severe complications yielding permanent damage is rare (0.000001%), the proportion associated with manipulation administered by those other than chiropractors is alarmingly high. With 94% of procedures performed by chiropractors, it would be expected that approximately 94% of serious complications are associated with their treatment and only 6% with nonchiropractic treatment. Examination of the literature, in fact, shows this to be false.[22] In Terrett's data, 10% of serious complications are from osteopaths, 9% are from MDs, and 20% are from therapists and others. In an additional 30 cases of complication incorrectly attributed to chiropractors, 13% were actually caused by physical therapists attempting manipulation. Used properly and for the appropriate patient, lumbar spine manipulations that are performed with maximum effort deemed clinically safe can generate loads consistent with those observed in common daily tasks on jobs requiring lifting and twisting movements.[23]

Future Research Opportunities and Priorities

The important research priorities for the chiropractic discipline relate to use and delivery options within the different delivery models (for example, direct access versus medical referral) and effectiveness studies for different chiropractic methods for common patient complaints. There is growing interest in studying the long-term effects of spinal manipulation on the prevention of musculoskeletal problems and whether spinal manipulation affects nonmusculoskeletal conditions.[7]

Self-Help versus Professional

Self-help is an important part of long-term recovery for patients with musculoskeletal complaints. The most effective means of treatment helps the patient relieve symptoms from injured tissues and promotes self-reliance to optimize the quality of life. The patient should rely on professional recommendations for short-term activity limitations and guidance for reactivation. Exercise for joint flexibility, strengthening, and endurance are the necessary tools.

Manipulation should not be attempted by an untrained individual as a part of self-help. The procedures themselves generally are not amenable to being performed by individuals on themselves. Serious complications have been reported in the literature from patients or unqualified persons attempting to perform spinal manipulation.

Visiting a Professional

A new patient appointment generally can be obtained with a chiropractor's office within 2 to 3 days and often on the same day in case of emergency. The initial visit is quite similar to a typical physician visit. Through a questionnaire or interview the necessary demographic data, as well as the basic history related to the presenting complaint, past medical history, and social and family information, is collected. General health information including vital signs (height, weight, blood pressure, pulse, temperature, respiration rate, and so on) and more detailed information about the effects of the main complaint, including location and severity as well as functional limitations are obtained.

The chiropractor performs a focused physical, orthopedic, neurologic, and biomechanic examination of the spine and related structures or systems. Based on the results the doctor may recommend additional tests, either by clinical laboratory exam (blood, urine), diagnostic imaging (radiograph, MRI, CT scan), or other specialized measurements. A diagnosis is made and a treatment plan is recommended. If necessary, consultation or referral with complementary medical specialists will be arranged. In most cases, appropriate treatment can commence on the first visit.

The follow-up visits include a brief reevaluation of the patient to gauge improvement and modify the treatment plan. If there is significant tissue inflammation and muscle tightness or spasm the manual therapy may be preceded with therapy modalities, such as ultrasound, electric stimulation, vibration, passive motion, stretch, cold or heat, and massage. And finally, the manipulation is applied.

The patient's experience of the manipulation begins with positioning of the joint (spine/extremity) near its end range. The patient often feels tension of the muscles and ligaments around the joint. If tolerated well, the segment is loaded quickly in the same direction. Besides the pressure used to position the patient, a "pinch" sensation and popping sound may occur and is a normal part of the process. Typically there is no additional pain with these maneuvers. Home and self-care recommendations and activity limitations may be explained for the patient to assist in recovery.

For most disorders, the treatment plan anticipates that the patient will receive care 2 to 5 times per week for the first week or two, depending on severity and complicating factors. Additional follow-up in the uncomplicated case occurs at a rate of 1 or 2 times per week for 2 or 3 weeks. The frequency of care decreases until the patient reaches maximum benefit or is resolved. Cases that are chronic or more complicated, including intervertebral disc syndromes, radiating extremity pain, degenerative disease, or postoperative cases, may take longer to manage. Their treatment may involve other manual therapy methods and involve comanagement with other health care providers. Cases unresolved after about 2 weeks should not continue with the same manual therapy and should be considered for interdisciplinary consultation.

Credentialing

The practice of chiropractic is regulated in all 50 states of the U.S. and in many countries worldwide. In all state jurisdictions there are state licensing boards that regulate education, experience, and moral character of candidates and also serve to protect the public health, safety, and welfare of its residents in matters of chiropractic practice. To varying degrees, state boards construct and administer licensure examinations to candidates or may require successful completion of the standardized series of examinations administered by the National Board of Chiropractic Examiners (NBCE).

The NBCE, established more than 35 years ago, functions similarly to the National Board of Medical Examiners. There are four parts plus a separate exam for physiotherapy.

Parts I and II cover basic sciences and clinical sciences respectively and are taken by students prior to graduation from chiropractic college. Part III is a written clinical competency examination that requires successful passing of Parts I and II. Part IV is a practical examination (objective structured clinical examination) that tests practical skills in radiograph interpretation and diagnosis, chiropractic technique, and case management.[25]

Consistent with other health professions, a new layer of credentialing is now in place through membership in health maintenance organization (HMO) programs, preferred provider organizations (PPOs), or independent physician associations (IPAs). Such organizations often are the first line of action to enforce or investigate problems regarding quality of care and patient satisfaction.

Training

There are sixteen chiropractic colleges in the U.S. and two in Canada. All those in the U.S. are now accredited and monitored by the federally recognized Council on Chiropractic Education (CCE). Most of the schools are also accredited by regional accrediting agencies for higher education. CCE standards and state licensing board requirements largely influence admission requirements of chiropractic colleges. A minimum of 2 academic years of undergraduate education is required with successful completion of courses in core sciences (biology, chemistry, physics), psychology, English or communications, and the humanities. Each required science course must include laboratories. Some colleges require more than the minimum 60 credit (semester) hours, and six states require a bachelor's degree in addition to the doctor of chiropractic degree for licensure. Most chiropractic colleges use a "rolling" admissions process, where qualified applicants are admitted on an ongoing basis (3 to 4 terms per year).

Chiropractic students receive about the same number of total hours of education as medical students. A chiropractic program consists of 4 academic years of professional training averaging a total of 4822 hours. Of this, approximately 1975 hours are in clinical sciences and 1405 hours are for clinical clerkship. There are five curricular areas of specialty that are emphasized in chiropractic education: adjustive (manipulative) techniques and spinal analysis (23% of the clinical program); principles and practice of chiropractic (10%); physiologic therapeutics (5%); and biomechanics (3%). There also is significant time spent in diagnosis, orthopedics, neurology, diagnostic imaging and radiology, and nutrition.

Specialty training is available through U.S. chiropractic colleges for part-time postgraduate education programs or full-time residency programs. These programs are available in family practice, applied chiropractic sciences, clinical neurology, orthopedics, sports injuries, pediatrics, nutrition, rehabilitation, and industrial consulting. Both the residency and postgraduate training programs lead to eligibility to sit for competency examinations offered by specialty boards recognized by the American Chiropractic Association, International Chiropractors Association, and the American Board of Chiropractic Specialties. Currently, orthopedics and sports chiropractic are the most prevalent specialty certifications.

There are some limited opportunities for chiropractors to participate in medical and multidisciplinary residencies. And some chiropractic schools are pursuing joint training opportunities with other universities in the areas of public health, epidemiology, and health care administration.[26]

What to Look for in a Provider

When choosing a chiropractic provider within the community, care should be taken to ask questions of colleagues, patients, and payors. If other health providers in the community recommend the chiropractor, then it is likely that chiropractor provides competent care and respects interprofessional courtesies and protocols. If a chiropractor is credentialed with a number of managed care plans, then that chiropractor probably has made a commitment to provide quality care without excesses in the use of radiology, diagnostic devices, or prolonged treatment plans.

Barriers and Key Issues

Scientific and clinical advancement of chiropractic has been hindered by its systematic exclusion by political medicine from access to social sources of funding resources. Because of their historical exclusion from participation in the mainstream of health care delivery, chiropractors have functioned outside of medical referral networks, institutional settings, multidisciplinary group practices and co-ownership, and federal and research foundation funding opportunities. Chiropractors historically have relied on individual patient referrals and marketing efforts to gain community presence and attract patients. Colleges have been strapped for resources by their reliance on tuition-based revenue systems. Only in the past 20 years has the profession been able to develop sufficient infrastructure to participate in the scientific debates on health and the prevention and treatment of disease.

Early efforts are underway to define and optimize the role of chiropractic in the health care system. As health reform efforts address the concerns of variations of practice, costs of care, and appropriate use of resources for all of the health disciplines, chiropractic is finding itself challenged with the same demands for accountability. A cadre of clinical scientists and a research culture has begun to form. The immediate issues include questions on the nature of subluxation and its role in health and disease; the dosage and duration of therapy to reach maximum benefit for specific disorders; and the optimization of clinical outcome. Like all of medicine, chiropractic must define its value in health care to reestablish its moral authority within the social system.[7]

Associations

American Chiropractic Association
1701 Clarendon Blvd.
Arlington, VA 22209
Tel: (800) 986-4636
www.amerchiro.org

International Chiropractors Association
1110 N. Glebe Rd. #1000
Arlington, VA 22201
Tel: (800) 423-4690
www.chiropractic.org

World Federation of Chiropractic
3080 Yonge St. #5065
Toronto, ON, CAN M4N 3N1
Tel: (416) 484-9978
www.wfc.org

Suggested Reading

1. Cherkin DC, Mootz RD, editors: *Chiropractic in the United States: training, practice, and research*, US Department of Health and Human Services, Agency for Health Care Policy and Research, Rockville, Md, 1997, AHCPR Pub No 98-N002.

   This monograph, funded and published as a part of the Medical Treatment Effectiveness Program (MEDTEP) of the Agency for Health Care Policy and Research, is the first concise expert appraisal of chiropractic practice, education, and research. It can be found at www.ahcpr.gov/clinic/chirop/.

2. Haldeman S, editor: *Principles and practice of chiropractic*. Norwalk, NJ, 1992, Appleton & Lange.

   This the second edition of Dr. Haldeman's concise handbook on chiropractic. It continues to serve as an essential textbook in chiropractic training and is respected internationally as the source book on the chiropractic discipline.

3. Haldeman S, Chapman-Smith D, Petersen D, editors: *Guidelines for chiropractic quality assurance and practice parameters*, Gaithersburg, Md, 1993, Aspen.

   Often referred to as the "Mercy Center Guidelines," this book contains the results of an evidence-based, consensus-driven inventory of the science used to guide chiropractic practice. The process and format have been subsequently repeated in Canada and Australia with similar results.

References

1. Phillips RB: A brief history of chiropractic. In Cherkin DC, Mootz RD, editors: *Chiropractic in the United States: training, practice, and research*, US Department of Health and Human Services, Agency for Health Care Policy and Research, Rockville, Md, 1997, AHCPR Pub No 98-N002.

2. Saal JS: The role of inflammation in lumbar pain, *Spine* 20(16):1821-1827, 1995.

3. Vernon HT: Biological rationale for possible benefits of spinal manipulation. In Cherkin DC, Mootz RD, editors: *Chiropractic in the United States: training, practice, and research*, US Department of Health and Human Services, Agency for Health Care Policy and Research, Rockville, Md, 1997, AHCPR Pub No 98-N002.

4. Triano JJ: The mechanics of spinal manipulation. In Herzog W, editor: Clinical biomechanics of the spine, St Louis, 1999, Mosby.

5. Federation of Chiropractic Licensing Boards: *Official directory: chiropractic licensure and practice statistics, 1996-97 edition*, Greeley, Colo, 1996, Federation of Licensing Boards.

6. Shekelle PG, Brook RH: A community-based study of the use of chiropractic services, *Am J Pub Health* 81:439-442, 1991.

7. Cherkin DC, Mootz RD: Synopsis, research priorities and policy issues. In Cherkin DC, Mootz RD, editors: *Chiropractic in the United States: training, practice, and research*, US Department of Health and Human Services, Agency for Health Care Policy and Research, Rockville, Md, 1997, AHCPR Pub No 98-N002.

8. Mootz RD: Content of practice. In Cherkin DC, Mootz RD, editors: *Chiropractic in the United States: training, practice, and research*, US Department of Health and Human Services, Agency for Health Care Policy and Research, Rockville, Md, 1997, AHCPR Pub No 98-N002.

9. Shekelle PG et al: Benefits and risks of spinal manipulation. In Cherkin DC, Mootz RD, editors: *Chiropractic in the United States: training, practice, and research*, US Department of Health and Human Services, Agency for Health Care Policy and Research, Rockville, Md, 1997, AHCPR Pub No 98-N002.

10. Triano JJ, Rashbaum RF, Hansen DT: Opening access to spine care in the evolving market: integlation and communication, *Top Clin Chiropr* 5(4): 44-52, 1998.

11. Bigos SJ, chair: Acute low back problems in adults. Clinical Practice Guideline No. 14. US Department of Health and Human Services, Public Health Service, Agency for Health Care Policy and Research, Rockville, Md, 1994.

12. Shekelle PG et al: The appropriateness of spinal manipulation for low back pain: indications and ratings by a multidisciplinary expert panel, Santa Monica, Calif, 1991, The RAND Corporation, R-4025/2-CCR/FCER.

13. Shekelle PG et al: Spinal manipulation for low-back pain, *Ann Intern Med* 117(7):590-598, 1992.

14. van Tulder MW, Koes BW, Bouter LM: Conservative treatment of acute and chronic nonspecific low back pain: a systematic review of randomized controlled trials of the most common interventions, *Spine* 22(18):2128-2156, 1997.

15. Triano JJ et al: Manipulation therapy versus education programs in chronic low back pain, *Spine* 20(8):948-955, 1995.

16. Hurwitz EL et al: Manipulation and mobilization of the cervical spine, *Spine* 21(15):1746-1760, 1996.

17. Cassidy JD, Lopes AA, Yong-Hing K: The immediate effect of manipulation versus mobilization on pain and range of motion in the cervical spine: a randomized controlled trial, *J Manipulative Physiol Ther* 15(9):570-575, 1992.

18. Spitzer WO et al: Scientific monograph of the Quebec Task Force on whiplash-associated disorders: redefining "whiplash" and its management, *Spine* 20(8S):21S, 1995 (suppl).

19. Triano JJ: Interaction of spinal biomechanics and physiology. In Haldeman S, editor: *Principles and practice of chiropractic*, Norwalk, NJ, 1992, Appleton & Lange.

20. Brennan PC et al: Enhanced neutrophil respiratory burst as a biological marker for manipulation forces: duration of the effect and association with substance P and tumor necrosis factor, *J Manipulative Physiol Ther* 15(2):83-89, 1992.

21. Haldeman S, editor: *Principles and practice of chiropractic*, Norwalk, NJ, 1992, Appleton & Lange.

22. Terrett AG: Misuse of the literature by medical authors in discussing spinal manipulative therapy injury, *J Manipulative Physiol Ther* 18(4):203-210, 1996.

23. Triano J, Schultz AB: Loads transmitted during lumbosacral spinal manipulative therapy, *Spine* 22(17):1955-1964, 1997.

24. Christiansen M, Morgan D, editors: *Job analysis of chiropractic: a project report, survey analysis and summary of the practice of chiropractic within the United States*, Greely, Colo, 1993, NBCE.

25. Sandefur R, Coulter ID: Licensure and legal scope of practice. In Cherkin DC, Mootz RD, editors: *Chiropractic in the United States: training, practice, and research*, US Department of Health and Human Services, Agency for Health Care Policy and Research, Rockville, Md, 1997, AHCPR Pub No 98-N002.

26. Coulter ID, Adams AH, Sandefur R: Chiropractic training. In Cherkin DC, Mootz RD, editors: *Chiropractic in the United States: training, practice, and research*, US Department of Health and Human Services, Agency for Health Care Policy and Research, Rockville, Md, 1997, AHCPR Pub No 98-N002.

Osteopathic Medicine

ROBERT KAPPLER

KENNETH A. RAMEY

KURT P. HEINKING

Origins and History

Osteopathic medicine, or *osteopathy*, as it is sometimes called, is a philosophy, a science, and an art. Its philosophy embraces the concept of body unity through structure and function in health and disease. Its science includes the chemical sciences, biologic sciences, and physical sciences that are related to the maintenance of health and the prevention, the cure, and the alleviation of disease. Its art is the application of the philosophy and the science in the practice of osteopathic medicine and osteopathic surgery in all its branches and specialties.

Osteopathic medicine was founded by Andrew Taylor Still, MD. Dr. Still was born in 1828. He served as a frontier physician in Kansas and Missouri and later on, he served as a surgeon for Union forces in the American Civil War. Dr. Still had an extensive knowledge of anatomy and physiology, and he used this knowledge to develop a method to both diagnose and treat the body through palpation and manipulation. His first attempt to present his ideas at Baker University in Kansas on June 22, 1874 was met with both adversity and ridicule. In 1875 Dr. Still moved to Kirksville, Missouri, where he later founded the American School of Osteopathy in 1892. Dr. Still refused to grant the MD degree to his graduates. Instead, he chose the DO (Diplomate in Osteopathy) degree in order to distinctly recognize his graduates as having a unique set of skills that distinguished them from conventional medical physicians. The Diplomate in Osteopathy degree was later changed to the Doctor of Osteopathy degree and eventually to the Doctor of Osteopathic Medicine degree. Dr. Still died in 1917. Today, DOs practice all branches of medicine and surgery, ranging from psychiatry to obstetrics, geriatrics, and emergency medicine. Interest in osteopathic medicine has grown over the years. The profession currently has a total of 19 different colleges of osteopathic medicine in the United States. More than 5000 students are enrolled in osteopathic medical schools, and at present there are more than 40,000 osteopathic physicians in the U.S.[1]

Mechanism of Action According to Its Own Theory

What makes osteopathic physicians different? There are the following four key principles to osteopathic philosophy:

1. The body is a unit. People are units of body, mind, and spirit. Every individual is regulated by and integrated through interdependent functions of associated anatomic, physiologic, and psychosocial systems. The circulatory, nervous, endocrine, immune, and musculoskeletal systems interact and respond to changes in both internal and external environments as an integrated whole.

   Imbalance in one area changes structure and function throughout the entire individual. If the imbalance persists, disease is the result. Disease is perceived as being the effect, not the cause. Osteopathic physicians strive to understand how the entire patient has deviated from health, with the end result being disease.

2. The body is capable of self-regulation, self-healing, and health maintenance. Our bodies normally have the natural capacity to meet the usual stresses of daily life. A person's present level of health depends on genetics, environmental influences, and adaptive responses to various stresses at that point in time. If any one factor exceeds the body's ability to adapt, disease is the result. The body is ultimately responsible for healing. Physicians only assist the body in the healing process.

3. Structure and function are reciprocally interrelated. Osteopathic physicians believe the entire individual is more than the sum total of individual parts. Systems are integrated and interrelated. Nothing exists in isolation. Each person is a complex integrated unit with various systems working interdependently to maintain the health of the entire individual. Structure affects function and vice versa. Separating one from the other only allows for a limited understanding of the entire individual.

4. Rational treatment is based on the basic principles of body unity, self-regulation, and the interrelationship of structure and function. Disease indicates a breakdown in the body's capacity for self-regulation. The neuromusculoskeletal system interacts interdependently with all aspects of structure and function. Osteopathic physicians use palpatory diagnosis and osteopathic manipulation to treat related somatic components. This helps normalize body physiology and allows homeostatic mechanisms to rebalance and return the individual to health. Depending on the condition, palpatory diagnosis and treatment may be used as the sole modality or combined with pharmaceutics, psychologic or physical therapy, and surgery.

The use of osteopathic manipulative medicine is a combination and integration of osteopathic philosophy, existing knowledge, diagnostic palpatory skills, and osteopathic manipulative treatment skills. This integration becomes osteopathic problem solving. Osteopathic physicians apply this theory in the clinical arena by asking the question: "Does the patient have a significant musculoskeletal component to the problem?" (Please note: The question is not: "Does the patient have some musculoskeletal findings?")

To answer this question, osteopathic physicians perform a screening musculoskeletal examination, a palpatory exam, and motion testing of various joints and tissues. Palpation for tissue texture abnormality is a screening procedure often used by experienced clinicians. When the tissue feels abnormal the examination focuses on this area to further define the problem.

Component parts of the osteopathic musculoskeletal examination can be classified by T.A.R.T.

Tissue Texture Abnormality: Feel, palpate

Asymmetry (Structure): Look

Restriction of Motion: Move, test motion

Tenderness: Palpate for tenderness (sensitivity)

These parameters apply whether the examination involves the entire musculoskeletal system or a region. The quality of a musculoskeletal examination can be evaluated by assessing the presence (or absence) of these four components. When the examination contains all four components, it is likely that somatic dysfunction is present. Somatic dysfunction is defined as impaired or altered function of related components of the somatic system, including the skeletal, arthrodial, myofascial, vascular, lymphatic, and neural elements.

Ultimately the physician must come to a conclusion regarding the musculoskeletal findings. Are they significant? Are they related to the patient's problem? What is the probable etiology? Are they related to other findings? What are the probable effects of this dysfunction? Somatic dysfunction that the physician determines to be related to the patient's problem is treated with osteopathic manipulative treatment (OMT). These techniques are applied by the physician. Osteopathic treatment specifically applied to the somatic component assists in the interruption of this cycle and may lead to a profound therapeutic effect.[1]

Biologic Mechanism of Action

Experienced osteopathic physicians detect palpable change in muscles and tissues. These changes appear to result from increased sympathetic tone and local inflammatory mediators. These palpatory changes reflect a stiff, tense muscle with taught overlying fascia and cool, sweaty skin. Osteopathic researchers believe that aberrant reporting of information to and from muscle spindles is related to the motion restriction found with somatic dysfunction. The other characteristics of these palpatory findings are similar to those seen with local increases in sympathetic tone and inflammatory processes.

Somatic dysfunction in the musculoskeletal system will lead to aberrant afferent signals to the central nervous system. These afferent impulses may lead to facilitation of segmentally related areas of the spinal cord. These facilitated areas of the spinal cord affect the autonomics supplying the viscera. Visceral dysfunction may be produced through somatic dysfunction (somatovisceral reflex).

Just as somatic dysfunction can lead to visceral dysfunction, disturbances in visceral organs are reflected in segmentally related areas of the musculoskeletal system (viscerosomatic reflexes). Visceral sensory information is conducted through the same ascending spinal tracts to the brainstem and hypothalamus as is somatic nociceptive information.

Which organs or blood vessels will be affected? This depends on the site of musculoskeletal dysfunction and the part(s) of the central nervous system (spinal segments) into which the aberrant signals are carried. The communication is bidirectional. The viscera and the musculoskeletal system become connected in an abnormal cycle of afferent and efferent impulses, which maintain and exacerbate the disturbance.

The mechanisms behind these reflex arcs are complex. The autonomic nervous system is not strictly an efferent system. All nerves carrying autonomic efferent axons also carry primary afferent fibers to the dorsal horns of the spinal cord.[1] The primary afferent fibers of the B-afferent system are present in both somatic and visceral tissues. Stimulation of these fibers releases substance P locally and increases the central activity of the hypothalamic-pituitary-adrenal axis. In response to this the sympathetics release norepinephrine and the adrenal gland releases cortical hormones. In summary, reflex arcs, local mediators, and the release of stress hormones are involved in the bidirectional communication between the somatic and visceral systems.

Through these mechanisms, neurologic, visceral, metabolic, and endocrine activity is constantly tuned to requirements of the musculoskeletal system. Because a large percentage of the total body's energy requirement is consumed by the musculoskeletal system, treatment affecting these mechanisms is of paramount importance when considering the interrelationship of the body's structure and function.[1]

Forms of Therapy

The physician must have an objective to be accomplished by the treatment. Treatments should be outcome-oriented. The chosen technique must be safe and potentially effective. The physician's ability to effectively execute a technique is a major factor in determining which technique to use. The objective of the treatment is constant and the method of treatment is variable. There are many different technique approaches. Physicians must choose from the various techniques that are effective in their hands. The dose of treatment is limited by the patient's ability to respond to the treatment. The physician may want very much to do more and go faster; however, the patient's body must make the necessary changes toward health and recovery. Risk-benefit relationships must always be considered. The physician must be able to effectively execute the technique. The technique must be modified to meet the needs of the patient and the physician.

There are a number of different types of OMT available. The *Glossary of Osteopathic Terminology* lists over 30 types of OMT. In general, osteopathic treatment can be broken down into two categories: direct and indirect techniques.

Direct osteopathic manipulative techniques involve the identification of a motion restriction and initial positioning into the restrictive barrier. The restrictive barrier is a functional limitation of normal physiologic motion. More simply, it is an area of the body exhibiting a reduction in normal motion. Examples of direct osteopathic manipulative techniques include high velocity-low amplitude techniques (HVLA), direct isometric muscle energy (postisometric relaxation), and direct myofascial release. The principle for HVLA is to engage a solid barrier and apply a short, quick thrust. The principle for direct isometric muscle energy is to engage the barrier; hold; instruct the patient to contract 3 to 5 seconds against your holding force; relax (postisometric relaxation); engage a new barrier; repeat this process several times; and retest. The principle for direct myofascial release is to load (apply a force) and hold. As release occurs the tight tissues stretch and lengthen. Soft tissue and articulatory techniques are designed to relax muscles and improve motion.

Indirect osteopathic manipulative techniques involve initial positioning away from the restrictive barrier. Release is through inherent forces. Counterstrain, functional, balanced ligamentous-membranous tension, and indirect myofascial release are examples. Perhaps the term "spontaneous release by positioning" describes these techniques. The critical factor in indirect techniques is to find that point of balance or position in which release will occur. Counterstrain uses tender points. The part being treated is positioned in a direction of ease or positioned in the position of original injury. When the proper position is obtained, tenderness in the tender point is significantly decreased or absent. The physician holds this position for 90 seconds, releases slowly, and reevaluates for tenderness. Functional technique uses percussion or palpation surrounding the joint to achieve balanced tension and release. Balanced ligamentous tension can be approached mechanically, but there is also a certain feeling that is present when the proper position is obtained.

Demographics

Osteopathic physicians are complete physicians and are fully licensed to practice all areas of medicine and surgery in all 50 states. Many foreign countries allow for the licensure of osteopathic physicians. The American Osteopathic Association estimates that this year, more than 45,000 osteopathic physicians will be in practice in the U.S. More than 64% of all DOs practice in primary care areas of family practice, internal medicine, obstetrics-gynecology, and pediatrics. DOs represent 6% of the total U.S. physician population and 18% of all military physicians. DOs represent 15% of physicians in small towns and rural areas. Each year, more than 100 million patient visits are made to DOs.

Indications and Reasons for Referral

The first question becomes: Does the patient have a significant musculoskeletal component to the problem? If the physician identifies musculoskeletal dysfunction (somatic dysfunction, code 739), and concludes that this dysfunction is associated with a patient problem or symptoms, the indication for OMT has been established.

Osteopathic referral is often indicated for the following reasons:

- The patient has a musculoskeletal component and the case is beyond the physician's expertise.
- The patient has a musculoskeletal component and there is failure of conservative treatment.
- The treatment is in conjunction with physical therapy.

The application of OMT in the clinical arena is only limited by the skill of the physician. OMT is effective as a primary or adjunctive treatment for the following populations and conditions:

Children: feeding difficulties (such as sucking abnormalities, vomiting, and diarrhea); colic; headaches; chronic sinus and middle ear infections; certain learning disabilities (such as attention deficit hyperactivity disorder); asthma; plagiocephaly; and strabismus

Adults: migraine, tension and cluster headaches; cervicothoracic and lumbosacral strains; sciatica; herniated discs; psoasitis; sacroiliitis; pain associated with whiplash; carpal tunnel syndrome; Bell's palsy; trigeminal neuralgia; fibromyalgia; asthma; premenstrual syndrome; irritable bowel syndrome; tinnitus; vertigo; and hypertension

OMT also can assist in the recovery from otitis media, sinusitis, and upper respiratory tract infections. It may provide some relief to patients with rheumatoid arthritis and degenerative joint disease.

Athletes: tarsal tunnel syndrome; Sever's disease; achilles tendonitis; posterior tibial stress syndrome (shin splints); Osgood Schlatter's disease; patellar tendonitis; piriformis syndrome; hip pain; bursitis; iliotibial band syndrome; rotator cuff tendonitis; lateral and medial epicondylitis; wrist pain; DeQuervan's tenosynovitis; overuse injuries; spondylolisthesis; and plantar fascitis

Geriatrics: osteoarthritis; rheumatoid arthritis; chronic obstructive lung disease; spinal stenosis; bursitis; and adhesive capsulitis

Office Applications

A patient's clinical condition or disease process may have somatic dysfunction associated with it. OMT treats the somatic dysfunction with a secondary influence on the pathophysiology. If the somatic dysfunction is an integral part of the patient's pathophysiology, then OMT is usually beneficial for the patient. Certain patients respond more favorably to OMT than do other patients. The following list is a ranking of patient presentations or conditions that usually respond favorably to OMT. As with all alternative therapies, the use of OMT does not preclude the use of mainstream medical therapies in addition.

Top level: *A therapy ideally suited for these conditions*

Cervical strain and sprain; facet syndrome; hamstring strain; lumbar strain and sprain; migraine; muscle spasm; myofascial strain; myositis; piriformis syndrome; rib sprain and strain; sacral sprain; stress; tension cephalgia; and thoracic sprain and strain

Second level: *One of the better therapies for these conditions*

Adhesive capsulitis; anterior knee pain; asthma; carpal tunnel syndrome; epicondylitis; impingement syndrome; irritable bowel syndrome; plantar fascitis; rotator cuff tendonitis; tendonitis; thoracic outlet syndrome; temporomandibular joint syndrome; and vertigo

Third level: *A valuable adjunctive therapy for these conditions*
URI or sinusitis; anxiety; depression; fibromyalgia; osteoarthritis; spondylolisthesis; degenerative disc disease; herniated disc; Bell's palsy; hypertension; chronic obstructive lung disease; gastrointestinal disorders; pneumonia; reflex sympathetic dystrophy; dysmenorrhea; infant feeding difficulties; pregnancy and childbirth; otitis media; and premenstrual syndrome

Practical Applications

Osteopathic manipulation works for more than just back pain. Its therapeutic applications are innumerable. It is very effective for the treatment of common pediatric conditions including feeding difficulties, colic, headaches, and chronic sinus and middle ear infections. It can provide relief in adults for headaches, carpal tunnel syndrome, Bell's palsy, trigeminal neuralgia, and cervical and lumbar strain and sprain. It can augment the rate of recovery from athletic injuries. In the geriatric population it may be used to improve functional capacity in osteoarthritis, improve symptoms in chronic obstructive lung disease, and improve symptoms in fibromyalgia. Its application is only limited by the skill of the physician.

Research Base

Evidence Based

Osteopathic manipulative treatment has been studied for many clinical problems. Larson describes how decreasing sympathetic tone through manipulation is used clinically in upper extremity complaints.[2] Somatic dysfunction of the upper thoracic spine with facilitation of the sympathetics is described as a mediator of paresthesia to the upper extremity.

In the hypertensive patient, OMT has been postulated to lower blood pressure by effecting neurogenic, humoral, and vascular factors. OMT is believed to break the cycle of increasingly frequent episodes of sympathicotonia and delay the stage of fixed hypertension.[3] Serum aldosterone levels have been shown to decrease 36 hours postOMT.[4] In a study of 100 hypertensive patients treated with OMT only, there was an average drop in pressure of 33 mmHg systolic (199 to 166 mmHg) and 9 mmHg diastolic (123 to 114 mmHg).[5]

Clinical studies on the beneficial effects of spinal manipulation and back pain are numerous and beyond the scope of this discussion. In the treatment of acute low back pain a joint commission by the U.S. Department of Health and Human Services reviewed randomized controlled trials focusing on patient-oriented clinical outcome measures by osteopathic, allopathic, and chiropractic physicians. They jointly supported spinal manipulation as an efficacious treatment for acute low back pain. Following these recommendations, federal guidelines endorse OMT for acute low back pain.[6]

Osteopathic treatment has been reported to decrease the symptoms and duration of the common cold and prevent complications and recurrence.[7] Research using rhinomanometry has shown that following OMT there is a reduction in the amount of work required by the nose during breathing.[8] Many patients report draining of the sinuses following manipulative techniques specifically addressing somatic dysfunction of the cranium.[9]

Basic Science

A tenet of the osteopathic profession is that palpable changes in the musculoskeletal system may signify or induce altered function in related visceral or somatic structures. Since the early 1940s researchers have observed that visceral stimulation results in localized responses in paravertebral musculature. A correlation between these palpable areas and related viscera has been reviewed by Beal.[10] Areas of the axial skeleton and soft tissues of the body that contain somatic dysfunction produce aberrant neural input from receptors to the segmental spinal cord. Inappropriate neural inputs result in segmental areas of the spinal cord undergoing facilitation and habituation.[11,12] The sympathetic neurons are in close proximity to somatic afferents and also undergo facilitation. Sustained sympathetic activity to muscle spindles alters the sensitivity of the spindle to a given stretch. This produces increases in muscle tension and responsiveness to stimuli.[13,14]

The facilitated segment is the physiologic cornerstone of somatic dysfunction. In *segmental facilitation* a spinal segment receives exaggerated input from somatic or visceral structures. Facilitation is the maintenance of a pool of neurons in a state of partial or subthreshold excitation. The neurons are basically in a state of hyperexcitability. Facilitation may be the result of a sustained increase in afferent input, aberrant patterns of afferent input, or changes within the effected neurons themselves or their environment. Facilitation involves the general somatic nerves as well as the autonomics. A condition of sustained and exaggerated neuronal activity occurs even under normal conditions of daily life. Both skeletal and visceral organs innervated by the facilitated segment can be influenced by neural overactivity.[15,16] Motor neuron pools in spinal cord segments related to areas of somatic dysfunction are maintained in a state of facilitation. Local sympathetic hyperactivity exaggerates the spindle's response to changes in length.[13,14] Muscles innervated by these segments are kept in a hypertonic state with subsequent impediment to spinal motion. Korr attributes this aberrant spindle discharge to a heightened level of gain from the gamma motor neurons. Etiologic factors that may contribute to this gamma-driven intrafusal fiber contraction are cerebral, emotional, and mechanical in origin, all involving some aspect of the autonomic nervous system.[16] Once facilitated, neural input to the segmental spinal cord may become fixated and learned.[11] Chronic facilitation and motion restrictions have structural and functional implications. Facilitation of the sympathetic neurons has been implicated as an etiologic factor in many disease states.[16] Effective treatment centers around creating a balance between sympathetic and parasympathetic tone.

Muscular activity, which functions through the stretch reflex, may be effected by sympathetic influences. This viscious cycle between inappropriate mechanoreceptor reporting and exaggerated response can maintain an inappropriate spinal reflex. Manipulative therapy applied to somatic areas involved in this response is thought to reset the spindle's gain, thereby reducing myofascial and arthrodial restrictions and restoring the tissue's motion and function. When restrictions of motion become chronic, muscle imbalance and substitution may ensue, producing faulty movement patterns and pain syndromes. Osteopathic treatment to spinal areas of somatic dysfunction decreases local tenderness and irritability of the tissues and improves motion restrictions.

Risk and Safety

Most adverse reactions from manipulative treatment are associated with high velocity-low amplitude thrust treatment. These are rare, and manipulation has a high degree of safety.[17] The most serious complication is the development of vertebral artery thrombosis following upper cervical manipulation. Juri Dvorak conducted a study in Switzerland and reported the incidence to be 1 in 400,000 manipulations (Personal communication with Dr. Kappler). H. D. Wolff, past president of the German Manual Medicine Society, conducted an investigation of 25 "accidents" in Germany. The manipulators involved the entire spectrum of practitioners. This study found that in all 25 cases, at least one of two errors of management existed: 1) a diagnosis of blockage (motion restriction) was not made; or 2) forces were not localized at the restriction and a general sweeping force was used instead (Personal communication with Dr. Kappler). Vick published a review of the literature from 1925 to 1993 citing 115 injuries in the U.S. relating to manipulation from a spectrum of practitioners.[17] Terrett listed 78 cerebrovascular manipulative injuries reported in the English language literature. Of these 78 cases, 8 were attributable to osteopaths.[18] Osteopathic physicians are aware of this rare possibility and usually chose alternative techniques if they feel that the patient is at risk for an adverse outcome.

Most studies in the literature deal with thrust manipulation irrespective of the type of practitioner. Patients with compromised skeletal structures (such as osteoporosis or metastatic malignancy) can sustain a pathologic fracture if excess force is used. Osteopathic physicians are able to diagnose these problems and treat the patient accordingly.

Other forms of osteopathic manipulative technique such as muscle energy (in which the patient controls the force), counterstrain, and indirect, are highly unlikely to produce an iatrogenic effect. In fact, Vick reports that no cases of injury were reported using muscle energy, indirect, or fascial techniques.[17] The patient may become sore after a very gentle treatment, but as the soreness resolves the patient is usually much improved.

Efficacy

It is virtually impossible to specify efficacy for specific diagnoses. Osteopathic physicians treat patients, not diagnoses. When musculoskeletal dysfunction contributes to patient problems, osteopathic manipulative treatment usually helps. If musculoskeletal dysfunction is unrelated to the patient's problem, manipulation is less effective. Generally musculoskeletal complaints respond to manipulative treatment. Inflammatory, degenerative, and traumatic changes to musculoskeletal tissues may have some temporary improvement, but the basic underlying pathology remains. For example, a hip joint with degenerative joint disease may exhibit some temporary improvement with manipulation, but the degenerative joint disease remains.

Future Research Opportunities and Priorities

Musculoskeletal complaints comprise a significant percentage of family physician office visits and place huge financial burdens on the nation's economy. Delineating the pathophysiology of these complaints is important for further research and more effective treatment. The researcher of as an independent variable must decide if a technique is to be evaluated, if OMT is to be tested, or if osteopathic health care is to be the subject of the study.

Self-Help versus Professional

Osteopathic manipulation must be applied by an osteopathic physician or similarly trained health care professional. Self-help might be in the form of specific exercises that help maintain freedom of motion and promote muscular strength, joint stability, and proprioception.

Visiting a Professional

The patient is asked a detailed history and a physical exam is performed. A musculoskeletal evaluation is also performed and, if clinically indicated, OMT is performed. The musculoskeletal evaluation involves palpation and motion testing to evaluate how well the joints and various tissues move. The manipulative treatment experience depends largely on the type of manipulative technique applied. High velocity-low amplitude thrust techniques usually produce a pop or click in the joint, and is usually the most vigorous form of treatment. Other forms of treatment involve small movements and gentle positioning. With this type of gentle approach the patient may wonder if the physician is actually performing a treatment. Once patients become accustomed to quality manipulative treatment, they appreciate the relief from symptoms and the increased freedom of motion.

Credentialing

Osteopathic physicians are licensed as physicians and surgeons in all 50 states. Osteopathic physicians may become board-certified in a number of specialties, including osteopathic family practice and osteopathic manipulative medicine.

Training

Osteopathic physicians are complete physicians and are licensed to practice all areas of medicine and surgery. To become an osteopathic physician, an individual must be a graduate of an osteopathic medical school. Each school is accredited by the Bureau of Professional Education of the AOA. Accreditation is recognized by the U.S. Department of Education and the council on postsecondary education. Applicants typically have a 4-year undergraduate degree and are required to take the Medical College Admissions Test (MCAT). The curriculum includes 4 years of academic study emphasizing basic science, clinical decision making, and additional training in osteopathic manipulative medicine. Osteopathic physicians must pass national board examinations to obtain state licenses. Most DOs complete a 1-year general rotating internship, which provides a foundation in primary care. Following this, DOs undertake a residency lasting 2 to 6 years in their particular field of interest. Board certification in the chosen area of specialty is gained through examination. Osteopathic physicians may complete postdoctoral training in any specialty; however, many osteopathic physicians choose primary care (family medicine, pediatrics, internal medicine) as a avenue to care for the entire individual. Most DOs hold hospital staff privileges.

What to Look for in a Provider

Unfortunately, many osteopathic physicians have reduced the application of osteopathic principles in their practice. The application of osteopathic principles will make the physician more effective regardless of specialty. Look for a physician that integrates osteopathic principles into the practice regardless of specialty. Word of mouth (person to person referral) is the best source of information. Find an osteopathic physician who has a reputation within the community of therapeutic effectiveness.

Barriers and Key Issues

The development of high level skills in using requires considerable time and practice. Some physicians are unwilling to make the investment of time and effort. The medical physician community is showing increasing interest in osteopathic manipulative techniques. This is especially true of those MDs who treat musculoskeletal problems and injuries. The Federation International of Manual Medicine (FIMM) is an international organization composed mostly of allopathic physicians (MD) who use manual medicine, a synonym for manipulative treatment. The American Academy of Orthopedic Medicine is the North American affiliate of FIMM.

Associations

American Osteopathic Association (AOA)
142 East Ontario St.
Chicago, IL 60611
Tel: (312) 202-8000
Toll-Free: (800) 621-1773, ext. 8252
www.am-osteo-assn.org

American Academy of Osteopathy (AAO)
3500 DePauw Blvd. Suite 1080
Indianapolis, IN 46268
Tel: (317) 879-1881
www.aao.medguide.net

American College of Osteopathic Family Physicians
330 East Algonquin Rd. Suite One
Arlington Heights, IL 60005
Tel: (847) 952-5100
Toll-Free: (800) 323-0794
www.acofp.org

The Cranial Academy
8202 Clearvista Pkwy., Bldg.#9, Suite D
Indianapolis, IN 46256
Tel: (317) 594-0411
www.CranAcad@aol.com

National Osteopathic Foundation
5773 Peachtree-Dunwoody Drive Suite 500-6
Atlanta, GA 30342
Tel: (404) 705-9999

Suggested Reading

1. Ward RC, editor: *Foundations for osteopathic medicine*, Baltimore, 1997, Williams & Wilkins.
   This is the standard textbook used in osteopathic medical schools throughout the U.S. It includes an in-depth discussion of osteopathic philosophy, history, basic sciences, and application to various clinical specialties. An extensive section on palpatory diagnosis and manipulative treatment is included.
2. Kuchera M, Kuchera W: *Osteopathic considerations in systemic dysfunction*, Kirksville, Mo, 1991, KCOM Press.
   This textbook summarizes the clinical application of osteopathic manipulative medicine in disorders of the HEENT, cardiovascular, pulmonary, gastrointestinal and genitourinary systems. A section on rheumatologic disorders is included.
3. Frymann V: *The collected papers of Viola M. Frymann, DO: legacy of osteopathy to children*, Ann Arbor, Mich, 1998, Edward Brothers.
   This series of collected papers summarizes the lifework of Viola M. Frymann, DO. It is especially applicable to the osteopathic treatment of children. The integration of osteopathy in the cranial field into the total treatment protocol is emphasized.
4. Greenman P: *Principles of manual medicine*, ed 2, Baltimore, 1996, Williams & Wilkins.
   This textbook summarizes osteopathic diagnosis, treatment techniques, and therapeutic exercise principles and prescription. The section on exercise is especially applicable in the rehabilitation of patients.

References

1. Ward RB, editor: *Foundations for osteopathic medicine*, Baltimore, 1997, Williams & Wilkins.
2. Larson NJ: Osteopathic manipulation for syndromes of the brachial plexus, *JAOA* 72:378-384, 1972.

3. Kuchera M, Kuchera W: *Osteopathic considerations in systemic dysfunction*, Kirksville, Mo, 1991, KCOM Press.

4. Mannino JR: The application of neurologic reflexes to the treatment of hypertension, JAOA 79:225-231, 1979.

5. Northup TL: Manipulative management of hypertension, JAOA 60:973-978, 1961.

6. Bigos SJ et al: *Acute low back problems in adults: assessment and treatment*, Rockville, Md, US Dept Health and Human Services, Public Health Service, Agency For Health Care Policy and Research, pub no. 95-0643, Dec. 1994.

7. Schmidt IC: As a primary factor in the management of upper, middle, and pararespiratory infections, JAOA 81:382-388, 1982.

8. Kaluza SM: The physiologic response of the nose to osteopathic manipulative treatment: preliminary report, JAOA 82:654-660, 1983.

9. Magoun HI: *Osteopathy in the cranial field*, ed 3, Kirksville, Mo, 1976, Journal Printing Co.

10. Beal MC: Viscerosomatic reflexes: a review, JAOA 85(12):786-801, 1983.

11. Patterson MM: A model mechanism for spinal segmental facilitation, JAOA 76:4-14, 1976.

12. Patterson MM: The spinal cord: active processor not passive transmitter, lecture, Louisa Burns Memorial, 1980.

13. Passatore M, Filippi GM, Grassi C: Cervical sympathetic nerve stimulation can induce an intrafusal muscle fiber contraction in the rabbit. In Boyd IA, Gladden MH, editors: *The muscle spindle*, London, 1985, Macmillan.

14. Passatore M, Grassi C, Flippi GM: Sympathetically-induced development of tension in jaw muscles: the possible contraction of intrafusal muscle fibers, *Pflugers Arch* 405:297-304, 1985.

15. Korr IM: Somatic dysfunction, osteopathic treatment and the nervous system: a few facts, some theories, many questions, JAOA 86(2):109-114, 1986.

16. Korr IM: Sustained sympathicotonia as a factor in disease. In Kiny N, editor: *The collected papers of Irvin M. Korr*, Indianapolis, 1997, American Academy of Osteopathy.

17. Vick DA: The safety of manipulative treatment: review of the literature from 1925 to 1993, JAOA 96(2):113-115, 1996.

18. Terrett AGJ: Misuse of the literature by medical authors in discussing spinal manipulative therapy injury, JMPT 18(4):203-210, 1995.

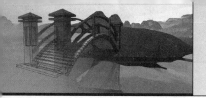

Massage Therapy

ELLIOT GREENE

Origins and History

Massage therapy is one of the oldest health care practices in existence. References to massage are found in Chinese medical texts that are more than 4000 years old. Massage has been advocated in Western health care practices since the time of Hippocrates, the "father of medicine." In the fourth century BCE Hippocrates wrote, "The physician must be acquainted with many things and assuredly with rubbing" (the ancient Greek term for massage was rubbing).

The roots of modern, scientific massage therapy go back to Per Henrik Ling (1776-1839). Ling was a Swede who developed an integrated system consisting of massage and exercises, a system that was both passive and active. He then established the Royal Central Gymnastic Institute in 1813 with the support and funding of the Swedish government to teach his methods to the public. *Medical gymnastics* and *Swedish movement cure* were the terms used then for Ling's methods, which later were termed *Swedish massage*.

Modern, scientific massage therapy was introduced in the United States in the 1850s by two New York physicians, brothers George and Charles Taylor, who had studied in Sweden. The first U.S. massage therapy clinics were opened by two Swedish physicians after the Civil War period. Baron Nils Posse ran the Posse Institute in Boston and Hartwig Nissen opened the Swedish Health Institute near the Capitol in Washington, D.C. In the period between 1880 and 1910, a considerable number of American physicians used massage in their practices.

As the health care system in the U.S. became influenced by new biomedicine and technologies in the early 1900s, and as physicians changed the way that they practiced, physicians began assigning time-intensive massage duties to assistants and nurses. In turn, by the 1930s and 1940s nurses and emergent physical therapists lost interest in massage therapy, virtually abandoning it in favor of "higher tech" equipment. However, a very small number of massage therapists carried on until the 1970s, when a new surge of interest in massage, an interest that continues to this day, revitalized the field, albeit in the realm of complementary and alternative medicine.

Mechanism of Action According to Its Own Theory

Massage therapy is the scientific manipulation of the soft tissues of the body for the purpose of normalizing those tissues and consists of manual techniques that include applying moving or fixed pressure and movement of the body. These techniques affect all body systems, in particular the musculoskeletal, circulatory-lymphatic, and nervous systems. The basic philosophy of massage therapy encompasses the concept of *vis medicatrix naturae*, aiding the ability of the body to heal itself and aimed at achieving or increasing health and well-being.

Touch is the fundamental medium of massage therapy. Although massage methods can be described in terms of techniques performed, touch is not used solely in a mechanistic way in massage therapy. Both scientific and artistic components are considered essential to effective practice of massage therapy. Because massage usually involves applying touch with some degree of pressure the massage therapist must use touch with sensitivity to determine the optimal amount of pressure to use for each person. Touch with sensitivity also allows perception of useful information about the body, such as locating areas of muscle tension and other soft tissue problems. Because touch is also a form of communication, sensitive touch can convey a sense of caring, an essential element in the therapeutic relationship, to the person receiving massage. Using the wrong kind of touch, sometimes thought of as "toxic touch," is counterproductive, renders a technique ineffective, and causes the body to defend or guard itself, introducing greater tension.

Biologic Mechanism of Action

The mechanism of action may differ depending on which technique or method is considered. Generally, massage is known to affect the circulation of blood and flow of blood and lymph, reduce muscular tension or flaccidity, affect the nervous system through stimulation or sedation, and enhance tissue healing.

Forms of Therapy

There are a fairly large number of different methods (about 100) that may be classified under massage therapy. Most of them (about 75%) are less than 20 years old. There are several reasons why this is so.

The period of the 1940s to the mid-1970s was a relatively dormant one for the massage therapy profession. Little standardization was established within the field. Then in the 1970s, changes in society, such as greater interest in fitness, healthier lifestyles, personal improvement, and alternatives methods of health care to complement biomedicine, stimulated a boom of renewed interest in massage therapy. An influx of new practitioners brought a wave of new ideas and creativity regarding ways to use "hands-on" techniques along with established ones. Because there was little standardization, these techniques sometimes developed into freestanding methods rather than being incorporated into an existing classification system. The many forms of massage native to most cultures around the world were another source of new techniques.

This proliferation of methods has slowed. It is expected, as has happened in the development of other professions, that there will be some consolidation and integration of these methods as the development of standards and credentials continues.

Descriptions of forms of massage therapy that are the most widely used or representative follow. In practice, many massage therapists use more than one technique or method in their work and sometimes combine several. Effective massage therapists ascertain each person's needs and then use the techniques that will meet those needs best.

Swedish massage uses a system of long gliding strokes, kneading, and friction techniques on the more superficial layers of muscles, generally in the direction of blood flow toward the heart and sometimes combined with active and passive movements of the joints. It is used to promote general relaxation, improve circulation and range of motion, and relieve muscle tension. Swedish massage is the most commonly used form of massage.

Deep tissue massage is used to release chronic patterns of muscular tension using slow strokes, direct pressure, or friction directed across the grain of the muscles. It is applied with greater pressure and to deeper layers of muscle than Swedish massage, which is why it is called deep tissue and is effective for chronic muscular tension.

Sports massage uses techniques that are similar to Swedish and deep tissue massages but are specially adapted to deal with the effects of athletic performance on the body and the needs of athletes regarding training, performing, and recovery from injury.

Neuromuscular massage is a form of deep massage that is applied to individual muscles. It is used primarily to release trigger points (intense knots of muscle tension that refer pain to other parts of the body) and also to increase blood flow. It often is used to reduce pain. Trigger point massage and myotherapy are similar forms.

Acupressure applies finger or thumb pressure to specific points located on the acupuncture meridians (channels of energy flow identified in Asian concepts of anatomy) to release blocked energy along these meridians that causes physical discomforts and rebalance the energy flow.

Shiatsu is a Japanese form of acupressure.

Manual lymph drainage improves the flow of lymph using light, rhythmic strokes. It is primarily used for conditions related to poor lymph flow, such as edema, inflammation, and neuropathies.

CranioSacral is a method for finding and correcting cranial and spinal imbalances or blockages that may cause sensory, motor, or intellectual dysfunction. There are two major approaches. Cranial osteopathy involves the manipulation of the bones and tissues of the cranium and spine. CranioSacral therapy is soft-tissue, fluid, and membrane-oriented and treats the head, spine, and sacrum as one continuous membranous sheath.

Zero balancing uses gentle pressure at key areas of the skeleton to balance the energy body with the structural body. This is based on a theory that an unseen energy body surrounds the physical body and when an injury or trauma occurs both bodies need to be healed.

The corresponding box shows a concept for organizing massage and bodywork methods into five groups. It also should be noted that there is a lack of a consensus about which methods should be included under massage therapy. Some of these methods have been categorized as bodywork, some as somatics, and some as somatic education.

FIVE CATEGORIES OF MASSAGE THERAPY AND BODYWORK

1. **Traditional European:** Methods based on traditional Western concepts of anatomy and physiology, using five basic categories of soft tissue manipulation: effleurage (gliding strokes); petrissage (kneading); friction (rubbing); tapotement (percussion); and vibration. Swedish massage is the main example.

2. **Contemporary Western:** Methods based on modern Western concepts of human functioning, using a wide variety of manipulative techniques. These may include broad applications for personal growth and balance of the mind, body, and spirit, in addition to traditional applications. These methods go beyond the original framework of Swedish massage and include Neuromuscular Massage, Sports Massage, Deep Tissue, Myofascial Release, Myotherapy, Bindegewebsmassage, Esalen, and Manual Lymph Drainage.

3. **Structural, Functional, and Movement Integration:** Methods that organize and integrate the body in relationship to gravity through manipulating the soft tissues and correcting inappropriate patterns of movement, as well as methods that bring about a more balanced use of the nervous system through creating new, integrated possibilities of movement. Examples are Rolfing, Hellerwork, Aston-Patterning, Trager, Feldenkrais, and Alexander.

4. **Oriental:** Methods of treatment using pressure and manipulation based on traditional Chinese and Asian medical principles for assessing, evaluating, and treating the energetic system to affect and balance the energetic system. Examples are Acupressure, Shiatsu, Tuina, AMMA Therapy, and Jin Shin Do.

5. **Energetic:** Methods affecting the biofield that surrounds and infuses the human body, by pressure and manipulation of the physical body or the passage or placement of the hands in or through that energetic field. These methods are based on Traditional Ayurvedic, Eastern or Western Esoteric, modern therapeutic, or other systems of healing. Examples are Polarity Therapy and Therapeutic Touch.

Demographics

The number of massage therapists in the U.S. can only be estimated, as no formal census has been taken. An estimate is affected by variables such as extent of training, full-time versus part-time work, and whether an individual uses methods considered to be forms of massage therapy. Consequently it is prudently estimated there are about 125,000 qualified massage therapists in the U.S., providing about 80,000,000 massage sessions (mostly 1 hour) per year. The number of massage therapists is increasing rapidly, with a corresponding increase in use by the American public. This forecast is supported by the Eisenberg study,[1] which found that, along with increased use of alternative medicine, use of massage increased 62% from 1990 to 1997.

Indications and Reasons for Referral

Massage is quite versatile. Its uses range from general relaxation, stress reduction, sports and fitness activities, health promotion, and first aid to treating specific maladies. From a wellness point of view, massage therapy can be part of a general plan to promote health and fitness. A simple ranking of conditions responsive to this form of treatment is as follows. As with all alternative therapies, use of massage therapy does not preclude the use of mainstream medical therapies in addition.

Top level: *A therapy ideally suited for these conditions*
Lymphedema (lymphatic massage) and stress

Second level: *One of the better therapies for these conditions*
Anxiety; back pain; colic; colitis and Crohn's disease; fibromyalgia; headaches (especially tension headaches); insomnia; irritable bowel syndrome; menstrual cramps; osteoarthritis; repetitive stress disorders; sprains (first and second degree); and strains (first and second degree)

Third level: *A valuable adjunctive therapy for these conditions*
AIDS; restless leg syndrome; arthritis; asthma; bronchitis; childbirth (recovery from); children's health; chronic fatigue syndrome; chronic pain; constipation; diabetes (if not contraindicated); diarrhea; diverticulosis and diverticulitis; female health; gastritis; gastrointestinal disorders; hypertension (if not contraindicated); male health; menorrhagia; mental health; postpartum care; pregnancy (if not contraindicated); pregnancy and childbirth (if not contraindicated); premenstrual syndrome; respiratory conditions; rheumatoid arthritis (if not locally contraindicated); sinusitis; sleep disorders; stomachache; and temporomandibular joint syndrome

Practical Applications

A physician has several options for integrating massage into the clinical setting: employ a massage therapist to work in the office, rent space within the office to a massage therapist, provide space and services for a massage therapist as an independent contractor, or refer to a massage therapist.

Research Base

From 1873, when the term *massage* first entered the Anglo-American medical lexicon, through 1939, more than 600 journal articles appeared in the mainline journals of medicine in English alone, including the *Journal of the AMA, Archives of Surgery,* and *British Medical Journal.* Research declined in parallel with the decline of interest that massage suffered until the 1970s.

More recently the pace has picked up again. Studies have been published on the effects of massage therapy for a variety of conditions, including the following: acute and chronic pain; chronic inflammation; lymphedema; muscle spasm; various soft tissue dysfunctions; anxiety; arthritis; autism; chronic fatigue syndrome; depression; diabetes; fibromyalgia; headache; hypertension; insomnia; lower back pain; nausea; premature infants; sleep; stress; and more. A number of studies have been done in Europe, particularly the former Soviet Union and East Germany, but many of these studies have not been translated yet into English.

Evidence Based

Premature infants treated with daily massage therapy gain more weight and have shorter hospital stays than infants who are not massaged. A study of 40 low birth weight babies found that the 20 massaged babies had a 47% greater weight gain per day and stayed in the hospital an average of 6 days less than 20 infants who did not receive massage, resulting a cost savings of approximately $3,000 per infant.[2] Cocaine-exposed preterm infants given massage three times daily for a 10 day period showed significant improvement. Results indicated that massaged infants had fewer postnatal complications and exhibited fewer stress behaviors during the 10-day period, had a 28% greater daily weight gain, and demonstrated more mature motor behaviors.[3]

A study comparing 52 hospitalized children and adolescents with depression and adjustment disorder with a control group that viewed relaxation videotapes found that massage therapy subjects were less depressed and anxious and had lower saliva cortisol levels (an indicator of less depression).[4]

A combination of massage techniques for 52 subjects with traumatically induced spinal pain led to significant improvements in acute and chronic pain and increased muscle flexibility and tone. This study also found massage therapy to be extremely cost-effective, with cost savings ranging from 15% to 50%.[5,6] Massage also has been shown to stimulate the body's ability to naturally control pain by stimulating the brain to produce endorphins.[7] Fibromyalgia is an example of a condition that may be favorably affected by this effect.

Lymph drainage massage has been shown to be more effective than mechanized methods or diuretic drugs to control lymphedema secondary to radical mastectomy; consequently, using massage to control lymphedema would significantly lower treatment costs.[8] A study found that massage therapy can have a powerful effect upon psychoemotional distress in persons suffering from chronic inflammatory bowel disease. Massage therapy was effective in reducing the frequency of episodes of pain and disability in these patients.[9]

Basic Science

Massage therapy produced relaxation in 18 older adult subjects, demonstrated in measures such as decreased blood pressure and heart rate and increased skin temperature.[10]

A pilot study of five subjects with symptoms of tension and anxiety found a significant response to massage therapy in one or more psychophysiological parameters of heart rate, frontalis and forearm extensor electromyograms (EMGs), and skin resistance, which demonstrate relaxation of muscle tension and reduced anxiety.[11]

Massage may enhance the immune system. A study suggests an increase in cytotoxic capacity associated with massage.[12] A study of chronic fatigue syndrome subjects found that a group receiving massage therapy had lower depression, emotional distress, and somatic symptom scores, more hours of sleep, and lower epinephrine and cortisol levels than a control group.[13]

Future Research Opportunities and Priorities

Regarding general questions, more efficacy, outcomes, and cost-effectiveness studies of massage are needed. Outcome studies should allow massage therapists to work in a manner that approximates actual working conditions as much as possible. With a few studies indicating substantial cost savings through using massage therapy, more studies should be done. Replication studies also are needed.

Regarding specific questions, because massage therapy is especially effective with soft tissue problems, it would be useful to study the effects of massage on muscle strains, sprains, tendinitis, problems related to acute and chronic muscle tension, and the tissue healing process. Because research evidence attributes a major percentage of health problems to stress and stress reduction is a powerful means to prevent or treat such stress-induced problems, studying the stress-reduction effects of massage therapy would be valuable.

Druglike Information

Warnings, Contraindications, and Precautions

Massage is comparatively safe. However, it is generally contraindicated for advanced heart diseases, phlebitis, thrombosis, embolism, kidney failure, cancer (if massage would accelerate metastasis or damage tissue that is fragile due to chemotherapy or other treatment), infectious diseases, contagious skin conditions, acute inflammation, infected injuries, unhealed fractures, conditions prone to hemorrhage, and psychosis.

Massage on affected areas (locally) is contraindicated for acute flare-ups of rheumatoid arthritis, eczema, goiter, and open skin lesions.

Precautions should be taken before using massage for pregnancy, high fevers, osteoporosis, diabetes, recent postoperative cases in which pain and muscular splinting would be increased, apprehensive patients, and mental conditions that may impair communication or perception.

Visiting a Professional

If it is the patient's first visit the massage therapist usually asks some questions about the reasons for getting a massage, current physical condition, medical history, lifestyle and stress level, experiences with specific areas of pain, and whether there is any specific need to be addressed during the massage. First, the massage therapist needs to screen for contraindications. Second, the massage therapist needs to be clear about what the expectations and goals are for the session. Third, the information provided helps the massage therapist determine what techniques to use and how to structure the session.

The therapist in most cases asks patients to remove as much clothing as they are comfortable removing. The therapist either leaves the room or otherwise provides privacy while the patient disrobes. A sheet or towel is provided for draping during the massage. The therapist will uncover only the part of the body being massaged, insuring that modesty is respected at all times. The draping also keeps the person receiving the massage warm.

The massage takes place on a comfortable, padded massage table. The massage therapist tells the patient what position to lie in on the table. The table may have some extra attachments or cushions, such as a face rest, which allows the patient to lie in a face-down position without turning the head and neck.

A peaceful and comfortable environment is provided. The massage therapist may play music during the massage if the patient approves. Some people find music to be relaxing but some find it distracting.

Before the massage begins the massage therapist may offer some advice that will improve the quality of the massage. A common one is to breathe, especially if a sensitive area is being massaged. Another is to communicate with the therapist about any needs or how the massage is going.

The massage therapist may use oil or lotion, which reduces drag on the skin while performing the massage strokes. If the patient informs the therapist of an allergy to some oils or lotions the therapist will use an alternative. Some forms of massage do not use oil. Depending on the patient's needs, the massage therapist will massage either the full body or only specific areas that need attention. For example, general relaxation or stress reduction sessions usually include all major areas of the body; a session for a localized injury, pain, or tightness focuses on a specific area. It is possible to spend most of an entire session on only one area.

After the massage is finished the patient once again is provided with privacy to get dressed. The usual length of a session is 1 hour. A massage session on a table generally should be a minimum of 30 minutes and maximum of 90 minutes.

An exception to this description is a seated massage. In this case the patient sits in a specially designed massage chair. The chair supports the front of the body, which allows access to most of the body. The patient remains clothed and oil or lotion is not used. Seated massages are usually shorter sessions that typically run from 10 to 30 minutes. Since the chairs are highly portable, seated massages take place in a variety of settings, especially the workplace. In addition, the patient may remain fully clothed for craniosacral or zero-balancing techniques.

The patient should let the massage therapist know in advance if an appointment needs to be canceled. Many massage therapists require a 24 hour notice.

Credentialing

The advancement of higher standards and professional credentials has paralleled the dynamic growth of the massage therapy profession. Massage therapists are currently licensed by 29 states, the District of Columbia, and a number of localities. Most states require 500 or more classroom hours of training from a recognized training program and passing an examination.

The National Certification Board for Therapeutic Massage and Bodywork (NCBTMB) inaugurated a national certification program in June 1992. The NCBTMB exam is accredited by the National Commission for Certifying Agencies, the chief outside agency for evaluating certification programs. Those certified can use the title National Certified in Therapeutic Massage and Bodywork (NCTMB). Most states have adopted this exam for their licensing examination.

A national accreditation agency, the Commission on Massage Therapy Accreditation, which was designed according to the guidelines established by the U.S. Department of Education, currently recognizes about 70 training programs for massage therapists. The Accrediting Commission of Career Schools and Colleges of Technology and the Accrediting Council for Continuing Education and Training also accredit massage training programs.

Training

The standard used in most licensing laws and generally accepted as a minimal level is 500 hours of classroom training. Training should include anatomy, physiology, pathology, massage theory and technique, and supervised practice. Although some states require continuing education, most massage therapists regularly take additional courses and workshops during their careers.

What to Look for in a Provider

Look for the following credentials for massage therapists:

1. State license if available (29 states and DC). Some localities may license massage therapists.
2. National certification by the National Certification Board for Therapeutic Massage and Bodywork (NCBTMB)
3. Certificate of graduation from a training program with a minimum of 500 hours of classroom training. An accredited program is desirable.
4. Membership in a recognized nonprofit professional association, such as the American Massage Therapy Association

An effective massage therapist also should have good communications skills and empathy.

Barriers and Key Issues

A key research related issue is the need for collaboration between researchers and massage therapists. Researchers would benefit by knowing more about interesting and promising possibilities for research, resources available from the massage therapy profession, and massage itself.

Researchers also need to work more closely with massage therapists while designing a study. Some studies have used massage in an inappropriate or ineffective manner. For example, a common error is to use massage sessions that are too brief in duration. Another is using undertrained individuals, which negatively affects results. Properly qualified massage therapists should be used for studies. Finally, the relative low level of funding for massage-related research also forms a barrier.

Regulations are another barrier. States and localities that do not effectively regulate massage therapy as a health care practice often unreasonably restrict the ability of massage therapists to practice with a highly structured web of health care regulations. Regulations that do not "make a place" for massage therapists only serve to deny the public access to massage therapy rather than protect the public or benefit the public's health.

Associations

The largest (more than 36,000 members) nonprofit association for massage therapists is the AMTA:

American Massage Therapy Association
820 Davis St., Suite 100
Evanston, IL 60201
Tel: (847) 864-0123
www.amtamassage.org

The AMTA has a Locator Service that can provide the names of qualified massage therapists. There are a number of much smaller associations devoted to specific methods. A few for-profit, privately owned trade organizations also exist; however, they mostly concentrate on marketing various services.

Suggested Reading

1. Beck MF: *Milady's theory and practice of therapeutic massage*, Albany, NY, 1994, Milady Publishing.
   Many massage schools use this as a text. It contains comprehensive information, including the growth and standardization currently taking place in the massage profession.
2. Loving JE: *Massage therapy: theory and practice*, New York, 1998, Appleton & Lange.
   This text presents the principles and techniques of massage and emphasizes the implementation of therapeutic skills to practice.

References

1. Eisenberg et al: Trends in alternative medicine use in the United States, 1990-1997, *JAMA* 280:1569-1575, 1998.

2. Field T et al: Tactile/kinesthetic stimulation effects on preterm neonates, *Pediatrics* 77(5):654-658, 1986.

3. Scafidi F et al: Cocaine exposed preterm neonates show behavioral and hormonal differences, *Pediatrics* 97(6):851-855, 1996.

4. Field T et al: Massage reduces anxiety in child and adolescent psychiatric patients, *J Am Acad Child Adolesc Psychiatry* 31(1):125-131, 1982.

5. Weintraub M: Shiatsu, Swedish muscle massage, and trigger point suppression in spinal pain syndrome, *Am Massage Ther J* 31(3):99-109, 1992.

6. Weintraub M: Alternative medical care: shiatsu, Swedish muscle massage, and trigger point suppression in spinal pain syndrome, *Am J Pain Mgmt* 2(2):74-78, 1992.

7. Kaarda B, Tosteinbo O: Increase of plasma beta-endorphins in connective tissue massage, *Gen Pharmacol* 20(4):487-489, 1989.

8. Zanolla R, Mizeglio C, Balzarini A: Evaluation of the results of three different methods of postmastectomy lymphedema treatment, *J Surg Oncol* 26:210-213, 1984.

9. Joachim G: The effects of two stress management techniques on feelings of well-being in patients with inflammatory bowel disease, *Nurs Papers* 15(4):5-18, 1983.

10. Fakouri C, Jones P: Relaxation Rx. Slow stroke back rub, *J Gerontol Nurs* 13(2):32-35, 1987.

11. McKechnie A et al: Anxiety states: a preliminary report on the value of connective tissue massage, *J Psychosom Res* 27(2)125-129, 1983.

12. Ironson G et al: Massage therapy is associated with enhancement of the immune system's cytotoxic capacity, *Int J Neurosci* 84(1-4):205-217, 1996.

13. Field T et al: Chronic fatigue syndrome: massage therapy effects on depression and somatic symptoms in chronic fatigue syndrome, *J Chron Fatigue Syndr* 3:43-51, 1997.

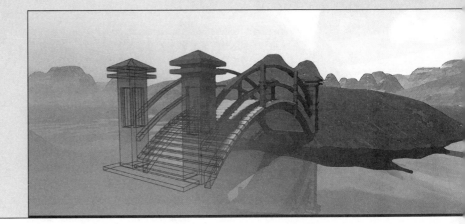

Bodywork

Alexander Technique, 350

Aston-Pattering®, 359

Bowen Technique, 371

CranioSacral Therapy, 381

Feldenkrais Method®, 393

Hellerwork Structural Integration, 407

Bonnie Audden Myotherapy, 417

Polarity Therapy, 423

Reiki, 435

Rolfing® Structural Integration, 444

Rosen Method, 453

Therapeutic Touch, 462

Trager® Approach, 472

Exploring the Concept of Energy in Touch-
   Based Healing, 483

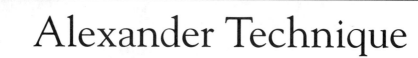

Alexander Technique

JUDITH C. STERN

"Change involves carrying out an activity against the habits of a lifetime."
F.M. Alexander

Origins and History

The Alexander Technique was developed a century ago by F.M. Alexander (1869-1955), an Australian actor who lost his voice while reciting Shakespeare. Through self-observation he noted his postural habit of "pulling his head back and down" while speaking and concluded that this "misuse" was the cause of his vocal problem. By correcting the relationship of the head, neck, and spine in activity, he solved his vocal problems. The medical community was intrigued by his discovery and encouraged Alexander to take his technique to London where doctors and scientists in the *Lancet* (1937) and the *British Medical Journal* testified to the efficacy of the Alexander Technique. In the 1930s he began training teachers to carry on his work, and the principles are still taught today throughout the world.

The Alexander Technique is a process of psychophysical reeducation that engages the mind and the body. Application of the technique improves postural balance and coordination and enhances mental alertness. In contrast to traditional medical approaches the Alexander Technique addresses the person as a "whole." It teaches the integration of the mind and the body, allowing the individual to become more aware of his internal and external worlds and therefore to be more present. This process develops an individual's ability to carry out life's activities with minimal strain and maximum ease and coordination. This state of optimal functioning increases mobility, decreases musculoskeletal pain, and improves health.

Mechanism of Action According to Its Own Theory

The theoretic principles of the Alexander Technique state that: 1) use affects function; 2) an organism functions as a whole; and 3) the relationship of the head, neck, and spine has a primary and crucial influence on an organism's ability to function as a whole.

F.M. Alexander observed that human movement is most fluid when the head leads and the spine follows. The operational concepts that developed from this observation are called *primary control, awareness, inhibition,* and *direction.* The experience of primary control involves the head leading and the spine following, thereby developing a new understanding of balance and ease in activity. To acquire this new experience as a skill and eventually as a habit the student takes lessons repeating the new experience under the hands-on direction of an Alexander Teacher. Repetition creates new motor pathways, new musculoskeletal patterns of behavior and the student learns to elicit new motor patterns independently. A student's proprioception and upright posture is improved. General coordination and balance are enhanced. The experience is one of greater energy and ease in activity.

Operational Definitions

Primary control is the inherent, balanced relationship between the head-neck-spine that comes first in every movement. This sequence determines the quality of human movement. When the head leads and the spine follows, movement is balanced, coordinated, and at ease.

Awareness means an increased and more subtle proprioceptive sense that allows an individual to notice postural habits that interfere with balance and poise. This is a moment-to-moment awareness integrated into daily life.

Inhibition is the practice of consciously pausing before acting, which allows time for releasing unnecessary habitual tension. It is a decision to respond mindfully and allow the right (expansive) direction to lead the activity.

Directions allow the neck to release; allow the head to release forward and up; allow the torso to lengthen and widen; allow the legs to release away from the torso; allow the shoulders to release away from the torso. After the inhibitory pause, the head and spine lengthen and widen into activity. Directions are conscious suggestions that encourage the natural poise of upright posture.

Biologic Mechanism of Action

The biologic mechanism that best explains Alexander's principles is the theory that the mind modulates the physiology of the autonomic nervous system. This theory has been researched by such scientists as Hans Selye, Herbert Benson, and Frank Pierce Jones. Selye defined the "stress-reaction" and observed the dynamic changes in the autonomic nervous system (ANS) when the "fight or flight" response was elicited. Increased blood pressure, heart rate, and digestion, rapid firing of the central nervous system, and increased mental alertness were the result of the stressful stimulus.[1] Benson studied the ANS using meditation skills and discovered the mind's ability to elicit the "relaxation-response" that lowers blood pressure, heart rate, and respiratory rate.[2] Jones studied the Alexander Technique specifically and validated the concept that the mind can modulate human movement using *Inhibition*. His studies demonstrated more efficient movement from sitting to standing position when using *Primary Control*.[3] The biology of the A.T. is the mind's ability to consciously change harmful, habitual physiologic reactions.

Demographics

There are 2000 Alexander Teachers worldwide and 1000 teachers in training programs. The United States has approximately 700 trained teachers located in 50 states and clustered in major cities. Alexander Technique teachers traditionally have come from the performing arts, dance, theatre, and music. More recently they come from the medical world, physical and occupational therapy, and massage.

People of all ages, genders, and professions will find the Alexander Technique beneficial. The Technique improves posture and coordination, relieves tension and pain, and alleviates persistent fatigue. It optimizes function in any activity at any level. The Alexander Technique is most frequently used by the following groups: performing artists; athletes; body workers; computer users; public speakers; pregnant women; fitness enthusiasts; dentists; psychotherapists; and architects.

Indications and Reasons for Referral

The Alexander Technique produces significant benefits as a primary approach to self-care. A course of lessons gives the student a new index of postural awareness. This allows the student to effectively modulate muscular responses to pain. Muscle tension diminishes and is often eliminated, flexibility and strength improve, endurance improves, and respiratory function is enhanced. These benefits are clear indications for referral for the following conditions:

1. The stress response: This is a "fight or flight" reaction marked by a tight neck and a contracted body. The Alexander Technique is a process that releases muscle tension and restores the organisms natural balance and coordination.
2. Chronic pain: The Technique can relieve the psychologic states of depression and anxiety that often accompany chronic pain disorder.
3. Back pain: The Technique is particularly effective for spinal dysfunction because of its emphasis on spinal decompression and rebalancing the musculature of the torso.
4. Osteoarthritis: The decompression benefits work when joint compression and deterioration are the major symptoms. Pain relief can be experienced immediately.
5. Postural problems: The Alexander Technique works effectively to restore balance and alignment in postural muscles. It is particularly effective with scoliosis and other abnormal spinal curvatures.
6. Asthma and breathing disorders: The Alexander Technique increases vital capacity and restores natural respiratory patterns to the ribcage, reeducating the diaphragm.
7. Repetitive strain injury and carpal tunnel syndrome: These diagnoses respond to the principles of the Alexander Technique because they are caused by poor postural habits.

8. Neurologic disorders: The disruption of the neurologic function often is accompanied by incoordination and balance problems that respond well to Alexander lessons.

Office Applications

A simple ranking of conditions responsive to this form of therapy is as follows. As with all alternative therapies, use of Alexander Technique does not preclude the use of mainstream medical therapies in addition.

Top level: A therapy ideally suited for these conditions

Arthritis; asthma; back pain; chronic pain; headaches; osteoarthritis; repetitive strain injury; respiratory conditions; and stress syndromes

Second level: One of the better therapies for these conditions

Chronic fatigue syndrome; emphysema; fibromyalgia; Lyme disease; multiple sclerosis; osteoporosis; postpartum syndrome; and rheumatoid arthritis

Third level: A valuable adjunctive therapy for these conditions

Scoliosis; Parkinson's disease; dystonia; stroke; brain damage; hypertension; lupus; mental health; neurologic diagnoses; pregnancy and childbirth; sleep disorders; and traumatic injury

Practical Application

The Alexander Technique is used as a rehabilitative process to address issues of pain, tension, weakness, poor coordination, and poor breathing patterns. Patients are referred for a series of lessons to address a specific problem or symptom. The skills of observation, light touch, verbal instruction, and guided movement are used to assess the problem. The student is then taught to develop an increased awareness of the postural habits that create or contribute to the symptoms. Alexander lessons strip away poor postural habits and teach new positive patterns of behavior that enhances a student's health and well-being. Symptoms are often modified or eliminated using the principles of the Alexander Technique.

Research Base

Evidence Based

The studies that confirm the effectiveness of the Alexander Technique have been published in medical and psychologic journals, as well as monographs. The most significant studies indicate that respiratory function improves in adults who studied the Alexander Technique as indicated by significant increases in all spirometry test parameters.[4]

Postural habits are profoundly affected by the Alexander Technique, specifically by learning and applying the concept of *Inhibition*, one of the basic principles of the Alexander Technique.[5]

Chronic pain sufferers that were studied and followed in England for 3 months to 1 year found the Alexander Technique the most effective treatment modality for relieving chronic pain when compared to other more traditional modalities.[6]

Performance stress can be as effectively treated with the Alexander Technique as with beta blocker medications. A study was carried out in Denmark with orchestral musicians during performance. The results of this study indicate the efficacy of the Alexander Technique in treating performance anxiety.[7]

Patients with scoliosis can significantly improve their physical appearance, strengthen their spinal musculature, and achieve their maximum spinal support by using the Alexander Technique.[8]

Risk and Safety

There are no known contraindications to the study of the Alexander Technique at this time. Students must be conscious, willing, and beyond the level of pain or injury that precludes learning.

Efficacy

Alexander Technique teachers report a high rate of efficacy in the use of the Alexander Technique when treating spinal pain, repetitive strain syndrome, asthma, and stress-related conditions. The author's experience includes 30 years as a physical therapist, practicing only the Alexander Technique for the past 14 years. Comparing the Alexander Technique to traditional physical therapy modalities, the author has found the Technique more effective for rehabilitation and health maintenance. When an individual is treated as a whole and taught a wellness skill, health is restored and maintained with greater efficacy.

Future Research Opportunities and Priorities

The Alexander community and the allopathic community would learn a great deal from long-range comparative studies done throughout the country comparing the treatment of low-back pain and asthma, as well as repetitive strain injury with the Alexander Technique and traditional medical modalities. This kind of study would objectively evaluate our clinical experience, and it could lead to a more effective integrated patient care.

Self-Help versus Professional

The Alexander Technique is an experiential learning process taught by highly skilled teachers. The skill of "good use" is acquired from expert mentors during three years of extensive, focused, hands-on training. The unique touch of an Alexander Technique teacher transmits the kinesthetic learning. An individual is able to learn best with the guidance of the supportive, trained, and nonjudgmental hands of a professional teacher.

Visiting a Professional

In an Alexander lesson the student is encouraged to wear loose, comfortable clothing that facilitates easy movement. The Alexander studio is a quiet, supportive, low-tech environment with a chair, a body work table and a mirror. Sessions are 45 to 60 minutes long and instruction is individually tailored to the student. Lesson time is used to explore the mind-body interaction. The teacher guides the Alexander process, imparting new kinesthetic awareness in both the resting state on the table and in activity, such as sitting, standing, walking, and bending. Supportive coaching develops the first Alexander concept of *Awareness*. Students observes their patterns of poor use (the pulling back and down of the head on the spine that creates unhealthy compression). The student is taught the second Alexander concept *Inhibition* (to pause after the stimulus and before the habitual response to compress). Now the student is ready to learn the third Alexander concept of the *Direction*.

With gentle hands-on skills, the student is guided into activity with the head leading and the spine following. The student experiences an expansive quality of movement that Alexander referred to as *poise*. Within the first five to 10 lessons the repeated experience of poise in activity becomes a skill that students can recreate on their own. This skill is applied to refined specialized activities. Students can bring musical instruments or even golf clubs to a lesson and apply the skills of *Awareness, Inhibition,* and *Direction* with the hands-on direction of the teacher. The Alexander Technique develops a level of skill that is based on a student's interest. Thirty lessons are recommended in order to learn the basic concepts of the Alexander Technique.

Credentialing

In the United States there are two credentialing organizations for teachers of the Alexander Technique.

The American Society for the Alexander Technique (ASAT) is the largest professional association of board-certified Alexander Technique teachers. It is affiliated internationally with similar credentialing bodies with similar training requirements and standards. It was formed in 1987, and more than 600 teachers have been trained and received ASAT certification. Teaching quality is monitored by the Training Approval Committee (TAC) and the Professional Conduct Committee.

Alexander Technique International (ATI) is an organization with nine regional offices worldwide. It acts as a membership organization and certifies teachers of the Alexander Technique. Certification is a process of sponsorship and evaluation. Training directors and senior teachers assess each individual.

Training

In the U.S. there are 18 ASAT-approved teacher training courses and five training courses affiliated with ATI.

To become a certified ASAT teacher an individual must complete 1600 hours of training over a minimum of 3 years at an ASAT-approved teacher training course. A board-certified teacher must meet the curriculum requirements of the organization's peer review panel (as previously defined) and be recommended by the training course director. There are no specific levels of training delineated by the TAC.

What to Look for in a Provider

An Alexander Technique teacher should be evaluated like all professionals. Training and certification, teaching experiences, and areas of specialty should be assessed. It is wise to take an introductory lesson before committing to a series of lessons and to speak with a student of that teacher. Both ASAT and ATI have referral networks and 800 numbers that are listed in this chapter.

Barriers and Key Issues

The barriers and issues that limit the use of the Alexander Technique by mainstream medical personnel are a lack of knowledge and experience with process, as well as fearful attitudes regarding complementary and alternative approaches to health care. Complementary modalities challenge today's health care belief systems. An expanded understanding of the mind-body connection and the approaches that address this connection are the key to opening these barriers.

Associations

The American Society for the Alexander Technique (ASAT)
3010 Hennepin Ave. South Suite 10
Minneapolis, MN 55408
Tel: (612) 824-5066
Toll-Free: (800) 473-0620
E-mail: ASAT@ix.netcom.com
www.alexandertech.com

Alexander Technique International (ATI)
USA Regional Office
1692 Massachusetts Ave.
Cambridge, MA 02138
Tel: (617) 497-2342
Fax: (617) 497-2615
E-mail: USG@ati-net.com
membership@ati.net.com

Suggested Reading

1. Caplan D: *Back trouble*, Gainesville, Fla, 1987, Triad.
   This book is an excellent paperback introduction for medical practitioners and people suffering from back pain and related medical conditions.
2. Gelb M: *Body learning*, New York, 1996, Henry Holt.
   Body Learning is an introduction to the Alexander Technique and includes beautiful photographs and a final chapter that addresses the most commonly asked questions about the Alexander Technique. This author strongly recommends this book as a wonderful introduction to philosophy and principles.
3. Jones FP: *Freedom to change: the development and science of the Alexander Technique*, London, 1997, Mauritz.
   This book is a scholarly work written by and including the research of Frank Pierce Jones at Tufts University in the 1950s. It is an excellent scientific introduction to the Alexander Technique.
4. Alexander FM: *The use of the self*, London, 1996, Gollancz.
   This is Alexander's book exploring his discovery of the Alexander Technique. It is a short paperback documenting how Alexander developed his technique and the basic principles and theories behind the technique.
5. McDonald G: *The complete illustrated guide to the Alexander Technique*, Boston, 1998, Element Books.
   This is the newest book on the market and the most complete book to date on the Alexander Technique. It is beautifully illustrated and beautifully written and provides access to history, principles, and application of the Alexander Technique.
6. De Alcantara P: Indirect procedures: a musician's guide to the Alexander Technique, Oxford, 1997, Oxford University Press.
   This book is an application book demonstrating how musicians use the Alexander Technique to enhance their skill and work directly with performance.

Bibliography

Alexander FM: *The use of the self*, London, 1996, Gollancz.

Brown R: *Authorized Summaries of F.M. Alexander's four books*, London, 1992, Stat Books.

Caplan D: *Back trouble: a new approach to prevention and recovery*, Gainesville, Fla, 1987, Triad.

Caplan D: *Postural management of scoliosis in the adolescent and adult based on the Alexander Technique*, Minneapolis, 1980, American Center for the Alexander Technique.

Gelb M: *Body learning*, ed 2, New York, 1995, Henry Holt.

Macdonald G: *The complete illustrated guide to Alexander Technique*, Boston, 1998, Element Books.

Nielsen M: Study of stress amongst professional musicians, Medical School, University of Aarhus, Denmark. In Stevens C, editor: *The Alexander Technique: medical and physiological aspects*, London, 1994, STAT Books.

Stern J: The Alexander Technique: an approach to pain control, *Lifeline* 3(4), 1992.

Tinbergen N: Ethology and stress diseases, *Science* 185(5):20-27, 1974.

References

1. Selye H: *Stress without distress*, New York, 1994, Lippincott.
2. Benson H: *The relaxation response*, New York, 1975, Morrow.
3. Jones FP: *Freedom to change*, London, 1997, Mauritz.
4. Austin MD, John HM: Enhanced muscular function in normal adults after lessons in proprioceptive musculoskeletal education without exercise, *Chest* 102:486-490, 1992.
5. Jones FP: Method for changing stereotyped response patterns by the inhibition of certain postural sets, *Psychol Rev* 72:196-214, 1965.
6. Fischer K: Early experienced of a multi-disciplinary pain management programme, *Holistic Med* 3(1), 1988.
7. Stevens C: *Medical and physiologic aspects*, London, 1994, Stat Books.
8. Caplan D: *Back trouble: a new approach to prevention and recovery based on the Alexander Technique*, Gainesville, Fla, 1987, Triad Communications.

Aston-Patterning®

LAURA SERVID

JENNA WOODS

JUDITH ASTON

Origins and History

The *Aston paradigm* is an evolution of realizations by Judith Aston about the nature of human existence. It includes perceptions about our bodies' natural form and function, our processes of learning and self-expression, and our interaction with the physical properties of the planet and our environment.

Key to the paradigm is the recognition that the human body is asymmetrically constructed, that its motion and structure take on three-dimensional asymmetric spiral forms, and that each human body is unique.

Judith Aston, founder of Aston-Patterning, is a former college instructor of movement and dance for performing artists and athletes, which she practiced between 1963 and 1972. She also worked in the field of psychology, assisting in identifying and processing patterns of physical and emotional expression. At the request of Dr. Ida Rolf, she developed and taught the pilot movement program for the Rolf Institute. As Judith Aston more closely observed the differences in people, she began to develop Neuro-kinetics, or movement education, to accommodate asymmetry and individual uniqueness. This identified a new model for standing balance, recognition, and use of each body's natural asymmetries and full three-dimensional structural support and movement, which is characterized by its ease and efficiency through the use of the forces of gravity and ground reaction force. The theories of the Aston paradigm as they are applied to movement is now known as Aston-Mechanics. This form of movement and movement education is the essence of the Aston work. It has evolved to include sophisticated forms of bodywork, as well as fitness training, teaching techniques, ergonomics, and product design.

Judith Aston now maintains schedules of training throughout the U.S. and New Zealand. She is a valued consultant in athletics, industry, and education. She continues to refine the Aston-Patterning system, develop ergonomic designs, and investigate further applications for her work.

Mechanism of Action According to Its Own Theory

Aston-Patterning is the application of the Aston paradigm to human movement, bodywork, and ergonomics, matching human function to its environment. As a form of therapy, its uniqueness lies partly in its comprehensive approach to the whole individual rather than seeing the body as separate parts. The understanding of a specific problem or interest is evaluated in relationship to the whole, taking into consideration the entire person, including the body, character expressions, personal beliefs, and movement habits. There is no set recipe for managing a problem.

A second distinction is its educational focus. Its goal is to teach people an awareness of themselves as dynamic structural beings, accessing the best available use of their bodies in efficient and less effortful movement to support a full expression of themselves as unique individuals.

Aston-Patterning is based on the belief that each body has a natural integrity of dimension and proportion in which all parts are allowed their own best three-dimensional shape and work together in cooperation for efficient function. The internal volume of each segment is addressed as well as the outer shape. This system uses spiral patterns in asymmetric three-dimensional forms to understand the human structure and its movement on the earth. This varies from the more mechanistic right angle planes that are commonly applied in traditional contexts.

The Aston alignment of the body hinges 2 to 4 degrees forward from the ankle, distributing the weight of the body over the whole foot. The position of the legs is matched to the hip joint such that there is an open stance with some external rotation of the whole leg. The pelvis then rests directly over the femurs in a few degrees of anterior tilt supporting the natural lumbar curve of the spine. In this posture the lower body provides a base of support for the upper body, the shoulder girdles hang easily on the ribcage, and the head is directly supported by the neck and chest. The angle of this posture provides the structure with its most optimal support and adds the dynamic quality that facilitates motion.

The view through the body from inside to out reveals the basis for the asymmetry that is honored in Aston-Patterning. After repeated observation, Judith Aston came to realize that our external shape reflects our internal body structure. The placement and size of the organs in the body is not even or symmetric and in a subtle way this asymmetry is seen in the outer body structure as well. To impose an external symmetry over an asymmetric core necessitates excessive tension at some level, which then compromises optimal function. Being bipedal creatures, in walking we balance our bodies over one leg and then the other. Aston-Patterning works to uncover the best structural support available through each side of the body and negotiates the asymmetries through movement between one side and the other. In this way tension is released and function is enhanced because of the absence of tensional stresses. Where more obvious asymmetry occurs because of accidents, illnesses, or surgeries, movement patterns are taught to include the asymmetric pattern rather than allowing a tension pattern to be created around it.

The Aston alignment guideline focuses on the interfaces between body segments that are viewed as apertures. When two segments are accurately aligned the overlap of the segments creates an open aperture that allows fuller functional communication between the segments. When the segments are displaced in relationship to each other the aperture is narrowed and the space for communication is decreased. This can result from sheer force or rotational tension creating a restriction between the two segments.

Motion is essential to our existence. Although this is an accepted fact, the traditional model of standing posture is static. Tension is associated with the notion of erect posture, thus initiation of movement requires effort. Tension leads to relative stillness, compromising the quality of the musculoskeletal, physiologic, and even psychologic function. The Aston model minimizes tension and effort needed to set the body in motion. Unique to the Aston system is a dynamic postural alignment using gravity and ground reaction force (GRF) to facilitate human movement.

In this system all movement is believed to occur in asymmetric three-dimensional spiral patterns or arcs of these spirals. Gravity assists to set the body weight in motion and GRF carries the body to the next segment of the movement through a push off the ground. GRF takes the body to the height of an arc, creating a *moment of suspension* in which the force of gravity on the body is reduced. Our experience of gravity can lead to a sense of heaviness or restriction weighing on our movements and psyches. The inclusion of this *moment of suspension* in each movement sequence allows a split second of freedom and expansion in which we can experience the sensation of being unweighted. This is an unparalleled benefit of Aston-Mechanics.

For work with patients, several factors distinguish the Aston-Patterning treatment from traditional forms of therapy. First, as previously mentioned, is the consideration of the person as a whole. The work is a cooperative collaboration between the practitioner and the patient. Essential to the work is the education of patients about themselves, distinguishing between habitual movement patterns and the unique asymmetric patterns of their own bodies, which allows movement with reduced tension and greater ease.

Second is the determination of the relationship between the patient's focus and the overall patterns of posture and movement that are observed. This problem-solving is key to the Aston-Patterning work. Dysfunction of a particular part often is the result of shifts in alignment or tension of adjacent segments. Resolution is achieved through integration of function through the whole, versus specific attention to just one part.

Third, in both the movement and bodywork *the sequence determines the result*. The bodywork for each individual is sequenced in a careful plan to determine the holding patterns that most control the overall structural patterns, so that release of one segment facilitates the reduction of the overall tension pattern. Movement education supports the changes that occur and assists in ongoing changes. Attention to how the patient learns is of key importance. The movement lessons are grounded in practical application, such as sitting or standing postures, bending, reaching, lifting, and walking. This brings the work into daily life rather than being an exercise that remains separate from normal function. Elements of the Aston fitness training that address loosening, stretching, and strengthening are tailored to the individual's patterns, activities, and lifestyle. Aston ergonomics teaches patients to adapt their environment to support their three-dimensional posture.

Fourth, the bodywork in Aston-Patterning is unique. Every person has an individual set of holding patterns based on varying combinations of intellectual, physical, and emotional habits. These holding patterns can be felt in the fascial tissues and have a directionality that occurs in three-dimensional spiral forms. When these patterns are matched in direction, speed, and amount of movement in the tissue, change occurs rather readily and with-

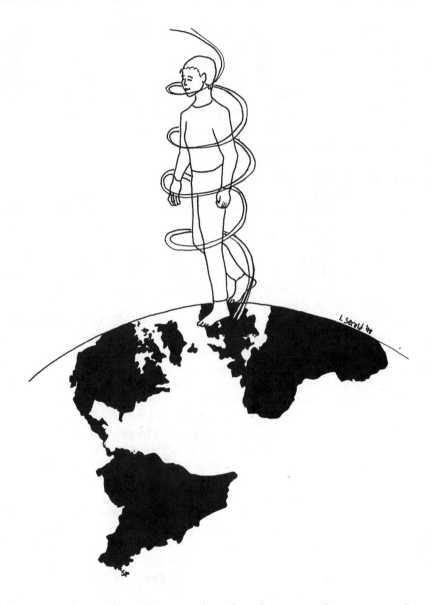

out discomfort. Using a three-dimensional touch and Aston mechanics, Aston-Patterning practitioners are taught a form of bodywork that is perceived by the patient to be very subtle and yet is profoundly effective. Changes are sustained by newly learned movement patterns and can enhance the whole system for a less stressful, healthier lifestyle.

Biologic Mechanism of Action

Empirically, the benefits of Aston-Patterning are seen again and again in clinical practice. To date there have not been scientific studies that measure and prove its effectiveness.

There are, however, biologic mechanisms that in theory and clinical experience respond well to Aston-Patterning.

The fundamental concept of spiral movement as described by the Aston paradigm matches the basic design of the human form, from its molecular structure to the wrapping of the muscles supporting the skeleton. It seems appropriate to apply these spiral forms to soft tissue work and movement, reflecting the natural structure and function as it exists in our bodies. Aston-Patterning uses this spiral system in all its bodywork and movement designs, accounting at least in part for its exceptional effectiveness.

It is generally recognized that bodywork can be an effective means of promoting the movement of fluid through our systems. Movement of fluids is essential to the body's processes. The study of fluid and elastic continuums recognize that all fluids move three-dimensionally with constant irregularities of flow caused by random turbulence. In the body the observable results of these irregularities are the asymmetric spirals ingrained in the form and function of tissues. The Aston training teaches the ability to "read" the dimensional grain of the tissue and discern its preferred direction for movement using three-dimensional touch. This consistently produces profound results in the tissue.

The mechanism of fluid exchange is an essential part of our physiology. The exchange of fluid across membranes is restricted where the membranes are stretched too tightly or lack appropriate mobility. Because all organs are suspended in tissue, the compromise of their space may adversely effect their function. Fluid exchange enhanced by application of the Aston principles enhances physiologic function and promotes a healthier state of being.

Aston-Patterning also has been effective in enhancing nervous system function. Proprioceptors monitor the changes needed to keep the body in balance and motion. Afferent information from both the Golgi tendon organs and the muscles spindle are based on stretch and tension. In a balanced body this allows for optimal function of the proprioceptors and enhanced communication between the skeletal structures and the brain as they work together to control human movement. The benefits of Aston bodywork and movement education have been seen in work with patients' neurologic deficits where proprioceptive and kinesthetic awareness has been restored beyond what was believed possible, allowing improved movement control and function.

In the musculoskeletal system, joint nutrition and fluid exchange occurs with intermittent compression and distraction. Aston-Patterning helps to achieve the most accurate alignment of the joint surfaces with respect to the individual's unique system, balancing tensions around the joints and promoting direct transmission of the forces sustained in movement through the weight bearing joints. Using gravity and GRF to assist in movement, a continuous system of alternating compression and distraction of the joints occurs, facilitating fluid exchange. Patients find that this healing occurs commonly as a result of Aston-Patterning, when the alignment and movement patterns are changed to eliminate the stresses.

Of increasing interest is the body-mind-spirit connection in relationship to disease and dysfunction of the human system. In Aston-Patterning the tissue is thought to be an ongoing record of our emotional, psychologic, and intellectual patterns. Changes in the tissues and in the carriage and movement of the structure allow change in attitude and emotional states. Where the body language and the emotion do not match, neither is fully honored and the differing messages are held in tension. While Aston-Patterning is not a psychologic form of treatment, this is certainly a consideration in its holistic approach. Options of expression can be offered to patients for their own exploration, and coordination with other therapists and practitioners is encouraged.

With regard to other alternative systems of treatment, Aston-Patterning can be considered a beneficial adjunct in many cases. The tensions of connective tissue that perpetuate the need for ongoing chiropractic adjustments may be eased, allowing those adjustments to be held longer. Energy flow facilitated in acupuncture may be more easily achieved in a body less held by inefficient movement habits or postural tensions. It can be imagined that the energies of the chakras as described in Indian traditions could be enhanced by the direct alignment of those energy wheels in a balanced body system. Certainly, the ergonomic and postural work can be beneficial to those practicing yoga or meditation.

The benefits of Aston-Patterning are far-reaching and comprehensive. These are only a few ways in which the Aston system is thought to be supported in scientific thought. The paradigm itself is a departure from the traditional models applied to the structure and alignment of the human form, but this departure is thought to be accurate to the function of the human system in the presence of the forces of gravity and GRF as they exist on our planet.

Forms of Therapy

Aston-Patterning is a system comprised of several integrated forms, including the following:

- *Aston movement education:* This teaches body mechanics based on Aston principles. Lessons begin with very basic actions and can progress to any kind of specialized, complex activity.
- *Aston massage:* A gentle three-dimensional form of tissue work, this massage focuses on more even body tone, relief from every day tensions, and assimilation of change.
- *Aston myokinetics:* This Aston-based myofascial work is used strategically with precision to sequentially release tensions in tissues that have become structurally ingrained through habitual use, overuse, or trauma.
- *Aston arthrokinetics:* Requiring advanced training, this form works most deeply to release structurally ingrained tensions in the joints, along bones, and in tissues that act like bone because of hardening.
- *Aston fitness training:* Here the principles of Aston-Mechanics are applied to exercises designed specifically for the individual. All exercises work to emphasize the cooperation of the whole body, even when targeting specific muscle groups. Honoring asymmetry, exercises may vary from one side of the body to the other, both in focus and number of repetitions. The system includes loosening, stretching, and toning to meet individual needs, as well as cardiovascular fitness.
- *Aston facial fitness:* This work combines the massage, myokinetic, and arthokinetic forms with some lymphatic drainage techniques and Aston-based isometric exercises for specific application to facial tone and expression.

- *Aston ergonomics:* Learning to arrange or modify objects in the environment (tools, furniture, equipment, and others) to support optimal body mechanics for any given activity is essential to support the rest of the Aston work.

Demographics

At present, there are certified Aston-Patterning practitioners in 15 states, with concentrations in California, Colorado, and Washington. There are certified Aston Movement practitioners in New Zealand. A list of practitioners is available at the Aston Training Center, listed in "Training."

People seeking Aston-Patterning are generally active with an interest in self-help and a commitment to active participation in their well-being. Although a majority of them may be women between the ages of 25 and 50 years, there is a full spectrum of people who have benefited from this work.

Indications and Reasons for Referral

The most common medical referrals are for musculoskeletal conditions and myofascial dysfunction resulting from injury, accidents, or surgeries. There often is a component of pain or limitation of function. Many are referred to Aston-Patterning when the conventional methods have been exhausted and the problem persists. In these cases it often is effective where other forms of therapy have reached an impasse because of its comprehensive approach to understanding the specific problem. Patients are also referred when there is an obvious postural component to their particular dysfunction and where movement education is recommended.

In the nonmedical context, Aston-Patterning offers assistance with basic activities of daily living and specialized work activities of any kind. Health professionals involved in physical contact with patients can find improved touch sensitivity, transfer, and handling skills, and personal physical safety. In sports and recreational activities, Aston-Patterning can contribute significantly to safety and performance. In dance, it can improve distribution of effort in the body, reducing risk of injury and enhancing the appearance of ease in performance. In vocal or instrumental music, it can improve the quality of resonance and tone. Actors can develop greater postural adaptability and hone characterization skills. Small children experiencing difficulties in basic activities may respond quickly and effectively to this work. Older adults have found it very beneficial in reclaiming their ease of movement and function. People of any age who are dissatisfied with their posture or their bodies for some reason may find way for positive change.

Patients are also referred by psychotherapists as a adjunct modality to their psychologic work. Here the aim is to work with changes in physical expression to complement their psychologic and emotional process.

Another major source of referral is word of mouth. People are generally impressed with the results achieved and are eager to send their friends and family for treatment.

Office Applications

Basic indications for this form of therapy fall into five categories. As with all alternative therapies, use of Aston Patterning does not preclude the use of mainstream medical therapies in addition.

1. Musculoskeletal disorders resulting from injury, accidents, or aging; back and neck pain and degenerative disc disease; knee and hip pain related to injury, trauma, or wear and tear; shoulder girdle dysfunction with associated bursitis or tendonitis; and overuse or repetitive strain injuries

   For these conditions the assessment of the individual posture and movement patterns, systematic sequenced release of fascial holding that maintains those dysfunctional patterns, and the movement education for more efficient body usage is extremely effective in restoring healthy function. The focus of treatment is to understand why the stress is occurring in the system and provide the necessary support through the structure and function to reduce the stress and allow healing to occur.

2. Myofascial pain related to the previous conditions

   The techniques in Aston Patterning bodywork are very effective in reducing myofascial pain and addressing trigger point restriction. Again, the strain of the tissue in one segment is often related to the balance of the whole, and when this is addressed the pain is reduced and often eliminated.

3. Chronic pain and dysfunction following a motor vehicle accident (MVA)

   The injury to soft tissue resulting from a MVA is present throughout the body tissues. This approach can sequence the unwinding of these strains by systematic evaluation of the position of the person in the car, the direction and sequence of the forces sustained by the body, and a determination of the body's likely protective response to this impact. Many times postures are sustained that match the pattern of the accident without the awareness on the part of the patient. They only know they are uncomfortable. Once the holding patterns in the tissues are released and the body is allowed to resume a more normal alignment, much of the ongoing discomfort is alleviated.

4. Decreased function due to neurologic deficits in cerebral palsy, multiple sclerosis, or stroke

   In the treatment of neurologic dysfunction, Aston-Patterning offers long-range assistance in efficient movement patterns and skeletal alignment, which enhances optimal available function. It can provide energy-saving techniques and reduce strain and stress on the system from abnormal movement patterns. Long-term benefits have been noted in the way of improved movement control, balance, and coordination.

5. Developmental disabilities

   The application of Aston-Patterning in the treatment of children with developmental disabilities is less common. Its use in conjunction with traditional neurodevelopmental treatment (NDT) techniques is believed to have extensive possibilities for positive outcomes. As with patients with neurologic deficits, these children can benefit from a balancing of alignment, education in most optimal movement patterns, and treatment that offers an organization to their systems facilitating their best function.

Practical Applications

Aston-Patterning is generally used in a manner similar to physical, occupational, or massage therapy. It is prescribed by physicians for management of injury and in rehabilitation.

Research Base

Unfortunately, there is not a scientific research base to confirm the effectiveness of Aston-Patterning. Empirically, it is known to be effective, and anecdotal or individual case history evidence abounds. There is a strong need for research studies that would provide scientific backing for its theory and test its effectiveness as a treatment modality, primarily of musculoskeletal conditions but in other arenas as well.

Druglike Information

Safety

Generally, this is a very safe form of therapy. Practitioners are cautioned to err on the side of too little change versus too much change, and the change is always checked for accommodation through the whole system. Risks occur if too much work is done too quickly. Possible risk also is present where bodywork is performed but left without the support of movement education or ergonomic changes. In this case the structures may be more vulnerable to injury because of a new resilience used with the stresses of old movement patterns.

Warnings, Contraindications, and Precautions

This form of therapy requires a commitment to participation on the part of the patient and is not effective in persons whose attitude is passive or wanting a fix without any personal involvement. It is more challenging with people whose body awareness and kinesthetic senses have not been developed. The learning of movement patterns and understanding of the work requires normal cognitive function. Tissue changes may be effected without this, but the memory and ability to repeat movement sequences is essential to sustaining these changes.

Drug or Other Interactions

Drugs that could interfere with balance are a contraindication in the use of this therapy.

Adverse Reactions

Release of holding in tissue can bring up emotional and psychologic issues that may be unexpected in the course of this form of treatment.

Pregnancy and Lactation

Because of the increased extensibility of tissues in pregnant women, caution must be observed and changes made slowly. Care is taken to maintain the stability of the pelvic floor and the safety of the fetus. Communication with the physician is advised, especially in cases where risk is thought to be present. Most often, however, this treatment has been found to be beneficial in pregnancy, reducing tension patterns that may inhibit the movements of the baby in the womb and increasing comfort for the mother. Aston-Mechanics can be very useful in labor and delivery.

Trade Products, Administration, and Dosage

Ergonomic products designed by Judith Aston are available through the Aston Line. These are cushions that enhance the support of the body structure for use in cars, offices, and other furniture. The use of these supports is most accurate when the assessment and education by a practitioner assures proper benefit for the specific individual.

Self-Help versus Professional

Training in Aston-Patterning is extensive and thorough, the basic course being 100 days of training over 2 years. It is taught only to licensed health practitioners. The practitioner not only requires an understanding of the work but must be able to embody the work for it to be effective. Although many therapists are introduced to the work in beginning prerequisite classes, the totality of the work cannot be appreciated in parts. It simply cannot be done without training.

Visiting a Professional

The Aston-Patterning office is likely to be comfortable and relaxed, with a massage table and an open area for movement, mat work, or use of some simple resistive exercise equipment. Clothing for the appointment should be comfortable. Shorts and a T-shirt or tank top allow the practitioner to better observe postural and movement patterns, but personal comfort levels and privacy are of utmost importance.

In a self-evaluation form or on your first visit, you likely will be asked for your history and to outline your habitual activities, physical traumas, chronic problems, surgeries, and current goals of treatment. Observation of standing posture and some basic movement pattern begin the visual assessment that helps determine general alignment patterns, areas of tension, and movement versus stillness. Palpation is done usually through clothing or a drape to create a body map of graded tension areas. Based on this information the practitioner will probably discuss with you their observations and propose a hypothesis about how the patterns might be able to change to assist you in reaching your stated goal. Choosing one of the Aston forms, you will be taken through a brief period of treatment to check to see if the hypothesis will produce the desired effect. The work is then continued to reach the desired amount of change, and the rest of the session is dedicated toward balance with the rest of the body and integration of the change into functional movement. The Aston-Patterning belief is that change and learning require comfort and ease without excessive self-consciousness. For this reason the practitioners work to accommodate you as a person working around chronic or painful limitations and make it your session.

By the end of the session you will have specific homework that applies to your daily movement patterns with a cue to help you remember it. The practitioner will work with you to discover the cue you find most helpful, whether verbal, kinesthetic, visual imagery, or a combination of these.

Frequency of sessions can be variable. Every session is self-contained to a degree, and the goal is to leave each session with something that will assist in ongoing change. Difficult or more acute situations may demand more frequent visits (1 or 2 times per week) but much of the work is cumulative and can be learned with less frequency and over a longer period of time (1 to 4 times per month). It takes time to integrate new movement into daily activity and persistence can result in continued progress.

Credentialing

All Aston-Patterning trainees are required to be licensed health care practitioners in practice. Judith Aston and senior faculty members train them through the Aston Training Center. Quality is insured by requirements for annual renewal of certification and continuing education classes.

Training

Prospective trainees for Aston-Patterning certification must complete prerequisite course before application. Application requirements include licensure as a health care practitioner, working knowledge of anatomy and kinesiology, evidence of ability to succeed in the training environment, and a detailed statement of purpose. Training consists of five 3-week segments that teach myokinetics, movement education, assessment, and problem-solving skills, with both classroom instruction and supervised clinical practice. After the first two segments there are requirements for practicing the material learned before the next classes. The evaluation includes a written and practical examination, at which time trainees sign a licensing agreement to become a certified Aston-Patterning practitioner.

The Aston Movement certification course consists of four 2-week segments teaching the Aston Massage, movement education, and assessment and problem-solving skills.

Active status as a practitioner is maintained by payment of an annual licensing fee and continuing education.

Aston Training Center
PO Box 3568
Incline Village, NV 89450
Tel: (775) 831-8228
Fax: 775-831-8955
E-mail: AstonPat@aol.com
www.AstonPatterning.com

What to Look for in a Provider

The provider must be a certified Aston-Patterning practitioner. Should there be a selection of practitioners available, look for personal rapport and compatibility or someone with a specialized interest that matches the specific needs. Because the therapeutic and educational relationship will be a cooperative effort, the choice is important.

Barriers and Key Issues

The extensive scope of this work is both its success and its limitation. The theory of Aston-Patterning can become a way of life and requires awareness and commitment to the use of its principles through everyday activity. Although it can be enormously beneficial, its comprehensive approach makes it difficult to access simply and quickly. This limits the number of trained practitioners. It also encumbers its understanding by the general public.

The application of this system to conditions that are thought of in medical terms can have very successful results, but as it did not originate from a medical model, its appreciation by the medical community has evolved more slowly. Lack of research has limited its credibility in the scientific realm. Studies that measure its effectiveness are needed and would greatly encourage its use.

The most helpful efforts to improve acceptance by the mainstream medical community might include the following steps: 1) initiate research to provide needed statistic evidence of effectiveness; 2) promote publication of Aston-Patterning articles in medical journals where medical professionals will be more likely to learn of the work; and 3) secure funding to manufacture Aston ergonomic design prototypes, particularly those for medical and athletic equipment.

Bowen Technique

PATRIK ROUSSELOT

Origins and History

The *Bowen Technique* (BT) is an original system of gentle but powerful soft tissue mobilization that affects the body both structurally and energetically to restore its self-healing mechanisms. It is painless, noninvasive, safe to use on anyone, ranging from newborns to the elderly, and provides lasting relief from a wide variety of acute or chronic conditions.

The BT was developed in Australia by the late Tom Bowen (1916-1982) a very intuitive, gifted, and self-taught healer who devoted a lifetime to develop his original technique independent of any previous training in medicine or any other modality. He claimed that he could sense minute variations of tension in the muscles that helped him find the precise places to mobilize. By 1975, he was seeing a remarkable 13,000 patients a year, as documented by the Victorian Government. Considering that treatments were usually 7 days apart and that most people only needed 2 or 3 visits, that was an amazing number of patients per year for a one-person clinic.

Bowen taught only a few therapists. In 1974 he met one of them, Oswald Rentsch, a natural therapist practicing massage and osteopathy. Over the next two and a half years Rentsch became Bowen's apprentice and scribe, documenting his treatment protocols. He started using Bowen's unique technique in Hamilton, where he and his wife Elaine operated their own clinic. It was not until Bowen's death in 1982 that the Rentsches started teaching what would be known as the Bowen technique. By 1990 they were teaching full-time and introduced the Bowen technique throughout Australia and New Zealand, then North America and the United Kingdom.

Mechanism of Action According to Its Own Theory

Tom Bowen never wrote anything about his work nor explained how and why it worked so well. We are left with several theories and Rentsch's observations during his apprenticeship at Bowen's clinic.

The Bowen technique is a system of subtle and precise mobilizations called *Bowen moves* that are applied over muscles, tendons, nerves, and fascia. The moves are performed using the thumbs and fingers, applying only gentle, noninvasive pressure. A treatment consists of a series of specific sequences of moves called *procedures*, with frequent pauses to allow time for the body to respond. To get a sense of what a move done over a muscle feels like, place your right thumb over the center of your left biceps.

1. Moving the thumb horizontally, draw the skin slack gently from the center of the muscle to its medial edge.
2. The muscle is challenged for several seconds by applying a gentle lateral pressure against its medial edge. Here the muscle fibers and its fascia are disturbed from their neutral position and slightly stretched.
3. Pressing gently towards the core of the muscle and using the skin slack available, roll your thumb laterally across the biceps just like a bicycle wheel rolling over a speed bump. After the thumb rolls over and across the muscle gently compressing it, it will react by springing back to its neutral position.

This typical Bowen move is the core of the BT and can be applied with some adaptations throughout the body in specific locations and in prescribed sequences to affect specific body systems (digestion, lymph circulation, respiratory apparatus, and so on) or body parts (pelvis, temporomandibular joint, shoulder, and so on). As simple as the technique sounds, the practitioner must develop with practice a keen sense of tissue tension. This will tell exactly where stress has built up in the tissue, how much pressure to use, and where and when to do a move to release that stress. The practitioner strives to do a minimum of moves or procedures to trigger in the body the desired self-healing response. The sicker the patient or the more acute the condition, the less is done during the session and the less pressure will be used to do the moves, and the more profound the effect will be on the body. One motto of the technique is "Less is more!"

Bowen believed his goal was to assist the body's natural ability to repair and regulate itself. He further believed that bodily dysfunction was the result of disturbances in the tissues. His underlying assumption was that structure governs function and that disturbances of structure in whatever tissue within the body will lead to disturbances of functioning in that structure and in turn of the function of the body as a whole. His goal was to restore the structural integrity in the body in order to restore its optimum function. He also believed in the universal life energy called *Qi* (pronounced "chi"). In Traditional Chinese Medicine, this energy must flow freely throughout the body to assure a state of maximum health. Bowen's gift was to discover a system of mobilizations that rebalances this natural flow of energy.

Biologic Mechanism of Action

Most likely there is an overlap of all the following mechanisms being activated at the same time with each Bowen move, as well as others yet undiscovered.

Stretch reflex: Most moves are done either at the origin, insertion, or belly of muscles where the golgi and spindle cells' receptors are located, informing the nervous system on the state of tension, length, or stretch in the musculotendinous tissue. These receptors are stimulated during the "challenge" and the "rolling" part of the move. In case of a pain-muscle spasm loop, we can break this vicious circle by changing the stimulus received by the nervous system.

Joint proprioreceptors: All moves done around a joint directly affect the joint capsule and ligaments that are richly enervated with proprioreceptors. Here again, stimulus will be received by the central nervous system, inviting normalization of the joint function without the need for forceful manipulation.

Fascia: Each Bowen move is done at the level of the superficial fascia and affects the relation between the fascia and the nerve, muscle, or tendon being mobilized. Fascia plays a major role in muscle coordination, postural alignment, and overall structural and functional integrity. All these will be negatively affected because following injuries the fascia will stiffen, contract, torque, and dehydrate, as shown by the work of Ida Rolf[1] and many osteopaths, including William Sutherland and John Upledger.[2,3] Following a Bowen session it is not uncommon to see adhesions loosen up, scar tissue soften, and posture and mobility improve without harsh mobilization or stretching.

Segmental viscerosomatic spinal reflexes: These reflexes are engaged in most basic procedures to produce referred reactions to the internal organs through stimulation of skin and muscles.[4]

Autonomic nervous system (ANS) rebalancing: The BT may have its most profound and important effect here where the body's self-healing mechanisms are governed. The ANS controls over 80% of bodily functions and is very susceptible to external stressors. Most people today live in a constant state of high stress and sympathetic ANS overstimulation. Healing occurs after the ANS shift from sympathetic to parasympathetic dominance. The BT seems to catalyze that shift: during sessions, patients often quickly fall asleep or drop in deep relaxation and loud peristalsis sounds can be heard. This indicates a shift towards parasympathetic dominance with release of stress at a deep level. This could explain why a few Bowen sessions frequently reactivate the recovery process, where healing from trauma, sickness, or surgery has stalled or reached a plateau.

Trigger points: Several Bowen moves overlap with recognized trigger points locations. By clearing these trigger points, referred pain will be relieved and joint mobility and muscle coordination will be improved.[5]

Acupuncture points and meridians: Most moves overlap acupuncture points and some actually cross over two or three acupuncture meridians at once. Acupuncturists have correlated the indications and effects of Bowen moves with the corresponding acupuncture points. They also commented on the immediate changes of the acupuncture pulses in response to moves or procedures. The overlap of these two systems could explain the very strong energetic component of the BT and its effect on the internal organs.

Neurolymphatic points and lymphatic circulation: Bowen moves overlap the location of many neurolymphatic reflex points that regulate the lymphatic system.[4] This explains detoxifying reactions, improved circulation, and drainage following sessions. These neurolymphatic reflex points also have shown a stimulating and strengthening effect on specific muscles as used in *Touch for Health*.[6]

Demographics

Because the technique is so effective, it has been embraced by a broad spectrum of health practitioners. To this date around 8000 people have taken Bowen Therapy Academy of Australia (BTAA) seminars, including 2000 in the U.S. Instructors are regularly offering seminars in Australia, New Zealand, the U.S., Canada, Quebec, England, Scotland, Northern Ireland, Austria, France, Italy, and Israel. Other countries certainly will be added to this list in the near future, such as Mexico, Brazil, and South Africa.

In North America, most practitioners tend to be concentrated on the west and east coasts of the U.S. and Canada, although there are several Bowen nucleus centers in between coasts.

The BT has been helpful to a wide range of patients of both sexes, from newborns to older adults, and from the disabled and chronically ill patient to the competitive athlete.

Indications and Reasons for Referral

The most common reasons why people consult a Bowen practitioner are for any condition affecting the musculoskeletal system, including back, neck, hip, and shoulder pain, to just name a few. As the main goal of the BT is to stimulate the body to engage in its own healing, it can be used effectively to reduce rehabilitation time after any illness, surgery or injury regardless of how old or recent it may be. Because of its gentleness it is recommended for painful conditions and is easily applied during pregnancy and to newborns or older adults. Because of the balancing effects of the BT on the ANS, any condition related to stress or tension and the internal organs are good indications. Patients with chronic illnesses or disabilities such as chronic fatigue, fibromyalgia, polio, cerebral palsy, multiple sclerosis, muscular dystrophy, and severe forms of arthritis have shown gradual improvement of their condition and quality of life. Often patients come to the BT after having tried many other modalities to no avail. If a patient has not responded to other forms of therapy, it is always worth giving the BT a try because in many patients it has shown to trigger sometimes surprising and unexpected recovery when nothing else had worked.

Office Applications

The BT does not seek to treat specific conditions or diseases but rather to gently stimulate the body to heal itself. The following list of diagnosed conditions comes from claims of patients worldwide who found relief from such conditions. As with all alternative therapies, use of this form of therapy does not preclude the use of mainstream medical therapies in addition. The policy of the BTAA is to seek medical opinion whenever necessary.

Top level: *A therapy ideally suited for these conditions*
Ankle sprains and strains; arthritis; bed wetting; breast pain (premenstrual syndrome, mastitis, lactation, engorgement); carpal tunnel syndrome; repetitive stress injury; chest wall pain; chronic pain syndrome; coccyx pain; cold and flu; concussion; dys-

menorrhea; elbow overuse syndromes; fibromyalgia; hamstring and adductor strain; hamstring tension; herniated disks; knee pain; loss of joint mobility; migraine and headaches; muscular back pain; newborn colic or irritability; pain and limitation postsurgery; pelvic imbalances (tilt, leg length, hip pain and imbalance, secondary inguinal and groin pain); premenstrual syndrome; pregnancy-related low back pain; rotator cuff problems; sacroiliac pain and imbalances (posttraumatic or related to pregnancy); sciatica; secondary foot pain (hammer toes, hallux valgus, plantar fasciatis); shin splints; shoulder adhesive capsulitis; sleep disorders; stress and tension; tennis elbow; temporomandibular joint pain; and whiplash injuries

Second level: *One of the better therapies for these conditions*

Kidney stone; infertility; constipation; diarrhea; asthma; hay fever allergies; emphysema; bronchitis; sinus congestion; chronic fatigue syndrome; AIDS-related pain; scoliosis; severe forms of arthritis; Bell's palsy; cerebral palsy; polio; multiple sclerosis; stroke; muscular dystrophy; Parkinson's disease; torticollis; hyperactivity; and attention deficit hyperactivity disorder

Third level: *A valuable adjunctive therapy for these conditions*

Addictions and drug detoxification; anginal chest pain; and incontinence (adult)

Practical Applications

The BT is a complementary modality, meaning it will enhance and complement, not interfere with other medical attention. Ideally, three sessions, once per week, should be enough to show benefit and response to the BT. After that and with severe chronic conditions, other modalities can be introduced effectively on an alternating weekly schedule.

Research Base

Evidence Based

Seba[7] showed the positive effect of the BT on patients diagnosed with fibromyalgia. They all experienced various degrees of relief, which lasted from a few days to several weeks. The measurements of shifts in the ANS by heart rate variability (HRV) studies fully complemented the clinical assessments.

Pritchard[8] showed that the BT consistently reduced subjects' level of anxiety and enhanced individuals' positive feelings by reducing tension, anger, depression, fatigue, and confusion. Objective measures of decrease in HRV and muscle tension correlate with subjective feelings of relaxation.

Bauman[9] assessed masseter tension by biofeedback, measured bite, and assessed subjective symptoms before and after BT treatment. Immediately after the first treatment, one-third of patients felt dramatic relief in some of their symptoms and 20 of the 22 patients showed significant improvement on the postbiofeedback assessment.

Basic Science

Whitaker[10] has shown that the BT affects the ANS by measuring changes in value and pattern in HRV before and after treatment.

Risk, Safety, and Efficacy

Tom Bowen estimated his own success rate to be about 88%. Based on the extensive patient volume of Bowen and many other practitioners, BT appears to be safe to use regardless of age or diagnosis. The only unpleasant possible and occasional reaction that some patients experience is a temporary discomfort or flu-like illness due to the body *detoxifying* itself.

Norman[11] in a thesis presentation compared practitioner and patient responses in a survey evaluating the efficacy of the BT in the treatment of pain. Practitioners rated the BT effective in 85% for back pain with an average of 4.3 sessions, 88% for neck pain with 4.5 sessions, 83% for stress and tension with 4 sessions, 83% for other conditions with 5.8 sessions, and 80% for fibromyalgia requiring longer treatments. The average length of infirmity for the patients involved in the survey was 7.9 years; many of these patients had tried several other forms of treatment that failed to produce satisfying results. Patients rated the effectiveness of the BT to be 85% for back pain, 80% for stress and tension, 95% for temporomandibular joint pain, 80% for hip pain, and 75.6% for other conditions. This study showed the BT to be more effective for acute conditions than for chronic conditions. Patients' satisfaction with the results that they received from the BT ranged from 77% to 100%.

This study parallels the author's seven years of clinical experience where relief is usually obtained immediately in about 75% to 85% of the time; if not, it will gradually happen in the days following treatment and where most conditions can be improved (if not resolved) in a few sessions. Complex chronic conditions may require ongoing treatment.

Studies in Progress

Studies are underway by Dr. Bernie Carter at the Metropolitan University of Manchester with leading Bowen therapist Rick Minnery. The study will follow patients with frozen shoulder and response to BT.

A study at Hugh Chatham Memorial Hospital in North Carolina will compare outcomes between patients who received standard modalities and those treated with the BT for acute and chronic patients that have not responded to traditional treatment for myofascial pain syndrome, back pain, TMJ, fibromyalgia, arthritis, fractures, soft tissue trauma, and gynecologic dysfunction.

Another study in England involving midwife and Bowen therapist Rick Minnery and Dr. Bernie Carter (senior lecturer in Health Care Studies of Manchester Metropolitan University) will be based at Royal Lancaster Infirmary, Women's and Children's Unit. The study will investigate antenatal problems in pregnancy, such as morning sickness, heartburn, low back pain, symphyseal pain, and breast discomfort.

Self-Help versus Professional

A Bowen treatment is the essence of simplicity but this apparent simplicity in its application is misleading because the subtleties of the technique must be gained from years of practice. Learning the BT must be done through BTAA seminars from a registered instructor; it cannot be learned from a manual. A few simple procedures can be shown to patients for self-help purposes.

Visiting a Professional

Usually the treatment is done on a massage table and can be administrated through light clothing. A typical session starts with three general procedures that address the whole body. Specific procedures can be added to address particular problems. All the mobilizations are gentle and noninvasive. Patients frequently remark on the gentleness and economy of mobilizations. The entire process is so soothing they often report feelings of relief following a move or fall asleep during the session.

There are measured pauses between sets of moves to allow the body time to respond during which the practitioner will leave the room to encourage quiet relaxation. A session may run from 20 to 50 minutes with occasional shorter session using advanced procedures. The patient is invited to walk for a few minutes at the end of the treatment to help alleviate possible residual pain experienced when standing up from the table. Substantial if not total relief may be experienced by the end of the session or in the following hours or days as the body continues to rebalance itself. To support this process and help integrate new movement patterns, patients will be asked to follow specific recommendations, including drinking more water than usual and walking regularly. Typical follow-up visits, if needed, will be scheduled 5 to 10 days apart.

Credentialing

Most Bowen practitioners already have some kind of license and are already practicing massage therapists, physical therapists, nurses, osteopaths, chiropractors, acupuncturists or medical doctors. The Bowen Academy is the credentialing body. In the U.S., starting in 1999 the practitioners will have to pass a written and practical test to become certified. A similar process is in place in the U.K. and Australia.

Training

In the U.S. the training consist of three seminars (level 1-2-3) to learn all the basic procedures before certification (level 4, see "Credentialing"). To maintain certification status, practitioners are required to do continuing education. Advanced seminars are offered to certified experienced practitioners.

Training programs differ slightly in Australia and the U.K. but are all approved by the BTAA. The BT is taught at naturopathic colleges in Oregon and Canada. It is also offered as continuing education courses for nurses at Dominican College School of Nursing in California. The U.K. branch of the BTAA is a member of the British Complementary Medical Association.

Bowen Technique also has veterinary applications, and a special training endorsed by the BTAA is offered to veterinarians and horse owners.

What to Look for in a Provider

Patients looking for a Bowen practitioner can ask practitioners how long they have been practicing the technique, how many level 3 refreshers they have attended, and the date of their last refresher. The author's experience as a BT instructor is that it takes an average of two to three refreshers to know how to perform well all the basic procedures. The finesse and art of knowing how to choose and combine the different procedures can take years of practice. On the other hand, new practitioners obtain frequently outstanding results even before having completed their training.

Barriers and Key Issues

BT is still a relatively new modality that is not yet widely known in the U.S. The studies validating the safety and mechanisms of operation of the BT are in progress. In addition, BT challenges belief systems with the experience of a minimal stimulus invoking such a powerful healing response. As Gene Dobkin, a U.S. instructor, puts it: "The magic of Bowen is not so much that it works, but that it works doing so little."

Associations

In 1987 the Rentsches established the Bowen Therapy Academy of Australia (BTAA) as a governing body and in 1994 they implemented a teacher's training program in Australia, North America, and the U.K. to satisfy the increasing demand for new seminars. Bowtech is the trade name of the BT.

For information regarding instructors, seminars, or practitioners, contact the following organizations:

The International Head Office in Australia:
Kath Nagorcka
PO Box 733
Hamilton, Vic. 3300
Tel: (03) 5572-3000
Fax: (03) 5572-3144
E-mail: bowtech@h140.aone.net.au
www.bowtech.com

Allison Powers, North American Coordinator
PO Box 20217
Boulder, CO 80308
Tel: (303) 665-2667
Fax: (303) 665-2557
E-mail: usabowen@aol.com

Web site in French: A source of information for Quebec that will be expanded to serve all other French speaking countries: www.bigfoot.com/~bowenquebec

England Coordinator:
Bowen Association UK
122 High St., Earl Shilton
Leicestershire LE9 7LQ
Tel: 01455 841-800
Fax: 04155 851-384
E-mail: powerpoint@pipemedia.co.uk
www.bowtech.com/uk

Daphne Olsen, New Zealand Coordinator
58 Kapiti Road, Paraparaumu
Tel: (4) 298-6595
Fax: (4) 298-5333

Dr. Jaimini Raniga, South Africa Coordinator
PO Box 3774, 8000 Cape Town
Tel: 21-438 0421 083 440 6300
E-mail: quancorp@iafrica.com

Suggested Reading

1. Interested individuals can receive *Bowen Hands,* the quarterly journal of the BTAA, by contacting the country coordinator or the Australian head office.

   Besides the BTAA training manual and the "Bowen Home Companion" by Gene Dobkin, reserved for the BT students and practitioners, there are to this day no books written on the technique available to the general public.

Bibliography

Schultz LR et al: *The endless web: fascial anatomy and physical reality,* Berkeley, Calif, 1996, North Atlantic Books.
Presents fascia as a weblike network connecting and affecting every structure in the body.

References

1. Rolf IP: *Rolfing: the integration of human structures,* 1977, Dennis Landman.

2. Upledger JE, Vredevoogd J: *CranioSacral therapy,* Seattle, 1983, Eastland Press.

3. Upledger JE: *CranioSacral therapy II: beyond the dura,* Seattle, 1987, Eastland Press.

4. Chaitow L: *Soft-tissue manipulation: a practitioner's guide to the diagnosis and treatment of soft tissue dysfunction and reflex activity,* 1990, Astrologers Library.

5. Travell J, Simons D: *Myofascial pain and dysfunction: the trigger point manual,* vol 1, Baltimore, 1983, Williams & Wilkins; and Travell J: *Myofascial pain and dysfunction: the trigger point manual: the lower extremities,* vol 2, Baltimore, 1991, Williams & Wilkins.

6. Thie J: *Touch for health: a practical guide to natural health using acupressure touch and massage,* Marina del Ray, Calif. 1979, Devorss.

7. Seba D: *The Bowen technique, a potential treatment for fibromyalgia.* Paper presented at the American Academy of Environmental Medicine, La Roya, Calif, 1997. The full report can be obtained from the AEHF, PO Box 29874, Dallas, TX 75229.

8. Pritchard A: *The psychophysiological effects of the Bowen Technique.* Department of Psychophysiology, Melbourne, Australia, 1993, Swinburne University. Submitted as a Psychophysiology Major Research Project, Semester 2.

9. Bowen Therapy Academy of Australia, *Bowen Hands,* BTAA Newsletter, Dec 95.

10. Whitaker JA: *The Bowen Technique: a gentle hands-on healing method that affects the autonomic nervous system as measured by heart rate variability and clinical assessment.* Paper presented at the American Academy of Environmental Medicine meeting, La Jolla, Calif, December 1997. The full report can be obtained from the AEHF, PO Box 29874, Dallas TX 75229.

11. Norman A: *The Bowen Technique: a study of its prevalence and effectiveness.* University of North Carolina at Chapel Hill, Department of Physical Education, Exercise and Sport Science, 1988, undergraduate honor's thesis.

CranioSacral Therapy

JOHN E. UPLEDGER

Origins and History

CranioSacral therapy is a hands-on modality that concentrates on normalizing body functions, which are either part of or related to a physiologic system called the *craniosacral system*. This body system is composed of the watertight compartment formed by the dura mater membrane and the cerebrospinal fluid it contains, as well as the bones to which the dura mater attaches, the joints or sutures that interconnect these bones, and other bones that are indirectly connected to the dura mater.

CranioSacral therapy today represents the refinement of concepts originally put forth by William G. Sutherland, DO, in the 1930s. John E. Upledger, DO, OMM, worked with Richard Roppell, PhD (Biophysics), Ernest W. Retzlaff, PhD (Physiology), Zvi Karni, PhD (Biophysics) and DSc (Bioengineering), Yoram Lanir, DSc (Bioengineering), Frederick Becker, PhD (Anatomy), and Jon D. Vredevoogd, MFA (Design) from 1975 through 1983 in the Department of Biomechanics at Michigan State University, College of Osteopathic Medicine, to research Dr. Upledger's clinical observations and those of other osteopathic physicians. The research produced—much of it published—formed the basis for the modality Dr. Upledger developed and named CranioSacral therapy.

Mechanism of Action According to Its Own Theory

The craniosacral system strongly influences the physiologic environment of its contents, which include the brain, spinal cord, cranial nerves, spinal nerve roots, and several of the ganglia that are enclosed within the dura mater membrane compartment. Also affected are the pituitary gland and its related structures, the pineal gland, the ventricular system of the brain, the enclosed blood vascular structures including the arterial system, the venous system, and some lymphatic drainage subsystems.

When there is impairment of the natural mobility of the dura mater or any of its attached bones, the function of the craniosacral system is compromised to some degree. More peripherally located bones and connective tissues that attach to the craniosacral system also may impair its function. These conditions can result in dysfunction of any of the structures within the craniosacral system or their related systems.

Generally using about five grams of pressure, the CranioSacral therapy practitioner evaluates the body's craniosacral system by testing for its ease of motion and rhythm. Treatment techniques are based on the release of motion restrictions in sutures, fasciae, membranes, and any other tissues that may influence the craniosacral system.

Biologic Mechanism of Action

The concept of a functioning craniosacral system is based on the rhythmic rise and fall of cerebrospinal fluid volume and pressure within the dura mater compartment, which is regulated by related inflow and outflow control mechanisms. Changes in fluid volume and pressure cause corresponding changes in dura mater membrane tensions that induce small accommodative movement patterns in these membranes. Research at Michigan State University showed that the bones that directly relate to the dura mater must be in continual, minute motion to accommodate the constant fluid pressure changes within the membrane compartment. This finding is consistent with those published in *Anatomica Humanica* by Italian professor Guiseppi Sperino, who noted that cranial sutures fuse before death only under pathologic circumstances. The 30th American Edition of *Gray's Anatomy* acknowledges that some cranial sutures possess potential for movement throughout life.

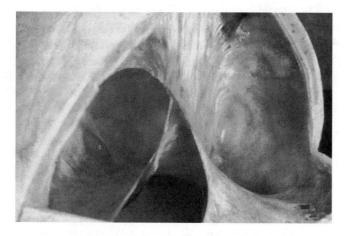

The intracranial membrane system is revealed by carefully removing brain tissue with a gloved hand to ensure that the membranes remain intact. This view from an anterior-lateral perspective illustrates the manner in which the falx cerebri separates to form the two leaves of the tentorium cerebelli. Also shown is the nerve tract that communicates with the sagittal suture and ventricular spaces.

Forms of Therapy

The methods of treatment always focus on the gentle, hands-on CranioSacral therapy approach. Within this context there are a number of techniques that the practitioner may employ based on the patient's condition. The techniques that are in the repertoire of most CranioSacral therapists and most frequently used are the following:

Energy cyst release: This technique is a hands-on method of releasing foreign or disruptive and obstructive energies from the patient's body. Energy cysts may cause dysfunction of the tissues and organs where they are located. This intention is usually derived from the patient's body; it is less often formulated by the therapist.

Direction of energy: This technique is done by intending energy to be passed from one hand of the therapist to the other through part of the patient's body. Dr. Sutherland first wrote about this concept in the 1930s. In the 1970s Dr. Upledger began advocating this technique for any part of the body that was injured, dysfunctional, or painful. It differs from polarity therapy in that its positioning and direction of energy is responsive almost en toto to the intention of the therapist or facilitator.

Myofascial release: An integral part of every CranioSacral therapist's repertoire, this technique is a manipulative form of bodywork, which seeks to restore balance to the body by releasing tension in the fascia.

Position of release: This technique involves following the patient's body into the position in which the original injury occurred, then holding that position until the traumatic experience is released. The correct position of release is dictated by the memory of the tissues. It is signified by a sudden cessation of the rhythmic activity of the craniosacral system.

Somatoemotional release: An offshoot of CranioSacral therapy, this technique developed by Dr. Upledger in the late 1970s is used to rid the mind and body of residual effects of past injuries and negative experiences locked in the tissues. Once energy cysts are released and the compensatory activities are no longer required, the body's self-correcting abilities take over allowing for more efficient use of body energy and neurologic function. It differs from energy cyst release and position of release techniques in that these two approaches are focused on a known or suspected problem, whereas somatoemotional release has no preconceived direction.

Demographics

CranioSacral therapy practitioners include osteopathic physicians, medical doctors, doctors of chiropractic, doctors of oriental medicine, naturopathic physicians, psychiatric specialists, psychologists, dentists, physical therapists, occupational therapists, nurses, acupuncturists, massage therapists, and other professional bodyworkers. There are practitioners in 56 countries around the world, with the largest concentration in the United States and Canada.

Patients range from newborns to older adults. They tend to be prior or current users of other manual therapies or advocates of noninvasive treatment modalities.

Indications and Reasons for Referral

CranioSacral therapy is very useful both as a primary and adjunct treatment modality. Because it enhances the body's own self-corrective mechanisms the therapy has been useful for a wide variety of problems that result from physiologic imbalances and obstructions, such as many types of visceral dysfunction. It works well to balance autonomic function and reduce sympathetic nervous system tonus. Substantial positive effects have been shown for chronic fatigue syndrome, chronic headaches, temporomandibular joint problems, whiplash, and an assortment of chronic pain syndromes.

CranioSacral therapy has been used effectively for children in cases of spastic cerebral palsy, seizure disorders, Down's syndrome, and a variety of central nervous system disorders and autonomic dysfunction.

Although there currently are no formal clinical studies, CranioSacral therapy also has been very effective in cases of endogenous depression, often in conjunction with treatment for endocrine imbalance. In combination with other body-mind therapies, it has shown to be efficacious in cases of posttraumatic stress disorder that is secondary to a wide range of causes.

Office Applications

A simple ranking of conditions responsive to this form of therapy is as follows. As with all alternative therapies, use of CranioSacral therapy does not preclude the use of mainstream medical therapies in addition.

Top level: *A therapy ideally suited for these conditions*
- Attention deficit disorder: CranioSacral therapy is used extensively with a high percentage of success.
- Headache: The CranioSacral therapy approach is excellent at identifying and effectively treating a wide variety of underlying causes for headaches.
- Otitis media: Temporal bone mobilization by CranioSacral therapy often is beneficial in otitis media, especially in prevention of its reoccurrence in chronic patients.
- Pain: CranioSacral therapy, by its effects on the autonomics, desensitizes facilitated segments and enhances fluid exchange throughout the body and psychoemotional effects.
- Wellness and health maintenance: An evaluation of the craniosacral system can reveal clues to very early onset problems that could be otherwise overlooked. In addition, good craniosacral system function is essential to higher levels of good health.

Second level: *One of the better therapies for these conditions*

- Autism: After CranioSacral therapy, patients generally inflict much less pain upon themselves, display affection toward others, and show greatly improved social behavior.
- Fibromyalgia: Results depend upon the underlying causes. However, good results usually are expected.
- Gastroenteritis: Best effects of CranioSacral therapy are obtained through the autonomic nervous system and related spinal cord segments.
- Heart disease: Excellent effects have been seen in angina patients, probably because of the positive effect of CranioSacral therapy on both the autonomics and related spinal cord segments, as well as its ability to reduce stress and anxiety.
- Osteoarthritis: CranioSacral therapy enhances fluid motion, releases muscle tonus, and desensitizes facilitated segments, all of which contribute to joint rejuvenation.
- Pneumonia: CranioSacral therapy enhances immune function, lymphatic drainage, tissue relaxation, and fluid exchange, and it desensitizes related facilitated segments. It also helps resolve fear and hysteria.
- Rheumatoid arthritis: Excellent responses have been reported as singular cases. Some reports state that blood studies have normalized.
- Sinusitis: CranioSacral therapy enhances blood flow to and lymphatic drainage from the involved areas, as well as improving mucus drainage, autonomic function, and immune function. It also reduces pain sensitivity.

Third level: *A valuable adjunctive therapy for these conditions*

- Chronic Fatigue Syndrome: Whether CranioSacral therapy is used as a primary or adjunctive treatment depends on the cause of this condition. Most therapists report improvement in about half the cases.
- Back pain: Once the underlying cause is determined, CranioSacral therapy is effective in biomechanical, neurogenic, and facilitated segment problems.
- Menstrual irregularity: CranioSacral therapy enhances the mobilization of fluids and autonomic balancing, improves endocrine control, and relieves neuromusculoskeletal and psychoemotional symptoms.

Practical Applications

CranioSacral therapy is useful as both a primary treatment modality and an adjunctive therapy. Many CranioSacral therapy practitioners may also incorporate acupuncture, manipulation, chakra balancing, Reiki, Alexander work, Feldenkreis work, general medicine, homeopathy, dentistry, psychotherapy, hypnotherapy, and spiritual counseling into the therapy session. Other health care providers may refer their patients to clinicians who practice CranioSacral therapy.

Research Base

Evidence Based

As a stepping stone toward clinical application of CranioSacral therapy, an interrater reliability study was devised. Twenty-five nursery school children were examined by two of four examiners on each of 19 evaluation parameters. The parameters, however, did not include the rate or amplitude of the craniosacral rhythm because these vary with examiner touch, intention, sharing of energy, and spontaneous "still points." The percentage of agreement varied from 72% to 92%, depending on the examiners and the allowed variance of either 0% or 0.5%.[1]

In a subsequent study, Dr. Upledger used this 19-parameter evaluation protocol to examine 203 schoolchildren. A technician recorded the orally reported data for a statistician, who collected information from each child's school file and historical data from interviews with the parents. This information was compared with the craniosacral system examination findings. The study results showed that the standardized quantifiable craniosacral system motion examination represents a practical approach to the study of relationships between craniosacral system dysfunctions and a variety of health, behavior, and performance problems.[2]

Other researchers have done similar studies related to psychiatric disorders[3] and symptomatology in newborns.[4]

Basic Science

Although Dr. Sutherland had theorized that human sutures were capable of movement through life, Dr. Upledger worked with Ernest W. Retzlaff, PhD, to find a scientific basis for this belief. Studying bone specimens taken from live surgical patients between the ages of 7 through 57 years, they were able to demonstrate definite potential for movement between the cranial sutures.[5-10]

Several initial studies laid the foundation for developing a model to explain the mechanism for the craniosacral system. An important factor was Dr. Upledger's discovery of what appeared to be fascia hanging from the free border of the falx cerebri on some cranium dissections of both embalmed and unembalmed cadavers. Under the microscope, these tissues appeared to be nerve tracts running out of the falx cerebri with brain tissue attached to their free end. Further research indicated that they were indeed the components of a nerve impulse and message delivery system between these intrasutural receptors and walls of the ventricles of the brain, wherein the choroid plexuses were located.[7,8]

Drs. Karni, Retzlaff, and Upledger named their explanation of the craniosacral system's function the *Pressurestat Model*. In this model the tough outer layer of the meningeal membranes (dura mater) forms a water-tight container. The cerebrospinal fluid contained within the system is extracted from the blood through a system called the choroid plexus, which is located largely within the lateral ventricles of the brain. The production or inflow of cerebrospinal fluid from the blood is rhythmic and is most likely controlled by fluctuations in the volume and pressure of cerebrospinal fluid within the dura mater (see "Suggested Reading").

The outflow of cerebrospinal fluid from the craniosacral system is through the arachnoid villae and granulation bodies, which are located within the venous sinuses of the intracranial membrane. These sinuses are a part of the path that the blood uses to return to the heart after its supply of oxygen has been delivered to the tissues. The resorption of cerebrospinal fluid back into the blood is constant rather than rhythmic as in the inflow of fluid into the system. In essence, the craniosacral system functions as a semi-closed hydraulic system (see "Suggested Reading").

Risk and Safety

Treatment techniques are based on gradual reestablishment of motion of all tissues that influence the craniosacral system. The CranioSacral therapy practitioner uses light touch—generally about five grams of pressure, which is about the weight of a nickel—to follow the movement patterns of the bones and tissues. This indirect method enhances natural corrective forces upon the bones, sutures, meningeal membranes, and related fasciae. When the therapist follows this gentle approach the method is extremely safe in most situations.

Efficacy

CranioSacral therapy aims to establish motion where stasis exists and enhances motion where partial restriction is present. The motion referred to ranges from gross joint motion to intracellular fluid and particle motion and all things in between. Clinical experience has demonstrated that CranioSacral therapy is helpful in at least 90% of patients. This does *not* mean that 90% of specific diseases are helped; it means that 90% of the time natural healing processes are facilitated.

The number of sessions required to achieve results is extremely variable, depending on the complexity of the layers of adaptation, patient defense mechanisms, and other factors. After an initial hands-on evaluation is conducted by a CranioSacral therapy practitioner, a recommendation can be made for that individual. In general, if there is no change in condition after six sessions, CranioSacral therapy may not be effective for that individual.

Future Research Opportunities and Priorities

Clinical outcome studies would be a high research priority. Some studies currently underway involve pain patients, juvenile offenders, and infants in a hospital neonatal intensive care unit.

Druglike Information

Safety

Generally using about five grams of pressure, the CranioSacral therapy practitioner evaluates the body's craniosacral system by testing for the craniosacral rhythm in various parts of the body, with the skull and sacrum most easily palpated. The practitioner uses light touch to follow the movement patterns of the bones and tissue. This indirect method enhances the natural corrective properties of the fascia and membranes. When the therapist follows this gentle approach the method is extremely safe and effective.

Warnings, Contraindications, and Precautions

Contraindications to CranioSacral therapy include any condition wherein a subtle change in intracranial fluid pressure could be deleterious. Among these are acute intracranial aneurysm with threat of rupture, cerebral hemorrhage for other reasons, subdural or subarachnoid bleeding, and increased intracranial pressure that could precipitate a medullary or brain stem herniation through the foramen magnum.

Drug or Other Interactions

Because CranioSacral therapy does not involve the use of drugs, these interactions do not occur. However, CranioSacral therapy may potentiate the effect of injected insulin in diabetic patients. Therefore close monitoring of blood sugar levels and appropriate modification of insulin doses should be carried out while a diabetic patient is undergoing CranioSacral therapy treatment. CranioSacral therapy also has been seen to potentiate the effects of antiseizure medications and psychopharmaceuticals. Therefore appropriate adjustments in dosages may be required.

Adverse Reactions

Some patients may experience mild posttreatment discomfort. One reason may be that their bodies are reexperiencing a previous trauma or injury as they are releasing from the tissues. These processes may require a few days to resolve. Another temporarily unpleasant reaction may occur when areas of "numbness" come back to "life" and are more sensitive. Also, just as the body has adapted to a malfunction, when the adaptation is removed, suppressed pain may resurface. There are many individual reasons for temporary worsening of symptoms following an effective treatment.

Pregnancy and Lactation

There are no contraindications to CranioSacral therapy. In fact, these conditions are indications as the therapy can help maintain a good hormone balance, alleviate postpartum depression, and restore normal pelvic function, thus eliminating many postdelivery back problems.

Trade Products, Administration, and Dosage

The term *CranioSacral therapy* was coined by Upledger and his fellow researchers Karni and Retzlaff to describe the therapy developed from research at Michigan State University. Previously the only type of cranial work that existed was Cranial Osteopathy, which was developed by William Sutherland and practiced by a select group of osteopathic physicians. Although there are other types of cranial work taught and practiced today the majority of practitioners have undertaken postgraduate study of CranioSacral therapy with The Up-ledger Institute, a health resource center established in 1985.

Self-Help versus Professional

Although the best results can be obtained through a skilled professional practitioner, there are some techniques that a layperson can be taught that may be used to supplement clinical sessions by a professional practitioner.

ShareCare, a 1-day workshop open to anyone, offers hands-on training and experience in palpating the rhythmical activity of the craniosacral system throughout the body. Workshop attendees are taught how to alleviate a wide variety of pain and symptoms by bringing the craniosacral system to a "still point" wherein the system readjusts itself and by using direction of energy techniques on an affected area of the body.

A self-help device called a "Stillpoint Inducer" also can bring about a therapeutic pause in the craniosacral system activity. It can be used by most people for approximately 15 minutes any time, up to four times per day.

Visiting a Professional

In CranioSacral therapy the usual sequence of events as carried out in conventional medicine is reversed. Rather than beginning patient evaluation by taking a verbal history as is the conventional approach, the CranioSacral therapist begins the evaluation through touch or palpation. The patient, who is fully clothed, rests on a padded table. Most often the therapist gently requests that the patient not talk about the complaints and medical and surgical histories until after the completion of the initial hands-on evaluation. Patients subjectively report an increased sense of well-being, improved sleep patterns, reduced manifestation of stress, normalization of blood pressure, reduction or disappearance of pain, increased energy levels, and fewer incidences of transitory illness.

Credentialing

CranioSacral therapy was originally brought forth as an additional treatment modality for practicing health care professionals. Since that time, the method has grown so rapidly that development of a specific certification for CranioSacral therapy became apparent. The Up-ledger Institute offers two levels of national certification for professional practitioners of CranioSacral therapy, involving a stringent three-part examination process of written, oral, and hands-on testing.

Training

Training in CranioSacral therapy for health care practitioners is conducted worldwide by The Upledger Institute. The training consists of postgraduate instruction comprised of lecture, demonstration, and practice. Continuing education units often are granted for these courses; professionals are advised to check with the appropriate licensing board.

The Upledger Institute
11211 Prosperity Farms Rd.
Palm Beach Gardens, FL 33410
Tel: (561) 622-4334
Toll-Free: (800) 233-5880
Fax: (561) 622-4771
www.upledger.com/acsta

What to Look for in a Provider

One requirement for practitioners is that they are licensed to practice in a health care profession that legally allows them to do CranioSacral therapy or they are practicing according to local laws, which vary widely. In general, we recommend a practitioner who has had advanced training or is certified in CranioSacral therapy. That person could be a medical doctor, osteopathic physician, dentist, chiropractor, registered nurse, physical therapist, occupational therapist, massage therapist, Rolfer, Soma practitioner, another type of bodyworker, or acupuncturist. The main issue is hands-on skill in addition to your personal evaluation of that person as a health care provider.

Barriers and Key Issues

Perhaps the largest stumbling block remains the belief held by students of the British anatomic model that skull bones fuse and are not designed for movement. Health care professionals who subscribe to the Italian anatomic model based on studies of unembalmed cadavers have long appreciated the subtleties of skull bone movement. Medical training of other anatomic models would be helpful to defuse this dogma.

The length of a typical CranioSacral therapy session—30 to 90 minutes of uninterrupted time with a single patient—has caused some health professionals to shy away from its use. However, those who recognize the potential benefits of the therapy may incorporate one or two techniques into their usual treatment time. Other health care providers refer their patients to CranioSacral therapy practitioners within their offices or outside their practices for adjunctive therapy.

Associations

The American CranioSacral Therapy Association, a nonprofit organization, was founded by a group of therapists and concerned laypersons in 1994. Its stated objectives are to bring CranioSacral therapy into public awareness, enhance networking between practitioners who use CranioSacral therapy, develop and institute the use of a certification program that will result in recognition of CranioSacral therapy as a specialty for persons who are licensed as health care practitioners in other fields, and ultimately develop CranioSacral therapy as an independently licensed and free-standing profession.

The American CranioSacral Therapy Association
c/o The Upledger Institute
11211 Prosperity Farms Rd.
Palm Beach Gardens, FL 33410
Tel: (561) 622-4334
Toll-Free: (800) 233-5880
Fax: (561) 622-4771
www.upledger.com/acsta

Suggested Reading

1. Cohen D: *An introduction to CranioSacral therapy*, Berkeley, Calif, 1995, North Atlantic Books.
   The book presents an overview of the various diagnostic, evaluative, and therapeutic approaches to the cranium, sacrum, dura mater envelope, and cerebrospinal fluid.
2. Upledger JE, Vredevoogd JD: *CranioSacral therapy*, Seattle, 1983, Eastland Press.
   In this book the authors define the physiology and anatomy of the craniosacral system, its function in health, and it relationship to disease processes.
3. Upledger JE: *Your inner physician and you*, Berkeley, Calif, 1991, Atlantic Books, and The Upledger Institute, Palm Beach Gardens, Fla.
   Dr. Upledger recounts his experiences investigating and developing CranioSacral Therapy. He describes today's applications of the therapy and his further explorations relating to the method.
4. Upledger JE: *A brain is born: exploring the birth and development of the central nervous system*, Berkeley, Calif, 1996, North Atlantic Books, and The Upledger Institute, Palm Beach Gardens, Fla.
   This in-depth, practical guide is helpful for professionals or parents interested in how the brain is formed and how its functioning affects health.

Bibliography

Gilmore NJ: Right brain, left brain asymmetry, *ACLD Newsbriefs*, July-August 1978.

Upledger JE, Vredevoogd JD: *CranioSacral therapy*, Seattle, 1983, Eastland Press.

Upledger JE: Craniosacral function in brain dysfunction, *Osteopath Ann* 11:318-324, 1983.

Upledger JE, Vredevoogd JD: Management of autogenic headache, *Osteopath Ann* 1979.

References

1. Upledger JE: Reproducibility of craniosacral examination findings: a statistical analysis, *JAOA* 76:890-899, 1977.

2. Upledger JE: Relationship of craniosacral examination findings in grade school children with developmental problems, *JAOA* 77:760-776, 1978.

3. Woods JM, Woods RH: Physical finding related to psychiatric disorder, *JAOA* 60:988-993, 1961.

4. Frymann VM: Relation of disturbances of craniosacral mechanisms to symptomatology of the newborn: a study of 1250 infants, *JAOA* 65:1059, 1966.

5. Retzlaff EW et al: Possible functional significance of cranial bone sutures. Report presented at the 88th Session of the American Association of Anatomists, 1975.

6. Retzlaff EW et al: Structure of cranial bone sutures, research report, *JAOA* 75:607-608, 1976.

7. Retzlaff EW et al: Sutural collagenous and their innervation in saimiri sciureus, *Anat Rec* 187:692, 1977.

8. Retzlaff EW et al: Nerve fibers and endings in cranial sutures, research report, *JAOA* 77:474-475, 1978.

9. Retzlaff EW, Mitchell FL Jr: *The cranium and its sutures,* Heidelberg, 1987, Springer-Verlag Berlin.

10. Upledger JE: Research and observations support the existence of a craniosacral system, *Alt Med J* 2:31-43, 1995.

Feldenkrais Method®

FRANK WILDMAN

JAMES STEPHENS

LEYA AUM

Origins and History

In our society, we do, by the promise of great reward or intense punishment, so distort the even development of the system, that many acts become excluded or restricted. The result is that we have to provide special conditions for furthering adult maturation of many arrested functions. The majority of people need to re-form patterns of motions and attitudes that should never have been excluded or neglected.

The method is named after the Israeli scientist Moshe Feldenkrais, DSc (1904-1984). Feldenkrais worked as a nuclear physicist with the Nobel laureate Joliot-Curie. After injuring his knee in a soccer game, Dr. Feldenkrais learned that a surgery had only a 50% chance of improving his condition, but if the surgery were unsuccessful it would confine him to a wheelchair for the rest of his life. Unsatisfied with these prospects, he proceeded to learn anatomy, kinesiology, and physiology and combined these with his knowledge of mechanics, physics, electrical engineering, and martial arts (he wrote several books on Judo and was the first non-Japanese to earn a black belt in this discipline). This endeavor not only restored most of the function to his injured knee but also marked the beginning of his investigation into human function, development, and learning that was to occupy him for the rest of his life and eventually lead to the development of the Feldenkrais Method. From the 1970s on he taught the method throughout the world. He directed the Feldenkrais Institute in Tel Aviv until his death in 1984.

Mechanisms of Action According to Its Own Theory

Many of our failings, physical and mental, need not be considered as diseases to be cured, but rather as an acquired result of a learned faulty mode of doing. Actions repeated innumerable times for years on end, such as all our habitual actions, mould even the bones, let alone the muscular envelope. The physical faults that appear in our body long after we were born are mainly the result of activity we have im-

posed on it. Faulty modes of standing and walking produce faulty feet, and it is the mode of standing and walking that must be corrected and not the feet.

Moshe Feldenkrais

Unlike other animals, which are preprogrammed to survive, human children must *learn* to move. Although a cat is born with the knowledge of how to move gracefully, it takes years for humans to learn movement well enough to function independently in the world. The necessity and ability to learn individual patterns of movement leads to a variety in human movement and posture unknown in other species and can be considered the most distinguishing feature of mankind.

Once they have reached a level of proficiency sufficient for walking, jumping, or playing sports, most people stop learning new movements and improving their body awareness. Whatever style of movement has been learned at this point, mostly through trial and error and imitation of models in the social environment, then begins to form a personal set of movement habits. These movement habits tend to overuse certain muscles and joints while neglecting or ignoring the use of others, thus leading to a limited range of movement and gross inefficiency.

Many people find they are simply unable to improve at activities that interest them, be they sports, dance, or music. They avoid engaging in activities where they could be confronted with a lack of coordination and awareness and never learn to ski or dance because they feel uncomfortable doing so.

Feldenkrais observed, "Through the first years of life, we organize our entire system in a direction which will forever after guide us in that direction. We end up being restricted, we don't do music, we don't do other things. What is more important, we find ourselves capable of only doing those things that we already know."

In the long run these limitations in awareness and coordination lead to physical difficulties, such as recurring pain, repetitive stress injuries. or problems recovering from injuries.

"This great ability to form individual nervous paths and muscular patterns makes it possible for faulty functioning to be learned. The earlier the fault occurs, the more engrained it appears, and is. Faulty behavior will appear in the executive motor mechanisms which will seem later, when the nervous system has grown fitted to the undesirable motility, to be inherent in the person and unalterable. It will remain largely so unless the nervous paths producing the undesirable pattern of motility are undone and reshuffled into a better configuration."

Moshe Feldenkrais, *Body and Mature Behavior*

No other animal has the ability to change and reorganize the way it performs familiar activities the way human beings can. People have the capacity to make each walk they take a different walk, completely new in style; to make each movement a new experience.

Yet this amazing capacity to learn is rarely used; most people find one way of doing something and stick to it until finally a knee or a back breaks down. Then they assume that their distress was caused by the activity they performed rather than their particular way of performing the activity.

The Feldenkrais Method sees problems as a consequence of arrested or incomplete learning that leaves its mark on all biologic functions, from digestion, breathing, and muscular control to the sexual act and social adjustment.

By recapitulating the exploratory style of learning natural to infants, patients of the Feldenkrais Method discover new ways to sense and move that expand awareness and develop more efficient and comfortable movement.

Biologic Mechanism of Action

Personal experience reduces the initially unlimited number of possible combinations of nervous interconnections to a few preferred and active patterns of moving and acting. Once an adequate and socially acceptable level of motor functioning is achieved, the process of exploratory learning and development of the body image is suspended. The acquired movement patterns grow so familiar through repeated use that they create a seemingly unalterable body image (for example, a person's walk or manner of speaking is as fixed as a signature). The body image, bound by motor habits and perceptions, becomes the basis for an individual's sense of self. Infants have a theoretically unlimited ability to change and reorganize the way they perform familiar activities. Growing into adults, they progressively restrict their repertoire of movements, using an ever-smaller part of potential human functioning.

Inefficient movement habits overwork certain muscles and joints while neglecting or ignoring the use of others, thus leading to a limited range of movement and gross inefficiency. In the long run these limitations in awareness and coordination can lead to severe physical difficulties. Parts of articulations can fill with fibrous tissues, especially between vertebrae where there is little movement in general. Ligaments shorten or become hyperelastic; some muscle fibers become too strong. Others in the same muscle group will atrophy. In the long run deformation sets in.

Forms of Therapy

The Feldenkrais Method uses two approaches in working with patients: Awareness Through Movement (ATM) lessons and Functional Integration (FI).

Awareness Through Movement

ATMs are verbally directed movement sequences presented in a group setting. Lessons generally last from 20 to 60 minutes. There are hundreds of ATMs to choose from in the Feldenkrais Method. The mechanisms of breathing, speaking and all aspects of postural control are explored and improved while perceptual capacities are increased. The aim of these lessons is not relaxation but healthy, powerful, easy, and pleasurable action.

Participants engage in precisely structured movement explorations that involve thinking, sensing, moving, and imagining. The lessons are often based on developmental movements, like rolling, crawling, or moving from lying to sitting or explorations of joint, muscle, and postural relationships. Minute, barely perceptible movements are used extensively to reduce latent tonus (degree of involuntary contractions) in the muscles. The gradual reduction of useless effort increases the kinesthetic sensitivity.

The lessons begin with comfortable, easy movements that gradually evolve into movements of greater range and complexity, recapitulating the childhood experience of originally learning to organize and control movements. Functions that require repetition to learn are taught through numerous variations that maintain the novelty of the situation. Once novelty wears off, awareness is dulled and no learning takes place.

The lessons are so arranged that they require concentration to sense kinaesthetic differences. Without real attention it is impossible to follow to the next stage in the lesson. Mechanical repetition without attention is discouraged and often impossible.

An important goal of ATM lessons is to learn how the most basic movement functions are organized and to teach awareness of the skeleton and its orientation. The participants have the opportunity to learn to eliminate unnecessary energy expenditure and efficiently mobilize their intentions into actions. Since learning is a highly individual matter, students are encouraged to learn at their own pace in a noncompetitive manner. This is why the same lesson often may benefit people of diverse ages, backgrounds, and abilities.

Functional Integration

For patients desiring more individual attention, Feldenkrais created a hands-on technique called Functional Integration (FI). Each FI lesson is tailored for the needs of the particular student; it is usually performed with the patient in a horizontal position to reduce as much as possible the influence of gravity on the body and thus free the nervous system. The reaction of the nervous system to the gravitational field has become a habit, and although this remains so, it is difficult to bring the muscles to respond differently to the same stimulus. Obviously then it is difficult to bring about any real change in the nervous system without reducing or eliminating the gravity effect.

The practitioner communicates through gentle and noninvasive touch the experience of comfort, pleasure and ease of movement, while the patient learns how to reorganize the body and behavior in new and more effective ways. The practitioner's touch is instructive and informative, not corrective. Patients are encouraged to explore new, more expanded functional motor patterns that they can then translate into new abilities.

The Feldenkrais Method offers patients new movement choices by allowing them to experience differences between effortful and effortless, efficient and inefficient, neutral and pleasurable movements. Unless individuals can sense these distinctions, they have no choice over the quality of their movements and are reduced to acting like a machine. Once they learn to differentiate movements and their qualities, they acquire alternative ways of performing the same task and regain a broader range of their possibilities.

Demographics

Feldenkrais practitioners can be found worldwide. In the United States they are concentrated along the east and west Coasts and the greater Chicago area. Countries that use the method most heavily are Australia, Germany, Sweden, Switzerland, The Netherlands, and France.

The work is used with infant, adolescent, adult, and geriatric patients.

Indications and Reasons for Referral

The Feldenkrais Method is applied to restore function lost through accident or degenerative diseases as well as to improve function in people who need to improve high-level skills.

It is used with all types of clinical disorders, from hemiplegia and cerebral palsy to acute or chronic back and other pain problems. It is used by professional athletes, dancers and musicians who have recurring injuries or stress symptoms and by coaches and physical education teachers in movement analysis and teaching technique. Other major areas of application include older adults with motor limitations, people with breathing disorders, and those suffering from chronic anxiety and psychosomatic disorders.

Office Applications

A simple ranking of conditions responsive to this form of therapy is as follows. As with all alternative therapies, use of the Feldenkrais Method does not preclude the use of mainstream medical therapies in addition.

Top level: *A therapy ideally suited for these conditions*

Autism; back pain; balance problems; cerebral palsy; chronic anxiety; chronic
. fatigue syndrome; chronic pain; closed head injuries; CVA (stroke); dystonia; fibromyalgia; head and neck pain; irritable bowel syndrome; motor limitations; multiple sclerosis; muscular dystrophy; neurologic disorders; open head injuries; orthopedic injuries; postpartum care; postsurgical tissue trauma; psychosomatic disorders; repetitive stress injuries; stress; temporomandibular joint pain; and whiplash

Second level: *One of the better therapies for these conditions*

Hypertension; insomnia; lazy eye; osteoarthritis; osteoporosis; periodic leg movement syndrome; sleep disorders; and tinnitus

Third level: *A valuable adjunctive therapy for these conditions*

Arthritis; cancer; constipation; emphysema; menstrual cramps; and vision

Research Base

Evidence Based

The first research study involving Feldenkrais Method (FM) was published in 1977 with several more appearing in the next decade. Since 1988 there has been an increasing amount of research done and recently this has been increasing each year. Because FM has such a wide range of effects, a wide range of outcomes has been looked at and reported. Most of the clinical studies to date have involved a very small number of subjects (6 or fewer). Some are larger, using control group designs. The areas of outcome break down into the following four general themes:

1. **Pain management:** Case studies describing the resolution of chronic back pain following the failure of other methods to ameliorate the problems have been published by Lake[1] and Panarello-Black.[2] A retrospective study of 34 patients using FM as an adjunct to treatment in a chronic pain management clinic showed that FM helped to reduce the pain and improve function and still was used independently by patients 2 years postdischarge.[3] Dennenberg[4] showed decreased pain and increased functional mobility using FM as a component of treatment for 15 pain patients. The primary result of this study was to show that there were changes in the pattern of health locus of control in patients participating in FM. A study using a group ATM intervention with five fibromyalgia patients showed significant decrease in pain and improved posture, gait, sleep, and body awareness.[5] Lake[6] showed changes in posture in patients with chronic back pain following FM. Chinn et al[7] showed improvements in functional reach in symptomatic subjects. Ideberg[8] showed significant changes in pelvic rotation and pelvic obliquity during rapid walking in 10 patients with back pain compared to normal controls, following a series of Functional Integration lessons. Narula showed decreased pain and improved function, including improved biomechanic efficiency, measured by motion analysis, in a sit-to-stand transfer from a chair, in several people with rheumatoid arthritis following 6 weeks of ATM lessons.[9]

2. **Functional performance and motor control:** Function is a result of movement. Changes in the process of control of movement therefore influence function. As noted above in relation to pain patients, there were changes in movement pattern leading to reduction of pain. These were patterns involved in the activities of walking[8], transfers[9,10] posture, reaching, and general activities of daily living.[11,12]

   As well as with orthopedic pain patients, functional improvements have been described in people with neurologic diagnoses. Although there was no formal quantitative assessment of balance, four women with multiple sclerosis reported improvements in balance in daily activities and improved walking and transfers, as assessed by video motion analysis.[13]

   Shenkman described improvements in posture in individuals with Parkinson's disease using FM as part of the intervention strategy.[14] Shelhav-Silberbush has reported case studies of two children with cerebral palsy who made major functional gains during several years of FM work.[15] Ginsburg has anecdotally described functional and motor control improvements in young people with spinal cord injuries who were involved in the "Shake a Leg" program.[16] Gilman has reported improved control of stuttering in two patients.[43]

   As well as improving function in people with impairments, FM also is used to improve athletic function. At this time the evidence for this is mostly anecdotal for skiiing[17] and kayaking. Jackson-Wyatt[18] has reported a case study of improved jumping following a Feldenkrais intervention.

   There also is interest in athletic injury prevention using ATM to improve flexibility and control. An initial study published in this area showed no increase in hamstring length following a single ATM lesson.[19] However, this study has several important design problems and further work is underway as follow-up.

3. **Psychologic effects:** Feldenkrais' initial intentions in the application of his work were to improve a person's awareness of the body in action (Awareness through Movement), improving the integration of functions (Functional Integration) and thereby effect a process of change leading to greater emotional maturity.[20,21] This has been studied very little. Dennenberg[4] has noted changes in health locus of control. Self-efficacy has been shown to be a significant correlate of successful rehabilitation, but there have been no studies published on this to date. Several studies are under way with patients with diagnoses of multiple sclerosis and fibromyalgia.

In an interesting study using analysis of clay figures, Deig described expansion in the detail and form of body image after a series of ATM lessons.[22] Shelhav-Silberbush has shown improvements in mobility skills, social function and IQ scores in a class of learning impaired children.[23] Recently, in a matched control group study with 30 children with eating disorders, Laumer concluded that a course of ATM facilitated an acceptance of the body and self, decreased feelings of helplessness and dependence, increased self-confidence, and a general process of maturation of the whole personality.[24]

4. **Quality of life:** Quality of life and its associated measures of perceived health status is becoming an increasingly important and widely used construct in assessing the overall outcome of a process of rehabilitation. In a problematic study that showed no significant functional or physiologic changes, Gutman[25] showed a trend toward improvement in overall perception of health status in a healthy older adult population. This finding has been corroborated in a similar population by improvements in vitality and mental health as measured by the SF-36[26] and in a group of women with multiple sclerosis using the Index of Well-Being.[13,27]

Basic Science

Theory underlying the Feldenkrais Method assumes a process of learning that is based in hard changes in the nervous system. Through this process an image of the body is constructed that corresponds to movement. In movement a person then interacts with the environment in a loop of perception and action that further refines movement and the sensory-perceptual processes. Dynamic systems theory as described by Thelen[28] and Kelso[29] best fits the observed processes of the Feldenkrais Method. This theory accounts for the process of skill acquisition, functional development, and organization change resulting from changes in posture and coordination[30] and relies on an understanding of the body as having a modifiable internal representation of body scheme[31] that includes the shape of the body surface, limb length, sequence of linkage, and position in space.[32] The process of skill acquisition, coordination change, or functional or motor development is driven by a process of active exploration involving awareness.[27,33]

Over the last 15 years, research in the area of neuroplasticity has built a solid foundation for the concept that interaction with the environment and changes in the structure of the body are represented by measurable changes in the process of representation in the cortex.[34,35] These changes may underlie and be related to basic processes of learning.[36,37] This plasticity of the central nervous system may be both the source of chronic functional problems and the means to recovery from them.[38,39]

Although none of the research on Feldenkrais Method addresses this basic level of physiologic function, physiologic changes do occur that fit within this theoretic framework. Some functional changes have been mentioned in the previous section. Others include changes in function of trunk and cervical muscles reflected by changes in EMG activity,[40,41] changes in muscle function and posture related to improvements in abdominal breathing,[42] and changes in body image or scheme.[21,23] Narula[43] also has reported increases in EMG activity in cases of low back pain where it appears that painful muscles had become inactive. It may be that reintegration of these muscles into normal movement patterns stimulates blood flow and thus a normal healing process.

Risk and Safety

There is very little risk involved in the use of this method. It is both conservative and safe. People are instructed to stay generally within the bounds of pain-free ranges of motion and use as little effort as possible to perform a movement. Comfort and ease and the explicit guides are understood to be part of the optimal conditions for learning. It is still possible for a person who has fibromyalgia or adhesive capsulitis to do too much and have pain as a result. However, if this should occur, limits are learned that then can be applied to future sessions. This kind of outcome happens infrequently and most often in home sessions not supervised by a practitioner, in which the student reverts back to a "more is better" philosophy so common in our culture. Often as a result of a slow and comfortable approach, people learn that they can do much more with much greater safety and comfort than they had imagined possible.

Efficacy

Generally, no statistics are known or published on the efficacy of this method. All conclusions about this are based on hearsay and general impressions. One of the authors (JS) takes the liberty here to report on the efficacy of using Feldenkrais Method as part of a rehabilitation process with 166 patients over the last 5 years in his private practice. Outcome has been judged on percentage of the original goals established at the initial visit that were achieved by the time of discharge. Four levels of outcome were used: 1) 100% achieved; 2) 75% to 90% achieved; 3) 50% to 75% achieved; and 4) less than 50% achieved.

Orthopedic cases made up 84% and neurologic cases made up 16% of the population. Age range was from 8 to 84 years, with most people being between 30 and 60 years. In 35 cases of back pain, 77% reached level 1 outcome and 91% reached a level 1 or 2. Of 20 cases of osteoarthritis, 80% reached level 1 and 95% reached level 1 or 2. 76% of 17 people with a primary diagnosis of neck pain reached level 1 and 88% reached at least level 2. In 13 shoulder diagnoses, 69% achieved level 1 and 92% reached at least level 2. Of 6 people with fibromyalgia, 83% reached level 1 and all reached at least level 2. Of 14 people with tendonitis or bursitis or other hip and knee problems, 85% reached level 1, an additional 7% reached level 2, and another 7% reached level 3. Of 8 people with back and leg pain from spinal stenosis of spondylolisthesis, 63% achieved level 1, an additional 12% reached level 2, and 25% achieved level 3 or 4. Of 3 TMJ cases, 2 reached level 1 and the other reached level 2. And of 5 people with scoliosis, 80% reached level 1 and 20% reached level 3. Reaching level 1 does not mean that the scoliosis was reversed. It means that pain was significantly reduced and function improved with long-term success.

Of the 27 neurologic cases, 60% were people with multiple sclerosis or stroke. Of the people with stroke, 50% achieved level 1 and 50% achieved level 2. Of the multiple sclerosis cases, 50% reached level 1 and only 17% were discharged below level 2.

Overall, out of 166 patients, 70% reached level 1, 22% reached level 2, 6.6% reached level 3, and 1.2% were at level 4 at discharge.

Future or Ongoing Research

As we stated at the beginning of this section, research on the Feldenkrais Method has just started in the last 10 years. Several studies now are in progress related to balance and self-efficacy in people with multiple sclerosis; function and length of the hamstrings; pain, function, and self-efficacy in people with fibromyalgia; the efficacy of ATM as an adjunct to cardiac rehabilitation; and back pain related to postural and motor control variables. The Feldenkrais Guild also is in the process of establishing a procedure for systematic collection of outcome data by all practitioners across the U.S. who want to participate in a multisite outcome study.

Other areas for future research include: injury prevention and performance enhancement in athletes, dancers, and musicians; controlled outcome studies with people who have had strokes, head injuries, and cerebral palsy; introduction of ATM into elementary schools to enhance self-image, attention capacity, and learning; study of other psychologic dimensions, such as body scheme, self-esteem, self-efficacy, anxiety, and learning; and inquiry into physiologic mechanisms of action, including balance and postural control, proprioception, and timing and sequencing on muscle activity in movements.

Visiting a Professional

The Feldenkrais Method is a learning experience, and people learn best when comfortable. Awareness Through Movement classes are taught on a floor with a carpet or mats, on chairs, or in standing position. Students pay attention to their own sensations and movements as the teacher guides them to explore a basic subject, such as how to improve turning so students can see farther around themselves with less effort and more integrated movement.

For Functional Integration, the Feldenkrais hands-on work, the practitioner takes a functional movement history and inquires as to duration and possible causes of the complaint. The practitioner explains that Feldenkrais work is not a medical procedure or substitute for medical attention. During the initial interview the practitioner observes the postural habits of the student. Then the clothed student lies, sits, or stands in one of about 30 different positions. The practitioner supports the student's postural habits with pillows so that the student is most comfortable and able to breathe. This means a person who is significantly bent forward in standing will require ample pillows behind the head when reclined, so the habitual curvature is supported. The student is asked to pay attention and neither help nor hinder. The practitioner works gently. Each hands-on lesson and class develops several basic functional subjects, such as balance, breathing, turning, or finding the relationship between the head and the pelvis.

Credentialing

Initial certification is granted by the educational director of training programs after students have passed a supervised clinic. Certification must be maintained through continuing education requirements on a biannual basis.

The Guild of Certified Feldenkrais Practitioners sets standards for Training Programs and certification.

Training

The training required to be a certified Feldenkrais practitioner requires 160 days of training spread over a period of over 3 years. The trainings are usually taught in segments meeting two or three times per year. The trainings prepare students to teach Awareness Through Movement lessons to groups and develop a private practice in Functional Integration. Competence and achievement are addressed on a continual basis throughout the duration of the program on an individual basis. Students enter trainings in this method from a wide variety of backgrounds.

What to Look for in a Provider

As with any art or craft, the longer practitioners have worked, the more sure are their hands and the greater levels of expertise and mastery they have developed. The directory of practitioners from the Feldenkrais Guild indicates the year in which each practitioner completed professional training.

The patient should feel trust for and rapport with the practitioner, particularly for Functional Integration, in which the patient will be physically touched.

Barriers and Key Issues

As physicians are recognizing the brain-body relationship and the importance of learning, interest in this scientifically-based system continues to grow.

Associations and Training Institutions

Feldenkrais Guild of North America
524 Ellsworth St. SW
PO Box 489
Albany, OR 97321
Tel: (541) 926-0981
Fax: (541) 926-0572
E-mail: feldngld@peak.org
www.feldenkrais.com

Movement Studies Institute
1832 Second St.
Berkeley, CA 94707
Tel: (800) 342-3424
Fax: (510) 548-4349
E-mail and Website: www.movementstudies.com

Suggested Reading

1. Feldenkrais M: *Body and mature behavior*, New York, 1970, International Universities Press.
   This technical book presents the theory of the Feldenkrais Method with supporting references drawn from physics, physiology, and psychology.
2. Feldenkrais M: *Awareness through movement*, New York, 1972, Harper & Row.
   Dr. Feldenkrais gives a 60-page introduction to his theory, written in an easy-to-understand style, then presents 12 Awareness Through Movement lessons, which readers can explore on their own.
3. Feldenkrais M: *The elusive obvious*, Cupertino, Calif, 1981, Meta Publications.
4. Feldenkrais M: *Adventures in the jungle of the brain; the case of Nora*, New York, 1977, Harper & Row.
5. Wildman F: *Feldenkrais: a guide for physical intelligence*, Berkeley, Calif, 1999, Intelligent Body Press.

Additional Resources

1. *The Intelligent Body:* Feldenkrais Professional audio and video tapes for home or hospital use are available through the Movement Studies Institute, 1832 Second St., Berkeley, CA 94707.

This company is directed by the author.

References

1. Lake B: Acute back pain: treatment by the application of Feldenkrais principles, *Austra Fam Physician* 14(11):1175-1178, 1985.

2. Panarello-Black D: PT's own back pain leads her to start Feldenkrais training, *PT Bull,* April 8, 1992: 9.

3. Phipps A et al: A functional outcome study on the use of movement re-education in chronic pain management, master's thesis, Forest Grove, Ore, May 1997, Pacific University, School of Physical Therapy.

4. Dennenberg N, Reeves GD: Changes in health locus of control and activities of daily living in a physical therapy clinic using the Feldenkrais method of sensory motor education, master's thesis, Rochester, Mich, 1995, Oakland University, Program in Physical Therapy.

5. Dean JR, Yuen SA, Barrows SA: Effects of a Feldenkrais ATM sequence on fibromyalgia patients. Abstract presented at the North American Feldenkrais Guild Conference, Los Angeles, September 1998.

6. Lake B: Photoanalysis of standing posture in controls and low back pain: effects of kinesthetic processing (Feldenkrais method) in posture and gait: control mechanisms VII, Eugene, 1992, University of Oregon Press.

7. Chinn J et al: Effect of a Feldenkrais intervention on symptomatic subjects performing a functional reach, *Isokinetics Exer Sci* 4(4):131-136, 1994.

8. Ideberg G, Werner M: Gait assessment by three-dimensional motion analysis in subjects with chronic low back pain treated according to Feldenkrais principles. An exploratory study. Unpublished Manuscript, Lund, 1995, Lund University, Department of Physical Therapy.

9. Narula M, Jackson O, Kulig K: The effects of six week Feldenkrais method on selected functional parameters in a subject with rheumatoid arthritis, *Phys Ther* (suppl) 72:S86, 1992.

10. Stephens JL et al: Changes in coordination, economy of movement and well-being resulting from a 2-day workshop in Awareness Through Movement. Abstract and presentation at APTA, Combined Sections Meeting, Boston, Mass, February 1998.

11. Bennett JL et al: Effects of a Feldenkrais-based mobility program on function of a healthy elderly sample. Abstract in *Geriatrics* (American Physical Therapy Association). Presented at Combined Sections Meeting, Boston, Mass, February 1998.

12. Phipps A et al: A functional outcome study on the use of movement re-education in chronic pain management, master's thesis, Forest Grove, Ore, May 1997, Pacific University, School of Physical Therapy.

13. Stephens JL et al: Responses to 10 Feldenkrais Awareness Through Movement lessons by 4 women with multiple sclerosis: improved quality of life, *Phys Ther Case Reports,* 1999 (in press).

14. Shenkman M et al: Management of individuals with Parkinson's disease: rationale and case studies, *Phys Ther* 69:944-955, 1989.

15. Shelhav-Silberbush C: The Feldenkrais method for children with cerebral palsy, master's thesis, Berkeley, Calif, 1988, Boston University School of Education, Feldenkrais Resources.

16. Ginsburg C: The Shake-a-Leg body awareness training program: dealing with spinal injury and recovery in a new setting, *Somatics* Spring/Summer:31-42, 1986.

17. McIntyre M: Unlock the trunk, *Skiing Magazine* October, 1992.

18. Jackson-Wyatt O et al: Effects of Feldenkrais practitioner training program on motor ability: a videoanalysis, *Phys Ther* (suppl) 72:S86, 1992.

19. James ML et al: The effects of a Feldenkrais program and relaxation procedures on hamstring length, *Austra J Physiother* 44:49-54.

20. Feldenkrais M: *Body and mature behavior: a study of anxiety, sex, gravitation, and learning*, New York, 1949, International Universities Press.

21. Feldenkrais M: Awareness through movement: health exercises for personal growth, New York, 1972, Harper and Row.

22. Deig D: Self-image in relationship to Feldenkrais Awareness Through Movement classes, independent study project, Indianapolis, 1994, University of Indianapolis, Krannert Graduate School of Physical Therapy.

23. Shelhav-Silberbush C: Movement and learning: the Feldenkrais method as a learning model, doctoral dissertation, Heidelberg, 1998, Heidelberg University, Faculty of Sociology and Behavioral Sciences (in German).

24. Laumer U et al: Therapeutic effects of Feldenkrais method "Awareness Through Movement" in patients with eating disorder (in German), *Psychother Psychosom Med Psychol* 47(5):170-180, 1997.

25. Gutman G, Herbert C, Brown S: Feldenkrais versus conventional exercise for the elderly, *J Gerontol* 32(5):562-572, 1977.

26. Stephens JL et al: Changes in coordination, economy of movement and well-being resulting from a 2-day workshop in Awareness Through Movement. Abstract and presentation at the American Physical Therapy Association, Combined Sections Meeting, Boston, Mass, February 1998.

27. Bost H et al: Feldstudie zur wiiksamkeit der Feldenkrais-methode bei MS—betroffenen. deutsche multiple sklerose gesellschaft, Saarbrucken, Germany, 1994.

28. Thelen E: Motor development: a new synthesis, *Am Psychol* 50:79-95.

29. Kelso JAS: *Dynamic patterns: the self-organization of brain and behavior*, Cambridge, Mass, 1995, The MIT Press.

30. Newell KM et al: Search strategies and the acquisition of coordination. In Wallace SA, editor: *Perspectives on the coordination of movement*, North Holland, The Netherlands, 1989, Elsevier Science Publishers B.V.

31. Maisson J: Movement, posture, and equilibrium: interaction and coordination, *Progress Neurobio* 38:35-56, 1992.

32. Gurfinkel VS et al: Body scheme in the control of postural activity. In Gurfinkel VS et al, editors: *Stance and motion: facts and concepts*, New York, 1988, Plenum Press.

33. Newell KM: Motor skill acquisition, *Ann Rev Psychol* 42:213-237, 1991.

34. Kaas J: Plasticity of sensory and motor maps in adult mammals, *Ann Rev Neurosci* 14:137-167, 1991.

35. Edelman GM: *Neural darwinism: the theory of neuronal group selection*, New York, 1987, Basic Books.

36. Kandel ER, Hawkins RD: The biological basis of learning and individuality, *Sci American* 267:78-88, 1992.

37. Thach WT, Goodkin HP, Keating JG: The cerebellum and the adaptive coordination of movement, *Ann Rev Neurosci* 15:403-442, 1992.

38. Jenkins WM et al: Functional reorganization of primary somatosensory cortex in adult owl monkeys after behaviorally controlled tactile stimulation, *J Neurophys* 63:82-104, 1990.

39. Byl NN et al: A primate model for studying focal dystonia and repetitive strain injury: effects on the primary somatosensory cortex, *Phys Ther* 77:269-284, 1997.

40. Brown E, Kegerris S: Electromyographic activity of trunk musculature during a Feldenkrais Awareness through Movement lesson, *Isokinetics Exer Sci* 1(4):216-221, 1991.

41. Ruth S, Kegerreis S: Facilitating cervical flexion using a Feldenkrais method: Awareness through Movement, *J Sports Phys Ther* 16(1):25-29, 1992.

42. Saraswati S: Investigation of human postural muscles and respiratory movements, master's thesis, 1989, University of New South Wales.

43. Narula M: Effect of Awareness through Movement lesson on motor unit activity in a painful muscle. Abstract, Annual Conference of the North American Feldenkrais Guild, Berkeley, Calif, 1994.

44. Gilman M: *Reduction of tension in stuttering through somatic re-education,* master's thesis, Northwestern University, Department of Communication Sciences and Disorders, Evanston, Ill, 1997.

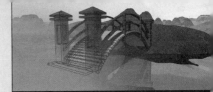

Hellerwork Structural Integration

JOSEPH HELLER

LINDA KANELAKOS FIKE

DANIEL BIENENFELD

DOUGLAS B. DRUCKER

Origins and History

Habit. Attitude. Gravity. Injury. Accommodation to discomfort or pain. These factors sculpt the body over time. We get used to them, but they eventually become noticeable in the body's structure, creating compression and restriction, and affecting our well-being in subtle ways.

Hellerwork Structural Integration is a wellness and preventive modality that consists of the following:

1. **Deep tissue bodywork:** Reduces tension and rigidity that accumulate in myofascial tissues. The bodywork releases tightness to improve body alignment, resulting in enhanced well-being.
2. **Movement reeducation:** Teaches patients how to use their bodies in keeping with its design and avoid putting unnecessary stress on their structure.
3. **Dialogue:** Enhances patients' awareness of how their attitudes affect their structure and movement patterns.

Hellerwork is a series of one-on-one sessions that address sleeve (near the surface) tissue, core tissue, and integration and balance of the core and sleeve. Through guided touch and education the body is reorganized along the line of gravity. This bodywork process is based upon the work of Dr. Ida Rolf.

Joseph Heller, a former aerospace engineer for NASA, founded Hellerwork in 1978. Heller first trained with Dr. Rolf in 1972 and became the first president of the Rolf Institute. As a result of his unique combination of expertise in structural integration, movement education, and his engineering background and perspective, Heller began to synthesize a new form of bodywork. In 1978 he left the Institute and began training his first practitioners. Thus Hellerwork is an evolution of Rolfing, adding movement reeducation and dialogue to the basic structural bodywork. This gives patients a more comprehensive exploration of their body-mind for long-lasting results.

The Hellerwork website includes an introduction to these fundamental concepts at www.Hellerwork.com.

Mechanism of Action According to Its Own Theory

The connective tissues of the body are a continuous tensegrity structure. This means that the bony tissues act as discontinuous compressional struts while the continuity of the structure is through the tensional fascial tissues. Being mostly fluid, the tensional elements are designed to be elastic and flexible. But because of physical and emotional trauma or structural, physical, or psychologic stress the connective tissues become increasingly dehydrated and rigid, causing reduced flexibility, impaired blood and lymph flow, and increasing tension. This can result in mild to severe myofascial pain.

Any tissue having a connecting function is regarded as connective tissue, including tendons, ligaments, and even blood. The connective tissue that Hellerwork primarily affects is fascia, a plastic-like tissue that wraps all organs, vessels, nerves, bones, and muscles, including the fibers and bundles. Fascia meets at the end of a muscle to create its tendon and attaches the muscle to the bone. It continues into other structures adjacent to the joint, providing stability. The fascial system is like a continuous multilayer body stocking woven throughout the body. Because of this interpenetration and interconnectivity, stress in any area can travel through the fascial network to affect other parts of the body.

In a balanced body the fascia is loose, moist, and very mobile, facilitating movement. However, under continued stress, restriction, or lack of movement, fascia becomes rigid. Layers begin to glue together, causing "knots" people experience in their backs or necks, for example. Although people associate tension and stiffness with muscles, it is actually the connective tissue that causes their discomfort. Hellerwork's bodywork component addresses this condition.

Gravity is the force that pulls together earth and the human body. If a body or structure is vertically aligned, gravity is a benign and positive force: it supports the structure in its balance. An imbalanced body, however, feels gravity as a stress, as a demand to hold on, and feels a need to tense up against it.

We give little attention to the effect of gravity on the body. Any aspect of our posture that takes us out of alignment—a sunken chest, a protruding head, a high shoulder, an inwardly shifted knee or ankle—makes us more vulnerable to gravity's effects, which in turn can affect our health and how we feel physically and emotionally. Body misalignment and its resulting imbalances cause us to be more accident-prone or more vulnerable to injury when confronted with rapidly changing conditions or surprise. It also may affect our wellness in ways that are subtler than our current level of science can measure or even detect.

The effectiveness of Hellerwork bodywork comes from restoration of alignment and release of tension and rigidity. Movement feels easier, pain is reduced, and less energy is spent maintaining tightened muscles. As a result, patients report a sense of increased energy and well-being.

The second component of Hellerwork is movement reeducation. Most people overexert in mundane body movements, such as walking, standing, lifting, driving, and even sitting. All of these actions, when habitually performed inefficiently, contribute to the stress we experience in our bodies. Ergonomic movement patterns are suggested as a way of discovering more effective, less stressful ways of using our body. Movement reeducation teaches ways of moving that follow the body's structural design and support the benefits obtained from the bodywork.

If patients continue their old habitual movement patterns, they will eventually reestablish their old tensions and misalignments. Hellerwork's movement reeducation reduces that likelihood through feedback and enhanced self-awareness. Usually the recommended movement changes are easier to make because of the bodywork, and the patient is more "tuned in" to what feels better as well.

Movement coaching also enhances a subtle body awareness that strengthens a sense of self-presence. This awareness makes it less likely that future tension and disease can enter the body unnoticed.

The basis of the dialogue work, Hellerwork's third component, is a fundamental body-mind principle. When a person represses the expression of a feeling or emotion (such as anger or fear) that they believe is not acceptable in their home or social environment, they attempt to mask its presence. They typically do this by automatically and unconsciously tightening the musculature that would be used in its expression. Temporomandibular joint dysfunction (TMJ) can be the result of an unconsciously clenched jaw from not speaking up or repressing angry words, for example.

The body also expresses habitual emotional attitudes. The sunken chest, characteristic of depression, is an example of an attitude that can become etched into tissue. If these experiences are ongoing, they accumulate in the myofascia as rigidity, and the body eventually becomes glued into this predominant posture with all of its resultant effects.

Using bodywork, movement awareness, and dialogue, the Hellerwork practitioner helps patients become more aware of their patterns, bring the holding to a conscious awareness, and release the tight muscles.

Biologic Mechanism of Action

The biologic mechanism of action for Hellerwork relates to the self-organizing characteristics of connective tissue. Connective tissue shares with many other gels a phenomenon called *thixotropy*: it becomes more fluid when it is stirred up and more solid when it sits without being disturbed. The pressure and movement of the practitioner's hands seem to rehydrate the tissue and change the thixotropy of the collagen, connective tissue's major component, toward a more fluid state. This allows the "ungluing" of the tissues that have adhered to each other, freeing the body for a new postural and movement potential.

Aligning the whole body structure in the field of gravity yields a number of results. These results can include less stress on the tissues, more breath capacity, and less compression of the abdominal organs caused by a slumping ribcage, as well as enhanced blood circulation to the brain by aligning a forward-jutting neck and head back over the supportive core of the body.

Forms of Therapy

There is only one form of Hellerwork Structural Integration. Hellerwork shares a common legacy with other modalities, which are also based upon the 10-session series of Dr. Rolf. Our routes may differ from each other but the goals for our work are very much the same. However, we each have our individual training and certification programs, reflecting our specialized approaches.

Demographics

There are more than 300 active Hellerwork Structural Integration practitioners in 28 states of the U.S. and in Canada, Japan, New Zealand, England, Germany, Australia, Spain, and Austria. Most practitioners are in private practice. A small percentage practice in doctors' offices or health care centers.

A list of certified practitioners, including locations, phone numbers and e-mail addresses where applicable, is available at the Hellerwork webpage, www.Hellerwork.com.

The Hellerwork patient base is widely varied, ranging in age from infants to octogenarians. The majority of these patients are in their late 30s to 50s, when people begin to feel the effects of past habits or injuries or are not looking or feeling as well as they think they could or should.

Indications and Reasons for Referral

Although not a treatment for any specific condition, Hellerwork reliably reduces or eliminates musculoskeletal pain caused by trauma and stress. It is also effective for releasing rigidity caused by past trauma, as first aid after injury to the musculoskeletal tissues, and reducing scar tissue or adhesions from injuries and surgeries. It is particularly helpful in balancing the structure of the body. It is most effective in reducing the impact of stress on the total body system and as preventive maintenance.

Patients regularly report the following benefits: increased energy, vitality, and fitness; improved athletic performance; deeper awareness of the body and sense of well-being; less rigidity; greater flexibility and ease of movement; and improved posture and body shape.

Office Applications

Hellerwork Structural Integration could be a valuable part of the treatment plan for patients who are experiencing the following conditions. As with all alternative therapies, use of Hellerwork does not preclude the use of mainstream medical therapies in addition.

Hellerwork is particularly useful for postural back pain, chronic musculoskeletal pain, chronic tension headaches, stress reduction, poor posture, tissue recovery after injury or surgery, and recovery from childbirth. It also is useful as adjunctive therapy for asthma (by relieving chest wall muscle tension), constipation or hemorrhoids (by relieving tension in pelvic floor musculature), and menstrual cramps (by relieving muscle tension in abdomen, hips, and legs). It also serves as a valuable adjunctive therapy for arthritis, irritable bowel syndrome, hyperactivity, and to assist normal processes such as pregnancy, childbirth, and children's health.

It is important to emphasize that Hellerwork practitioners believe that pain and tension are usually the result of an overall pattern of imbalance in the body. Therefore rather than treating the pain or tension "symptom," Hellerwork focuses on rebalancing the entire body, allowing the "symptoms" to resolve themselves during the course of the series.

Research Base

Evidence Based

Two studies of the psychologic effects of Hellerwork Structural Integration may be of interest: *The Psychological Effects of Hellerwork: A Phenomenological Study* by Doug Drucker, PhD,[1] and *Psychological Correlates of Hellerwork Intensive* by Carol Walker, PhD.[2] The Drucker study showed Hellerwork to be an effective provider of symptom relief and educational medium. Another study by Valerie V. Hunt demonstrated that in structural integration work the myofascial tissues themselves become more efficient and show a reduction of state trait anxiety.[3] A similar study by Julian Silverman established that this type of work helps the central nervous system process information more effectively. Subjects who received structural integration work were more capable of focusing both on one stimulus or effectively holding many stimuli at once. When the body and its structural system are working more efficiently, apparently the mind does as well. This implies that patients become able to handle stress more proficiently in its varied forms.[4]

As yet there are no studies on the physiologic effects of Hellerwork per se. However, the Valerie Hunt study previously referenced would be applicable.

Efficacy

Hellerwork almost always produces results that the patient can feel and others can often observe. Joseph Heller estimates the series efficacy rate to be more than 90%.

Future Research Opportunities and Priorities

Scientific studies of definable and measurable results experienced in Hellerwork would enhance its regard within the medical community. But when contrasted to typical studies, Hellerwork can appear very "slippery." It appears so even to practitioners; that is part of its "art." Often initial goals change midstream, yielding results much richer than those first expected. A defined, measurable path could stifle the very process it is designed to profile. When studies can embrace this level of flexibility and creativity, then there can be scientific validation that is representative the work. Until then, there is likely to be frustration on both sides.

Druglike Information

Safety

Hellerwork Structural Integration is not a treatment for disease, conditions of organs, or symptoms of the nervous system. Most results that people generally associate with medical intervention occur within Hellerwork Structural Integration by releasing basic tension in the connective tissue and by bringing the body back into its proper alignment.

Hellerwork is contraindicated only when pressure on the soft tissues cannot be tolerated. Otherwise, Hellerwork is a very safe modality.

As a matter of course all patients are encouraged by the practitioner to speak about the experience of their session as it progresses. Rapport between the practitioner and patient is exceedingly important and is meticulously attended by the practitioner. It is important for the patient to feel safe in speaking up about what is comfortable and what is not as the session proceeds. If the work is becoming uncomfortable the patient is encouraged to speak about that. "Stop" is always honored. Work never proceeds until the patient is ready, and it continues in a manner supportive to the patient's experience. This is not "no pain, no gain" work.

Also, the patient and the practitioner work together to strategize the quantity of sessions that is needed to complete the work. The traditional 10 sessions are usually adequate for the patient's goals. However, when a particular area does not feel complete or if additional sessions would continue a momentum of change, the decision is made mutually by the patient and practitioner, and it is often made at the suggestion of the patient. Also, beginning the Hellerwork series does not require its completion; the patient can end the work at any time.

The Hellerwork Code of Ethics and Standards of Professional Practice are available on the Hellerwork website, www.Hellerwork.com.

Adverse Reactions

Occasionally muscular soreness is experienced after the session. Temporary rashes caused by released toxins sometimes occur, as does mild fatigue. Each of these and any other potential side effects occur less than 5% of the time and typically disappear within 24 to 36 hours. Increased water intake after a session can help lessen any possible postsession discomfort.

Self-Help versus Professional

Hellerwork requires working with a trained practitioner. It cannot be self-administered. The crucial mix of bodywork, movement, and dialogue in combination with the trained eye and intuition of an experienced, creative practitioner cannot be replicated by individuals on their own.

Visiting a Professional

Every patient is different. Each person begins the series with a different reason for being there, a different body than any other patient, and a different road of history. So no two Hellerwork series are ever alike. Some patients have little body-mind awareness; others have been increasing this awareness for many years. The series can start at a different place for each and go farther with some than with others. There are patients who are not yet in tune with the potentialities that Hellerwork holds; thus their series might look more like massage for individual body areas given in a logical sequence.

All patients are assessed in a way that addresses where they are, where they want to go, at what speed they want to go there, and how much scenery they want to see along the way. Some can be gently coaxed into stretching their scope. Some are there to drink in all they can. For others, the practitioner perceptively does not offer anything beyond what patients ask for and trusts that their experience awakens something within.

At the start of the first session the practitioner takes a health history and establishes with the patient the goals for the series. After rapport has been established the patient typically removes outerwear for "before" pictures to determine the baseline alignment for use in future comparison. If the patient prefers, pictures can be taken with clothing rather than without. During the course of their session, the practitioner observes the patient's body for structural imbalance and restrictions in movement. The patient, still in undergarments, then lies down on a bodywork (standard massage) table as the practitioner proceeds to work with the hands on and around the patient's body tissues.

Especially characteristic of the work is its bilateral approach. During a session's initial stages the patient shares the subjective experience of that session's body area of focus. Combined with the practitioner's observations and intuition the work begins exclusively on the most symptomatic side. Once work on that side feels complete the bodywork is paused to allow the patient to get up and move around to compare how each side feels in function and explore the effects of the work.

This process is a rich source of data for the nervous system; the body and mind learn much from this experience. Frequently the just-worked side that initially felt worse is now functioning smoothly, while the side that "felt fine" now feels troublesome: the mundane stickiness of the body that has previously been silent has now been revealed. This somatic experience helps the body learn how to discern the presence of tension. This is a valuable skill for the patient in preventing not only the return of old tightness but also the establishment of new tensions that the patient's unfolding life may have in store.

Once this experience has been sufficiently explored the bodywork resumes, now focusing on the other side to bring both into functional balance. Through pressure, movement, and stretching the practitioner restores fluidity to the tissues and subtly rearranges them to fit and function better in their alignment with gravity. Bodywork can also be done as the patient sits or stands.

The practitioner shares observations with the patient and they visit casually about the theme of the session associated with that area of the body. The practitioner highlights the more common attitudes and emotions associated with that area. As the patient becomes more aware of personal attitudes and emotions, the patient becomes more responsible for them. Thus they are less likely to "run in the background," out of reach of the patient's awareness.

When the structural work is finished, the practitioner works with the patient in establishing relevant new movement patterns that support the new alignment. Sometimes video feedback is used when it can complement the work. Often what our body feels like it is doing is not what it is observably doing, and so video feedback can be valuable feedback.

When the patient has become organically aware of the changes in structure, coupled with new movement patterns and attitude awareness, the session is complete and the patient dresses to return to daily life. The richness of the session's content typically feeds further reflection as the new material and awarenesses integrate into the patient's body and daily life, especially during the next few days.

The series as a whole is divided into three groups of sessions based on areas of the body addressed. The superficial tissue sessions, a minimum of three that address the torso, legs, and arms, focus on the layers of connective tissue near the surface of the body, also called the "sleeve." The session themes deal with issues of infancy and childhood: breathing, standing up independently, and reaching out.

The core sessions, a minimum of four, deal with the deeper musculature and connective tissues (upper legs, front and back of torso, and head or neck), which assist in fine motor movement. These sessions focus on the issues of adolescence: control and surrender (such as fear and trust), gut feelings, holding back emotions, and the balance of reason and passion.

The integrative sessions balance the core and the sleeve, and they also address rotational patterns of the body. They focus on issues of maturity: masculine and feminine (such as "doingness" and "beingness") styles and values, integration, and coming out into the world.

An excerpt from the *Hellerwork Patient Handbook* outlining the scope of content for the first session may be reviewed at the Hellerwork website (www.Hellerwork.com).

The length of each session varies among practitioners from 45 minutes to 2 hours; cost ranges from $60 to $120 per session. Both factors reflect the practitioner's experience, personal style, and geographic location. Typically sessions are scheduled weekly, but this can vary for the patient's convenience.

Credentialing, Training, and What to Look for in a Provider

All practitioners are certified by Hellerwork International after completing an extensive 1250-hour training program that includes anatomy, movement, psychology, and the body's subtle energetic systems. This rigorous training program requires 18 months to 2 years to complete. No state licensing is available for Hellerwork, but all practitioners comply with local licensing required for touch therapies in their area.

Hellerwork Structural Integration schools are located in North America, New Zealand, and Europe. Information regarding the training program and regarding specific locations for training is available at the Hellerwork website; please see www.Hellerwork.com.

Barriers and Key Issues

A difficulty in explaining the art of Hellerwork is the richness of the experience. Because Hellerwork directly and indirectly addresses many aspects of the patient's *beingness* and the practitioner has many levels of approach, it is difficult, if not impossible, to neatly summarize the Hellerwork experience in two or three sentences. Because each series is customized to the individual patient and each practitioner has a large skill palette from which to draw, generalizations are difficult.

Also, health care has traditionally been defined as treatment of disease or injury. Since Hellerwork is a wellness program, it has not fit the traditional health care model. Recent shifts in priorities of the public will allow Hellerwork and other similar programs to gain more exposure as their relevance is better understood and appreciated.

Many health care consumers will not consider or explore any modalities whose cost will not be reimbursed by their health insurance. As alternative modalities become better understood and their value comprehended, and as insurance consumers insist on their coverage, the visibility and use of modalities such as Hellerwork will increase.

Associations

Hellerwork is represented worldwide by Hellerwork International. The Associated Bodywork and Massage Professionals (ABMP) recognizes Hellerwork International and its practitioners.

Hellerwork International
406 Berry St.
Mt. Shasta, CA 96067
Tel: (800) 392-3900
E-mail: Hellerwork@Hellerwork.com
www.Hellerwork.com

Associated Bodywork and Massage Professionals (ABMP)
28677 Buffalo Park Rd.
Evergreen, CO 80439
Tel: (800) 458-2267
E-mail: expectmore@abmp.com
www.abmp.com

Suggested Reading

1. Heller J, Henkin WA: *Bodywise*, Oakland, Calif, 1991, Wingbow Press.
2. Heller J, Hanson J: *The patient's handbook*, Mt. Shasta, Calif, 1981, Hellerwork International.
3. An extensive list of articles about Hellerwork is available at the Hellerwork website, www.Hellerwork.com.

References

1. Drucker D: The psychological effects of Hellerwork: a phenomenological study, San Diego, 1990, United States International University. Available through Dissertations International.
2. Walker C: Psychological correlates of Hellerwork intensive Malibu, 1995, Pepperdine University. Available through Dissertations International.
3. Hunt VV et al: *A study of structural integration from neuromuscular, energy field, and emotional approaches*, Boulder, Colo, 1997, Rolf Institute.
4. Silverman J et al: Stress, stimulus intensity control, and the structural integration technique, *Confina Psychiatrica* 16:201-219, 1973.

Bonnie Prudden Myotherapy

BONNIE PRUDDEN

ENID WHITTAKER

Origins and History

> MYOTHERAPY *is a method of relaxing muscle spasm, improving circulation and alleviating pain. To defuse "trigger points," pressure is applied to the muscle for several seconds by means of fingers, knuckles and elbows. The success of this method depends on the use of specific corrective exercise for the freed muscles. The method was developed by Bonnie Prudden in 1976.*
>
> **Taber's Cyclopedic Dictionary**

Bonnie Prudden myotherapy is a hands-on, drugless, noninvasive method of relieving muscle related pain, which emphasizes speedy, cost-effective recovery and active patient participation for long-term relief. It relaxes muscles, improves circulation, and alleviates pain in all parts of the body while it increases strength, flexibility, coordination, stamina, and energy and improves posture, gait, sleep patterns, and work and play performance quickly, effectively, and lastingly. The patient, shoeless and wearing loose clothing, lies relaxed on a table as the body is checked for areas of potentially active "trigger points," highly irritable spots that remain in the muscle after it has been damaged. Although Bonnie Prudden myotherapy has its origins in the medical discipline of trigger point injection therapy developed by Janet Travell, MD, it is noninvasive and very teachable, which has encouraged widespread use by the ordinary person through Bonnie Prudden's books, videos, self-help tools, and television and radio appearances. The chronology of myotherapy is as follows:

1930s, Germany: Dr. Hans Lange uses a sclerometer to prove that tender areas in muscles are 50% harder than surrounding areas.

1930s, Austria: Orthopedist Hans Kraus develops therapeutic exercise with Austria's Olympic Trainer, Heinz Kowalski, and emigrates to America.

1940s, United States: Janet Travell, MD, develops trigger point injection therapy. Lange's "tender areas" become known as "trigger points." The two valid medical disciplines complement each other as trigger point injections are followed by muscle stretching exercise facilitated by muscle relaxing coolant sprays, ethyl-chloride and fluorimethane.

1976, United States: Bonnie Prudden, exercise specialist, researcher, author, and television and radio personality, discovers that noninvasive pressure to trigger points by fingers, knuckles, and elbows, followed by specific corrective exercise, produces superior results to those engendered by injection, followed by "spray and stretch."

1978, United States: London University graduate and internist Desmond Tivy, MD, coins the name my*otherapy*.

1980, United States: Bonnie Prudden authors her first book, *Pain Erasure the Bonnie Prudden Way*.

1985, United States: Bonnie Prudden authors *Myotherapy: Bonnie Prudden's Complete Guide to Pain Free Living*. These two books, with forwards and afterword by Dr. Desmond Tivy, put myotherapy into the capable hands of the general public.

For a more complete history, read *Pain Erasure* and *Myotherapy*.

Mechanism of Action According to Its Own Theory

Bonnie Prudden myotherapy is the noninvasive offshoot of two medical disciplines, trigger point injection therapy (Travell) and therapeutic exercise (Kraus). Travell holds that injecting procaine and saline into trigger points denies them oxygen and in effect defuses them, allowing painful muscles to relax. Stretch exercises are then used as a coolant spray is applied to the painful area.

Bonnie Prudden discovered, serendipitously, that defusing trigger points by injection was unnecessary, as was the coolant spray. Manual pressure applied to trigger points is noninvasive, far less painful, and covers much larger areas and also distant areas of referred pain. Specific therapeutic exercises used immediately following trigger point defusing by simple pressure erases the pain. A daily program of the same simple exercises makes recovery sure and lasting.

Forms of Therapy

Because there is only one Bonnie Prudden School of Physical Fitness and Myotherapy, there is only one form of the therapy, and treatments are typically consistent between practitioners.

Demographics

Typically, certified Bonnie Prudden myotherapist practitioners choose myotherapy as a second career. They come from all over the U.S. as the Bonnie Prudden School is the only one of its kind in the world. About 75% of practitioners have been in pain themselves and have been helped by myotherapy through the use of Ms. Prudden's books, videos, and self-help tools or as a result of having visited a practitioner.

Users of Bonnie Prudden myotherapy range in age from newborns through old age and include the handicapped. The typical patient is 40 to 70 years, has had pain for many years, has tried traditional medicine, and wants to take a more active role in health care.

Indications and Reasons for Referral

Bonnie Prudden myotherapy is effective for muscle-related pain. Examples include back pain; headaches; sciatica; shoulder and neck pain; repetitive motion injuries such as carpal tunnel syndrome; sports injuries; temporomandibular joint syndrome; hip, knee, and foot pain; menstrual cramps; and pain associated with pregnancy. It can relieve the pain that is associated with arthritis, fibromyalgia, chronic fatigue, multiple sclerosis, and lupus. Although myotherapy does not cure disease, it relieves pain and provides a better climate for recovery.

All patients require medical clearance that assures that the pain is not due to anatomic pathology. As with all alternative therapies, use of myotherapy does not preclude the use of mainstream medical therapies in addition. Pain associated with the following conditions can be eliminated or greatly alleviated using myotherapy:

Top level: *A therapy ideally suited for these conditions*
Back pain; chronic pain; headaches; and menstrual cramps

Second level: *One of the better therapies for these conditions*
Asthma; childbirth; hemorrhoids; and osteoarthritis

Third level: *A valuable adjunctive therapy for these conditions*
Arthritis; well child care; chronic fatigue syndrome; colic; colitis and Crohn's disease; constipation; diabetes; female health; hypertension; impotence; multiple sclerosis; pregnancy; pregnancy and childbirth; premenstrual syndrome; respiratory conditions; restless leg syndrome; rheumatoid arthritis; and stress

Druglike Information

Warnings, Contraindications, and Precautions

Myotherapy concentrates solely on functional muscle anatomy and has virtually no side effects other than occasional bruising. Myotherapy almost always works very quickly; therefore the myotherapist usually knows after one treatment whether or not it will be effective. Most patients require fewer than 10 treatments to erase the pain and learn the corrective exercises and self-help myotherapy necessary to prevent its return. A contraindication would be the presence of a pathologic condition. This must be addressed by the physician before embarking on a series of myotherapy treatments.

Visiting a Professional

Because there is only one Bonnie Prudden School of Myotherapy, treatments are typically consistent from one practitioner to another. A Bonnie Prudden myotherapy treatment is 90 minutes for the first session (which includes a vital history) and 60 minutes for subsequent sessions. Depending on geography, sessions range in cost from $40.00 to $150.00.

Objectives are to erase muscle spasm and pain, increase range of motion, and prevent the return of pain by reeducating the muscle into its normal resting relaxed condition with specific exercises designed for each individual problem.

There are typically four components to an initial myotherapy session. First, a history is taken to help determine when and where the trigger points were laid down in the patient's muscles. Patients are asked about their birth, past and present occupations, sports, accidents, operations, injuries, and whether or not they have a disease such as multiple sclerosis.

The patient is given the Kraus-Weber test to determine the strength and flexibility of key posture muscles. The myotherapist then locates (based on the history) and erases the trigger points believed to be most directly responsible for the pain, limited range of motion, nerve or circulatory problems, and muscle fatigue and weakness.

To defuse trigger points, pressure is applied to the muscle for several seconds by means of fingers, knuckles, and elbows. The treatment is considered to be a partnership and the patient is instructed to direct the force of the pressure by letting the therapist know when a trigger point is found and the level of pain on a scale of one to ten.

The newly relaxed muscles are then passively stretched and the patient is given corrective exercises to do at home. These keep the muscles free of spasm and are the key to the success of the treatment.

Subsequent sessions focus on erasing the patient's individual trigger points using a combination of techniques. Corrective exercises are reevaluated and the patient learns how to maintain the pain-free state and prevent the reoccurrence of pain through the use of self-help myotherapy and exercise.

After an initial 1-hour treatment, patients usually are very relaxed and use words like *looser, lighter,* and *warmer* to describe how they feel. It is normal to note what would seem to be a remarkable reduction of pain and increased flexibility after the first treatment. Patients also report improved sleeping patterns following the reduction of pain. These immediate changes usually hold until the next treatment and become long-term changes, especially if the patient faithfully performs the homework exercise and self-help techniques as prescribed.

Credentialing

Following graduation from the Bonnie Prudden School for Physical Fitness and Myotherapy, graduates may sit for board exams administered by Bonnie Prudden Pain Erasure, L.L.C. These consist of approximately 25 hours of practical, written, and oral testing. In some states, myotherapists must pass a massage exam to practice myotherapy.

Training

Certified Bonnie Prudden myotherapists train for 1300 hours at the Bonnie Prudden School for Physical Fitness and Myotherapy. This course of study, established by Bonnie Prudden, is the only school of its kind in the world; therefore all receive the same consistent level of training.

Bonnie Prudden Pain Erasure L.L.C. offers weekend training seminars, professional treatments, self-help classes, exercise classes, and Bonnie Prudden products, such as books, videos, and equipment. The Bonnie Prudden School for Physical Fitness and Myotherapy is a state-licensed 1300 (33-week) program that prepares students for a career as Certified Bonnie Prudden myotherapists.

What to Look for in a Provider

Bonnie Prudden myotherapists do not diagnose and are required to obtain medical clearance before treating a patient. Look for current Bonnie Prudden certification displayed on wall. To maintain certification, Bonnie Prudden myotherapists must update with 45 hours of training every 2 years. Those wishing to find a CBPM or verify current certification may contact Bonnie Prudden Pain Erasure at:

Bonnie Prudden Pain Erasure, LLC
4725 E. Sunrise Drive, #346
Tucson, AZ 85718
Tel: (800) 221-4634
Fax: (520) 529-6679
E-mail: info@bonnie prudden.com
www.bonnieprudden.com

Associations

The International Myotherapy Association (IMA) is made up of certified Bonnie Prudden myotherapists. It serves as a trade organization of individuals who have the common interest of promoting the practice and improvement of myotherapy, develops and enforce rules of professional and ethical conduct among practitioners, and provides scholarships to worthy candidates for the study of myotherapy

International Myotherapy Association
E-mail: dham2@swlink.net
www.myotherapy.org/index

Suggested Reading

1. Prudden B: *Pain erasure the Bonnie Prudden way*, New York, 1980, Ballantine Books.
2. Prudden B: *Myotherapy: Bonnie Prudden's complete guide to pain free living*, New York, 1985, Ballantine Books.

References

The following books by Bonnie Prudden contain chapters on myotherapy as it pertains to each particular age group.

1. Prudden B: *How to keep your child fit from birth to six*, New York, 1986, Ballantine Books.
2. Prudden B: *Fitness from six to twelve*, New York, 1987, Ballantine Books.
3. Prudden B: *Teenage fitness*, New York, 1988, Ballantine Books.
4. Prudden B: *Bonnie Prudden's after fifty fitness guide*, New York, 1987, Ballantine Books.

Polarity Therapy

LESLIE KORN

Origins and History

Randolph Stone (1890-1981) originally conceived of Polarity Therapy, a philosophy and method of health care, education, and healing based on electromagnetic and subtle energy fields and their flow or disruption in the human or animal body. Stone's work reflected a lifetime of scholarship and clinical practice that was infused with a deep respect for the practice of spiritual awareness and service to others. He received his degrees in osteopathy, chiropractic, naturopathy, naprapathy, and neuropathy. In 1914 he was granted an OP (Other Practitioner) license by the state Board of Examiners in Chicago, granting him the right to practice all methods of drugless healing without surgery.

Trained in the manipulative therapies of early twentieth century European-American medicine, Stone believed there was a missing link underlying the cause and effect of health and illness. His annual visits to India (where he made his home later in life) provided him an opportunity to practice medicine among the poor as well as people referred to as "incurable." Ayurvedic medical principles, with their emphasis on energy centers or *nadis*, influenced his practice, as did acupuncture. These healing traditions led Stone to synthesize Western and Eastern "drugless" healing practices, which he called Polarity Therapy. Unlike acupuncture, which used needles to stimulate the life force, he believed that the artful application of hands, with consciousness and intention behind them, could create even more beneficial effects. He thus transformed the mechanical approaches to the manipulative therapies by advancing the following thesis: if the energy blockage(s) underlying disease could be released, structure and function would find their own level and return the individual to balance and optimal health.

Mechanism of Action According to Its Own Theory

Polarity Therapy is the science and art of healing that brings balance to the human energy field by hands-on manipulation of bone, soft tissue, and energy points; vegetarian, nutritional, and attitudinal counseling; and specific stretching exercises using sound and movement called *Polarity Yoga*.

Polarity Therapy addresses the physical, mental, emotional, and spiritual well-being of the individual, suggesting that energy blockages in one field are reflected in all fields. The goal of Polarity is to trace (by palpation) and release (by skilled touch) those energy blockages that manifest as pain. To do this, the practitioner applies three depths of touch depending on whether the energy blockage reflects a hyperactive, hypoactive, or neutral state of activity. These include a very light touch (off the body or gentle hands-on), a medium touch (meeting tissue resistance), and deep pressure used to break up crystalline deposits and scar tissue. A major emphasis is placed on understanding how poor nutritional habits and poor digestion lead to energy blockages that manifest as pain, gas, and discomfort. Pressure on energy points, rocking, bone manipulation, stretching, and rotation of joints are some of the methods used to help the patient achieve deep relaxation, improve digestive function, gain greater self-awareness of behavioral and cognitive impacts on health, and take an increasingly responsible role in creating a healthier lifestyle. Because Polarity Therapy has its roots in both chiropractic and cranial osteopathy, a major principle is to make structural adjustments or manipulations only *after* the energy underlying the structural balance is addressed.

The theory of Polarity Therapy suggests that all forms and processes arise from a universal source of life energy and, like the function of the atom, all life energies revolve around a neutral core, reflecting attraction and repulsion as well as positive and negative action and reactions. The physical and subtle energies of the body and mind are comprised of both functional and structural relationships that can be assessed, interpreted, and responded to therapeutically based on these principles of attraction and repulsion.

In clinical practice, this attraction and repulsion is manifested in obvious ways such as physical compensatory strategies found in the geometric structures of the spine, or more subtle symptoms such as inhibition of respiratory processes and restriction of diaphragmatic function following emotional trauma. It is the practitioner's responsibility to "trace" these imbalances through thorough assessment and evaluation, a refined proprioceptive sense of palpation and therapeutic touch, history-taking, and communication to develop a plan for managing the helping and healing process.

The practitioner assesses imbalances and helps the patient achieve a state of balance through artful and specific strategies whereby the innate wisdom and restorative capacities of the whole being can bring about improved health and well-being. Imbalances in one area (physical function) are reflected in imbalances in other reciprocal areas (reflexes). Reflexes may be functional, structural, mental, or emotional. These reflexes may be acute or latent, consciously known, or unknown to the patient.

Neck pain, for example, would be assessed as it relates to structural stressors, such as genetics, posture, occupational ergonomics, or acute changes resulting from an accident, as well as for chronic restrictions that may result from poor digestion and fecal elimination. Generally, the interrelationships among several variables are evaluated. This theory of Polarity suggests that by releasing energy blockages, whether they are manifested as physical pain, restricted range of motion, mental negativity, or autonomic hyperarousal, deep relaxation is affected. Energy is also balanced and flows throughout constricted or flaccid areas; as a result, the patient feels better kinesthetically, release fears, or reframes negative belief systems, and the whole organism moves toward its potential.

The theory of Polarity Therapy emphasizes the importance of the practitioner's role in modeling a healthy lifestyle. A vital part of the theory of Polarity involves engaging patients to act positively on their own behalf and to assume a vital role in healing. The theory and practice of intention also plays a strong role, and many practitioners develop a non-denominational meditation practice to focus the power of intention for healing and bioenergies. The role of love and compassion, or unconditional positive regard, coupled with the role of positive intention, facilitates the work of the practitioner with the patient.

Biologic Mechanism of Action

Polarity Therapy is a unique bridge between the purely energetic-based methods, such as Reiki and acupuncture, and the physical-based methods such as massage, chiropractic, and osteopathy. Because Polarity Therapy integrates energy methods with physical manipulation of soft tissue and postural alignment of bony structures (with the addition of lifestyle counseling), practitioners draw from many disciplines to link research with clinically observed patient responses.

Psychobiologic responses based on research in massage and acupuncture and clinical observations of response to Polarity Therapy suggest increased levels of endogenous endorphins and the neurotransmitter serotonin result.

Psychophysiologic responses are observed as autonomic alterations in states of consciousness, such as deep relaxation associated with brain hemispheric synchrony and parasympathetic dominance. Anecdotal reports of hypnagogic imagery associated with theta states and increased creativity are common. Krieger[1] has reported increased levels of anomalous cognition resulting from the practice of therapeutic touch, and this has been observed among practitioners. It may result from the effects of increased blood flow into the right hemisphere in response to meditation. Korn has postulated that Polarity Therapy is a form of meditative touch.[2]

Psychologic effects have been observed or reported in Polarity Therapy patients.[2,3] These effects have a potential to decondition cognitive belief systems and affective states. Polarity Therapy facilitates sensory-motor biofeedback and awareness. The Polarity session also facilitates states of consciousness associated with alpha and theta wave states and serves as a deconditioning strategy for state-dependent memories held in body tissues.[3]

Polarity Therapy helps to define and improve body image by enhancing kinesthetic and proprioceptive recognition of boundaries. This feature is useful when working with people with body image-related disorders such as bulimia, anorexia, alexythymia, and changes arising from loss of limb or chronic illness.

Polarity Therapy helps regulate complex neurobiologic rhythms within the body and between people, and it facilitates the capacity for attachment among healthy individuals and people suffering from attachment-related disorders. Axt[4] has published her clinical research on the application of Polarity Therapy for the treatment of autism and of children with special developmental needs. To date, the only controlled experimental research directly using the modality of Polarity Therapy involved pilot studies at The Ohio State Medical School.[5]

Scientific research in bioelectromagnetics and bioenergy fields has proliferated significantly in the past 20 years (Becker,[6] Green,[7] Adey,[8] and Oschman[9]). This research provides the foundation for understanding the effects of electromagnetic and subtle energy fields on human function. This research provides theoretic and conceptual links for research in the fields of Polarity and related touch therapy fields.

Demographics

Approximately 1200 practitioners are members of the American Polarity Therapy Association (many others practice professionally but are unregistered) located throughout the United States, Canada, Mexico, and Europe. Some individuals primarily practice Polarity Therapy while other clinicians, such as chiropractors, massage therapists, psychologists, and somatic educators, are dual-trained and incorporate Polarity Therapy as an adjunctive part of their profession. Patients are drawn from a broad spectrum of individuals seeking to improve their health or recover from acute and chronic illnesses.

Women seek treatments from Polarity therapists in greater numbers than men. This reflects a woman's general tendency to seek alternative forms of healing more often[10] and because women are more likely to seek touch therapies.

People of all ages receive Polarity Therapy. Individuals from middle class and European-American backgrounds use Polarity Therapy most frequently. Increasingly, though, practitioners in other countries (Poland, Spain, Germany, Switzerland, Mexico), as well as the inner cities and rural areas of the US, are reaching out in public health settings to bring Polarity Therapy to more diverse groups of people.

Forms of Therapy

Criteria for the practice of Polarity Therapy (615 hours of training) are outlined in the Standards for Practice. These standards form the core foundation for practice that is expanded upon by individual practitioners, who may emphasize their own methods and idiosyncratic approaches to practice.

Some practitioners emphasize exploring nutritional changes, such as a vegetarian diet, while others emphasize bodywork more. Others may integrate the use of tuning forks (music energetics) and craniosacral therapies. Following the 615-hour training, which includes clinical practice sessions and supervision, the practitioner is proficient in Polarity Therapy and is able to develop and implement an appropriate plan for the patient. Registration as a Polarity practitioner requires competency in the main areas of bodywork, evaluation, nutrition, exercise, and communication.

The practice of Polarity Therapy has always included practitioners from other modalities. In recent years, practitioners have expanded their practices with additional or advanced training in other modalities or have specialized within their practices. These methods include craniosacral therapies, music or sound energetics, Polarity Yoga, and posttrauma therapy.

Indications and Reasons for Referral

Individuals seek Polarity practitioners for a variety of reasons at different stages in their lives or during the course of their illness. Chronic or acute pain, stress, a lack of success with conventional therapies, referral from a friend or relative who has been helped, curiosity, or not wanting to use drugs or see a physician are some reasons people seek a Polarity practitioner. Individuals may have been referred by another practitioner for adjunctive work (for example, a psychotherapist for trauma resolution, a surgeon for preoperative relaxation or postoperative healing) or to assist in reduction of pain medications or drug and alcohol detoxification.

There are numerous health conditions and disorders that result in patient referrals to Polarity Therapists. Main conditions for referral include the following:

- Somatization disorders
- Chronic and acute pain
- Temporomandibular joint pain
- Depression
- Chronic fatigue and fibromyalgia
- Stress-related disorders, including organic dysfunction related to autonomic hyperarousal
- Psychologic distress, such as anxiety
- General feelings of malaise

Polarity Therapy has also been used for postsurgical recovery; to increase lymphatic (edema) and circulatory flow; and to treat sinusitis, asthma and allergies, osteoarthritis, and rheumatoid arthritis. Polarity Therapy has been used widely during early, middle, and later stages of pregnancy; during delivery; and for postpartum care of mothers and infants. Digestive complaints, including irritable bowel, Crohn's disease, constipation, and poor peristalsis in adults and older adults are common reasons for referral. Specialized treatments that are not often found in other modalities include prostate drain and perineal treatment to release tissue congestion in the prostate and to release spasm or chronic contraction in the perineal area and anal sphincter. Polarity Therapy also is used by practitioners trained in appropriate methods of touch for resolution of traumatic stress, associated phobias, and traumatic memories.

Anecdotal evidence suggests that—as with many complementary therapies—people often seek help through Polarity Therapy as a "last resort." Those seeking treatment include individuals diagnosed with neurologic conditions such as multiple sclerosis, peripheral neuropathy, and sequelae of stroke. Children and adults with autism and attention deficit disorder[11] also receive treatment.

Individuals already using holistic approaches for recovery from various forms of cancer, heart disease, and diabetes also undertake treatment. For example, individuals may undertake treatment for breast cancer to improve energy flow as an adjunct to comprehensive nutritional and metabolic modalities, or to militate against the side effects of radiation or chemotherapy. Polarity Therapy techniques may be used to aid the postsurgical wound healing process, decrease adhesion formation, and regain range of motion and reduce pain (as in the case of mastectomies).

Polarity Therapy has been applied in crosscultural settings for treatment of culture-bound syndromes such as *susto* (fright) and *mal de ojo* (evil eye). Because Polarity Therapy is rooted in touch, a nonverbal language that can be found in similar forms in most cultures, it can facilitate crosscultural communication.

Polarity Therapy also helps maintain well-being as well as fostering optimal health and performance among athletes.

Office Applications

The following is an alphabetic list of conditions that respond to Polarity Therapy. As with all alternative therapies, the use of Polarity Therapy does not preclude the use of mainstream medical therapies in addition.

Abortion-related trauma; acute pain; anxiety; asthma (including exercise-induced asthma); autonomic hyperarousal; benign prostatic hyperplasia; carpal tunnel syndrome; chronic pain; colitis; constipation; decompression illness (postchamber); digestive disorders associated with autonomic hyperarousal; dysmenorrhea; edema associated with pregnancy and premenstrual condition; fatigue; fibromyalgia; hypoxia due to shallow breathing; muscle tension including respiratory diaphragm constriction; nerve impingement disorders; premenstrual pain; sacroiliac joint pain; sinusitis; situational depression; soft tissue pain; temporomandibular joint dysfunction; tension headaches; thoracic outlet and tinnitus; torticollis; traumatic stress; and whiplash

Practical Applications

Licensed clinicians may undertake study at the associate level or registered level to integrate methods into their practice. Otherwise, they can refer to a Polarity Therapy practitioner.

Licensed health care clinicians typically refer patients to a Polarity Therapy practitioner to integrate a *bodyworker* into the team of providers already working on behalf of the patient. This also may take place in the growing number of group "integrative" medicine practices.

Polarity is ideal for patients with stress-related disorders. Enhancing self-regulation capacities significantly relieves both affectively and psychophysiologically stress-related disorders. The ability to relax deeply and develop awareness about how cognition and behavior contributes to illness is an important part of a lifestyle change and home self-care program.

Polarity Therapy is beneficial for patients suffering from chronic pain and the despair it may bring. Polarity Therapy has the capacity to provide a respite from pain and restore simple bodily pleasures. In addition, it activates and renews patients' hopes that their body is not merely a source of suffering. Chronic pain is a complex syndrome requiring a comprehensive approach. Polarity Therapy provides a structured approach to gaining awareness into proprioceptive sensations and increased self-regulation of mental and physical functions. Increased levels of endorphins and serotonin, improved circulation and lymphatic drainage, and an enhanced sense of pleasure and well-being all promote the healing process.

Research Base

Risk and Safety

No authoritative studies have been done on the risks and safety issues associated with Polarity Therapy. However, based on information gleaned from insurance or malpractice claims, no claims have been made against practitioners. Some claims have been filed and settled with regard to ethical misconduct. These involved practitioners who were dually trained and licensed in another specialty. There is an active ethics board that reviews and responds to complaints. By all accounts, Polarity Therapy is a very safe, gentle technique.

Efficacy

Benefit probabilities vary according to the goals and objectives that are set by patients and practitioners. Polarity practitioners do not diagnose or label themselves "healers." They believe that by restoring balance to the energy fields, the body and mind can help individuals regain their health and their well-being. A distinction is made between *healing* and *cure*. Polarity Therapy can and does bring about "healing," but it may not cure. At a basic level, Polarity Therapy can help almost everyone achieve a state of deep relaxation and (at least temporary) peace of mind. Because Polarity Therapy is as much a philosophy of balanced living as it is a therapeutic intervention, there is a wide variation in effects.

From a long-term standpoint, Polarity Therapy is very effective for many people and conditions. The positive effects are cumulative when applied correctly. Many practitioners would agree that changing disease processes rooted in poor lifestyle habits takes time, strong patient motivation, compliance, and self-care at home between visits. In this regard, Polarity Therapy is as much an education process as a treatment program.

There are few people who cannot or do not benefit from regular skilled touch, exercise, improved nutrition, and mental attitudes. For example, health problems experienced by older adults (such as constipation, poor circulation, insomnia, loneliness, and depression) are especially responsive to the skilled, caring, and therapeutic touch of a compassionate practitioner. While the focus may be on stimulating peristaltic rhythm and ensuring adequate and correct nutrition and water intake, the synergetic effects of the whole experience are difficult to reduce into separate variables.

Anecdotal reports indicate a majority of patients received positive benefits that increase with time. When Polarity Therapy is viewed as a method that increases awareness and consciousness about the self and body-mind functions, logic suggests a range of positive benefits that increase in direct proportion to the increased levels of awareness. This is not to say that all benefits depend on either belief or long-term sessions alone. One, two, or more Polarity sessions have alleviated conditions such as chronic headaches, osteoarthritic pain, and lower back pain.

Druglike Information

The use of nutrition and herbs is a vital part of Polarity Therapy practice.

The herbal formula *polarity tea* is comprised of equal parts of fenugreek seed, fennel seed, licorice root, and double the amount of flax seed. Combine these seeds and roots, and simmer 1 teaspoon of the mixture in boiling water for approximately 15 minutes. Strain after boiling. Drink two cups daily.

The liver flush or the "Orange Randolph" also is part of the morning drink. This consists of 4 to 6 ounces of fresh squeezed citrus juice (orange or lemon) in a glass with 1 to 2 tablespoons of cold pressed virgin olive oil. Add one clove of fresh garlic or ginger. Mix in blender, then drink the liver flush in alternating sips with the hot polarity tea as a breakfast drink. Eat nothing else for 2 hours.

The following is a brief review of some of the herbs just mentioned:

Flax (*Linum usitatissimum L*) is rich in unsaturated fatty acids containing from 39% to 41% linoleic acid.[12] The seed is traditionally used throughout India and Mexico, either as a tea or soaked in water and allowed to swell as an aid to intestinal function.

Fennel (*Foeniculum vulgare mill*) contains essential oils and is used as a carminative.[12]

Licorice is used in Ayurveda (India) as a tonic demulcent, expectorant, diuretic, emmenagogue, and gentle laxative.[13] People with hypertension or edema should not drink large quantities of licorice root tea.

Fenugreek is used traditionally to regulate blood sugar. Folk reports suggest efficacy for allergies.

Self-Help versus Professional

The practice of Polarity Therapy is divided into self-applied and professional practice. The practitioner's goal is to help the patient integrate lifestyle practices that include the philosophy and self-help exercises, nutrition, relaxation strategies, and pressure points in different body areas.

A professional practitioner is required for application of the complete program (tailored to each individual) and for administration of full bodywork sessions.

Visiting a Professional

A Polarity practitioner is a professional skilled in the art of touch and health education for therapeutic purposes. The practitioner will ask what the patient hopes to obtain from a session or a series of sessions; take a history; and use methods of touch, exercise, and nutritional and attitudinal counseling. Because Polarity involves a commitment to a healthy lifestyle, the practitioner will present options for improving health through behavioral changes. However, the practitioner should not be dogmatic when making these suggestions. The practitioner should gently assist patients in making the changes that feel right for them. A Polarity session generally involves lying on a treatment (massage) table with light cotton clothes (or without, as the patient prefers). The patient then receives an hour-long session with an experience of deep relaxation and varying pressures from light to moderate or deep. The session should not hurt, but it should be both be stimulating and relaxing. During the session, the patient can talk or remain silent as desired, and the practitioner will help the patient to focus on breathing and learning how to relax and achieve a healthy balance of body and mind. Because Polarity also supports the role of spirituality in health and healing, the patient is welcome to talk about spiritual interests and to ask health-related questions. The results of Polarity Therapy sessions vary and may include profound relaxation, new insight into energetic patterns and their implications, and relief from numerous specific problematic situations.

Credentialing

The APTA maintains a registry of registered practitioners. There are no states that license Polarity Therapy by itself.

Training

The APTA oversees the development of standards for training at two levels and for continuing education. Currently, the first level of Associate Practitioner (155 required course hours) provides a basis for beginning to practice, with an additional 460 hours required for achieving the status of Registered Polarity Practitioner.

Training for students is available from both schools and individuals. A yearly conference is also available that provides seminars for practitioners and interested individuals. A list of registered schools and membership can be obtained from the APTA.

What to Look for in a Provider

Word of mouth often is the best form of referral in any therapy. Speaking with friends or colleagues about their experiences with particular practitioners is considered the best way to find a competent, artful, and caring practitioner. Patients often hear of practitioners when they take a course in a community setting or attend a Polarity Yoga class. This allows them to view the work of the teacher or practitioner. The APTA also maintains a directory of practitioners organized by name, location, and practitioner status. Practitioners should provide a clear description of their scope of practice in their state and the benefits and limitations of their treatment, while maintaining professional boundaries. To better understand the scope of practice, the patient can request to review a code of ethics as well as a book of standards for the practice of Polarity Therapy.

Many people who practice Polarity Therapy are also licensed in other modalities (such as chiropractic, medicine, osteopathy, physical therapy, naturopathy, pharmaceuticals, nursing, or social work). Others, for one reason or another, have chosen not to register with the Association. Many of these people have successful and competent practices and are also good referral sources. A clinical relationship with a Polarity practitioner should be viewed in the same light as a relationship with any health care professional. The ingredients for success are the same—practitioner competence, patient compliance, and good interpersonal "chemistry."

Barriers and Key Issues

A more widespread acceptance of Polarity Therapy is limited by several barriers. The first barrier relates to patient access, which is limited by the number of practitioners. Currently there are only about 1200 practitioners in the organization. The second barrier concerns the need for compliance. Polarity Therapy is a very specialized form of bodywork therapy, and unlike many forms such as massage, it strongly suggests or even requires good patient compliance. The third barrier is cost. Insurance generally does not cover Polarity Therapy services. As a result, a Polarity Therapy patient faces sessions that cost anywhere from $25 to $150 an hour. Polarity Therapy is also a labor-intensive modality that managed care and modern allopathic practice most often cannot accommodate. It has been used by allied health professionals such as physical therapists or others who segment their clinical practice into 30-, 60-, and 90-minute appointments.

The fourth barrier is the general lack of understanding of Polarity Therapy by the mainstream medical community. Training is focused on developing good skills with an emphasis on touch and sensitivity to human energy fields. Because Polarity Therapy has until recently only been viewed as an esoteric science by mainstream allopathic medicine, it has been a neglected modality.

However, during the last 20 years, the mainstream medical community has accepted Polarity Therapy to a larger degree for many reasons. Because of the growing acceptance of complementary practices and because mainstream medical personnel themselves have sought complementary treatments for their own health, they have passed this knowledge to their own patients. Many practitioners who are dually trained integrate Polarity Therapy into public health, community health, and social service settings as well as private group practice settings. During the past 20 years, universities have begun to offer Polarity courses for credit, and medical schools have offered lectures and courses in primary care, geriatrics, and psychiatric departments.

Associations

American Polarity Therapy Association
2888 Bluff St. #149
Boulder, CO 80301
Tel: (303) 545-2080
Fax: (303) 545-2161
E-mail: hq@polaritytherapy.org
www.polaritytherapy.org

Suggested Reading

1. Stone R: *Polarity Therapy: the complete collected works*, vol 1, Sebastopol, Calif, 1986, CRCS Publications.
2. Stone R: *Polarity Therapy*, vol 2, Summertown, Tenn, 1999, Book Publishing.
   The seminal, two-volume work by Dr. Stone provides theory and principles of practice for the professional and advanced student.
3. Stone R: *Health building: the conscious art of living well*, Sebastopol, Calif, 1986, CRCS Publications.
   An outline to the self-care and nutritional program of the Polarity diet. Useful for students and patients.
4. Gordon R: *Your healing hands: the Polarity experience*, Berkeley, Calif, 1984, Wingbow Press.
   A clearly illustrated text that provides simple Polarity principles and methods for self, friends, and family.
5. Chitty J, Muller ML: *Energy exercises*, Boulder, Colo, 1990, Polarity Press.
   A comprehensive approach to Polarity Yoga. Includes illustrations and detailed directions.
6. Beaulieu J: *Polarity Therapy workbook*, New York, 1994, Bionsonic Enterprises.
   A comprehensive text based on APTA standards for students who are studying Polarity Therapy (available directly from the APTA).
7. Korn L: *Somatic empathy*, Olympia, Wash, 1996, DayKeeper Press.
   An integrative text that provides a rationale for the use of Polarity Therapy and psychotherapy for treating posttraumatic stress.

References

1. Krieger D, Peper E, Ancoli S: Therapeutic touch: searching for evidence of physiological change, *Am J Nurs* 79(4):660-662, 1979.
2. Korn L: *To touch the heart of (the) matter: Polarity Therapy in somatics*, spring-summer, 1985.
3. Korn L: *Somatic empathy*, Olympia, Wash, 1996, DayKeeper Press.
4. Axt A: Autism viewed as a consequence of pineal gland dysfunction, *Farmakoterapia W Pyschiatrii I Neurologii* 1: 112-134, 1998.

5. Benford S: *Identification and measurement of alternative healing energies*, Unpublished correspondence, Dublin, Ohio, 1998.

6. Becker RO: *Evidence for a primitive DC electrical analog system controlling brain function, subtle energies*, 2(1): 71-88, 1990.

7. Green E: *Consciousness psychophysiology and psychophysics: an overview*, Topeka, 1990, The Menninger Clinic.

8. Adey WR: Whispering between cells: electromagnetic fields and regulatory mechanisms, *Frontier Perspective* 3(2): 21-25, 1993.

9. Oschman J: What is healing energy?: the scientific basis of energy medicine, *J Bodywork Movement Ther*, 1997.

10. Eisenberg DM et al: Trends in alternative medicine use in the United States, 1990-1997: results of a follow-up national survey, *JAMA* 280(18):1569-1575, Nov. 1998.

11. Axt A: Autism viewed as a consequence of pineal gland dysfunction, *Farmakoterapia W Psychiatrii I Neurologii* 1: 112-134, 1998.

12. Morton J: *Major medicinal plants: botany culture and uses*, Springfield, Ill, 1977, Charles C. Thomas.

13. Snow J: Glycyrrhiza glabra L, *Protocol J Botanical Med* 1(3), 1996.

Reiki

JACQUELINE FAIRBRASS

Origins and History

Reiki is an ancient natural healing art. Using "laying on of hands," Reiki is a touch healing system. Truly holistic in nature, Reiki healing sessions promote healing on all levels: physical, mental, emotional, and spiritual. This system of "laying on of hands" is documented as being discovered and practiced in Japan in the mid-1800s, although it is commonly believed to be traced back to early Tibetan teachings from around 3000 BCE. In addition, it is considered by many to be the healing method employed by Buddha and Jesus Christ.

Dr. Mikao Usui, a Christian theologian and teacher, is revered as the founder of the practice of Reiki. Accordingly, Reiki is sometimes labeled "the Usui system of natural healing" or *Usui Shiki Ryoho*, which translates into "natural healing by the Usui method." The history of Reiki has been handed down by word of mouth and therefore often is short of factual evidence. Even so, the story is quite consistent, and although most teachers write their own version the details have remained very similar. Traditionally it is told as follows: After being questioned by his students at Doshisha University in Kyoto, Japan about the healing Jesus performed, Dr. Usui began a quest to find the answer to how Christ was able to heal by touch. His travels took him to North America and back to Japan, where he studied both Christianity and Buddhism and learned to communicate in English, Chinese, and Sanskrit, as well as his native Japanese, which took 14 years of his life.

Although he had found the intellectual knowledge, it took a spiritual revelation to enable Dr. Usui to actually be able to practice Reiki and teach others. Before his death, Dr. Usui passed on the title "Grand Master of Reiki" to Chujiro Hayashi. Hayashi formalized the teachings and training of others and documented numerous healing sessions performed by his students. Reiki still is practiced in Japan today, where there are established clinics. From Japan, Reiki was brought to North America, originally introduced into Hawaii in 1937 by Hawaya Takarta, a Japanese-American woman. Takarta established a clinic in Hawaii, working as a practitioner while teaching and training other practitioners. Takarta died in 1980, having passed the Reiki teachings to 22 Reiki Masters in North America. From here Reiki has spread over the globe and is practiced in most Western cultures. There is no longer a "Grand Master of Reiki" and each teacher or Master is considered an equal.

There are many different Reiki training establishments around the world, but the teachings remain basically the same.

Mechanism of Action According to Its Own Theory

Reiki is pronounced as "ray key." *Rei* means "universal" and refers to the energy of the spiritual dimension and soul. Some would refer to it as "God" or "Goddess." *Ki* refers to the vital life force energy that flows through all that is alive. The concept of ki energy is common in most religious and cultural histories, including some current psychotherapy schools and quantum physics. Commonly it also is known as *chi, prana,* and *holy spirit.* Reiki presents the concept of "universal life-force energy." It is the coming together of the spiritual dimension and living energies to awaken a dynamic healing process to release the cause of stress in the body, mind, emotions, and spirit.

Because of the spiritual component of Reiki, it is important to note that Reiki is not a religion and holds no doctrines or creeds. However, Reiki practitioners and students undertake to live by the following guidelines:

> *Just for today I will live the attitude of gratitude*
> *Just for today I will not worry*
> *Just for today I will not anger*
> *Just for today I will do my work honestly*
> *Just for today I will show love and respect for every living thing*

The art or technique of Reiki is energy focus. *Webster's Dictionary* describes *energy* as an inherent power; therefore anyone can learn Reiki. The skill of the practitioner or therapist depends on training and commitment to practice. The practitioner focuses the Reiki energy through the hands. The act of touch, laying hands on the body to relieve pain and to comfort, is as old as time itself. When we experience pain the most natural thing to do is to place our hands on it. The touch of a human hand conveys a feeling of peacefulness, warmth, and healing. Our natural instinct is to reach out and touch another human being who is hurting, whether the pain be physical, mental, or emotional. The Reiki practitioner takes this a step further. By laying the hands on a person or an animal, the practitioner awakens the ability to heal, both in the self and others. The practitioners have been attuned to channel healing energy by being connected to the Reiki energy by a Reiki Master or teacher. The attunement process only can be passed on by a Reiki Master or teacher who has studied and has the ability to connect the student to the Reiki energy. Therefore Reiki cannot be studied just from books. It takes a trained professional to make the energy connection. A Reiki therapist will be certified by the Master, which conveys proof to others that Reiki is the energy healing the therapist is using.

Forms of Therapy

In addition to the basic Reiki path a number of teachers have introduced branches of interest. Sai Baba or Tera Mai Reiki has a focus toward collective planetary healing as opposed to individual healing. Mari-El is another spin-off from Reiki, with a more female perspective, where patients are encouraged to explore past lives to facilitate understanding of current life situations. New branches of Reiki are springing up and may be considered carefully by the individual interested in pursuing Reiki as part of a wellness program. One new branch is Karuna Reiki, which has been trademarked in the United States. Prerequisite to studying Karuna Reiki is the traditional three levels of Reiki.

Demographics

In the early 1990s Reiki practitioners were numbered in the hundreds. To date, there are hundreds of thousands throughout the world. Most urban centers in North America and Canada have numerous Reiki practitioners and teachers. However, most people trained in Reiki use it for their own personal benefit. It is one of the few therapies that is equally effective in self-care as in the treatment of others.

Indications and Reasons for Referral

Obviously with something as elusive as Reiki and the lack of scientific background, claims for Reiki healings must be considered carefully. The one area that results can be guaranteed is in stress management. Many stress-related disorders may benefit from Reiki treatments. A Reiki session performed by a skilled and qualified practitioner will result in stress release. The recipient becomes relaxed, breathing deepens, and the parasympathetic nervous system is stimulated.

A simple ranking of conditions responsive to Reiki treatments is as follows. As with all alternative therapies, Reiki does not preclude mainstream medical therapies in addition.

Top level: *A therapy ideally suited for these conditions*

Addictions; amenorrhea; asthma; childbirth; chronic fatigue syndrome; chronic pain; constipation; discomfort during pregnancy; female health; gastroenteritis (including diarrhea and vomiting); gastric ulcers; general discomfort and pain from disease processes; headaches; high blood pressure; impotence; menstrual cramps; menopause; muscular aches and pains; pain management; Parkinson's disease; pregnancy; psoriasis; some psychiatric disorders; and stress and stress-related disorders

Second level: *One of the better therapies for these conditions*

AIDS; Alzheimer's disease; arthritis; asthma; back pain; cancer; cervical cancer; children's health; colic; colitis and Crohn's disease; endometriosis; general ear pain; heart disease; hemorrhoids; hyperactivity; hypertension; insomnia; lung cancer; male health; mental health; osteoarthritis; osteoporosis; ovarian cancer; ovarian cysts; postpartum care; prostatic cancer; rheumatoid arthritis; sinusitis; and stomach ache

Third level: *A valuable adjunctive therapy for these conditions*

Bronchitis; conjunctivitis; diverticulosis and diverticulitis; fibrocystic breast disease; herpes; irritable bowel syndrome; periodic leg movement syndrome; preconception; prostatitis; respiratory conditions; sleep disorders; uterine fibroids; vaginal infection; and viral and bacterial infections

The use of Reiki also has been successful as a treatment for a variety of chronic conditions. Problems that are more chronic in nature require treatments over a longer time. In particular, there are numerous testimonials about the efficiency of Reiki treatments with palliative care and pain management.

Reiki is very effective when used as first aid for cuts, burns, sprains, and others. The Reiki practitioner on these occasions obviously does not place the hands on the recipient but works in the subtle anatomy or *aura* (the electromagnetic field that surrounds and permeates all life forms). It also is valuable during times of serious accidents and injury. An individual does not have to be sick to benefit from Reiki. Practice promotes mental clarity, emotional balance, and general well-being. Reiki accelerates healing, brings about a state of deep relaxation, and is an impetus to spiritual growth.

Druglike Information

Safety

Reiki does not conflict with other health care but enhances its results. It does not interfere with traditional medical treatment but facilitates the benefits and speeds the recovery from toxic side effects. It also may be used in conjunction with other complementary healing modalities, including massage, craniosacral, reflexology, and others. Reiki speeds the healing process and provides a source for restoring energy while an individual is ill, under medical treatment, or in recovery. Often with only one treatment, Reiki can relieve the physical symptoms and emotional upset associated with stress, headaches, backaches, digestive disorders, and general irritability. Most minor aches and pains can be relieved within just a few minutes.

Research Base

Evidence Based

For some time, scientific studies have been conducted in the area of laying on of hands; however, proven clinically validated studies are limited. The most well known Reiki study was conducted in 1997 by Karin Olson, RN, PhD, from Edmonton, Alberta. The purpose of the study was to explore the usefulness of Reiki as an adjuvant to opioid therapy in the management of pain. A pilot study was conducted involving 20 volunteers experiencing pain at 55 sites for a variety of reasons, including cancer. A second-degree certified Reiki therapist performed all treatments. Pain was measured using a visual analogue scale and a Likert scale immediately before and after treatment. Both instruments showed a highly significant ($p < 0.001$) reduction in pain following the Reiki treatment.[1] Laying on hands to relieve anxiety has been validated by experiments carried out at St. Vincent's Medical Centre in New York.[2] Extensive testing has been conducted in Japan, but the records have not been made available in the West.[3]

Most Reiki healing stories are testimonials by those who believe in its potency. These range from stories telling of relief from minor headaches, which a practitioner can demonstrate within 5 minutes, to claims to healing from HIV and cancer. At its simplest, Reiki relieves stress, and this can be guaranteed. As various studies indicate that stress is the major component of disease in 75% to 85% of incidences, Reiki often can be an important tool in leading to wellness. At its most complicated, people claim that Reiki has transformed their lives by bringing awareness and healing on many levels.

Basic Science

Little traditional scientific evidence exists. However, Dr. John Zimmerman of the University of Colorado has established that magnetic fields around the hands of healers are up to several hundred times stronger than those fields around nonhealers, using a superconducting quantum interference device.[2]

Risk and Safety

Reiki is completely safe. There is no danger involved in using or receiving a Reiki treatment. Reiki has no contraindications, and it has been shown to be efficacious in cases when there is no belief in it. The recipient does not have to believe in Reiki for it to work; the recipient only has to be open to receive a treatment.

Efficacy

The only guarantee that can be made for a Reiki session is that stress and anxiety will be lessened. Testimonials are personal, varying with people from slight improvement in disease symptoms to complete wellness. Using Reiki is a personal experience.

As the use of alternative or complementary therapies becomes more widespread, we are sure to see more clinical studies undertaken.

Future Research Opportunities and Priorities

Further pain management studies are being considered at this time. Validating through clinical research therapeutic applications of Reiki has proven difficult because of the lack of control of variables, in particular the surroundings and settings as preferred by individual therapists.

Self-Help versus Professional

Reiki is often used for self-help. The first degree is primarily for personal use, and individuals often train in it for this purpose.

Visiting a Professional

Reiki therapists have learned a series of hand positions, which cover the entire body, both front and back. Traditionally the treatment begins with the recipient lying on the back on a massage-type table. The practitioner places the hands gently on the head of the patient for around 2 to 5 minutes. Starting at the head, the practitioner moves down the entire body to the feet. The hand movements are passive, and there is no massaging or rubbing involved. Around halfway through the session the therapist asks the recipient to turn and lie on the front. The therapist then places the hands on the back, lifting and replacing to cover the entire back of the body in the same way. At no time does the recipient feel any discomfort. If the recipient is unable to lie in a position comfortably, adjustments are made to facilitate comfort. Lying down facilitates complete relaxation, allowing the body and mind to shift into a parasympathetic state, and bringing rest and repair.

Hands are positioned lightly on the recipient, and the feeling of Reiki flowing into the body is as if someone had placed a hot water bottle on the spot where the hands are placed. The recipient normally remains fully clothed throughout the treatment. There is no reason for the recipient to undress because the energy flows through clothing. However, loose clothing is recommended so that the recipient may be as comfortable as possible and able to breathe deeply. The practitioner's hands are not placed on the breasts or genitals. Sensitivity to patient comfort is an essential component in the Reiki treatment. This type of session would last around 1 hour to 1.5 hours. However, short spot treatments are used and Reiki can be performed with someone sitting in a chair. More controversial is the *distant healing method*. Taught at the second (practitioner) level, distant healing involves using symbols drawn in the air to send healing Reiki energy to people at a distance. There rarely is a charge for this service.

Most Reiki healing sessions are performed quietly. Silence is preferable because it enables the practitioner to focus and use the intuitive abilities. It also facilitates relaxation on the part of the recipient. Most Reiki healers play soft music throughout the session, keep lighting to a minimum, and most importantly they do not disturb the session by taking phone calls, for example. Reiki practitioners center themselves and calm their minds before beginning a session, and they encourage the recipient to relax and breathe deeply. Some therapists "scan" the body for disturbances in the energetic field. This is performed once the recipient is on the table and consists of the therapist placing the hands about 4 inches from the body and feeling for variations in temperature. When a hot or cold spot is ascertained the therapist may ask for feedback from the recipient or just note the imbalance and spend some extra time at those places during the treatment. When asked for feedback a patient may respond with a physical disorder or discomfort in the area, or it may be a blockage on the emotional or mental energetic levels. For the patient a Reiki session brings a sense of harmony to the whole subtle anatomy.

The Reiki recipient usually enters a deep state of relaxation comparable to a meditative state. During a session the recipient may feel the usual warmth from the therapist's hands placed on the body, as well as tingling sensations, occasional coolness, vibrations, and extreme heat from the hands. After the session, recipients may feel as though they have woken from a deep sleep, or they may be aware of being in a dream state through the entire session, including seeing colors and the sense of "past life" recall. Often the Reiki therapist may encourage the patient to discuss these sensations and attempt to facilitate an interpretation, but it is up to the patient to decide whether they are personally significant. The feeling of deep relaxation stays with patients for some time afterwards, depending on the personal stress level they return to in their lives. The patient may begin a detoxification process, such as an increase in the size or number of bowel movements for the next few days. Regular treatments strengthen the relaxation response and the time in which the patient releases from stress and tension.

Credentialing

The therapy is not regulated anywhere in the world and there are no registration processes. There are numerous individual organizations that have attempted to formalize training, but the general consensus is that of freedom in the training process. Therefore the most effective way of finding a Reiki practitioner is through referral. Because of Reiki's nonscientific background and lack of formalized registration, many Reiki therapists do not advertise but rely on networking.

Training

There are three traditional levels of Reiki. The first degree is primarily for personal use. At the first degree level the student is attuned to the Reiki energy through a ceremonial process. The student learns basic hand positions for self-healing and treating others in both lying and sitting positions and begins studying energy healing concepts. At the second degree or practitioner level the student focuses more on working with others. The use of symbols, including the distant healing symbol, to strengthen the Reiki energy is the main focus of the second degree. The third level of Reiki is traditionally that of Reiki Master or teacher. With accelerated learning, many teachers offer an interim course, that of a third degree without the teacher training. This enables students to gradually move into a teaching position if desired. The Reiki Master is both a practitioner and teacher and usually has studied and worked with Reiki extensively. An apprenticeship to a Reiki Master is a common way in which the teachings are passed on. During this apprenticeship, students study Reiki and apply the Reiki principles to their lives, making changes in lifestyle to enhance personal wellness on all levels.

What to Look for in a Provider

Occasionally, Reiki Masters have taken "quickie" courses and are not particularly experienced or well-versed in the therapy. Accordingly, it is customary to ask therapists how long they have practiced and what other qualifications they bring to their practice. Because Reiki is used in conjunction with numerous healing modalities, Reiki therapists often are versed in other therapies, which can be very useful if assisting patients through the healing process.

Associations and Teaching Establishments

Although some Reiki associations have been established, the general consensus in the field is that Reiki is not a "regulated" profession. A Reiki Master does not have to belong to any organization.

For more information, contact one of the following:
In the United States:

Center for Reiki Training
Tel: (810) 948-8112
Toll-free: (800) 332-8112
Fax: (810) 948-9534
E-mail: center@reiki.org
www.reiki.org

The Reiki Alliance
PO Box 41
Cataldo, ID 83810

In Canada:

Fairbrass School of Complementary Therapies*
PO Box 47082
2638 Innes Road
Gloucester, ON K1B 5S0
Tel: (613) 834-7519
Fax: (613) 834-4103
E-mail: fairbras@comnet.ca

Worldwide:

Reiki Outreach International
PO Box 609
Fair Oaks, CA 95628
Tel: (916) 863-1500
Fax: (916) 863-6464

Suggested Reading

1. Baginski BJ, Sharamon S: *Reiki universal life energy,* Mendocino, Calif, 1988, Life Rhythm.
   Easy to read and understand, this book covers how Reiki works, self-treatment, and starting up a home-based professional practice.
2. Horan P: *Empowerment through Reiki,* Twin Lakes, Wis, 1992, Lotus Light.
   Description of how Reiki works and the ways it can be used to effect positive changes in health and well-being.

---

*This company is owned by the author.

3. Stein D: *Essential Reiki, a complete guide to an ancient healing art*, Freedom, Calif, 1996, The Crossing Press.

Understanding the metaphysical principles of how Reiki works, its teachings and practice, and why individuals should get to know Reiki.

4. Lubeck W: *Reiki, way of the heart*, Twin Lakes, Wis, 1996, Lotus Light.

Describes how Reiki works and the possibilities that open through the experience of Reiki energy.

References

1. Olson K, Hanson J: *Using Reiki to manage pain: a preliminary report, Cancer Prevent Control* 1(2):108-113, 1997.
2. Rand WL: Reiki research, *Reiki News* (summer):1-9, 1995.
3. Petter FA: *Reiki fire*, Twin Lakes, Wis, 1997, Lotus Light.

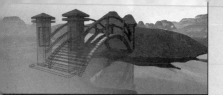

Rolfing® Structural Integration

ALINE NEWTON

BRET NYE

RUSSELL STOLZOFF

Origins and History

Rolfing Structural Integration was developed by Ida P. Rolf, PhD (1896-1979). Dr. Rolf was born in New York in 1896, graduated from Barnard College in 1916, and received her doctorate in biological chemistry from the College of Physicians and Surgeons of Columbia University. Until the late 1920s she worked as a researcher at the Rockefeller Institute. Dr. Rolf evolved her methods over several decades and was profoundly influenced by the theories and practices of yoga, osteopathy, and homeopathy, which she used for her own health. Initially, Dr. Rolf was attracted to yoga because its theories were aimed at evoking human potential—physically, mentally, and emotionally.

In her early work she used various yoga and other movement exercises to create length across the joints of the body. Dr. Rolf also subscribed to a core concept from osteopathy— that body structure determines its function—and she adopted this principle in the creation of her methods of manipulation. However, she disagreed with the osteopathic emphasis that focused solely on freeing joint restrictions because it left out the crucial role that soft tissues play in determining body structure and function. Instead, Rolf developed the idea that bones are held in place by the body's pervasive network of soft tissues: muscles, fascia, ligaments, and tendons. She saw that chronic shortening in the body's soft tissues from strain, injury, and faulty habits creates compensatory adjustments throughout the body structure, including the misalignment of bones and their joints. She also pioneered the viewpoint that bodies are only balanced to the extent that they are organized vertically with respect to gravity. Imbalances are exacerbated by the compressive effects of gravity.

In the 1950s, after many years of experimentation with her patients, Rolf created and refined a 10-session sequence of myofascial manipulations that could be used to teach students to organize and balance misaligned body structure and thereby improve its function. In the mid-1960s, during the burgeoning human potential movement at the Esalen Institute in Big Sur, California, Rolf's methods became famous for transformational change. Dr. Rolf founded the Rolf Institute in 1971 in Boulder, Colorado, choosing some of her students from that time to teach and carry on her work. Today the Rolf Institute is a flourishing teaching and research center with its international headquarters in Boulder, Colorado and training centers in Washington, D.C., Germany, Brazil, and Australia.

Since Ida Rolf's death in 1979 the work of Rolfing structural integration has evolved to include a variety of soft tissue techniques (for example, deep connective tissue, craniosacral, visceral, and nonthrust joint techniques), all used in service of the principle of freeing compensations and organizing a body in gravity. Along with the original sequence of 10 sessions, principles have evolved that enable a more individualized and effective approach to changing a person's patterns of structure and function. Some Rolfers also are trained in Rolf Movement Integration, a method that enables them to assist patients in developing more effective habits of movement to support the structural changes that occur in the course of a Rolfing series.

Mechanism of Action According to Its Own Theory

The objectives of Rolfing—integration of human structure and improvement in human functioning—are accomplished primarily by a systematic manipulation of the connective tissues of the body. These connective tissues contain various proportions of collagenous fibers and fluid matrix. Selective deposition and resorption of connective tissue elements in response to internal and external environmental influences allows for the plasticity inherent in the human shape. Random, disruptive events of life (injuries, prolonged sitting, poor movement patterns, postural manifestations of psychologic stressors, and so on) can result in dysfunctional fixations and structural relationships with consequent loss of ease and range of motion. However, this plasticity of connective tissue also enables a Rolfer to selectively alter connective tissue structures in support of greater structural integration. By selective release and alteration of connective tissue structures the Rolfer accomplishes the task of structural integration. Dr. Rolf theorized that through the careful application of energy (in the form of pressure exerted by the practitioner's fingertips, knuckles, or elbow), it was possible to fundamentally change the tension matrix in these connective tissues. The release of fixations in the connective tissue network (what Dr. Rolf called "the organ of shape") and the resultant increased continuity and balance are primary goals of Rolfing.

From the outset, Dr. Rolf stressed that structural integration was an educational process. The relationship between connective tissue structures and the nervous system is not completely understood. It was apparent to Dr. Rolf that there is significant interaction between these two systems and that that change in one would manifest as corresponding change in the other. As Rolfing changes the shape of a patient's body, integrating its segments by releasing connective tissue fixations, it often elicits pronounced shifts in awareness of bodily sensations, proprioception, and emotions. The mechanism by which this happens is not known, but the integrin system, which links the extracellular matrix (connective tissue) to the biochemistry and behavior of individual cells, represents a promising pathway.[1]

As the theory and practice of Rolfing has evolved over the years, there have been many techniques developed that take advantage of the concept of motility. Whereas mobility is voluntary bodily motion used primarily in locomotion, *motility* describes more subtle and involuntary motion in the body's tissues. Although the concept of motility was first described in the osteopathic literature and still is used in many osteopathic manipulative techniques, Rolfers have developed many uniquely Rolfing-based manipulative techniques that acknowledge and use the body's inherent motility and thus can evoke structural change with a minimum of effort and patient discomfort.

Biologic Mechanism of Action

Given these evolutions in the theory and practice of Rolfing, it is unclear at this point to what extent the changes elicited by Rolfing are a result of the following three proposed mechanisms:

1. Physically elongating the patient's connective tissues and freeing fixations in the patient's structures by application of direct pressure and movement;
2. "Educating" the neuromuscular network to operate more efficiently and at a lower level of tonus; and
3. Evoking an inherent negentropic organizational process by contacting and facilitating the restoration of the patient's own motility.

In all likelihood, all three mechanisms are at play in varying proportions depending on the unique needs of each patient and the aptitudes and inclinations that both the patient and Rolfer bring to the process.

Forms of Therapy

Rolfing is a service mark of the Rolf Institute of Structural Integration. The generic work is known as Structural Integration. Several schools of Structural Integration have evolved, all deriving from the work of Dr. Rolf, and each with a slightly different emphasis (for example, more psychologic or stricter adherence to the original 10 session sequence) and different educational prerequisites and training. The Rolf Institute training program is the most extensive and requires mandatory continuing education.

Demographics

Practitioners of Rolfing-Structural Integration can be found worldwide. In the U.S., Rolfers practice in nearly all 50 states, with concentrations on the East and West Coast and in Colorado. Patient population ranges from infancy to old age and is distributed equally between genders. It is estimated that more than 1 million people have received Rolfing work.

Indications and Reasons for Referral

People seek Rolfing as a way to improve posture, ease chronic musculoskeletal pain and stress, and improve performance in their professional and daily activities. Classic reasons for referral include the following:

- Postural conditions such as poor posture, hyperlordosis, kyphosis, and scoliosis
- Chronic musculoskeletal conditions such as back pain, neck pain, joint restrictions, and chronic tension
- Cervicogenic (stress or tension) headaches
- Radicular pain such as sciatica, carpal tunnel, and neck-shoulder-arm syndromes
- Stress
- Limited range of motion and flexibility
- Poor coordination
- Postinjury or postsurgery rehabilation
- Aftereffects of old physical and emotional trauma (the "never-quite-right again" syndrome)
- Occupational injuries such as repetitive strain injuries (RSI), carpal tunnel, and back problems
- Improvement in athletic performance

Typically Rolfers see patients who have already consulted an MD and may have tried a pharmacologic approach or treatments such as chiropractic, massage, and a variety of physical therapy modalities, with little or no abatement in their symptoms.

The Rolfing model suggests that a wide variety of symptoms actually may reflect general structural imbalances or bad habits of movement and posture held in place by restrictions in the connective tissue "web." These problems, which tend not to respond to local treatment, often are effectively addressed by identifying and releasing the overall imbalances and restrictions in the soft tissue network.

Office Applications

A simple ranking of conditions responsive to this form of therapy is as follows. As with all alternative therapies, use of Rolfing does not preclude the use of mainstream medical therapies in addition.

Top level: A *therapy ideally suited for these conditions*

Back pain; carpal tunnel; hyperlordosis; joint restrictions; kyphosis; limited range of motion and flexibility; musculoskeletal tension; neck pain; poor coordination; poor posture; pregnancy (musculoskeletal complaints during and after); rehabilitation (postinjury or postsurgery, including orthopedic intervention or mastectomy); repetitive strain injuries; sciatica; scoliosis; and stress

Second level: *One of the better therapies for these conditions*

Arthritis; chronic pain (musculoskeletal); foot pain; headaches; osteoarthritis; post-partum care; and temporomandibular joint pain syndrome

Third level: *A valuable adjunctive therapy for these conditions*

Asthma; chronic fatigue syndrome; insomnia; and menstrual cramps

Research Base

Evidence Based

Early research in the effects of Rolfing goes back to Dr. Rolf's tenure at the Rockefeller Institute from 1918 to 1927. She published a total of 13 papers, including *Project Breakthrough* at the Foundation for Brain-Injured Children in 1963. The subjects were children with poor coordination and disorganized, immature movement patterns for their age level. They exhibited better muscle tone, better alignment, improved language skills, and social responsiveness after Rolfing. A study of other neurologically compromised subjects, cerebral palsy in this case, published by Perry et al in 1981, documented significant changes in lower extremity passive range of motion, muscle strength, balance, and gait with Rolfing.[2]

Dr. Valerie Hunt, collaborating with Robert Wagner and Wayne Massey at the University of California-Los Angeles in the late 1970s, published papers that documented, among other things, electromyographic evidence of improved reciprocal inhibition in paired muscle groups after Rolfing; for example, when the biceps flex the elbow, the triceps passively lengthen with diminished resistance to the desired motion.[3-5] This was considered a hallmark finding that documented what Dr. Rolf had observed empirically: That Rolfing resulted in greater ease of motion. In 1988 Rolfer and physical therapist John Cottingham was able to demonstrate increased parasympathetic (and therefore relatively decreased sympathetic) tone following Rolfing[6] and its relationship to improved pelvic inclination following Rolfing.[7] In 1997, Cottingham and Rolfer Jeff Maitland, PhD, published a case study illustrating Rolfing's integrative "third paradigm" approach in the treatment of people with chronic, idiopathic low back pain.[8]

Studies in Progress

Based on the remarkable results of a pilot project that reduced worker compensation costs in one manufacturing plant by 88% (primarily by reducing the incidence of and disability from repetitive stress injuries like carpal tunnel syndrome) the Rolf Institute is applying for funding for a larger study in three to five companies. In 1992 at the pilot study plant with 1650 employees, workers' compensation costs were approximately $1.3 million. In 1996, as a result of implementing an innovative program featuring Rolfing by Siana Goodwin, the figure dropped below $150,000 with 2400 employees. Another pending research project by John Cottinghamn will evaluate the effects of Rolfing and Rolfing Movement work on balance, posture, and parasympathetic tone in a group of older adults with balance dysfunction.

Self-Help versus Professional

It is not possible for individuals to "Rolf" themselves. However, Rolfers often are the source for self-help techniques based on an understanding of body function and exercise. It is the goal of the Rolfing practitioner to assist the patient in making lifestyle choices and integrating self-help techniques that will maintain the improvement resulting from the treatment.

Visiting a Professional

A typical first visit to a Rolfer usually involves talking about why the patient is interested in receiving Rolfing. Rolfers want to know the aspects of personal history that are likely to have an impact on body structure and function. Physical and emotional injuries, accidents, surgeries, and illnesses are among the most basic kinds of information needed. Additionally, current information including the type of work done, current levels of stress and pain and the way it is managed, and nutritional and exercise habits will help the Rolfer to further understand how daily life may affect the patient's body and how to proceed effectively. After an initial interview the Rolfer will want to observe the patient standing and in motion. This visual assessment of body structure and movement helps form a strategy that will address individual needs.

With the patient laying on a padded table, sessions begin with the Rolfer assessing the way the body's soft tissues are arranged around the skeletal structure. With the use of gentle yet penetrating manual manipulation of muscles and fascia, Rolfing systematically addresses the underlying causes of chronically tense muscles and motion restrictions in joints. By focusing on the structural relationships between adjacent areas and the body as a whole, these manipulations gradually organize tensional forces in the soft tissues and bring about shifts in body balance that translate into greater ease of posture and movement. Most Rolfers also verbally direct the patient's awareness to areas of the body and may ask the patient to move to help the body change. Most people discover that focusing their attention on the Rolfer's actions helps them to consciously participate in the process by allowing their bodies to respond to the suggestions their Rolfer's hands are making.

The benefits of Rolfing are best realized in a series of sessions. Each session is designed to focus on a particular set of structural relationships at varying levels of depth. In general the sessions proceed from surface structural relationships to deeper ones. As the sessions progress the patient's body structure becomes increasingly balanced and integrated.

An average basic series is comprised of 10 sessions; however, the exact number of sessions needed to for thoroughness can vary greatly depending on the nature and severity of structural issues and the ability of the body to adapt to change. After a basic series of sessions, periodic follow-up sessions may be needed or desired. Rolf Movement Integration sessions also may help to pattern new postural awareness and movement options that can augment the effects of the manipulations. After a period of integration in which the effects of Rolfing continue to unfold through the daily use of the patient's more efficient body, advanced series of sessions may be held to further address remaining structural imbalances and focus on applications of the changes to daily life.

Credentialing

The Rolf Institute is the sole certifying body for Rolfers. It is the organization that trains people as Rolfing practitioners and supports research and public awareness. The Institute sets high standards for its members by monitoring adherence to its code of ethics, standards of practice, and continuing education program.

Training

There are many imitators who provide various forms of work such as deep tissue massage and structural or postural integration. However, only certified Rolfers have gone through the rigorous training program and continuing education that enables Rolfing to maintain the high quality of the service mark. Certified Rolfers can be recognized by their listing in the Rolf Institute Directory for the current year, which is available through the Rolf Institute (see "Associations").

Barriers and Key Issues

Research

The complexity of the Rolfing Structural Integration model does not lend itself easily to the current standards in scientific research. It is difficult to isolate a single interventional factor when the connective tissue web as a whole is the primary means to change. Also, there is a powerful personal and psychologic dimension and an aspect of patient awareness that often plays a part.

Reputation

In the past, Rolfing has had a reputation for being painful. Developments in technique enable the Rolfing practitioner to accomplish the goals of structural integration with significantly less discomfort than was originally the case. However, the image persists somewhat in the public eye.

Lack of Insurance Coverage

Most patients do not receive insurance reimbursement for Rolfing treatments. A Rolfing series requires a significant investment of both time and money. Though it is very effective, it is not a "quick fix" technique.

Unfamiliarity

Rolfing Structural Integration is based on a complex model of structure and movement that is unfamiliar to practitioners of conventional therapies.

Associations

Rolf Institute of Structural Integration
205 Canyon Blvd.
Boulder, CO 80302
Tel: (303) 449-5903
Toll-Free: (800) 530-8875
Fax: (303) 449-5978
E-mail: RolfInst@aol.com
www.rolf.org

European Rolfing Association e.v.
Kapuzinerstr. 25
D-803307 Munich, Germany
Tel: 49 89 54 37 09 40
Fax: 49 89 54 37 09 42
E-mail: rolfingeurope@compuserve.com

Associacao Brasileira de Rolfistas
Caixa Postal 11299
05422-970 Sao Paulo-SP, Brazil
Tel/Fax: 55 11 887 0670
E-mail: rolfing@dialdata.com.br

Australian Rolfing Office
90 Plateau Rd.
Bilgola Plateau
NSW Australia 2107
Tel/Fax: 61 02 9918 2324
E-mail: JohnSmithSomatics@bigpond.com

Suggested Reading

1. Rolf IP: *Rolfing: reestablishing the natural alignment and structural integration of the human body*, Rochester, Vt, 1989, Healing Art Press.
   A fairly technical book by the originator of Rolfing Structural Integration. A thorough explanation of the original ideas behind the practice of Rolfing.
2. Feitis R: *Ida Rolf talks about Rolfing and physical reality*, New York, 1978, Harper and Row.
   A collection of epigrams and short pieces that give an idea of the breadth of Ida Rolf's work and thought.
3. Bond M: *Rolfing movement integration, a self-help approach to balancing the body*, Rochester, Vt, 1993, Healing Arts Press.
   A practical introduction to body awareness and Rolfing Movement Integration.
4. Maitland J: *Spacious bodies: explorations in somatic ontology*, Berkeley, Calif, 1995, North Atlantic Books.
   A theoretic exploration of some of the current developments in the Rolfing Structural Integration model.

References

1. Ingber D: The architecture of life, *Sci Am* 278(1):48-57, 1998.
2. Perry J, Jones MH, Thomas L: Functional evaluation of Rolfing in cerebral palsy, *Develop Med Child Neurol* 23(6):717-729, 1981.
3. Weinberg R, Hunt V: Effects of structural integration on strait-trait anxiety, *J Clin Psychol* 35(2):319-322, 1979.
4. Hunt V, Massey W: Electomyographic evaluation of structural integration techniques, Los Angeles, 1977, UCLA Press.
5. Hunt V, Massey W: A study of structural integration from neuromuscular, energy field, and emotional approaches, 1977.
6. Cottingham J: Effects of soft tissue mobilization on parasympathetic tone in two age groups, *JAPTA* 68:352-356, 1988.
7. Cottingham J: Shifts in pelvic inclination angle and parasympathetic tone produced by Rolfing soft tissue manipulation, *JAPTA* 68:1364-1370, 1988.
8. Cottingham J, Maitland J: A three-paradigm treatment model using soft tissue mobilization and guided movement-awareness techniques for patients with chronic back pain: a case study, *J Orthop Sports Phys Ther* 26(3):155-167, 1997.

Rosen Method

ANNE REIN

GLORIA HESSELLUND

MARION ROSEN

Origins and History

Rosen Method bodywork is an intuitive system of hands-on work developed by Marion Rosen through her work as a physical therapist over a period of 30 years. Rosen Method movement exercises are designed to move all of the joints in the body through their available range of motion and expand the chest to free up breathing capacity.

Rosen Method has tremendous power to transform, liberate, and restore. The work can induce a deep state of relaxation, relieve and clear chronic pain, release muscle tension, restore freedom of movement to the limbs, neck, and torso, and create an emotional container for unconscious thoughts, memories, and feelings to reveal themselves. It addresses the emotional causes of physical pain, and it works through the easing of muscle tension, the slowing down of the breath, and the unconscious associations arising from spoken words.

The basic concepts of Rosen Method can be easily explained to anyone having basic knowledge of human anatomy, but the true power of the work can be known only through experience—from receiving sessions on a table, participating in movement classes, or entering a Rosen Method training program. The authors encourage the reader to consider trying such a session, should an opportunity be available.

Rosen Method belongs to the field of somatic therapy, which, after more than 60 years of experimentation and refinement, is now coming into its maturity. Somatic therapies now enjoy widespread public awareness, increased attention from the popular media, and growing acceptance from physicians and other primary health care providers. These therapies generally address the integration of body, mind, and spirit with the purpose of creating greater awareness of the totality of the individual's experience and, especially with Rosen Method, restoring a sense of ease and well-being. Most work through hands-on bodywork, movement, subtle energy work, or some combination of these techniques.

Many somatic therapies, including Rosen Method, spring from a common source—the unique partnerships among physical therapists and psychoanalysts such as Wilhelm Reich and Karen Horney that flourished, primarily in Europe, between the two World Wars. As a young woman, Marion Rosen participated in such a partnership.

In her youth, Marion wanted to be a dancer but had been told she was too tall. In 1936 she became an apprentice to Lucy Heyer, herself a former dancer, who worked as a "breath therapist" in partnership with her husband, Dr. Gustav Heyer, a German medical doctor and psychoanalyst. Mrs. Heyer had been trained by Elsa Gindler, who is the founding mother of many contemporary somatic therapies.

In 1938 Marion fled Germany for Sweden and took her first course in physical therapy there while waiting for a U.S. visa. Arriving in San Francisco in 1939, Marion took a job as a physical therapist at Kaiser Permanente in Richmond, California. In 1944 she graduated from another physical therapy training program offered by the Mayo Clinic and received her physical therapy certificate.

Soon after, Marion opened a private physical therapy practice in Oakland. Over the years she treated a number of individuals who continued to experience chronic pain even though their injuries had occurred years earlier and there was no remaining evidence of injury or trauma. Through experimentation she discovered that people who talked about their injuries healed more quickly. Gradually Marion developed the theory that trauma of all kinds—physical, emotional, and mental—is held in the body as chronic muscle tension. In practice, she found that as the muscles relaxed and let go, her patients often experienced emotions, thoughts and feelings they had been holding unconsciously in their bodies, often for long periods of time.

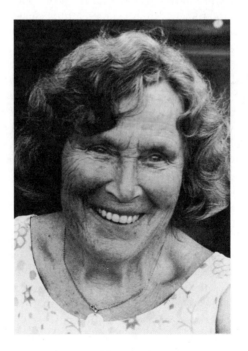

Marion Rosen, founder of Rosen Method.

Subtle changes in the breath also caught Marion's attention. She saw that when patients deeply relaxed (often as a result of remembering something they had "put away"), the diaphragm would let go. When the diaphragm relaxed, the patients entered a deep state of relaxation, which ushered in an enduring sense of ease, well-being, and peace. A number of Marion's patients reported having feelings of being at one with the universe.

Marion developed a reputation in the medical community as a professional who could successfully treat patients that failed to respond to conventional medical treatment. Doctors referred patients with asthma, chronic pain, and psychosomatic illnesses to her, and she developed a reputation for being able to treat these individuals successfully. Not completely satisfied with only treating injuries, Marion was also captivated by the restorative and transformational potential of her discoveries, and she began to wonder what her work could do for people who were basically healthy and well.

Marion created Rosen Method Movement in response to requests from former patients who asked for exercises that would help prevent injuries. Marion set to music the range-of-motion tests used by physical therapists and began conducting movement classes. This playful, low-impact form of movement is designed to move all the joints in the body and free up breathing capacity.

In 1972 Marion began teaching her method to others, first to individuals who sought her out; and in 1980 she began holding public classes. Approaching 20 years as a profession, Rosen Method now has 13 centers for training practitioners, who number approximately 600, from 15 countries in North America, Europe, and Australia.

Mechanism of Action According to Its Own Theory

At its best, Rosen Method bodywork is a means of contacting the unconscious through the body. A skilled practitioner can run the hand lightly over patients' bodies and "read" from their life experiences and know something of the pains they have suffered and the choices they have made as a result.

The practitioner's intention is to be engaged with a whole person, the totality of the person's being. Through this connection the practitioner can sometimes catch a glimpse of the totality of the person's life and essential truth as it presents itself in a moment in time. The practitioner may be able to hold a mirror at such an angle that patients can come into the experience of themselves as a whole being. This phenomenon makes it especially difficult to break the work down into steps or components.

Nevertheless, there are three principle techniques used in Rosen Method bodywork, presented here in the order in which they are usually taught to Rosen students:

1. Finding muscle tension in the body through hands-on touch and helping the patient to become aware of it
2. Observing and responding to subtle changes in the breath
3. Talking, which requires the practitioner to develop a vocabulary of bodily feelings and sensations, make observations to the patient about areas of holding, track the patient's actual words, and play off unconscious associations with those words.

We tense our bodies when we feel threatened, criticized, ashamed, angry, or in any other state that brings us into conflict with others. Children especially tend to contract in response to overwhelming demands, a frightening situation, or a critical presence. Repeated over time, these contractions become habitual and result in chronic muscle tension.

The theory of Rosen Method with respect to muscle tension is that chronic muscle tension has meaning for an individual through which it carries a clue to memories or feelings that the person has suppressed. Rosen practitioners refer to chronic muscle tension as a "holding," to convey that the person has chosen (albeit unconsciously) to tense a specific group of muscles in response to the unique situation, thereby "putting away" some of the memories and feelings about life experiences.

A boy who is told "big boys don't cry" tenses the neck muscles to squelch his tears until he no longer remembers he is tensing these muscles. Eventually, the man walks into the office of a physical therapist or a Rosen Method practitioner seeking relief from chronic neck pain. Or perhaps he walks into the office of a psychotherapist because he has lost touch with his feelings and is unhappy.

A child who has experienced harsh or frightening circumstances takes a stance of defiance by "digging in her heels," thereby locking the knees, tightening the hamstrings, squeezing the muscles around the pelvis, exaggerating the lumbar curve, and thrusting forward her rib cage as if to say "I can take care of myself." Aside from the risk of being pushed over in this unstable arrangement, she is a candidate for potentially serious back problems, and she cannot let anyone into her heart because she is so busy holding her position. Will she find Rosen work, or will she need surgery? And can she be happy in her life?

We learn to hold ourselves back, to keep our feelings to ourselves. Our choices shape our bodies, and then our bodies begin to shape our experience.

To the reader familiar with therapeutic massage, the touch in a Rosen session might feel, at first encounter, similar to massage. The similarity goes only so far, though, because Rosen Method has its own technique for contacting muscle tension. The practitioner may get the hands around the held area and exaggerate the muscle contraction to get the tense muscles to "wake up" and let go of their chronic holding. The intention is to meet the holding with approximately the same force it exerts on the body, and make a space—with the practitioner's hands and presence—for the emergence of any feelings or memories that have been put away in the form of muscle tension.

A Rosen Method practitioner often works with one *active* hand, contacting the muscle tension as described above, and one *listening* hand. What the practitioner is listening for are subtle changes in the body, perhaps a softening of the contracted muscles, and especially for changes in the breath.

A Rosen Method practitioner is a connoisseur of the breath. The practitioner can distinguish the "automatic" breath (rhythmic and regular) that walks in the door from the more personal breath (uneven and less regular) that arrives when the body allows itself to sink into the table and be met by the hands. The practitioner knows what a "performed breath" looks like—it may be deep, but it carries visible effort: a contraction of the accessory breathing muscles in the neck, shoulders, and rib cage; and a forced inhale or exhale. The practitioner awaits the "breath of ease," the breath that ripples up effortlessly through the musculature and accompanies deep relaxation. Tight muscles release, and if the patient is supine the freely swinging movement of the diaphragm is clearly visible. The whole body has breathed a sigh of relief.

Often the breath of ease follows a statement by the patient (or practitioner) that reveals something of the person's essence and resonates with the deepest nature. The breath arrives by way of confirmation, as if announcing "the truth has been spoken in this moment."

Sometimes only a few words are exchanged between patient and practitioner during the course of a Rosen session. Occasionally a session unfolds in near total silence. All of the physical benefits of Rosen—the easing of chronic tension, the lessening of pain, the deep relaxation—can occur without talking. But it is the words that pull what is felt into consciousness and thereby open a door to new possibilities.

Biologic Mechanism of Action

Rosen Method work is well-grounded in human anatomy and physiology. Understanding the mechanics of breathing and some anatomy is important to practicing Rosen because the action of the diaphragm is central to Rosen work. The Rosen practitioner works to release the diaphragm by gently rocking the rib cage, massaging the back muscles that attach to the vertebral column around T12, and moving the psoas muscle, which directly affects the diaphragm.

An understanding of the diaphragm can also bridge the gap between an intuitive system and the conventional body of medical knowledge. Through its vast attachments to the skeleton and viscera, connections to the central and peripheral nervous systems, and voluntary and involuntary regulation, the diaphragm is involved with a whole array of phenomena affecting relaxation.

Rosen theory, which supports Marion's clinical observations, says that these factors along with the diaphragm's location in the center of the body make the diaphragm key to understanding the connection between body, mind, and spirit. We also believe that the unique quality of sensory input to muscle tension through Rosen touch, verbal dialogue, and the deep relaxation of the skeletal muscles and diaphragm leads to a heightened state of physical and emotional awareness and results in a new range of possibilities for living.

Forms of Therapy

Rosen Method is offered in two forms: hands-on bodywork and movement.

People seek out Rosen Method bodywork because they have physical pain or discomfort with nonspecific diagnosis, muscle tension, and postural problems or feel generally stressed. Many patients come with a desire for emotional and spiritual growth. Patients receiving psychotherapy come to Rosen Method to enhance their work with their psychologist or counselor.

Participants in Rosen Method movement classes tend to come because they want to improve their range of motion, increase their breathing capacity, and develop an overall sense of ease in movement. The invigorating, low-impact movements can be especially beneficial for people recovering from injury or leading a sedentary lifestyle.

Demographics

There are 13 Rosen training centers in the U.S., Canada, Sweden, Norway, Finland, Denmark, Russia, Germany, Switzerland, France, and Australia. Rosen Method practitioners tend to be clustered around these centers. See "Associations."

Rosen Method movement classes are especially good for people who want to increase their mobility, and they tend to draw participants who are middle-aged and older. There is no other demographic data available on patients who tend to use this modality.

Indications and Reasons for Referral

Medical professionals refer patients to Rosen Method practitioners for conditions that have a stress-related component, chronic pain that has a nonspecific diagnosis, back pain, and neck pain. Psychotherapists and counselors refer patients who need help with relaxing and contacting emotions. Rosen Method has been highly effective with back pain, arthritis, asthma, chronic pain, headaches, chronic fatigue, and stress. Many psychology professionals and patients consider it a valuable complement to psychotherapy.

Office Applications

A simple ranking of conditions responsive to this form of therapy is as follows. As with all alternative therapies, Rosen Method does not preclude mainstream medical therapies in addition.

Top level: *A therapy ideally suited for these conditions*
Arthritis; back pain; chronic fatigue; headaches; and stress

Second level: *One of the better therapies for these conditions*
Asthma; colic; constipation; hypertension; insomnia; menstrual cramps; osteoarthritis; preconception; and restless leg syndrome

Third level: *A valuable adjunctive therapy for these conditions*
Allergies; colitis and Crohn's disease; emphysema; postpartum care; pregnancy and childbirth; and premenstrual syndrome

Research Base

No formal research exists for this form of therapy.

Druglike Information

Warnings, Contraindications, and Precautions

Patients with medical conditions should consult their physicians before receiving sessions. Likewise, psychotherapy patients should consult their therapists.

Rosen Method is contraindicated for anyone with a history of psychosis, serious mental illness, or any psychologic condition that requires an individual to maintain a rigid defense structure.

Rosen Method should not be used in the acute stage of any physical or emotional trauma because it could aggravate these conditions.

Rosen Method is not recommended for individuals in the early stages of recovery from alcohol or drug addiction, although it can be very effective in later stages (1 year of recovery or longer.)

Self-Help versus Professional

Because it is difficult to contact your own chronic tensions, Rosen *bodywork* cannot effectively be applied on yourself. Rosen *movement* as a daily practice is "self-help." However, a Rosen Method practitioner is required to learn it.

Visiting a Professional

Rosen Method bodywork sessions are conducted on a massage table with the patient partially clothed and covered with a blanket. Sessions last for 50 to 60 minutes and are received once per week or once every 2 weeks over a period of time, the length of which varies depending on the goal of the patient. Strict confidentiality is maintained. The Rosen practitioner may consult with other appropriate medical or psychologic professionals only with consent of the patient.

Rosen Method movement classes are conducted with groups of students in spacious rooms. Students wear comfortable clothing. Movements are done independently in a circle, in partnership, and on the floor with the accompaniment of music.

Training and Credentialing

The training of a Rosen Method practitioner requires 3 or more years; the length of study being determined by the time that it generally takes a student with no previous experience to learn both the observational skills required for Rosen Method (the ability to see and feel subtle changes in the breath and musculature) and also the intuitional skills (the ability to set the ego aside and trust the unconscious process to reveal itself through the patient or practitioner).

Rosen Method training requires 2 years and 350 hours of classroom instruction, followed by an internship that requires 350 patient hours, supervision, and periodic patient review sessions. There are two training tracks: the long-term training, which consists of weekly classes and hands-on practice; and the intensive track, which permits the student to participate in six 9-day intensives over a 2-year period. The internship common to both tracks requires at least 9 months and may take up to 18 months, depending on the intern's rate of progress.

The Rosen Institute, a nonprofit governance organization that holds the Rosen Method service mark, certifies practitioners at the recommendation of an intern's primary supervisor and the director of training for the intern's school. Rosen Method students are formally evaluated four times during their training: after each year of classroom training; midway through the internship; and at the end of the internship.

What to Look for in a Provider

Rosen Method certification is the most important qualification to look for in a Rosen practitioner. After that, years of experience can be a factor, as well as personal style. If there is more than one practitioner available in your area, it is a good idea for patients to have at least one session (and possibly several) before committing to a longer-term course of treatment.

Barriers and Key Issues

Individual Rosen practitioners do have relationships in which they refer to physicians and receive referrals from physicians. However, the scope of this mutually beneficial practice has been limited because Rosen Method is not well-known outside the metropolitan areas where practitioners are clustered. The authors certainly encourage physicians and other health professionals who have access to local practitioners to become familiar with the work, try out a session themselves, and make referrals where appropriate. The Rosen Institute is planning to increase efforts to publicize the effectiveness of Rosen Method to the medical community.

Lack of insurance coverage for somatic therapies is another key barrier that keeps Rosen Method (along with other somatic therapies) from being widely prescribed. A shift in policy in the medical insurance industry would be valuable because Rosen Method can play a very important role in "wellness" medicine and preventative health care.

Associations

The Rosen Institute
825 Bancroft Way
Berkeley, CA 94710
Tel: (510) 845-6606

Rosen Method Professional Association
PO Box 11144
Berkeley, CA 94712
Tel: (510) 644-4166 (administration)
Toll-Free: (800) 893-2622 (U.S. Referral Service)

Suggested Reading

1. Rosen M, Brenner S: *The Rosen method of movement*, Berkeley, Calif, 1991, North Atlantic Books.

    Outlines the theory and objectives of Rosen Movement, provides an overview of a Rosen Movement class, and gives illustrated descriptions of each of the movement exercises.
2. Mayland EL: *Rosen method: an approach to wholeness and well-being through the body*, Berkeley, Calif, 1984, The Berkeley Center (self-published).

    A concise summary of the theory of Rosen Method based on in-depth interviews with founder, Marion Rosen. Available through Rosen Method, c/o The Berkeley Center, 825 Bancroft Way, Berkeley, CA 94710; Tel: (510) 845-6606.

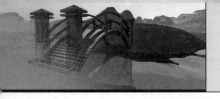

Therapeutic Touch

STUART LEDWITH

Origins and History

Therapeutic Touch (TT) can be defined as the exchange of life force energies between two or more people with the expressed purpose of healing, changing, communicating, and growing in a healthy spiritual and physical manner. It is a healing modality that involves touching with the conscious intent to help or heal. TT decreases anxiety, relieves pain, and facilitates the healing process. The process of TT has the following four basic phases:

1. Centering the self physically and psychologically; that is, finding within the self an inner reference of stability.
2. Exercising the natural sensitivity of the hand to assess the energy field of the patient for clues to differentiate the quality of energy flow.
3. Mobilizing areas in the patient's energy field that appear to be nonflowing (in other words, sluggish, congested, or static).
4. Directing excess energies to assist patients to repattern their own energies.[1]

Mechanism of Action According to Its Own Theory

Touch is a powerful, valuable tool; patients relax with and deeply trust a practitioner who touches appropriately and deftly. A practitioner can glean amazing amounts of information by listening with the hands. The therapeutic value of this modality is gained through the exchange of energies between the patient, whose body speaks to the practitioner, and the practitioner, who can return to the patient those energies most helpful in the healing process.

Body energies may be sensed by the practitioner as hot or cold, active and passive, blocked or free. Usually the practitioner senses a contrast between well and ill, and some feel the pain or tenseness of the patient. Energies sensed in return by the patient are usually voiced as relaxing, warm, soothing, eradicating pain, and life-giving.

Each region of the body contains specific, informative energy patterns and functions. The primary regions—head, throat, heart, gut, lower abdomen, sacral region of the spine, knees, and feet—each communicates its particular energy of health or nonhealth to the practitioner. In any disorder where energy can be viewed as outside normal limits, TT will be quite helpful in returning the patient to good health.

> *Your brain is extremely well integrated with the rest of your body at a molecular level, so much so that the term* mobile brain *is an apt description of the psychosomatic network through which intelligent information travels from one system to another. Every one of the zones, or systems, of the network—the neural, the hormonal, the gastrointestinal, and the immune—is set up to communicate with one another, via peptides and messenger-specific peptide receptors. Every second a massive information exchange is occurring in your body. Imagine each of these messenger systems possessing a specific tone, humming a signature tune, rising and falling, waxing and waning, binding and unbinding, and if we could hear this body music with our ears . . .*
>
> **Candace Pert, PhD**

Therapeutic touch practitioners have learned to hear this body music with their hands and respond to it with appropriate energy of healing actions.

Biologic Mechanism of Action

Physical symptoms of ill health manifest from some type of trauma and or insult to the body, whether it be an infecting agent, a blow to the head with a blunt instrument, or an anger-filled relationship. The brain is very willing to keep, available for recall, a sensate memory of that trauma or insult. However, it is not willing to feel the pain associated with that trauma. Instead, the body "parks" the pain chemically, delivered through the autonomic nervous system or a neuropeptide messenger system, to the body at the cellular level in gender-specific regions or zones. When blocks or trigger points are parked at the cellular level, the cells involved are no longer able to communicate well with surrounding cells. This eventually causes a larger organ or system dysfunction.

An understanding of how the brain or mind can park a block or trigger point in the body can be gained from the works of Candace Pert, PhD. Her research in the field of neurotransmitters, especially neuropeptides as mind-body messengers, is crucial. She writes in her book *Molecules of Emotion*, "Repressed traumas caused by overwhelming emotion can be stored in a body part, thereafter affecting our ability to feel that part or even move it." She describes peptides as informational substances that connect the brain or mind, the immune system, the endocrine system and our entire psychoemotional complex.[2]

Understanding cell biology will help define the phenomenon of therapeutic touch. An important factor is the gap junction of the cell, its regulation, and the building of larger junction complexes.[3] A *gap junction* is an opening in the cell wall through which it may communicate with neighboring cells. A *gap junction complex* is a large group of function-related cells, such as heart muscle tissue, a group of purkinje fibers, or a specific valve. Whether a gap junction is open, permeable (healthy), closed, or obstructed (part of a disease complex) depends on many factors.

In the human heart, factors that can close gap junction complexes, such as acidosis, sodium pump inhibition, or elevated intracellular calcium, may cause sudden heart failure.[4] Trauma, whether real or imagined, and body insult of any nature can cause a variety of similar cellular conditions that may cause gap junctions (trigger points) and whole junction complexes (blocks) to close.

Each gap junction complex has a specific function and signature energy. For example, the human heart as a whole complex functions to pump blood through the body. Normal sinus rhythm "feels" comfortable, uncongested, and contented. It has many subset complexes with very specific functions, such as heart muscle tissue, purkinje fibers, valves, and others. Closed gap junction complexes here would lead to heart malfunction; the distinctive "feel" of the heart as a whole for the practitioner would be congestion, panic, density, or cold. The greater heart region of the body has an emotional energy function dealing with matters of love.

In short, as a response to trauma or body insult, issue-specific gap junction complexes become closed. This adversely affects the flow of calcium, sodium, potassium, and neuropeptide messenger molecules through the localized cell walls, thus interrupting cellular communication. The energies exchanged through the process of TT open those gap junction complexes and allow a return of cellular communication followed by a return to a healthy status.

Forms of Therapy

Therapeutic touch has taken on two basic forms: those practitioners who touch, read, and change the energy field surrounding the body following the Krieger-Kunz method; and those practitioners who read, work, and deliver energies of healing directly to the body. Both forms use the same basic tenets of assessment, removal of blocks, and exchange of healing energy.

Demographics

According to statistics compiled by Nurse Healers-Professional Associates Cooperative, TT currently is taught in 90 colleges and universities in this country and abroad. It currently is practiced in more than 100 hospitals and health centers in the United States and Canada.[5]

A review of the literature indicates that there is no age, gender, or religious limitation on who uses TT. Some are seeking a cure, peace of mind, or a short, specific therapy; some are in tremendous pain; and many want help with surgery preparation—the types of patients are varied and wonderful.

Indications and Reason for Referral

Common reasons for referral from the medical mainstream is for treatment of chronic disorders, such as chronic pain, chronic fatigue syndrome, fibromyalgia, weight loss, stress, abuse, addictions, and for surgery preparation. Often cancer patients who have exhausted other forms of treatment indicate that TT may be their last hope.

Dynamic results are evident using TT in the preparation of patients for surgery. In a very relaxed state each functional system in the body can be easily trained to perform well under the effects of anesthesia. The tissues that will be cut can "allow" the scalpel to cut without seeing it as trauma or insult and thus heal with much less pain, requiring much less pain medication and fewer days in hospital. Many patients are ready to return to work days and weeks before their friends with similar problems.

The "energy" disorders, such as fibromyalgia, chronic fatigue syndrome, and chronic pain syndromes, tend to respond very well to TT. Although TT does not stop the effects of lupus, it is very effective at stopping the pain of an intense flair of joint pain.

Therapeutic touch has worked quite successfully with women enduring difficult pregnancies, which led to wonderful, live births. Fibrocystic breast disease responds well to the removal of blocks and trigger points from pectoral regions, enough so that repeat mammograms show the difference with many patients.

Chronically somatic patients benefit from TT because an understanding person is spending time and attention on them, listening to them, and offering energy solutions that seem to make sense to them. Many such patients are slow learners and need repetition of explanations of diagnoses, treatments, and care.

Office Applications

A simple ranking of conditions responsive to this form of therapy is as follows. As with all alternative therapies, TT does not preclude mainstream medical therapies in addition.

Top level: *A therapy ideally suited for these conditions*

Arthritis; back pain; chronic fatigue syndrome; chronic pain; female health; fibrocystic breast disease; headaches; hypertension; male health; menstrual cramps; ovarian cysts; preconception; difficult pregnancy; and stress

Second level: *One of the better therapies for these conditions*

Addictions; allergies; bronchitis; cancer; diverticulitis; endometriosis; heart disease; irritable bowel syndrome; menopause; ovarian cancer; periodic leg movement syndrome; premenstrual syndrome; restless leg syndrome; rheumatoid arthritis; and sleep apnea

Practical Applications

The practical applications of TT are many. In her book *Therapeutic Touch Inner Workbook*, Dolores Krieger cites numerous hospitals that are using TT in operating and treatment rooms and to calm patients, reduce pain levels, and help patients get through the many traumatic events of hospital stays. She also cites many treatment centers that use TT with children and adults, as well as several mental health settings.[5]

Because training is available at so many colleges and healing centers around the U.S. and Canada, it would be quite practical to have office nurses trained in TT to assist patients in office settings.

Research Base

Evidence Based

Research in TT began in the 1970s with Krieger,[6] who demonstrated an increase in the mean hemoglobin level in a group of patients who received TT compared to a group of patients who received routine nursing care.

Recently, Turner et al[7] at the University of Alabama tested the effect of TT on pain and anxiety levels in burn patients. Subjects who received TT reported significantly greater reduction in pain and anxiety. Lymphocyte subset analyses on blood from 11 subjects showed a decreasing total CD8+ lymphocyte concentration for the TT group.

A study by Daley[8] looked at TT and its effectiveness in treating full-thickness human dermal wounds. Although the results of the studies were inconsistent overall the series of experiments nonetheless significantly expanded the theoretic boundaries and understanding of the TT process.

A study by Gagne and Toye[9] tested the effects of TT and relaxation therapy in reducing anxiety. Results showed that whereas relaxation therapy provided significant reduction of anxiety on the self-report measure and the movement measure, the nursing intervention of TT resulted in significant reductions of reported anxiety.

A study by Samuel[10] found that for the participants receiving treatments, TT was a fulfilling multidimensional experience that facilitated personal growth.

Other studies have shown that people receiving healing touch have increased alpha brain waves, which is characteristic of a deep meditative state. Deep relaxation is associated with reduced stress, improved respiration, better hormonal balance, enhanced bowel function, lower cholesterol levels, and heightened immune responses.[11]

Basic Science

Many differing types of touch have been identified, such as functional, social, friendly, love, sexual, aggressive, and nurturing.[12] Each type of touch can be shown to have a different effect in the body as it is sensed and responded to through the actions of the autonomic nervous system and other messenger systems. Blood pressure can be raised or lowered; pulse rate can rise or fall; and skin temperature can rise or fall. Through differing messenger systems a love touch may elicit tears, excitement, laughter, or a sense of security and calmness. Aggressive touch may elicit an adrenaline response.

Therapeutic touch, which is mostly functional and nurturing in nature, elicits many responses in the body, such as increased white cell counts, relaxation, and lowered blood pressure, most of which are intentioned to heal or help.

Risk and Safety

Appropriate touch is imperative to developing safe, therapeutic rapport and trust. Many patients are coming in for safe touch again after being abused and do not need more distress.

Side effects are few. Many patients will be light-headed for up to fifteen minutes after a long session and require recovery time. If their issues were particularly difficult, they are given all the time they need to recover before they drive their cars. Also, their bladders will be full; apparently renal arteries relax well. Thirst for several days may persist after a session, especially if many trigger points were released.

Efficacy

A high percentage of patients state that they achieve an added value to their lives as a result of the healing work. Often there is a secondary benefit from the experience, such as increased self-confidence, self-control, and a deeper sense of who they are. A small portion of patients do receive the cure for which they are searching; others are happy with even the smallest of changes in their lives.

Most current research completed in single and double-blind studies consistently demonstrates that therapeutic touch is significantly effective.

Future Research Opportunities and Priorities

Therapeutic touch is new and research is needed in several areas. The connection between the autonomic nervous system, peptide messengers, and cellular gap junction complexes could be explored thoroughly. Detection devices are needed to test and identify specific energies as they pass through the hands A priority is that practitioners of TT continue to evaluate and test themselves and continue to teach others, especially in the medical mainstream, about the value of TT.

Druglike Information

Safety

Review of the literature suggests that the procedure is quite safe. However, much of the literature is anecdotal in nature, but none suggests danger. Safety needs to be provided in several ways. The patient needs to feel secure spatially, spiritually, physically, and psychologically. A trusting rapport is a must, just as appropriate touch is basic to patient safety.

Actions

In response to trauma or body insult, issue-specific gap junction complexes become closed, adversely affecting the flow of calcium, sodium, potassium, and neuropeptide messenger molecules through the localized cell walls, and thus interrupting cellular communication. The energies exchanged through the process of TT open those gap junction complexes and allow a return of cellular communication, followed by a return to a healthy status.

Warnings

From a review of the literature, change often accompanies the use of healing energies. Patients should be informed about the possibility of personal growth and change as a result of such therapy.

Interactions

Therapeutic touch has been found to interface well with all healing modalities both traditional and orthodox, as well as more recent therapies, such as biofeedback and massage. It is recommended that TT be a part of all bodywork.[5]

Adverse Reactions

From a review of the literature, adverse reactions are few; some light-headedness may follow a session, along with increased thirst.

Pregnancy and Lactation

The author has treated a number of pregnant patients without ill effects. However, no large-scale studies are available.

Self-Help versus Professional

For nurses and other bodywork professionals who would like to enhance their abilities or further educate themselves for their own benefit, there exists a wide range of self-help literature, such as *Therapeutic Touch Inner Workbook*[2] and *Therapeutic Touch, A Practical Guide*.[13]

For those nurses who wish to practice in hospitals, hospices, clinics, or private offices, there are classes of several varieties. Many nursing schools offer TT classes as part of their ongoing curriculum; some offer classes associated with clinical experiences; and still other schools teach therapeutic touch classes as part of their associated evening classes.

Visiting a Professional

A typical visit to a TT practitioner begins with the referral appointment call, during which information about the patient's diagnosis and desired treatment is discussed.

At the appointment the patient is asked for a complete medical history, emotional assessment, and personal desires from the encounter. During the interview the practitioner evaluates the patient's body language (both spoken and unspoken), mannerisms, and word choices. The practitioner searches for many possible causes for the symptoms presented.

Once this phase is completed the patient is offered the opportunity to be "touched." The patient may lay down on a work table or sit upright on a chair or stool. The patient is asked to relax. The practitioner begins the TT process by evaluating the patient's energies, either touching the patient's body or moving the hands close to the patient's body.

As each area of the body is explored the practitioner responds to the "feelings" in the hands with the appropriate energy responses. The patient may feel the energy exchanged if it is strong enough to be felt. Often the energies used are quite subtle. As the session ends the patient is given an opportunity for questions and answers and comments. If further appointments are needed, they are scheduled.

Credentialing

Although therapeutic touch was originally identified as a nursing function 20 years ago, other professionals who have patient contact have adopted it as well. TT is growing rapidly and training closely follows generally accepted norms, but it is not yet fully standardized.

Practitioners of TT may receive certificates of completion of classes and add that credential to their basic degree status as a nurse or physical or massage therapist. Many practitioners have advanced degrees in their field at the bachelor's, master's, and doctoral levels and may both teach and have private practices.

Organizations such as the National League for Nursing and the American Nurses' Association promote TT classes and publish TT articles; however, they do not certify TT training. The American Holistic Nurses Association offers certification in "healing touch," a TT variant. The Nurse Healers and Professional Associates Cooperative was formed to promote TT and offers training to those interested.

Training

Therapeutic touch is taught at beginning, intermediate, and advanced levels in continuing education programs, graduate nursing education, and summer intensive workshops. Self-teaching workbooks follow a similar path and leave the timing and level structure to the student.

Beginners (Level I) of the Krieger-Kunz method are taught basic TT and have the opportunity to practice it under supervision and receive feedback. They also learn the scientific basics and supporting research.

Level II participants are given the opportunity to deepen their knowledge and understanding of TT. They learn methods to enhance their ability to use therapeutic touch specifically and effectively. They are taught specific techniques for dealing with pain, interfacing emotions with physical fields, incorporating imagery, effectively using the body's energy, and counseling skills and finally learn to experience therapeutic touch as provider and recipient.

Level III participants explore in depth each part of the therapeutic touch process with even more complicated diagnoses. They are given time to discuss at length any issues raised in earlier training especially those centering around imagery, counseling, and living in that desired centered state. Often participants are required to read a number of sources on healing theories and psychologic methods.

What to Look for in a Provider

A TT practitioner will have at least a professional license as nurse, massage or physical therapist, or other medically associated degree. The practitioner will have completed formal (certificate) or informal therapeutic touch training. It would not be inappropriate to ask for a list of references. The practitioner will be knowledgeable, professional, warm, caring, and compassionate. You may find this practitioner in a hospital, clinic, or private office.

Finding an experienced practitioner may be important. One study reported in *American Journal of Nursing* (Mackey 1995) finds that much more effective results were obtained by a practitioner who was doing more than 60 treatments per month than a practitioner who was completing only 10 per month.[14]

Barriers and Key Issues

Education about TT in the medical community is the greatest barrier to greater cooperation. Our differences are this: The medical professionals and medical doctors use and work with the finest healing science in the world, whereas practitioners of therapeutic touch use the finest healing arts in the world. Mixing the arts and sciences makes for good healing medicine.

> *The Ptolemaic earth at the center of the universe can give way to the Copernican sun-centered theory— but not without considerable resistance. Witness Galileo, who was brought before the Inquisition for his role in promulgating that theory over a century after it was first proposed.*
> **Holistic Nursing: a Handbook for Practice, 1999**

Suggested Reading

1. Cowens D: *A gift for healing: how you can use therapeutic touch*, New York, 1996, Crown Trade Paperbacks.
   Easily brings therapeutic touch within the reach of everyone.
2. Dossey B et al: *Holistic nursing: a handbook for practice*, Gaithersburg, Md, 1995, Aspen.
   Covers a full range of healing modalities for healing the whole patient.
3. Krieger D: *Therapeutic touch inner workbook*, Santa Fe, 1997, Bear & Co.
   Learn how centering yourself and focusing your attention are at the core of all healing interventions.
4. Motz J: *Hands of life*, New York, 1998, Bantam Books.
   Learn the secrets of using your body's own energy medicine for healing, recovery, and transformation.
5. Pert C: *Molecules of emotion: why you feel the way you feel*, New York, 1997, Scribner.
   Discover how emotions and health are linked at the molecular level.

Bibliography

Heidt PR: Openness: a qualitative analysis of nurses' and patients' experiences of Therapeutic Touch, *Image: The Journal of Nursing Scholarship* 22(3):180-186, 1990.

References

1. Dossey B et al: *Holistic nursing: a handbook for practice*, Gaithersburg, Md, 1995, Aspen.

2. Pert C: *Molecules of emotion: why you feel the way you feel*, New York, 1997, Scribner.

3. Alberts B et al: *Molecular biology of the cell*, ed 3, New York, 1994, Garland.

4. Katz A: *Physiology of the heart*, ed 2, New York, 1992, Raven Press.

5. Krieger D: *Therapeutic touch inner workbook*, Santa Fe, 1997, Bear & Co.

6. Krieger D, Peper E, Ancoli S: Therapeutic touch: searching for evidence of physiological change, *Am J Nurs* 79(4):660-662, 1979.

7. Turner JG et al: *The effect of therapeutic touch on pain and anxiety in burn patients*, J Adv Nurs 28(1):10-20, 1998.

8. Daley B: Therapeutic touch, nursing practice and contemporary cutaneous wound healing research, *J Adv Nurs* 25(6):1123-1132, 1997.

9. Gagne D, Toye RC: The effects of therapeutic touch and relaxation therapy in reducing anxiety, *Arch Psychiatric Nurs* 8(3): 184-189, 1994.

10. Samuel N: The experience of receiving therapeutic touch, *J Adv Nurs* 17(6): 651-657, 1992.

11. Cowens D: *A gift for healing*, New York, 1996, Crown Trade Paperbacks.

12. Tovar MK, Cassmeyer VL: Touch: the beneficial effects for the surgical patient, *AORN* 49(5):1356-1361, 1989.

13. Macrae J: *Complementary modalities. Part 1: therapeutic touch, a practical guide*, New York, 1988, Knopf.

14. Mackey R: Discover the healing power of therapeutic touch, *Am J Nurs* 95(4):26-32, 1995.

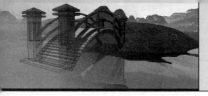

Trager® Approach

JACK LISKIN

Origins and History

The *Trager Approach* is named after Milton Trager, MD, who developed and practiced its principles for seven decades and taught his methods to students from the mid-1970s until his death in 1997. Like other individuals prominent in the field of bodywork whose names are synonymous with their methods, he was keenly observant of the human body, sensitive to the nuances of relationships between mind and body, and gifted with hands that could communicate with and make changes in the people he touched. He developed his guiding principles first through the personal exploration of movement as a beach acrobat, bodybuilder, boxer, and dancer. As he matured, he came to an increasingly subtle awareness of the mental correlates of musculoskeletal and movement patterns. Early on, he translated this knowledge into instinctive hands-on work with children with paralysis and palsy and people with chronic pain, successfully easing their bodies and also teaching them skills for improved balance and movement.

He built this work into a career, but it was not until his fifties that he formalized his education with medical studies, and it would be another 20 years before he began his teaching to health care and mental health professionals as well as massage therapists and lay people who realized the value and potential of his methods. His students early on formed an institute that today carries on Dr. Trager's work internationally through formal training and certification programs.

Mechanism of Action According to Its Own Theory

At the deepest level, healing potential is imminent in the universe. Entering a meditative state ("hook-up" in Trager parlance), the practitioner is in a better position to access this potential. The practitioner can transmit the peace and calm of the "hooked-up" state to the person receiving a Trager session. This mental state influences the nervous and musculoskeletal systems toward relaxation and improved physical mobility. That is, the *manner* in which the practitioner "approaches" the receiving person is fundamental and at least as important as any technique the practitioner may use.

The practitioner, while working with the body, seeks to affect the mind of the receiving person because physical patterns are conditioned, embedded, and perpetuated in the mind, and no permanent change is possible physically until the mind pattern changes. Patterns can be formed genetically through physical or emotional trauma, stress, or repeated unhealthy mental or physical activity. A Trager session is a *feeling* experience; patterns can change only when the receiving person has *felt* a new and different possibility.

Muscle, because of its presence and activity throughout skeletal and visceral systems, including the blood vessels, is necessarily a primary component of physical pattern development. The ability to tense and relax muscle as appropriate to meet varying needs is thus critical to developing beneficial and healthful patterns. The practitioner is trained to develop exquisite awareness of relaxation and tension of the tissues and then to train the receiving persons to improve their awareness and skill in altering their own tension patterns. This is accomplished through touch and gentle passive movement of joint areas (*tablework*), and movement education—in Trager jargon, *Mentastics* (mental gymnastics). The work is pleasurable to receive because it is rhythmic, gentle, and relaxing. By recalling the mental state associated with a session, receivers are able to both improve their mental state at will and elicit the free, easy, balanced, and pain-free movement that was experienced during the session.

Practitioners seek to effect long-term change. This is accomplished not by forcing the body to change but rather by repetitive influence, allowing the change to come from within the receiving person. If there is resistance, the practitioner backs away or gently overcomes it through the repetitive, rhythmic, pleasant motion. Practitioners set the receiving person's body in motion and use the weights and natural movement rhythms of the individual's body to sustain the motion. The wave of motion thus generated resonates through the body, integrates the parts of the body, and gently breaks up restrictive muscle patterns.

Biologic Mechanisms of Action

The overarching principle in Trager work can be stated as follows: *Physical patterns reflect mental patterns, and such patterns can be changed through special kinds of awareness, movement and skilled touch.* That is, neurologic and psychologic pathologies are perceptible in corresponding musculoskeletal or movement pattern pathologies. They can be repatterned through appropriate touch and movements, through neuronal and articular mechanoreceptor signals to the central nervous system, which concurrently elicit change in the mental state. Recent discoveries of new neuropeptides and their wide distribution in the nervous system lend credence to such mind-body links. Hubbard's EMG studies confirmed the autonomic system innervation of skeletal muscle, further establishing the connection between emotion and muscle tension (for example, in stress responses).[1]

Psychologic research into state-dependent learning and behavior helps to explain how specific mental states elicit behaviors previously learned while in such states. This opens possibilities for teaching healthy behavioral patterns by changing the person's mental state and then teaching people to change their mental state at will.[2] Relaxation training applied to a wide variety of diseases has repeatedly produced improvement in clinical conditions.[3]

Finally, Ornish has shown that change in mental state as accomplished through meditation is effective as a component of a program which has successfully reversed cardiovascular disease.[4] That meditation derives from spiritual traditions is relevant because the Trager Approach includes a spiritual orientation. Research on the positive health effects of spiritual practice is in its infancy, but early studies in this field have produced intriguing and positive findings.

Forms of Therapy

The two components of Trager work are tablework, during which the receiving person lies on a comfortably padded table, and movement education or Mentastics, which are taught before or after the tablework portion of the session. Although there are standardized movements that practitioners are trained to perform during tablework and typical Mentastic moves that may be shown to patients, there is much tailoring of the work to the specific conditions and needs of the receiver and therefore room for creativity in a session. What is always the same is the "approach," the manner of the practitioner: gentle, easy, light, soft, playful, rhythmic, and meditative, with much attention to the comfort and well-being of the receiver.

Most typically, Trager work is used to promote relaxation and reduce muscle tension, but the capacity to reduce tension implies the ability to increase it as well, and the work—a special form of it called *Reflex Response*, in which some practitioners are trained—can be used where weakness or paralysis is present in the receiver. In this form of the work the practitioner seeks to elicit and amplify muscle tone and movement.

Although most practitioners will take at least a brief focused history, those with health care or mental health training or special interest also may explore with patients aspects of their health behavior, helping people to increase their awareness and make connections between their mental state, behavior, physical responses or conditions, and personal development. Some practitioners who have studied other modalities may combine them with Trager work during a session. Although this is not condoned by the Trager Institute, it is not uncommon.

Demographics

The first class of students trained by Dr. Trager was composed of health care and mental health professionals, including several from France. This established the international scope of the Trager Approach early on; as of this writing, there are more than 1100 practitioners worldwide, with the largest concentrations in the U.S., Canada, and Europe. There are more than 800 students in training. Although practitioners continue to enter from the ranks of health care and mental health professionals, more students come from other massage or bodywork backgrounds, and others are lay people. Thus, although Trager work may be found in the occasional medical practice, it is mostly practiced outside the conventional medical environment, often in the home or private office of practitioners who may be primarily oriented toward the well-being and personal development of their patients rather than toward medical problems or conditions.

Those who avail themselves of the Trager Approach may be referred by a knowledgeable physician or psychologist, or they might visit a physical therapist who is also a Trager practitioner. More likely, they are referred by a friend, family member, or alternative medicine provider who has experienced Trager work and believes in its efficacy for a specific problem. Others receive sessions in order to maintain or enhance their current health, to de-stress and feel good, or to develop themselves personally and even spiritually.

Indications and Reasons for Referral

Without a history of controlled research, indications for referral cannot be specified with absolute confidence. But looking at commonalities in current empirical referral and usage patterns, the following four main categories for potential referral are observed: 1) pain; 2) movement or neurologic disorders; 3) relaxation training; and 4) health promotion and enhancement, disease prevention, health maintenance, and personal development.

Pain: Many manifestations of musculoskeletal or myofascial pain may be eased by Trager work, especially chronic pain. Examples include acute and chronic back pain, neck pain, shoulder pain, tension-type or mixed headache, and carpal tunnel syndrome. Generally the role of tension in musculoskeletal pain is underappreciated, and medical practice would be improved by incorporating modalities that address this problem. People with chronic fatigue, fibromyalgia, and other poorly understood conditions with a pain component are commonly referred to Trager practitioners. People with osteoarthritis may experience improved mobility. Postsurgical and postinjury rehabilitation may be enhanced with Trager work.

Movement or neurologic disorder: Problems involving spasm, tremor, dystonia, and weakness or paralysis (where movement and balance training may be beneficial) may be ameliorated with Trager work. Examples include the dystonias, Parkinson's disease, cerebral palsy, and multiple sclerosis. There also may be potential benefit for epilepsy.

Relaxation training: This category encompasses many problems, given our pressurized society. Examples include stress-related conditions, anxiety, panic attacks, and insomnia. There may be benefits for individuals with hypertension and other cardiovascular problems, asthma, and hyperactivity.

Health promotion and enhancement, disease prevention, health maintenance, and personal development: This broad category includes referrals (usually self-referrals) for people wishing to develop or maintain a healthy lifestyle. Incorporating body awareness and relaxation training into a health maintenance program—one that includes good nutrition, exercise, a balance of activity and rest, satisfying personal relations, and involvement in activities that transcend the ego—takes health care beyond disease treatment and into the realm of personal development.

A simple ranking of conditions is as follows:

Top level: *A therapy ideally suited for these conditions*
Myofascial syndromes

Second level: *One of the better therapies for these conditions*
Chronic pain; headaches; neck pain; back pain; and stress-related illnesses

Third level: *A valuable adjunctive therapy for these conditions*
Chronic fatigue; hyperactivity; insomnia; multiple sclerosis; Parkinson's disease; dystonia; carpal tunnel; fibromyalgia; and postsurgical rehabilitation

Office Applications

In clinical practice, Trager work has the advantages of being noninvasive, low risk (because of the gentleness of its application), without appreciable side effects, and pleasurable to patients. Further, it involves the patient in learning improved body awareness and better self care. It is a conservative treatment in the best sense and as such can be used confidently as a first-line approach or first-line adjunct to medical treatments. For people with chronic pain, particularly myofascial pain but also headache, jaw pain (TMJ), carpal tunnel problems, neck and shoulder pain, and back pain, an early trial of Trager work is warranted.

For people recovering from surgery, Trager work can be part of a mobilization program. For patients with stiffness, balance and movement difficulties, or neurologic problems manifesting those symptoms, such as Parkinson's disease, multiple sclerosis, and the dystonias, it can be a most useful adjunct.

Further, patients whose problems have an underlying or concomitant stress component and who have difficulty relaxing can benefit from Trager work. This also is true for patients with psychologic problems, such as anxiety, depression, and panic syndromes. For such patients, even a session or two at the right time can reorient patients toward more healthful patterns of living and help them take control of their health. Trager work thus offers not only therapeutic benefits for medical conditions but also wellness and health promotion components, which add value to the practice.

Practical Applications

Most multispecialty groups or large family, internal medicine, and neurology practices and health maintenance organizations can afford to have a Trager practitioner on staff full or part-time. This offers maximum convenience to patients and demonstrates the commitment of the practice to health-enhancing complementary methods. Other practices can establish a relationship with a practitioner in the area for referrals. The practitioner within the practice setting will require a quiet room, pleasantly appointed, with a padded massage-type table and cloth sheets and gowns. An area for movement training is helpful, although quiet hallways or areas outside the building also can be used.

Within a practice, complete Trager sessions can be scheduled for an hour; first sessions may take longer. Focused, problem-oriented sessions can be shorter; however, allowing ample, unrushed time is essential for effective work. There is no set number of required sessions. Many patients will benefit from a single session, but because the work is a teaching method, reinforcement is important for success, especially for patients with chronic, long-term problems. A typical format might involve five or six weekly sessions with evaluation of status during and at the end of that period. At that time the patient can be discharged, the continuation of sessions or an increase or decrease in the session interval might be recommended, or an as-needed revisit schedule can be established.

If the practitioner is outside the medical practice, periodic discussion of the patient's progress with the clinician is helpful. The time which the practitioner devotes to the patient and atmosphere of the session often stimulates patients to reveal important information about their health and life situation that clinicians will find valuable for their ongoing care. A practitioner who is not otherwise licensed and trained in a health care profession may need guidance from the clinician as to what kind of information is important to convey and how it should be presented.

Research Base

To date, Trager work has not had the benefit of controlled randomized clinical research to inform its development and use. Three small studies in the physical therapy literature[5-7] showed improvement in lung function in 12 patients with chronic lung disease,[5] pain relief in a patient with chronic back pain,[6] and improvement in trunk mobility in a child with cerebral palsy.[7] A case report in the occupational therapy literature[8] showed improvement in the postsurgical rehabilitation of a patient with severe tendon damage of the forearm.

Rising interest in alternative and complementary approaches has opened new opportunities for controlled clinical research. One proposed study would incorporate Trager work in the treatment of multiple sclerosis. Already funded is another controlled randomized study at an academic health center that will investigate the efficacy of Trager work for chronic headache. Other studies have been proposed relative to Parkinson's disease and other neurologic conditions. Not only symptom moderation but also function and quality of life changes are appropriate outcomes to be studied for any of the conditions and problems investigated in future studies. Conditions involving chronic pain are obvious candidates for study, but other conditions such as epilepsy, hypertension, and asthma would also be of interest.

Druglike Information

Although no research data are available regarding the safety of Trager work, the sensitivity required of practitioners and gentleness of the methods make it unlikely that patients would be harmed. In particular, practitioners do not use force where there is resistance to motion or excessive muscle tone. Furthermore the work is painless and practitioners advise their patients to tell them immediately if they experience pain or discomfort during a session. This active feedback mechanism reduces the potential for harm. Trager work can be used concurrently with pharmacologic treatment or physical therapy strengthening programs. In the latter instance, patients can be advised that the Trager work adds another skill that they can use as a complement to the therapy.

Precautions

Some patients may find relaxation threatening and will demonstrate a paradoxic reaction to Trager work, becoming anxious as relaxation deepens. In these cases there may be a history of abuse or other psychologic trauma or problem that should be considered, and patients should be encouraged to discuss their reactions. Exploring and overcoming these reactions may lead to rapid improvement in the patient's condition. Trager work can be adapted to sidewise and other positions when patients cannot be comfortable in the prone or supine position. It is conceivable that in the face of joint hypermobility there might be excessive stretch, and caution should be exercised in such an instance. People with prolonged continuous muscle tension may experience mild muscle soreness for up to 24 hours following a session. When this disappears it often gives way to significant symptom relief. Often, sleep depth and duration improved immediately following a session.

Contraindications

Trager practitioners are advised in training to not work on pregnant women in the first trimester. This is conservative and possibly undue caution because work in the abdomen is very gentle, and work peripheral to the abdomen certainly should not be harmful. Likewise, practitioners are advised to not work on people with thromboembolic risk or history. Here too, gentle work or work distant from the embolic source site is likely to be safe. Practitioners are taught to not work on people with potentially metastasizing cancer; this is conservatism based on lack of data. Finally, practitioners are advised to not work on joint areas where people are experiencing an acute flare-up of rheumatoid arthritis.

There is no contraindication to sessions more frequent than once per week and there may be advantages to a more concentrated series of sessions, at least early on, for patients with severe problems. If the gap between sessions is too long, particularly early in treatment, the benefits of reinforcement of learning may be diminished.

Visiting a Professional

If a practitioner is incorporated into a medical practice, front office staff must understand the particular time and scheduling needs of the practitioner and patient. The Trager session should be a personal, comfortable, and unpressured experience from beginning to end, including in the front office. If practitioners are in their own offices, that experience can be controlled more easily. It probably is a good idea for the patient and practitioner to have at least a brief phone conversation before the initial visit. The patient may have initial questions about Trager work, and this first contact personalizes the experience and breaks the ice.

Referring clinicians may, in their desire to direct the patient toward Trager work, overstate the benefits and the abilities of the practitioner. The whole issue of expectations, hopes, and fears, particularly for people with chronic and debilitating problems for which there is no known cure, is a delicate one. It is probably best for all concerned to expect positive outcomes without guaranteeing cures and miraculous changes. In referring a patient the clinician may wish to say something on the order of, "Other of my patients with this problem have found this approach to be extremely helpful, and I know that practitioner X is very capable." This assumes that the clinician knows the practitioner, and in fact, clinicians should at least be acquainted with practitioners if they plan to refer to them. This is particularly important when it comes to exchanging information about the patient's condition and progress.

The Trager Institute, for liability and other reasons, does not make medical claims for the Trager Approach and is careful not to use the word "therapy" in relation to it. At a practical level, however, patients, practitioners, and clinicians understand the therapeutic benefits of the work.

Credentialing

Trager practitioners are certified by the Trager Institute, which monitors the training and continued competency of practitioners. Once certified, the practitioner must have an annual tutorial from an Institute-approved tutor and a recommendation from that tutor to maintain certification. The practitioner must receive at least four Trager sessions annually and must attend at least 3 days of continuing education every 3 years (one class each year is required for practitioners in their first 3 years of practice). Trager practitioners are not regulated as such by any state. States or local jurisdictions may, however, have their own regulations for hands-on therapists. Some states or counties may require practitioners to obtain a massage license. If practitioners already are licensed in one of the health care professions, they may be able to do Trager work under that license.

Training

Trager trainings are conducted around the world by Institute-approved instructors. To become a practitioner, an individual must experience the work from a certified practitioner before entering the training track. After a week-long initial training the student must complete and log at least 30 practice sessions, receive at least 10 sessions, and attend additional tutorials to be eligible for the intermediate training. After that second training the student again completes and logs at least 30 sessions and receives additional tutorials and sessions. Anatomy training also is required during this period. After these requirements have been met, the student must conduct a complete session on a tutor to become a practitioner. The work must be of sufficient quality that the tutor recommends the student for practitioner status. If it is not, more practice sessions or more tutorials and classes may be recommended. Once practitioner status is achieved the practitioner then may charge for sessions. Achieving practitioner status typically takes 1 to 2 years.

What to Look for in a Provider

Trager practitioners who receive referrals from health care providers should understand the medical model. Some practitioners already have a health care background; for those who do not, there is a class currently available through the Trager Institute, which focuses specifically on Trager work in the medical context.

Good practitioners will model those attributes that they aim to teach to their patients. They will be gentle, calm, easy, and comfortable with their own bodies. They should notice and be able to communicate information about the patient, which the medical clinician may not have observed through conventional medical evaluation. A good provider will be highly sensitive to the needs and reactions of patients. Trager practitioners will look for mind-body connections and in the process may help referring clinicians better understand their patients.

The practitioner's demeanor should be at once warm and professional. Because of the intimate nature of the work the practitioner should evidence clear, strong, and appropriate boundaries. Avoid practitioners who make extravagant claims for the benefits of their work. Although such claims may originate from a sincere enthusiasm about the work, they ultimately may set up patients for future disappointment. The physical environment of the practice should be one that the referring clinician would consider appropriate, and there should be adequate provision for privacy. Many people receive Trager work wearing only underwear, but a good practitioner will be sensitive to and able to accommodate the varying modesty needs of their different patients.

Barriers and Key Issues

Barriers and issues vary by perspective; the practitioner, medical clinician, and patient have different concerns. Medical clinicians may have the most difficult obstacle to surmount, for they must integrate their ideal model of scientific, linear-causal medicine (with its actual uncertainties and gaps in scientific knowledge) with the holistic needs of patients and with the empiric pressures of practice. Faced with such a hurdle, the clinician might profitably exclaim, "Now that I've given up all hope, I feel much better." Such an admission allows the clinician to think "outside the box" and thus develop more creative solutions to patient problems.

Conventional medical training does not emphasize the mind-body connection. It is disease-oriented rather than health-oriented, and it does not train students in sensitive touch for diagnostic or therapeutic purposes. Conventional training does not adequately prepare doctors to assess muscle tension and the subtle restrictions in joint mobility that play an important role in many medical problems. Thus it may be difficult for medical clinicians to understand Trager principles and methods. Trager work assigns value and gives priority to feeling good. It trains people away from symptom obsession and toward positive body awareness.

From the patient's lay point of view, gentle and intimate touch for therapeutic purposes also may be outside society's governing paradigm and therefore suspect. It may be hard for patients to accept connections between mind and body processes or to accept that they can produce beneficial changes in health by developing awareness and the ability to relax and feel good. Further, it may be hard for a patient who values overwork, time pressure, and disregard for negative feedback from the body (symptoms) to develop balanced habits of self-care.

Trager practitioners without medical training may lack knowledge of the medical model and disease processes. They may find it difficult to communicate with clinicians, for Trager jargon is so spectacularly nonmedical as to be almost incomprehensible to medical people. Their training clearly conveys the therapeutic potential of Trager work while cautioning students not to call it therapy; practitioners may find it difficult to resolve this contradiction. Finally, practitioners may struggle with their relationship to the whole medical system. They are not licensed by governmental entities; they may have difficulty getting reimbursed by third-party payers; and their work may not be accorded the respect they believe it deserves.

Associations

The Trager Institute, based in Mill Valley, California, is the single international organization for practitioners and students. With the help of a full time Executive Director, staff, and Board of Directors, the Institute maintains a worldwide directory of practitioners and students and monitors the training, continuing education, and certification of practitioners. It is associated with a federation of bodywork organizations and monitors developments in the field. Institute-approved instructors and tutors are carefully selected after completing extensive preparation to attain those statuses, and each of these groups meets annually for training and discussion of key issues.

Trainings, although held at various locations worldwide, are all conducted under the auspices of the Institute and are announced in its periodic publications. In addition to the basic practitioner trainings, there are various other course offerings pertinent to the development of practitioners and students. Inquiries can be addressed to:

The Trager Institute
21 Locust Ave.
Mill Valley, CA 94941
Tel: (415) 388-2688.
E-mail: admin@trager.com
www.trager.com

Suggested Reading

1. Liskin J: *Moving medicine: the life and work of Milton Trager, MD,* Barrytown, N.Y., 1996, Station Hill Press.
   This book chronicles the development of the man and his work and explores the principles underlying the Trager Approach, as well as its place in medical practice.
2. Trager M: *Trager mentastics: movement as a way to agelessness,* Barrytown, N.Y., 1987, Station Hill Press.
   This book poetically explores the movements that Dr. Trager developed and taught to his students and patients.
3. Davis C, editor: *Complementary therapies in rehabilitation,* Thorofare, N.J., 1997, Slack.
   This compilation details a variety of modalities, including Trager work, as useful methods in rehabilitation.

References

1. Hubbard DR, Berkoff GM: Myofascial trigger points show spontaneous needle EMG activity, *Spine* 18(13):1803-1807, 1993.

2. Rossi EL: *The psychobiology of mind-body healing: new concepts of therapeutic hypnosis*, New York, 1986, W.W. Norton.

3. Engel JM et al: Long-term follow-up of relaxation training for pediatric headache disorders, *Headache* 32:152-156, 1992.

4. Gould K et al: Changes in myocardial perfusion abnormalities by positron emission tomography after long-term intense risk factor modification, *JAMA* 274(11):894-901, 1995.

5. Witt PL, MacKinnon J: Trager psychophysical integration: a method to improve chest mobility of patients with chronic lung disease, *Phys Ther* 66(2):214-216, 1986.

6. Witt PL: Trager psychophysical integration: an additional tool in the treatment of chronic spinal pain and dysfunction, *Whirlpool* (summer):24-26, 1986.

7. Witt PL: Effectiveness of Trager psychophysical integration in promoting trunk mobility in a child with cerebral palsy: a case report, *Phys Occup Ther Pediatr* 8(4):75-94, 1988.

8. Cooper C, Liskin J, Moorhead JF: Dyscoordinate co-contraction: impaired quality of movement in patients with hand disorders, *Occup Ther Prac* 4(3), 1999.

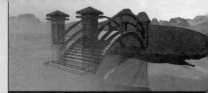

Exploring the Concept of Energy in Touch-Based Healing

M. SUE BENFORD

GARY E.R. SCHWARTZ

LINDA G.S. RUSSEK

SHANE BOOSEY

Origins and History

The term *bioenergy* is an elusive, if not completely foreign concept to most Western medical practitioners. However ill-defined and unrecognized, it often is implicated as an important component in many complementary and alternative therapies. This apparent dichotomy has been the focus of a great deal of research. Practitioners using hand-mediated energy techniques claim beneficial healing results through some type of interaction between the healer's energy field and the patient's energy field, yet Western medicine has called into question the efficacy of such practices.

In the April 1, 1998 issue of *Journal of the American Medical Association (JAMA)* the work of fourth-grader Emily Rosa et al made headlines by demonstrating that 21 therapeutic touch practitioners were unable in 280 trials to detect another human being's energy field (in other words, Emily's hand). The practitioners identified the correct location of Emily's hand just 44% of the time; if they had guessed at random, they would have been correct 50% of the time. The report on the study is accompanied by a note from the journal's editor, Dr. George Lundberg, who says, "Practitioners should disclose these results to patients, third-party payers should question whether they should pay for this procedure, and patients should save their money unless or until additional honest experimentation demonstrates an actual effect."

Part of the resistance on the part of Western practitioners such as Lundberg lies in the fact that science has never fully explained nor documented exactly what is the "cause and effect" within the various bioenergy healing methodologies. Although the existence of some type of electromagnetic energy field surrounding living organisms seems to have been accepted as a truth by allopathic medicine, the identification, interaction, mode of transference, and underlying reason for the occurrence of a therapeutic effect has remained undefined by rigorous scientific testing.

Among the bioenergy therapies, therapeutic touch has created the largest body of published research. Often practiced by nurses, this therapy has been shown to reduce anxiety in hospitalized cardiovascular patients[1] and in chemotherapy oncology patients[2] while reducing measured stress in premature newborns.[3] The practice also has been shown to reduce tension headache pain.[4] Research on the objective physiologic effects of therapeutic touch are presently inconclusive and difficult to interpret because of inconsistent methods among researchers.[5] However, therapeutic touch has been shown to dramatically increase the rate of healing of dermal punch wounds[6] and in one pilot study caused a decrease in the concentration of suppressor T cells, implying an increased immune response.[7]

A separate study involving the effects of another hand-mediated therapy, Reiki, showed significant changes in hemoglobin and hematocrit values after treatment.[8] Researchers are continually trying to explain the mechanism behind the healing process involved in these modalities.

In a series of papers, Schwartz and Russek[9-12] have demonstrated how the integration of general systems theory with contemporary concepts of energy (termed *dynamical energy systems theory*) provides a plausible scientific framework for addressing interactive cause-effect in both conventional and alternative medicine. Moreover, Schwartz et al[13] published two studies that predated the Rosa et al experimental method with substantially more trials, controls, subjects, and investigators. They obtained positive findings indicating that untrained college students could, in fact, detect another human being's energy field above chance. Schwartz et al[14] considered various potential bioelectromagnetic sources of energy, including infrared (heat) and electrostatic body-motion effects, to explain these findings.

However, in a recent experiment, Schwartz and Russek[15] discovered that college students could detect not only another human being's energy field above chance, but they could detect another individual's "intention" to interact with them above chance as well. Such findings challenge contemporary medical science to consider alternative modes of energetic interaction that go beyond traditional bioelectromagnetic signals (they also potentially explain why Rosa et al failed to obtained positive findings).

The question still remains: What does the trained healer do to effect changes within a human or nonhuman recipient? Part of the answer may be found in the discovery of large frequency-pulsing biomagnetic fields emanating from hands of therapeutic touch practitioners during therapy as measured by an extremely sensitive magnetometer called a SQUID (Superconducting Quantum Interference Device).[16] Similar frequency-pulsing biomagnetic fields were later measured and quantified from the hands of meditators and practitioners of yoga and Qi Gong using a simple magnetometer. These fields were 1000 times greater than the strongest human biomagnetic field[17] and were found to be in the same frequency range as those being tested in medical research laboratories for use in speeding the healing process of certain biological tissues.[16,18] This range is low energy and extremely low frequency, spanning from 2 Hz to 50 Hz.[18]

One hypothesis behind the therapeutic effects of magnetic energy is that specific frequencies trigger a multitude of specific biologic processes at the cellular and molecular level, initiating injury repair.[19] A second hypothesis suggests that magnetic fields actually clear the passageway within the body's matrix to allow the innate biologic energy to initiate its natural healing process.[20]

During the last 10 years, there has been an escalation of research in China on Qi Gong, the grandfather of bioenergy modalities. These research activities have primarily focused on the following three categories of experimental methodology: 1) investigation into the nature of the external Qi of Qi Gong and the mechanism by which it accomplishes its effects by directly applying the external Qi to the sensors or detectors of analytic instruments; 2) measurement of the changes in various physiologic parameters and tissues of human beings and other organisms during the emission of the external Qi and the circulation of the internal Qi of Qi Gong; and 3) the effect on organisms (such as cancer cells) and various bacteria in vitro through the application of the external Qi of Qi Gong with corresponding analysis of the mechanisms by which the external Qi accomplishes its effects, using analytic techniques.

From this research it is now clear that the effects of Qi Gong are manifested in many forms and that the levels of Qi Gong effects are complex and not well understood. In most of these experiments a system of "human to human" or "human to organism" is usually employed. For example, in many studies a Qi Gong Master emits external Qi to a human being or a nonhuman organism while the effects are monitored under controlled scientific conditions.

The matter-energy manipulation observed in these controlled Chinese trials demonstrated unexpected and unexplainable variations in the basic characteristics of most substances tested, ranging from radioactive materials to simple tap water.[21-28] Furthermore, these external Qi effects were noted at significant distances; for example, more than 10,000 miles between Qi transmitter and receptor has been recorded, indicating that the matter-energy manipulation phenomenon is not limited to close proximity. Thus bioenergetic effects appear to extend beyond hand-mediated practices to also include such well-known practices as prayer and remote visualization techniques.

Radiation Hormesis

Recent experiments by Benford et al[29,30] have suggested a new hypothesis for at least part of the beneficial effects induced by bioenergy techniques: low-dose ionizing radiation. In preliminary studies, Benford et al identified statistically significant decreases in extremely high-frequency electromagnetic fields, known as *gamma rays*, during Polarity therapy sessions with a therapist and subject. One hypothesis suggests that the fluctuations may occur because of increased gamma ray absorption by the subject during bioenergetic treatments and, like the low-frequency magnetic fields previously mentioned, result in the activation of specific cellular and molecular processes that are beneficial to healing.

Benford proposed that this effect is similar to the therapeutic health effects seen in low-dose radiation experiments where it is thought that just enough radiation is absorbed to induce the expression of repair genes without actually causing serious biologic damage.[31] Much research documents the positive health effects of low-dose radiation, which is often referred to as *hormesis*.[32-34]

Proposed Hormetic Effects of Low-Dose Ionizing Radiation

Biochemical	Cellular	Organismal
Stimulates DNA repair	Stimulates immune response	Decreases cancer risk in chronically exposed populations
Induces free radical detoxification and repair systems	Functions as a vital life force that may even be essential requirement	Extends average life-span in lightly exposed populations
	Functions as general metabolic catalyst and fertility enhancer	Produces evolutionarily favorable selection pressure that benefits species as a whole

The idea of hormesis goes back to ancient Greece, where it was thought that frequent small doses of a poison would fine-tune the body and cause positive health effects. The same idea has been thought to apply to radiation, such that small amounts of ionizing radiation, such as gamma rays, are actually beneficial, and that without it our health actually suffers.

Though not extensively documented in the medical literature, there is evidence for the existence of hormesis in carcinogenesis studies.[35-37] For several decades, increased longevity and decreased cancer mortality have been reported in populations exposed to high background radiation. Established radiation protection authorities consider such observations to be spurious or inconclusive because of unreliable public health data or confounding factors, such as pollution of air, water, and food, smoking, income, education, medical care, population density, and other socioeconomic variables. Recently, several epidemiologic studies have demonstrated a statistically significant correlation between positive health effects and exposure to low or intermediate radiation levels. Dr. Zbigniew Jaworowski, past chairman of the United Nations Scientific Committee on the Effects of Atomic Radiation (UNSCEAR), in his current review of hormesis cites recent data showing hormetic effects in humans from the former Soviet Union.[38]

One of the most remarkable studies related to radiation hormesis, with relevance to the Benford et al research, was conducted on seriously ill non-Hodgkin's lymphoma patients by Dr. K. Sakamoto of the Tohoku University in Japan. Fractionated doses of 10 centigray (cGy) 3 times per week or 15 cGy 2 times per week were given for 5 weeks for a cumulative dose of 150 cGy. Both whole body and half-body low-dose ionizing irradiation were tested. The results demonstrated that half-body irradiation (HBI) of the rib cage area (thorax from xyphoid process to suprasternal notch) was as effective as whole body irradiation (TBI). In some patients, tumors completely outside the HBI field disappeared after HBI alone. Analysis of peripheral lymphocytes demonstrated immune system stimulation. The 10-year survival of patients receiving only standard protocol local high-dose radiotherapy and chemotherapy is 65%, compared to 84% 10-year survival of patients receiving additional low-dose TBI or HBI ($P < 0.05$).[39]

Using Radiation for Bioenergy

According to the healing therapists, when the body's energy field is "blocked" their treatments serve to release the blockages and encourage the flow of energy into the body. Also observed by trained healers is the "pulling effect of universal energy" by subjects in a dis-

Documented Effects from Low-Dose Radiation that May Relate to Bioenergy Therapies Used by Alternative Therapy Practitioners	
Increased Effect	**Decreased Effect**
Cellular growth rate and wound healing	Cancer mortality
Developmental rate	Cardiovascular death rate
Acuity of senses	Respiratory mortality rate
Memory	Infection
Immunity	Neonatal death rate
Fecundity	Sterility
Mean life span	Total mortality rate

ease state. This pulling subsides as the patient's condition improves. If these are correct assessments of what is occurring, then a healing energy session should demonstrate absorption of gamma rays from the surrounding electromagnetic field and into the body itself. Moreover, once absorbed, the potential for dynamical energy system interaction becomes plausible.

In human cells, only 40% of the total potential energy in glucose is transferred to ATP. The remaining 60% of the energy is generated in the form of heat.[40] Given this inefficient energy cycle, it is not hard to imagine the cellular need for an alternative fuel supply other than food stuffs.

By comparison, plants are able to capture the energy in sunlight and use this energy to synthesize glucose by the complex, enigmatic process of photosynthesis. It is a well-known fact that all life is ultimately dependent on the energy derived from sunlight. But are human cells directly benefiting from radiant energy?

A crucial observation is that bacteria are considered a part of the plant kingdom. It is believed that mitochondria, the power-producers within the human cell, were once free-dwelling prokaryotes identical to bacteria. Subsequently, mitochondria are more closely aligned to organisms from the *plant* kingdom capable of photosynthetic processing of radiant energy than the eukaryotic cells with which they now share a symbiotic relationship. The theory of free-standing mitochondrial bacteria, originally championed by Dr. Lynn Margulis, suggests that today's mitochondria are the descendants of ancient prokaryotes that established a symbiotic relationship within eukaryotic cells.[41]

More recent research by Martin and Müller suggests that the archaebacterium host (the theoretic ancestor of the mitochondria) was strictly autotropic, which means it was self-feeding. This assumption further supports our theory that the primordial mitochondrial archaebacterium may have depended on the abundant ionizing radiation as a fuel source for its nutritional energy needs.[42]

If modern-day mitochondria are known to be capable of anaerobic energy generating processes and, like other plant organisms, can theoretically use radiant energy as a power source for energy production, is it not possible that this ability extends to the use of high-energy gammas to supply energy within the cell? After all, before an atmosphere rich in oxygen and their symbiotic relationship with the eukaryotic cells, these strict autotrophs required some energy source powerful enough to supply all their energy needs.

Renowned cell biologist and radiation hormesis expert Dr. T.D. Luckey coined the term for this gamma usage within living cells as radiogenic metabolism.[43] By Luckey's description, radiogenic metabolism is concerned with "the promotion of metabolic reactions by ionizing radiation and its products. It is hypothesized that radiogenic metabolism was involved in prephotosynthetic transformation of radiant energy into chemical energy. Metabolic adaptation to the utilization of free radicals from the radiolysis of water could be the evolutionary precursor to the use of active oxygen radicals in photosynthesis and respiration."[43]

His rationale for the existence of this phenomenon begins with readily accepted premises and ends with postulates that can be tested, as follows:

1. Ionizing radiation was a major energy source 3 to 4 billion years BP (Before Present) during the origin of life and development of early metabolic pathway;

2. The atmosphere at that time was highly reducing;

3. Volcanic dusts and water clouds made the sunlight an inconsistent force at the surface of the earth;

4. Warm pools contained adequate nurture for diverse fermentation;

5. In a few millennia, fermentation would have been expected to slow because of depletion of oxidants to accept protons and electrons from fermentation;

6. Discontinuous sources of oxidants included sporadic disgorgement of nitrates, sulfides, carbon dioxide, metals, and even small amounts of oxygen by geologic processes;

7. A continuous supply of oxidants was provided by the generation of free radicals by ionizing radiation, as exemplified by the simplest radiolysis products from water;

8. As exhaustive fermentation depleted other supplies, the radiolytic supply became qualitatively important. Regular association to transition metals and certain organic radicals with active oxygen radicals would reoccur to encourage their use by evolving organisms;

9. Organisms reacted positively to this supply of oxidants by concentrating intracellular potassium two hundredfold over seawater. Because ^{40}K (the radioactive isotope of K) was about 10 times more abundant then than now, this supplied Beta-radiation within the cell matrix. This constant supply of intracellular free radicals had survival value during periods of low availability of exogenous oxidants and allowed further evolution of metabolic machinery to use active oxygen radicals in a prephotosynthetic system;

10. The gradual decrease of radionuclide radiation was accompanied by an increased constancy of sunlight; this allowed the evolution of systems with efficient pigments that could use low-energy photons (photosynthesis with visible light).[43]

If high-energy gamma photons are being "digested" and used as an ongoing energy source by human cells, then there should be some identifiable byproduct of the metabolism. Recently published work by Dr. Fritz-Albert Popp of the International Institute of Biophysics suggests that low-energy biophotons are continuously emitted from human beings and other living organisms. In a long-term study with human subjects, Popp demonstrated that photon emissions from each of the skin areas tested followed the same biologic rhythms but were phase-shifted between various body parts, such as hands versus forehead. Popp also demonstrated that normal patterns are disrupted in people suffering from various illnesses and diseases.[44]

In a separate series of experiments, Popp discovered that one of the roles of biophotons involves "the growth of bacteria in their nutritional medium."[45] Bacterial nutritional mediums emit photons as a result of routine oxidative processes such that the photon output of the medium radiates uniformly for days. However, once bacteria are introduced to the medium the photon emission immediately decreases. Once the colonies have obtained a more highly concentrated population density, the unexplained absorbance dissipates.[45]

Additionally, the gamma ray studies of Benford et al may indicate that the body has a "self-regulation" mechanism, which works by absorbing only the amount of gamma energy needed at that time. At higher altitudes where naturally occurring ambient gamma rays are more abundant the need for these types of energy interventions may not be as great as in a lower elevation. Subsequently, the magnitude of the observed healing results also may be affected depending on the ambient background gamma radiation (see the table "Background Ionizing Radiation Exposures of Different Populations"). In other words, in the lowest place on earth, the Dead Sea region, many more "healing miracles" might be apparent than in the upper elevations of Colorado. Further research needs to be conducted to determine what limits and parameters of gamma radiation are required for a therapeutic effect to be achieved.

Background Ionizing Radiation Exposures of Different Populations[46]	
Centigray (cGy) Per Year	**Population**
0.26	United States
1.3	Guarapari, Brazil
2.3	Kerala, India
20.0	Kerala Beach, India
20.0	Guarapari Beach, Brazil
24.0	Ramasar, Iran

Integrating the Radiogenic Metabolism Hypothesis with Dynamical Energy Systems Theory

Dynamical energy systems theory, when integrated with the radiogenic metabolism hypothesis, leads to a set of novel hypotheses that can be put to empiric test. In a series of recent papers, Schwartz and Russek[10,15] have outlined the logic whereby dynamical interactions in material systems that involve recurrent feedback processes (the well-established explanation for self-regulation in systems) inherently store information and energy about the complex relationships that emerge over time between the components comprising the system. This mechanism, termed the *systemic memory hypothesis*, predicts that all dynamical systems store information and energy to various degrees.

As reviewed in the Schwartz and Russek papers, the logic of systemic memory was anticipated by a number of distinguished physicians and neuroscientists, including William James, Warren McCulloch, and Karl Pribram. However, these individuals limited their application of the logic to neural feedback systems, not feedback systems in general. The one individual who appreciated the generality of the logic was the distinguished anthropologist and systems theorist Gregory Bateson, who wrote "The simplest cybernetic circuit can be said to have memory of a dynamic kind—not based upon static storage but upon the travel of information around the circuit." According to quantum dynamics, physical systems are in continuous interactive resonance (even at the temperature of absolute zero); hence, information will perpetually travel around the circuit.

The general systems logic of recurrent feedback loops, a well-accepted mechanism for explaining how neural networks learn, applies to all dynamical network organizations, not just dynamical neural network organizations. Moreover, the logic of recurrent feedback applies to interactions within the "space" that exists between all "particles" of matter in dynamical networks.

These dynamical interactions have been described as being pure or "virtual" energy systems within material systems, or more precisely, informed energy systems. The systemic memory mechanism potentially explains the origin of holism and emergent processes in all systems, from the micro to the macro.

The systemic memory hypothesis predicts a spectrum of seemingly anomalous memory-like phenomena in nature, including cellular memory purportedly stored in donor organs as sometimes observed in heart transplant patients; muscular memory purportedly observed in kinesiology; and physical-chemical memory hypothesized to occur in homeopathy. The systemic memory hypothesis reflects a general and intrinsic systemic process that logically applies inexorably to all systems at all levels in nature. It not only predicts seemingly anomalous memory-like phenomena in physics, chemistry, physical chemistry, biochemistry, and cellular biology, it also predicts anomalous memory-like phenomena purported to occur in alternative healing practices and spirituality.

Comparisons Between Radiation Hormesis Effects and Bioenergy Mediated Effects

It is well known that large and small doses of the same agent can elicit opposite biologic effects. This hormetic or "reverse effect" has been shown to exist for drugs, hormones, vitamins, essential minerals, and ionizing radiation.[46] Numerous animal studies indicate a radiation-induced hormesis occurs in major physiologic functions[47,48] and at all levels ranging from biochemical to organismal[49] (see the table "Proposed Hormetic Effects of Low-Dose Ionizing Radiation"). Mechanisms include activated cellular repair systems, increased immune competence, and supplementation with an essential agent.[34,36,47-51]

Similarly, biophysiologic effects derived from both research and anecdotal reports on effects of hand-mediated bioenergy techniques provide a striking comparison with reported radiation hormesis effects.[46]

Conclusion

With more and more research into the field of energy medicine, it is becoming clearer why these therapies have proven themselves effective for many years. Credible theories backed by research are slowly filling in the scientific details behind these once mysterious methods of healing. However, future research is needed to test these hypotheses. It is important to know that these therapies work but also that we can measure their effectiveness using objective and controlled parameters. The day is coming in the near future when physicians will be able to not only recommend these therapies to their patients but precisely explain why and how they work.

References

1. Heidt P: Effect of therapeutic touch on anxiety level of hospitalized patients, *Nurs Res* 30:32-37, 1981.
2. Guerrero MS: The effects of therapeutic touch on state-trait anxiety level of oncology patients, *Masters Abstr Int* 42(24):3, 1985.
3. Fedoruk RB: Transfer of the relaxation response: therapeutic touch B as a method for reduction of stress in premature neonates, *Dissert Abstr Int* 46:978B, 1985.
4. Keller SK, Bzdek VM: Effects of therapeutic touch on tension headache pain, *Nurs Res* 35:101-108, 1986.
5. Slater VE: Healing touch. In Micozzi MS, editor: *Fundamentals of complementary and alternative medicine*, New York, 1996, Churchill Livingstone.
6. Wirth DP: The effect of noncontact therapeutic touch on the healing rate of full thickness dermal wounds, *Subt Energ* 1(1):1-20, 1992.
7. Quinn JF, Strelkauskas AJ: Psychoimmunologic effects of therapeutic touch on practitioners and recently bereaved recipients: a pilot study, *Adv Nurs Sci* 15(4);13-36, 1993.
8. Wetzel WS: Reiki healing: a physiologic perspective, *J Holistic Nurs* 7:47-54, 1989.
9. Russek LG, Schwartz GE: Energy cardiology: a dynamical energy systems approach for integrating conventional and alternative medicine, *Advances* 12(4):4-24, 1996.
10. Schwartz GE, Russek LG: Dynamical energy systems and modern physics: fostering the science and spirit of complementary and alternative medicine, *Alt Ther Health Med* 3(3):46-56, 1997.
11. Schwartz GE, Russek LG: Do all dynamical systems have memory? Implications of the systemic memory hypothesis for science and society. In Pribram KH, editor: *Brain and values*, Hillsdale, N.J., 1998, Lawrence Erlbaum.
12. Schwartz GER, Russek LGS: The plausibility of homeopathy: the systemic memory mechanism, *Integr Med* 1(2):53-59, 1998.
13. Schwartz GE, Russek LG, Beltran J: Interpersonal hand-energy registration: evidence for implicit performance and perception, *Subt Energ* 6(2):183-200, 1995.
14. Schwartz GER et al: Electrostatic body-motion registration and the human antenna-receiver effect: a new method for investigating interpersonal dynamical energy system interactions, *Subt Energ Energ Med* 7(2):149-184, 1996.
15. Schwartz GER, Russek LGS: Interpersonal registration of actual and intended eye gaze: relationship to openness to spiritual beliefs and experiences, *J Sci Explor*, 1998, in press.

16. Zimmerman J: Laying-on-of-hands healing and therapeutic touch: a testable theory, *BEMI Currents* 2:8-17, 1990.

17. Seto A et al: Detection of extraordinary large biomagnetic field strength from human hand, *Acupunct Electrother Res Int J* 17:75-94, 1992.

18. Sisken BF, Walder J: Therapeutic aspects of electromagnetic fields for soft tissue healing. In Blank M, editor: Electromagnetic fields. Biological interactions and mechanisms, *Adv Chem Ser* 250:277-285, 1995.

19. Bassett CA: Bioelectomagnetics in the service of medicine. In Blank M, editor: Electromagnetic fields. Biological interactions and mechanisms, *Adv Chem Ser* 250:261-275, 1995.

20. Oschman JL: A biophysical basis for acupuncture. Proceedings of the First Symposium of the Society for Acupuncture Research, Rockville, Md, 1993,

21. Yan X et al: The influence of the external qi of Qi Gong on the radioactive decay rate of 241Am, *Ziran Zazhi (Chinese Nature Journal)* 11:809-812, 1988.

22. Yan X et al: An experimental study on ultra-long distance (2000 km) effects of the external qi of Qi Gong on the molecular structure of matter, *Ziran Zazhi (Chinese Nature Journal)* 11:770-775, 1988.

23. Yan X et al: The external qi experiments from the United States to Beijing, China, *Zhongguo Qi Gong (China Qi Gong)* 1:4-6, 1993.

24. Yan X, Lu Z: Observations of the effect of external qi of Qi Gong on the ultraviolet absorption of nuclei acids, *Ziran Zazhi (Chinese Nature Journal)* 11:647-649, 1988.

25. Yan X, Li S, Yang Z: Observations of the bromination reaction in n-hexane and bromine system under the influence of the external qi of Qi Gong, *Ziran Zazhi (Chinese Nature Journal)* 11:653-655, 1988.

26. Yan X et al: The effect of external qi of Qi Gong on the liposome phase behavior, *Ziran Zazhi (Chinese Nature Journal)* 11:572-573, 1988.

27. Yan X et al: The observation of effect of external qi of Qi Gong on synthesis gas system, *Ziran Zazhi (Chinese Nature Journal)* 11:650-652, 1988.

28. Yan X et al: Laser raman observation on tap water saline, glucose, and medemycine solutions under the influence of the external qi of Qi Gong, *Ziran Zazhi (Chinese Nature Journal)* 11:567-571, 1988.

29. Benford MS et al: Gamma radiation fluctuations during alternative healing therapy, *Alt Ther Health Med* 1999, in press.

30. Unpublished data on file.

31. Benford MS: Biological nuclear reactions: empirical data describes unexplained SHC phenomenon, *J New Energ,* in press.

32. Luckey TD: *Radiation hormesis,* Boca Raton, Fla, 1991, CRC Press.

33. Cohen BL: Test of the linear-no threshold theory of radiation carcinogenesis for inhaled radon decay products, *Health Phys* 68:174-177, 1995.

34. Sugahara T, Sagan LA, Aoyama T: Low dose irradiation and biological defense mechanisms, *Excerpta Medica,* Amsterdam, 1992.

35. Howe GR, McLaughlin J: Breast cancer mortality between 1950 and 1987 after exposure to fractionated moderate-dose-rate ionizing radiation in the Canadian fluoroscopy cohort study and a comparison with breast cancer mortality in the atomic bomb survivors study, *Radiat Res* 149:694-707, 1996.

36. Kondo S: Health effects of low-level radiation, Osaka, Japan, 1993, Kinki University Press.

37. Calabrese EJ, Baldwin LA: The dose determine the stimulation (and poison): development of a chemical hormesis database, *Int J Toxicol* 16:545-569, 1997.

38. Jawarowski Z: Beneficial radiation, *Nukleonika* 40:3-12, 1995.

39. Sakamoto K: Fundamental and clinical studies on cancer control with total or upper half body irradiation, *Jpn J Cancer Chemother* 9:161-175, 1997.

40. Vander AJ: *Energy and cellular metabolism. Human physiology,* New York, 1970, McGraw-Hill.

41. Margulis L: *Symbiosis in cell evolution,* San Francisco, 1981, W. H. Freeman.

42. Martin W, Müller M: The hydrogen hypothesis for the first eukaryote, *Nature* 392(6671):37-41, 1998.

43. Luckey TD: Radiogenic metabolism, *Am J Clin Nutr* 33:2544, 1980.

44. Cohen S, Popp FA: Biophoton emission of the human body, *J Photochem Photobiol* B: Biology 40:187-189, 1997.

45. Popp FA: Biophotons and their regulatory role in cells, *Front Perspect* 7(2):19, 1998.

46. Luckey TD: Low-dose irradiation reduces cancer deaths, *Rad Protect Manag* (Nov/Dec):58-64, 1997.

47. Luckey TD: *Hormesis with ionizing radiation,* Boca Raton, Fla, 1980, CRC Press.

48. Luckey TD: *Radiation hormesis,* Boca Raton, 1991, CRC Press.

49. Macklis RM, Beresford B: Radiation hormesis, *J Nucl Med* 32(2):350-359, 1991.

50. Liu SZ: *Biological effects of low level ionizing radiation and molecular biology research,* Changchun, 1995, Norman Bethun University.

51. Brodsky A: Radiation risks and uranium toxicity with applications and decisions associated with decommissioning clean-up criteria, Hebron, Conn, 1996, RSA Publications.

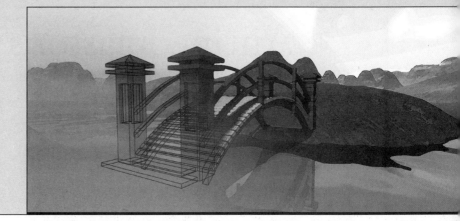

Pharmacologic and Biologic Treatments

Antineoplastons, **496**
Chelation Therapy, **508**
Enzyme Therapy, **517**
Flower Essences, **535**
Herbal Medicine, **545**

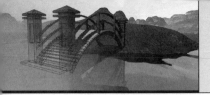

Antineoplastons

Antineoplastons A10®
and AS2-1® Injections

STANISLAW R. BURZYNSKI

Origins and History

Antineoplaston A10 (A10) is a mixture of sodium salts of phenylacetylglutamine (PG) and phenyacetylisoglutamine (isoPG) in a 4:1 ratio. Antineoplaston AS2-1 (AS2-1) is a mixture of the sodium salts of phenylacetic acid (PN) and PG in a 4:1 ratio.

Antineoplastons A10 and AS2-1 are the lead formulations in a new class of antitumor agents called *antineoplastons*. Chemically, antineoplastons are peptides, amino acid derivatives, and organic acids. The research into antineoplastons, which has developed over the last 30 years, is based on the theory of the existence of a system of expression modulators of oncogenes, tumor suppressor genes, and differentiation inducers. The main purpose of the components of this system, called antineoplastons, is the defense of the body against occurrence of defective cells. The mechanism of defense is based not on destruction, but on down-regulation of oncogenes or up-regulation of tumor suppressor genes and induction of differentiation in defective cells. Research into antineoplastons began in 1967 when significant deficiencies of the peptide content were noted in the serum of cancer patients compared with healthy people. Initially, antineoplastons were isolated from blood and later from urine. The first active component, Antineoplaston A10, was identified as 3-phenylacetylamino 2, 6-piperidinedione and was reproduced synthetically. A10 and AS2-1 injections are synthetic analogs of metabolites of 3-phenylacetylamino-2, 6-piperidinedione.[1]

Mechanism of Action According to Its Own Theory

The exciting aspect of the mechanism of action of antineoplastons is down-regulation of oncogenes and activation of tumor-suppressor genes. Neoplastic process results from increased activity of oncogenes and decreased expression of tumor suppressor genes. Effective cancer treatment requires reverse action on these genes.[2]

Biologic Mechanism of Action

Based on published data, PN works as a chemical microswitch that turns off signal transduction through the *ras* oncogene pathway by inhibition of farnesylation of the $p21^{ras}$ protein and causes downregulation of Bcl-2.[3,4] PN also increases the expression of the p53 tumor suppressor gene. Activation of the p53 system involves increasing both the expression of the WAF1 gene and formation of $p21^{WAF1}$ protein, which demethylate promotor sequences of tumor suppressor genes.[5] In vitro studies also have shown that PG and isoPG have antineoplastic activity and that their mechanisms appear to differ from that of PN.

Demographics

A10 and AS2-1 are available only in FDA-controlled Phase II studies. Currently 67 studies are conducted under IND # 43,742, involving more than 1000 physicians in the United States, Canada, The Netherlands, United Kingdom, Australia, and Japan. Such practitioners, usually oncologists and internists, are homogeneously distributed throughout the U.S. The additional physicians who would like to use antineoplastons in the treatment of their patients should contact Burzynski Clinic for further information. The treatment is used both for children as young as 3 months of age and adults with no upper age limit. Among the patients there is approximately an equal ratio between men and women. Antineoplastons have been applied to patients of all races and cultures, but most of the patients are middle-class Caucasians with a high school or university education.

Forms of Therapy

A10 and AS2-1 injections are administered intravenously and intraarterially. The injections are delivered through intravenous or intraarterial catheter and ambulatory infusion pump. The treatment does not require hospitalization.

Indications and Reasons for Referral

The classic reason for referring to this type of therapy is incurable cancer. The therapy is applied the best for primary brain tumors, especially anaplastic astrocytoma, low-grade astrocytoma, mixed glioma, brain stem glioma, and glioblastoma multiforme. The additional indications for Phase II studies in brain tumors include the following: oligodendroglioma; primitive neuroectodermal tumor (PNET); rhabdoid tumor; neurofibroma; schwannoma; visual pathway glioma; ependymoma; craniopharyngioma; choroid plexus carcinoma; germ cell tumor, and meningioma. The therapy also is best applied to non-Hodgkin's lymphoma, cancers of the esophagus, pancreas, prostate, and unknown origin, and neuroblastoma. Additional Phase II studies are conducted in breast, colon, lung, liver, kidney, ovary, and uterine cancers. Clinical studies also are conducted in multiple myeloma, mesothelioma, ma-

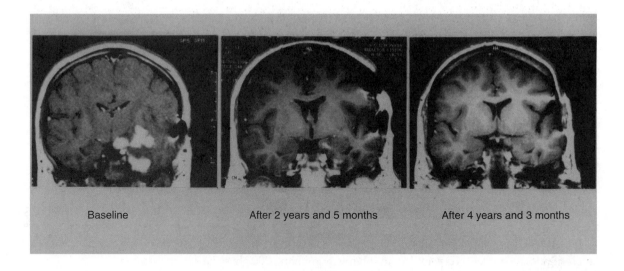

| Baseline | After 2 years and 5 months | After 4 years and 3 months |

MRIs of the head showing complete response during treatment with Antineoplaston A10 and AS2-1 injections in a 12-year-old patient with anaplastic astrocytoma.

lignant melanoma, soft tissue sarcoma, chronic leukemias, sarcoma, neuroendocrine tumors, and adrenal carcinoma.

Research Base

Basic Science

To prove anticancer activity, antineoplastons underwent numerous experiments done by researchers all over the world. Researchers at Kurume University of Japan and the Medical College of Georgia proved activity of A10 against lymphoma and breast cancer in tissue culture. Also the study at Kurume University with A10 injections to athymic mice with transplanted human breast cancer determined marked inhibitory activity. A team at the University of Turin observed marked inhibition of growth of colon adenocarcinoma by A10. Injections of A10 to mice implanted with sarcoma cells at Shandong Medical University in the People's Republic of China confirmed definite antitumor activity. Tissue culture experiments with AS2-1 in the HBL-100 breast cancer line have shown an inhibitory effect and a dose response. Additional studies confirmed that AS2-1 and PN promotes terminal differentiation in human promyelocytic leukemia HL-60, chronic lymphocytic leukemia, neuroblastoma, murine fibrosarcoma V7T, hormonally refractory prostate adenocarcinoma PC3, astrocytoma, medulloblastoma, malignant melanoma, and ovarian cancer.[2] Such studies were performed in a number of institutions including The National Cancer Institute, Memorial Sloan-Kettering Cancer Center, Mayo Clinic, M.D. Anderson Cancer Center, and UCLA.

Risk and Safety

Antineoplastons A10 and AS2-1 are basically nontoxic in animal tests. Phase I studies of A10 and AS2-1 began in April 1980 and proved lack of significant toxicity.[1,2] The incidence of adverse drug reactions is arrived from data on 1216 patients with various types of malignancies treated under IND #43,742. Most patients who participated in the clinical studies or were treated under Special Exceptions had advanced cancer with short life expectancies. In many patients it was difficult to identify whether the side effects were due to the advanced stage of the disease or to antineoplastons. The most important adverse reaction was serious hypernatremia, which occurred in 0.8% of patients.

Additional side effects were usually mild and included increased diuresis and slight thirst, hypochloremia, hypocalcemia, hypomagnesemia, hypokalemia, nausea and vomiting, anemia, leucopenia, thrombocytopenia, allergic reaction, febrile reaction, peripheral neuropathy, somnolence, confusion, headaches, vertigo, slurred speech, tinnitus and decreased hearing, and decreased and blurred vision.

Efficacy

The initial Phase II studies in astrocytoma and high-grade glioma began in 1988 and 1990 and were conducted outside IND process. Astrocytoma study included 20 patients and most of them (15) were diagnosed with Grade 3 astrocytoma. The complete and partial responses occurred in 30% of patients; stable disease, 50%; and progressive disease, 20%.[6] The study in high-grade glioma involved 12 patients diagnosed with glioblastoma multiforme and anaplastic astrocytoma. Thirty-three percent of patients obtained complete and partial responses. Stable disease and progressive disease were determined in 33% of patients.[7]

The first FDA-supervised Phase II study included 36 evaluable patients diagnosed with glioblastoma multiforme (39% of patients), anaplastic glioma (36%), low-grade glioma (14%), PNET (8%) and malignant meningioma (3%). Complete responses were documented in 25%; partial responses, 19.5%; stable disease, 33.3%; and progressive disease, 22.2%. The median survival time from the first day of treatment is approximately 3 years.

In FDA-controlled Phase II studies in astrocytoma in 80 evaluable patients complete and partial responses have been documented in 31%; stable disease, 41%; and progressive disease, 28%.

In a group of 37 evaluable patients with brain stem glioma, 30% obtained complete and partial responses; 40%, stable disease; and 30%, progressive disease. The responses were categorized as defined by the National Cancer Institute and required complete disappearance of all contrast-enhanced tumors on imaging studies for 4 weeks or longer for designation of complete response. More than 50% reduction was required in the sum of the products of the greatest perpendicular diameters of contrast-enhanced tumors for at least 4 weeks and no appearance of new lesions for designation of partial response. Stable disease was defined as less than 50% change (either greater or smaller) in the sum of the products of the greatest perpendicular diameters of the contrast-enhanced tumors for a minimum of 12 weeks. Progressive disease was defined as a greater than 50% increase in the sum of the products of the greatest perpendicular diameters of the contrast-enhanced tumors compared with the nadir evaluation or appearance of new lesions.

Other

Four additional Phase II studies with PN injections are sponsored by the National Cancer Institute (NCI) regarding primary malignant brain tumors, non-Hodgkin's lymphoma, chronic lymphocytic leukemia, multiple myeloma, adenocarcinoma of the pancreas, and malignant melanoma.[8]

Five studies with oral formulations of A10 and AS2-1 (capsules) in breast, colon, lung, and prostate cancer are in process at the Burzynski Clinic. Two Phase II studies with AS2-1 capsules (one in hepatoma and another in colon cancer with liver metastases) are conducted at Kurume University School of Medicine, Japan under the supervision of the Japanese government.[9,10] Two Phase II studies with AS2-1 capsules (one in HIV infection and another in autoimmune diseases) are conducted at the Burzynski Clinic.

Future Research Opportunities and Priorities

Only four FDA-supervised Phase II studies reached a final point, which allowed the conclusion that there is some antitumor activity in primary brain tumors. The priority is to complete the remaining Phase II studies. In addition, preclinical studies are conducted on a new generation of antineoplastons, which have an activity much higher than those currently used.

Office Applications

The illnesses that are most to least likely to be effectively treated based on the results of Phase II studies include the following: astrocytoma (low grade and anaplastic); mixed glioma; brain stem glioma; non-Hodgkin's lymphoma; oligodendroglioma; glioblastoma multiforme; adenocarcinoma of the pancreas; adenocarcinoma of the esophagus; adenocarcinoma of the prostate; carcinoma of unknown primary; rhabdoid tumor; PNET; and neuroblastoma.

Practical Applications

Antineoplastons are used in Phase II studies and under Special Exceptions (for patients who do not qualify for admission to Phase II studies). The physician or patient interested in this form of therapy should contact Burzynski Clinic at (281) 597-0111 or visit the web page at www.cancermed.com. The physician who would like to use antineoplastons will receive protocol and an informational brochure and will be required to fill out FDA Form 1572. There are no charges for pharmaceutic formulations of A10 and AS2-1, but there is a charge for services and equipment (such as the pump). The patient may receive the treatment under the care of a local physician or at Burzynski Clinic. After the initial review of the medical records, patients are then informed if they are qualified for admission to a clinical study. Such patients then are invited to Burzynski Clinic in Houston for a consultation. After 2 weeks of treatment at Burzynski Clinic they may return home and continue

Druglike Information

Description

Antineoplaston A10 injection is a mixture of the sodium salts of PG and iso-PG in a 4:1 ratio. Antineoplaston AS2-1 is a mixture of the sodium salts of PN and PG in a 4:1 ratio. The molecular weight of PG is 264.28, and its empiric formula is $C_{13}H_{16}N_2O_4$. Its structural formula is as follows:

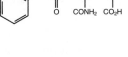

The molecular weight of isoPG is 264.28, and its empiric formula is $C_{13}H_{16}N_2O_4$. Its structural formula is as follows:

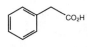

The molecular weight of phenylacetic acid is 136.14, and its empiric formula is $C_8H_8O_2$. Its structural formula is as follows:

The ingredients occur naturally in the human body but are produced synthetically for pharmaceutic use.

Safety

The treatment with A10 and AS2-1 is usually free from side effects. Special attention should be directed to monitoring of electrolytes in the patient's serum. The most important adverse reaction was serious hypernatremia, which occurred in 0.8% of the patients. Hypernatremia can be avoided and successfully treated with proper monitoring of electrolytes and hydration of patients.

Actions

A10 is a differentiation-inducing agent. The mechanism of the induction of terminal differentiation by A10 is unknown. It is postulated that abnormal cells under the influence of A10 transform into differentiating cells that ultimately enter the phase of irreversible senescence and cell death. When all cancerous or abnormal cells undergo differentiation and programmed cell death, the patient enters remission.

The basic mechanism of A10 seems to be the substitution of glutamine by PG. The relative excess of glutamine is essential for a cell entering the S phase of the cell cycle and cell division. Availability of glutamine to cells in the human organism is regulated through the well-known conjugation of glutamine with phenylacetic acid into PG. More than 90% of PN is bound with glutamine to form PG. Administration of A10 to patients introduces PG, which competes with glutamine. Isoglutamine and its derivatives have shown marked antitumor activity in tissue culture studies. The conditions after administration of A10 favor cellular differentiation and inhibition of neoplastic cell growth.

Antineoplaston AS2-1 is a gene-regulating and differentiation-inducing agent. The active ingredient of AS2-1, PN, is known to modulate the expression of *ras* oncogenes and tumor suppressor gene p53 (see "Biologic Mechanism of Action").

Pharmacokinetics

In patients with neoplastic disease, rapid A10 infusions produce plasma PG levels in the range required for in vitro antineoplastic activity. In these patients, A10 is rapidly cleared from plasma and PG and isoPG levels in plasma near preinfusion levels within 4 hours of infusion. Animal studies have shown that within 4 hours of drug administration, approximately 70% of the A10 is excreted in the urine in an unaltered form.

Oral AS2-1 in humans (22.0 to 36.0 mg/kg) produces a rapid (30 to 120 minutes) and dose-dependent increase in plasma PN levels that peak at 1.0 to 2.0 mmol. Patients receiving AS2-1 injections (total phenylacetate in ~10-min injections = 0.23 mmol/kg) immediately after A10 injection have mean peak plasma PN levels near 3.0 mmol. These levels are similar to levels required for in vitro antineoplastic activity. With both oral and intravenous treatment, plasma PN levels return to preinfusion levels 4 to 5 hours after drug administration. At this point, tissue levels of PN are highest in liver and kidney. In humans, 99% of infused PN is excreted in the urine as the glutamine conjugated form (for example, as PG).

Warnings, Contraindications, and Precautions

Serious hypernatremia was observed in 10 of 1216 cases (0.8%); however, only 3 cases were not resolved. One patient refused the treatment, and in two additional cases, hypernatremia was a premortal event for patients with terminal brain tumors. One of these patients died of intracerebral hemorrhage. It is unclear to what degree A10 contributed to hypernatremia in these patients. A10 was administered together with AS2-1, which also may contribute to hypernatremia. Serious hypernatremia was possibly related to brain tumor in 8 patients and liver disease in 2 patients. A high percentage of hypernatremia in patients can also be explained by the high sodium intake with A10 and AS2-1, because both ingredients are injected as sodium salts. Additional pharmacokinetic studies in patients receiving high dosages of A10 failed to reveal significant changes in levels of plasma electrolytes. It is recommended that patients receiving A10 have frequent monitoring of electrolytes, as described in "Administration and Dosage."

Antineoplastons A10 and AS2-1 are contraindicated in patients who have previously shown allergy to them.

Caution should be exercised and the dosage reduced when administering A10 to patients with kidney and liver impairment. Antineoplastons A10 and AS2-1 should not be used in patients who have either a leukocyte count below 1000/mm3 or a platelet count below 50,000/mm.[3] The average sodium content of A10 is 24.5 mg/mL. Because of the sodium content of A10, it is recommended that patients with hypertension and those with a history of congestive heart failure, cardiovascular disease, or renal disease that medically contraindicate administration of high doses of sodium not be treated with A10.

Drug or Other Interactions

Medications considered necessary for the patient's welfare may be given at the discretion of the treating physician. Drug interactions are not known.

Adverse Reactions

Almost all patients experience increased diuresis and slight thirst. The treatment is usually free from adverse reactions or associated only with mild side effects. Moderate side effects (Grade 2 by NCI criteria) included the following: fluid retention in 0.2% of patients; hypernatremia (1.6%); hypochloremia (1.6%); hyperchloremia (0.4%); hypocalcemia (0.2%); hypokalemia (2.5%); hypomagnesemia (0.7%); nausea and vomiting (0.6%); elevation of SGPT (0.1%); leucopenia (0.1%); allergic skin rash (0.7%); fever (2.9%); chills (0.1%); headaches (0.1%); tinnitus and decreased hearing (0.7%); and decreased and blurred vision (0.2%).

Serious adverse reactions (Grade 3 and 4 by NCI criteria) were observed only in a small number of cases and included the following: hypernatremia (0.8%); hypocalcemia (0.2%); hypomagnesemia (0.1%); hypokalemia (0.1%); elevation of serum bilirubin (0.1%); SGOT (0.1%) and SGPT (0.1%); and thrombocytopenia (0.1%). It is suspected that in many cases neurologic toxicity, visual toxicity, and ototoxicity resulted from brain tumors. Serious thrombocytopenia occurred in a single patient who received combination chemotherapy 6 weeks before administration of antineoplastons, which could have contributed to bone marrow suppression. Generally, adverse reactions were fully reversible.

Pregnancy and Lactation

There are no studies with A10 in pregnant women. Female patients must not be pregnant or breastfeeding and must be either incapable of becoming pregnant or currently using contraceptive methods. Male patients should use appropriate contraception during the treatment and at least 4 weeks after discontinuation of treatment.

Trade Products

Antineoplaston A10 injections are available in 500 mL and 1000 mL (300 mg/mL) plastic bags for single-dose injections.

Antineoplaston AS2-1 injections are available in 250 mL (80 mg/mL) plastic bags for single-dose injections. Antineoplaston A10 and AS2-1 are registered trademarks of this author.

Administration and Dosage

Antineoplaston A10 should be administered intravenously daily together with AS2-1 through a double channel infusion pump and intravenous catheter. A single-lumen Broviac, Groshong, or equivalent catheter is necessary for treatment.

The recommended dosage of A10 for intravenous injections for adults is from 5 to 15 g/kg/day and for children from 5 to 20 g/kg/day. The recommended dosage of AS2-1 for intravenous injections for adults is between 0.2 to 0.4 g/kg/day and for children from 0.2 to 0.6 g/kg/day.

For instructions on intraarterial administration, contact the Burzynski Clinic.

Self-Help versus Professional

The treatment should be applied by licensed physicians experienced in the treatment of cancer. A 3-day training session is offered by Burzynski Clinic but is not required.

Visiting a Professional

Before the consultation the patient is required to provide medical records, including films of radiographs and scans to determine the eligibility for Phase II studies. The eligible patients have consultations at Burzynski Clinic, which include history and physical examination, baseline laboratory testing (CBC, chem 27, urinalysis, and tumor markers). Baseline radiographic procedures are scheduled as required for the type of cancer and include MRI, CT, PET, and bone scan. Bone marrow and tumor biopsies are scheduled if necessary. Placement of subclavian vein catheter is usually done as an outpatient procedure, but placement of intraarterial catheter requires hospitalization. The patients are required to have daily visits at the Burzynski Clinic for the first 2 weeks of intravenous and 4 weeks of intraarterial treatment. The follow-up visits are scheduled monthly and follow-up radiographic procedures are scheduled from 4 to 8 weeks. The antitumor response of the treatment should be assessed by taking into consideration the demonstrable objective changes that are observed by physical examination and appropriate radiologic studies (CT, MRI, and PET). Tumor measurements by MRI and CT shall be recorded at least every 8 weeks during the first 2 years of treatment. Once an objective response is accomplished, it is recommended that treatment be continued until complete remission occurs and for 8 months thereafter. It is recommended that the patient have laboratory tests, including hematology and chemistry studies, performed weekly during the first 6 weeks and at least every 3 weeks thereafter during the course of treatment. Patients receiving A10 at a dosage of 5.5 g/kg/day should have their serum electrolytes checked at least once weekly. Patients receiving A10 at dosages in excess of 5.5 g/kg/d should have their serum electrolytes checked at least three times weekly (for example, Monday, Wednesday, and Friday) or more frequently as medically indicated. Testing for serum levels of sodium, potassium, chloride, and bicarbonate should always be included; testing for serum levels of magnesium, calcium, and phosphorus should be included in at least half of those determinations. During antineoplaston dose escalation, all patients should have these electrolyte determinations performed at least every other day. Patients who have been on antineoplastons injections for more than 60 days may have electrolyte levels determined twice per week, provided that they have been on a stable dosage for at least 2 weeks, have a normal serum sodium, and do not have any other serum electrolyte abnormalities.

Credentialing

There are no license requirements for this type of therapy. A10 and AS2-1 are available throughout the entire United States in Phase II studies that are supervised by the FDA. Administration of antineoplaston agents must be performed under the supervision of a physician.

Training

No special training is required.

What to Look for in a Provider

Burzynski Clinic is currently the only provider of antineoplastons.

Burzynski Clinic
12000 Richmond Ave.
Houston, TX 77082
Tel: (281) 597-0111
Fax: (281) 597-1166
www.cancermed.com

Barriers and Key Issues

The main issue, which has kept this therapy from receiving the visibility or credibility it deserves, was bias of medical establishment and governmental agencies. The main stumbling blocks that have kept it from being used by mainstream medical personnel is lack of understanding of the mechanism of treatment and the reticence on the part of mainstream medical personnel to consider alternative treatments.

Associations

There are no national and international associations for this type of therapy.

Suggested Reading

More than 400 publications on antineoplastons, their active ingredients, and prodrugs were published as of January 1, 1999. Approximately 40% of these publications were authored by S. R. Burzynski and associates and 60% were authored by researchers not associated with S. R. Burzynski. S. R. Burzynski has authored 120 patents that have been approved. For details regarding publications, please contact the Burzynski Clinic. It is suggested to read the following books and articles:

1. Burzynski SR: Antineoplastons in the treatment of malignant brain tumors. In Klatz RM, Goldman R, editors: *Anti-aging medical therapeutics*, vol 2, Marina del Ray, Calif, 1998, Health Quest Publications.
2. Burzynski SR, Kubove E, Burzynski B: Treatment of hormonally refractory cancer of the prostate with Antineoplaston AS2-1, *Drugs Exptl Clin Res* 16:361-369, 1990.
3. Elias T: *The Burzynski breakthrough*, Santa Monica, Calif, 1997, General Publishing Group.
4. Moss RW: The fiercest battle: Burzynski and antineoplastons. In *The cancer industry*, New York, 1991, Paragon House.
5. National Institutes of Health: Antineoplastons. In *Alternative medicine: expanding medical horizons*, Washington, D.C., 1994, U.S. Government Printing Office.
6. Samid D, Shack S, Sherman LT: Phenylacetate: a novel nontoxic inducer of tumor cell differentiation, *Cancer Res* 52:1988-1992, 1992.

References

1. Burzynski SR: Synthetic antineoplastons and analogs, *Drugs Future* 11:679-688. 1986.
2. Burzynski SR: Potential of antineoplastons in diseases of old age, *Drugs Aging* 7:157-167, 1995.
3. Shack S et al: Increased susceptibility of ras-transformed cells to phenylacetate is associated with inhibition of p21ras isoprenylation and phenotypic reversion, *Int J Cancer* 63:124-129, 1995.

4. Adam L et al: Sodium phenylacetate induces growth inhibition and Bcl-2 down-regulation and apoptosis in MCF7 ras cells in vitro and in nude mice, *Cancer Res* 55:5156-5160, 1995.

5. Gorospe M et al: Up-regulation and functional role of p21 Waf1/Cip1 during growth arrest of human breast carcinoma MCF-7 cells by phenylacetate, *Cell Growth Differ* 7:1609-1615, 1996.

6. Burzynski SR, Kubove E, Burzynski B: Phase II clinical trials of Antineoplaston A10 and AS2-1 infusions in astrocytoma. In Adam D, editor: *Recent advances in chemotherapy*, Munich, 1992, Futuramed.

7. Burzynski SR, Kubove E, Szymkowski B: Phase II clinical trials of Antineoplaston A10 and AS2-1 infusions in high grade glioma. Presented at the 18th International Congress of Chemotherapy, 1993, Stockholm.

8. Thibault A et al: A phase I and pharmacokinetic study of intravenous phenylacetate in patients with cancer, *Cancer Res* 54:1690-1694, 1994.

9. Tsuda H et al: Quick response of advanced cancer to chemoradiation therapy with antineoplastons, *Oncolog Rep* 5:597-600, 1998.

10. Kumabe T et al: Antineoplaston treatment for advanced hepatocellular carcinoma, *Oncolog Rep* 5:1363-1367, 1998.

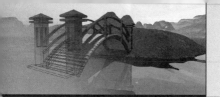

Chelation Therapy

MITCHELL J. GHEN

THEODORE C. ROZEMA

Origins and History

Chelation is defined as the incorporation of a metal ion into a heterocyclic ring structure. Chelation therapy is a subject well-documented and used widely around the world for removal of toxic metals that have found their way into the human body and are causing disruption of basic cellular chemistry.

Lead toxicity is still a great burden to infants and children, especially in third world countries that have not removed lead from their gasoline supplies. In India, more than 30 million people are poisoned with arsenic and great effort is being spent to clean up public water supplies that act as the source.[1] Iron overload from multiple blood transfusions, especially those with thallasemia, is found primarily around the Mediterranean basin.[2] Mercury intoxication is commonly seen from fish ingestion and possibly from amalgam filling leakage.[3] Mercury is methylated by algae and bacteria, which then move up the food chain. It is then ingested by large fish like salmon and tuna, which are then eaten by the general public. The heavy metals, including mercury, cadmium, lead, and arsenic, are considered sulfhydryl reactive metals.[4] Both mercury and cadmium are deposited in the kidneys. Lead is deposited primarily in bone, cadmium is deposited in peripheral nerves, and mercury is deposited primarily in the central nervous system. Consider that the half-life of these heavy metals in the human body may exceed 20 years.[5]

Early in the 1950s, Dr. Norman Clarke, Sr. at Providence Hospital in Detroit, Michigan was using disodium EDTA, a synthetic amino acid with chelating properties for the removal of lead from workers in the battery industry. Not only did this compound remove lead, but he also observed other changes in these patients. Angina was reduced or eliminated, intermittent claudication was relieved, and even radiographs demonstrated a reduction of calcium in calcified heart valves.

Patients who seek a physician trained in chelation therapy are usually those who have seen another patient who has improved by taking this therapy. There are those faced with the possibility of bypass surgery, amputation, or angina (that is unresponsive to modern medicines) who are seeking an alternative. Others are simply interested in improving their health status, realizing that the reduction of toxic metals is worth the effort to seek such therapy.

In summary, EDTA therapy has been used since the early 1950s for patients with toxic mineral poisoning, vascular diseases, (coronary, peripheral, and carotid), rheumatoid arthritis, scleroderma, osteoporosis, diabetes mellitus, porphyria, and digitalis intoxication.

The potential deleterious effects of heavy metal poisoning to humankind can be mitigated with chelation therapies.

Mechanism of Action According to Its Own Theory

Clinical experience has demonstrated that chelation has been used successfully in millions of patients with coronary artery and peripheral vascular disease. A weekly intravenous dose of EDTA can in many cases improved clogged arteries and relieved peripheral vascular and cardiovascular symptomotology.

Biologic Mechanism of Action

There is only one mechanism of action of EDTA when introduced into the body. It is a chelating agent that binds minerals and removes them from the body. EDTA is not a specific chelator. EDTA will remove lead, arsenic, cadmium, nickel, and aluminum, all known to be toxic in some amount to the human body. It also will remove calcium, zinc, copper, manganese, chromium, and other essential minerals to the body. DMSA (Meso-2, 3-dimercaptosuccinic acid) and DMPS (dimercaptopropane sulfonate) are sulfhydryl-containing compounds that may also effectively chelate heavy metals, particularly mercury. DMSA is an analogue of BAL (British Anti-Lewisite), another compound also used for heavy metal chelation. It also is worthy to note that sulfur-containing amino acids such as methionine and cysteine and related compounds such as N-acetylcysteine, S-adenosylmethionine, alphalipoic acid, and the compound glutathione (GSH) can help the chelation process and improve the elimination of heavy metals from the body. The balance achieved by removing toxins and supplementing the essential minerals at the appropriate time makes training in this therapy mandatory before attempting its use.

Because serum calcium is the most abundant and most easily chelated mineral in the blood, the IV introduction of disodium magnesium EDTA will immediately cause the release of the magnesium and the binding of calcium to this compound.[6] This has the effect of reducing serum ionized calcium, which causes an immediate increase in parathyroid hormone.[7] (This phenomenon is well-known as a specific test to check parathyroid functional integrity.)[8] The amount of soft tissue and blood calcium available for immediate replacement of that bound to EDTA is insufficient to accomplish this task, so there is a secondary effect on the soft bone pool of calcium that contributes to this replacement. The effect on bone is to stimulate bone-reforming centers to osteoclastic (calcium removal) for 21 days following which the center becomes osteoblastic (calcium acquisition) for 120 days, a net improvement of 100 days in bone calcium increase from this therapy.[9] This interestingly is what is attempted with the use of alendronate sodium for patients with osteoporosis.

The term *hardened arteries* or *arteriosclerosi* is involved with calcium deposition. EDTA has a marked effect on calcium and parathyroid hormone release. Repetitive treatments of EDTA might have the effect of softening arteries over time. This concept has been well-studied in animals and found to be effective.[10] Magnesium released during IV administration of EDTA has been shown to restore electromagnetic potential across cell membranes.[11] The effects of calcium and magnesium in the development of atherosclerosis have been studied extensively.[12] Because the same type of studies cannot be done in humans, extrapolation of the animal data to humans and observation of the clinical results in physicians' offices has kept this therapy alive over many years.

It is well known that there are minerals in the human body that are able to cause oxidative damage; iron and copper are the transitional metals that easily give up electrons and are the culprits in many oxidative reactions.[13] It has been shown that copper is an effective oxidizer of LDL cholesterol and that oxidized LDL is the form that accumulates in arterial plaque. Animal studies also have shown that antioxidants such as vitamin E, BHT, and EDTA prevent oxidation and therefore they would prevent LDL deposition in arterial walls.[14] Other studies report reduction in plaque size with the use of magnesium disodium EDTA.[15]

Forms of Therapy

Lead is removed with a number of chelating agents, including calcium disodium EDTA, DMSA (meso-2, 3-dimercaptosuccinic acid), or D-penicillamine.[16,17] DMSA also is used for arsenic and mercury poisoning. Note that DMSA will readily cross the blood brain barrier. DMPS (2,3 dimercaptopropane sulfonate) has been used classically to remove mercury from the periphery. Desferroximine is used routinely for persons with acute iron poisoning and iron overload syndromes.

Demographics

Practitioners are distributed throughout the U.S. With the exception of childhood lead poisoning, most patients are men and women in their fifth decade and older.

Indications and Reasons for Referral

Indications for chelation use include advanced atherosclerosis, cerebral vascular insufficiency,[18] coronary artery disease,[18-20] and peripheral vascular disease.[18] Patients with scleroderma and systemic sclerosis have benefited from chelation therapy.[21] Although there are no clinical studies, anecdotal reports suggest patients with rheumatoid arthritis, collagen vascular diseases, and multiple sclerosis have benefited from EDTA. Even the rare condition of calcinosis universalis has improved.[22] We have found that patients with osteoporosis gain an increase in bone calcium density after a series of treatments.[23] Diabetic patients usually demonstrate improvement after chelation therapy. Even the complications of diabetes are often addressed by this treatment, which includes vascular insufficiency. The need for insulin or oral hypoglycemic medications may be reduced or eliminated altogether.[14]

Patients with porphyria also have had improvement with this type of program. The relationship between zinc and copper is often normalized during a course of EDTA treatment. It is suggested that equilibrium will occur in several metalloenzyme systems.[24] Patients demonstrating intoxification of other heavy metals, such as mercury, cadmium, and arsenic, also should have the respective chelating agents to remove these deleterious substances.

Office Applications

A simple ranking of conditions responsive to this form of therapy is as follows. As with all alternative therapies, chelation therapy does not preclude mainstream medical therapies in addition.

Top level: *A therapy ideally suited for these conditions*

Arteriosclerotic occlusive disease (whether it be carotid arteries, cerebral arteries, coronary arteries, or peripheral vascular disease); Alzheimer's disease with proven heavy metal intoxication; hematomachrosis; and overt lead and arsenic or cadmium poisoning

Second level: *One of the better therapies for these conditions*

Diabetes mellitus, fatigue syndromes with proven heavy metal intoxications, and hypertension

Third level: *A valuable adjunctive therapy for these conditions*

Amyotrophic lateral sclerosis; collagen vascular diseases; hypertension; multiple sclerosis; osteoporosis; porphyria; restless leg syndrome; and rheumatoid arthritis

Practical Applications

Signs of heavy metal toxicity are numerous and similar to other conditions, making diagnosis a formidable challenge. Headaches, dizziness, memory impairment, hearing difficulties, irritability, weight loss, tremors, and allergy symptoms may be related to these metals.[25]

The need to remove a toxic mineral from the body has induced chemists to create more than 10,000 chelating agents. However, only about six or seven are in use today because the toxicity of many of these agents usually exceeds the toxicity of the metal being removed.

Research Base

Evidence Based

Large retrospective studies have shown marked improvement in patients with coronary artery disease (92.5%), peripheral vascular disease (97.5%), and cerebrovascular disease

(54%).[18] Other studies have shown that 58 out of 65 patients on the waiting list for bypass surgery were able to cancel the surgery and 24 of 27 patients on the waiting list for amputations were able to cancel surgery.[26]

Druglike Information

Drug or Other Interactions

EDTA has been clinically shown to have an effect on the vascular system, reducing the symptoms of angina and improving arteriosclerotic heart disease,[27] peripheral arterial occlusion and intermittent claudication,[28] improvement in brain circulation,[29] and in general improving the well-being of the patient. Physicians were curious as to why these benefits were happening. The earliest compound used was disodium EDTA. However, this compound was difficult to use as it lowered serum calcium and too much could cause tetany or death.[30] It was much safer to use the calcium disodium EDTA, but then the benefits to the vascular system were not shown to occur. Dr. Popovici, PhD, and others at Georgetown University in Washington, D.C. used a known lethal dose of disodium EDTA for rabbits. After magnesium was added to this compound, fatalities to the rabbits no longer occurred. This has led to the use of magnesium disodium EDTA for the present use in vascular disease.[30]

Actions and Pharmacokinetics

EDTA has been shown to transiently reduce platelet aggregability,[31] inhibit antibody formation,[32] lower blood cholesterol,[33] stimulate C-AMP,[34] and reduce oxidized metals to their more efficient states, thereby restoring enzymes to full activity. This affects many other cellular and physiochemical activities, which in turn affects proper metabolic functioning.

Most chelating agents, such as EDTA, DMPS, as well as desferroximine, are mainly bioavailable through the parental route. Although there are several oral agents that are used for heavy metal toxicity, it usually is best to administer the drugs intravenously for improved efficacy; for example, EDTA can be given orally, but it is only 5% absorbed and has been shown to have no effect on the serum calcium or the parathyroid hormone.[35]

Adverse Reactions

Like any other drug, EDTA can have side effects and it can cause toxicity. In early studies with EDTA, patients complained of the following side effects: nausea, occasional vomiting, and also a rare febrile systemic reaction. These reactions would occur between 4 to 8 hours after the infusion of EDTA.[36] These rare reactions usually have been associated with excessive doses of EDTA and with an overly rapid administration. The physiologic basis for these effects is unclear at the present time. These side effects typically are not seen if the established protocol is followed, but there is the possibility that they still can rarely occur. Allergic reactions are extremely rare.

Safety

If used correctly, chelating agents are extremely safe and reported adverse reactions are quite rare. The physician administering these substances should have proper training before using them. Refer to the *Physician's Desk Reference* for a full listing of side effects, adverse reactions, and contraindications.

Warnings, Contraindications, and Pregnancy

Because EDTA is cleared through the kidneys, physicians must monitor kidney function regularly. EDTA chelation therapy, when administered at the proper rate, dose, and frequency, is not nephrotoxic. In fact, during the course of chelation therapy, renal function usually improves compared to pretreatment levels.[37] The only true contraindication is poor renal function. Patients who are pregnant can be chelated but the risk versus reward must be carefully considered. Recognize that heavy metal toxicity in women usually is not seen until after menopause.

Self-Help versus Professional

The removal of heavy metals from the human body requires skilled, educated practitioners. Also note that the use of the chelating agents as described requires state licensure (MD, DO, or ND in some states) for usage.

Visiting a Professional

A professional will take a thorough history and physical examination and then order the necessary tests as diagnostic and baseline studies. The patient should be prepared to have blood drawn and the vascular system checked with a noninvasive doppler unit. The first treatment generally will not occur until all studies have returned and been evaluated by the practitioner.

Training, Associations, and Credentialing

Training in chelation therapy may be obtained by attending courses given by the American College for Advancement in Medicine or the Great Lakes College of Clinical Medicine. Written and oral exams are given by the American Board of Chelation Therapy to test competency. Each of the following organizations maintains a practitioner data bank:

The American College for Advancement in Medicine
23121 Verdugo Dr., Suite 204
Laguna Hills, CA 92653
Tel: (714) 583-7666
Toll-Free: (800) 532-3688
E-mail: acam@acam.org
www.acam.org

The Great Lakes College of Clinical Medicine
The American and International Board of Chelation Therapy
1407-B N. Wells St.
Chicago, IL 60610
Tel: (312) 787-2228
Toll-Free: (800) 286-6013
E-mail: info@glccm.org
www.glccm.org

What to Look for in a Provider

Call one of the organizations previously listed and ask for their list of physicians providing chelation in your area.

Barriers and Key Issues

Findings suggest many uses for the compound EDTA for other than strictly lead poisoning. In the "early days," patients were hospitalized and the treatment was administered for as many as 6 days in a row with Sunday being the day of rest. Physicians were experimenting because they did not know how much to administer, how often to give the therapy, and how fast to run the IV. There were a great number of studies done and the general consensus was that this therapy had promise for vascular disease.[38]

Abbott Laboratories had the patent rights to EDTA. It is possible that they did not do further research with EDTA because their patent rights to EDTA were expiring and they no longer would have exclusivity for this compound. Also, bypass surgery already had made its debut and the research on EDTA for vascular disease came nearly to a halt.

However, there were a few physicians using EDTA for vascular disease who were continuing to help their patients, even without a definite FDA indication listed on the package insert. Some of these physicians have been using this therapy continuously since 1962. These physicians were brought together through their interest in chelation therapy for vascular disease and formed the American Association of Medical Preventics in 1973. Since that time, this organization has grown, changed their name to the American College for Advancement in Medicine, includes more than 1000 active members, and has trained more than 5000 physicians in the safe and effective use of EDTA for vascular disease.

Suggested Reading

1. Seven MJ: *Metal binding in medicine,* Philadelphia, 1960, JB Lippencott.
   This was the first definitive symposium on the use of chelating agents in medicine.

2. Halstead B, Rozema T: *The scientific chelation therapy,* ed 2, Tyron, NC, 1997, TRC Publishing.
   This is probably the best text for complete understanding of chelation, related biochemistry, and clinical applications.

3. Rozema T: Protocols for chelation therapy, *J Adv Med* (special issue) 10(1), 1997.
   This is a manual for the safe application of EDTA.

4. McDonagh EW, Rudolph CJ: A collection of published papers showing the efficacy of EDTA chelation therapy, Gladstone, Mo, 1991, McDonagh Medical Center.
   This is a compilation of many studies to support the efficacy and use of EDTA.

References

1. Graziano JH: Role of 2,3 dimercaptosuccinic acid in the treatment of heavy metal poisoning, *Med Toxicol* l:155, 1986.

2. Flynn DM: Five year controlled trial of chelating agents in treatment of Thalassemia Major, *Arch Dis Child* 8:829, 1973.

3. Burton Goldberg Group: *Alternative medicine, the definitive guide,* Fife, Wash, 1995, Future Medicine.

4. Kuig D: Cysteine metabolism and metal toxicity, *Altern Med R* 3(4):262, 1998.

5. Herber RFM et al, editors: *Handbook on metals in clinical and analytical chemistry,* New York, 1994, Marcel Dekker.

6. Rubin M: *Magnesium EDTA chelation cardiovascular drug therapy,* ed 2, Philadelphia, 1988, W.B. Saunders.

7. Chen I et al: Radioimmunoassay of parathyroid hormone: peripheral plasma immunoreactive parathyroid hormone response to ethylene diamine tetraacetate, *J Nucl Med* 15:763, 1974.

8. Jones KH, Fourman P: Edetic acid test of parathyroid insufficiency, *Lancet* 2:119, 1963.

9. Rassmussen H, Bordier P: The physiological and cellular basis of metabolic bone disease, Baltimore, 1974, Williams and Wilkins.

10. Malinovska V et al: Ultrahistochemical study of the effect of glucagon and Chelation III on arterial wall structure after experimental calcification, *Folia Morphologica* 28:20, 1978.

11. Altura BM, Altura BT: Magnesium withdrawal and contraction of arterial smooth muscle effect of EDTA, EGTA, and divalent cations, *Proc Soc Exp Biol Med* 154(4):752, 1976.

12. Orimo H, Ouchi Y: The role of calcium and magnesium in the development of atherosclerosis; experimental and clinical evidence, *Ann NY Acad Sci* p. 441, 1991.

13. Dermopoulos H: Molecular oxygen in health and disease. Presented at the AAMP Tenth Annual Spring Meeting, May 21, 1983, Los Angeles.

14. Chisolm GM III: The oxidative modification of LDL implications in diabetes mellitus, *Lipid Letter* 5:5, 1988.

15. Wartman A et al: Plaque reversal with MgEDTA in experimental atherosclerosis: elastin and collagen metabolism, *J Atheros Res* 7:331, 1967.

16. Agerty HA: Lead poisoning in children, *Med Clin N Am* 36:1587, 1952.

17. Belknap EL: EDTA in the treatment of lead poisoning, *Industr Med Surg* 21:305, 1952.

18. Olszewer E, Carter JP: Chelation therapy: a retrospective study of 2870 patients, *J Adv Med* 2(5):197, 1989.

19. Casdorph HR: EDTA chelation therapy, efficacy in arteriosclerotic heart disease, *J Hol Med* 3(1):53, 1981.

20. McDonagh EW, Rudolph CJ: Noninvasive treatment for sequellae of failed coronary circulation: 100% occlusion of left anterior descending coronary artery, 30% stenosis right coronary artery and left ventricular contractility deficit, *J Neurol Orthop Med Surg* 12:169, 1993.

21. Birk RE, Rupe CE: The treatment of systemic sclerosis with disodium EDTA, pyridoxine, and reserpine, *Henry Ford Hosp Med Bull* 14:109, 1966.

22. Davis H, Moe PJ: Favorable response of calcinosis universalis to edatharnil disodium, *Pediatrics* 24:780, 1959.

23. Rudolph CJ, McDonagh EW, Wussow DG: The effect of intravenous ethylene diamine tetraacetic acid (EDTA) upon bone density levels, *J Adv Med* 1(2):79, 1988.

24. Painter JT, Morrow EJ: Porphyria. Its manifestations and treatment with chelating agents, *Texas State J Med* 55:811, 1959.

25. Haas E: *Staying healthy with nutrition,* Berkeley, Calif, 1992, Celestial Arts.

26. Hancke C, Flytlie K: Benefits of EDTA chelation therapy in arteriosclerosis: a retrospective study of 470 patients, *J Adv Med* 6(3):161, 1993.

27. Clarke NE, Clarke CN, Mosher RE: Treatment of angina pectoris with disodium ethylene diamine tetraacetic acid, *Am J Med Sci* 232:654, 1956.

28. Casdorph HR, Farr C: EDTA chelation therapy III: treatment of peripheral arterial occlusion, an alternative to amputation, *J Hol Med* 3(1):3, 1983.

29. Casdorph HR: EDTA chelation therapy II, efficacy in brain disorders, *J Hol Med* 3(2):101, 1981.

30. Popovici A et al: Experimental control of calcium levels in vivo, *Proc Soc Exp Biol Med* 74:415, 1950.

31. Kindness G, Frackelton JP: Effect of ethylene diamine tetraacetic acid (EDTA) on platelet aggregation in human blood, *J Adv Med* 2(4):519, 1989.

32. Kozlov VA, Novikova VM: Calcium ion dependent immunosuppressive effect of ethylene diamine tetraacetic acid (EDTA), *Zh Mikrobiol, Epidemiol Immunobiol* (Russian) 1:69, 1978.

33. McDonagh EW, Rudolph CJ, Cheraskin E: The effect of intravenous disodium ethylene diamine tetraacetic acid (EDTA) upon blood cholesterol levels in a private practice environment, *J Intern Acad Prev Med* 7:5, 1982.

34. Brachaet P, Klein C: Cell response to C-AMP during aggregation phase of dictyostelium discoideum. Comparison of the inhibitory effects of pregesterone and the stimulatory action of EDTA and ionophore A-23187, *Differentiation* 8(1):1, 1997.

35. Sidbury JB Jr, Bynum JC, Fetz LL: Effect of chlating agent on urinary lead excretion, comparison of oral and intravenous administration. *Proc Soc Exp Biol Med* 83:266, 1953.

36. *Goodman and Gillman's pharmacological basis of therapeutics: heavy metals and heavy metal antagonists,* 1980.

37. McDonagh EW, Rudolph CJ, Cheraskin E: The effect of EDTA chelation therapy plus supportive multivitamin-trace mineral supplementation upon renal function: a study in serum creatinine, *J Hol Med* 4:146, 1982.

38. Foreman H: Pharmacology of some useful chelating agents. In Seven MJ, Johnson LA, editors: *Metal-binding in medicine,* Philadelphia, 1960, JB Lippincott.

Enzyme Therapy

RALF KLEEF

OTTO PECHER

Origins and History

Enzymes are catalytically active polymer compounds made of amino acids. They are involved in virtually all vital metabolic processes. They facilitate metabolic conversions, control energetic processes, and regulate syntheses. Without enzymes, few, if any, metabolic processes can occur within an organism.

Enzymes have an active role in medical therapy. Ingestion of enzyme supplements is common in cases of intestinal enzyme deficiency. External use of enzymes for impaired wound healing (for example, in the presence of varicose ulcers) has been part of the armamentarium of medical practitioners for centuries. Parental thrombolytic therapy with streptokinase or urokinase for cardiac or cerebrovascular occlusive events is used commonly in medical centers worldwide.

For many years, enzymes were declared incapable of reaching the whole organism by virtue of an inability to be absorbed through the intestines. The reason for this belief is that enzymes are macromolecules with molecular weights between 16,000 and 60,000 per molecule. However, newborn babies receive antibodies from their mothers through breastmilk. These antibodies must cross the intestinal barrier to reach lymphatic vessels and the bloodstream. These antibodies, called *immunoglobulins*, also are macromolecules with a size comparable to that of the enzymes.

Professor Seifert of the Chirurgischen Universitat-Klinik in Kiel fed rats and dogs with equine gamma globulins radioactively marked to demonstrate on a scientific basis the absorption of these macromolecules. These equine gamma globulines are extremely large with a molecular weight up to 120,000 atoms. Surprisingly, these large molecules were absorbed and therefore could act systemically on the entire organism. As for the oral forms of proteolytic enzymes, their enteric absorption as biologically intact macromolecules has been described.[1-3] In this way, oral use of selected enzymes can have systemic applications.

Enzyme Therapy was developed originally by Max Wolf, MD in New York in the late 1930s. Wolf based his research on findings of Beard (1907) and Freund (1935). He investigated numerous enzymes and enzyme combinations for their antiinflammatory and oncolytic effects. Oral enzyme therapy is far more than merely supplementation for intestinal enzyme deficiencies. In medical applications, most enzymes derive from animals (such as trypsin and chymotrypsin) and plants (such as bromelain and papain) and often are used in combination with a flavonoid, such as rutosid. For the past 40 years, proteolytic enzyme combinations have been registered in Germany for therapeutic use in humans. Their efficacy has been assessed in various states of oncologic and viral diseases and traumatic and inflammatory conditions.[2,3]

Mechanism of Action According to Its Own Theory

A short description on the mechanics of immunology is required to explain the value of enzyme therapy. The body recognizes foreign agents, such as bacteria and viruses, as enemies by antigens on their surface. Other chemical substances and mutated cells also may be seen as foreign in the same way. In response to antigen presence the body produces antibodies, which couple with the antigen to form immune complexes. Large cells called *macrophages* exist to destroy these immune complexes enzymatically. But these macrophages "look" for large immune complexes, so sometimes the medium size immune complexes are "ignored." These smaller complexes can circulate throughout the lymphatic system and bloodstream until they adhere to and penetrate a tissue. Eventually they are stored there. From this moment on, these immune complexes become pathogenic; that is, they can cause a disease.

When the quantity of immune complexes exceeds a certain threshold, macrophages become less active as if overwhelmed. This high level of immune complexes triggers the second immune defense, the complement system. The complement system consists of a cascade of 9 enzymes, activated in sequence. When the entire enzymatic cascade has been activated, a huge dissolvent activity of albumins begins, causing an inflammatory reaction. In consequence the tissue is destroyed and suddenly that which we call an *autoimmune disease* arises; the organism attacks itself.

If, for example, the immune complexes are fixed in the renal tissue, then through the activation of the complement system an inflammation can occur in the kidney, resulting in what we know as *glomerulonephritis*. The disease process depends on where these immune complexes are deposited. For instance, if the lung is involved, then the result is pulmonary fibrosis. If the pancreas is involved, the result is pancreatitis. Joint involvement results in rheumatioid arthritis, and so on. Chronic inflammations of the intestines, such as Crohn's disease or ulcerative colitis, stem from immune complexes in the intestinal tissues. Infections by certain bacteria, viruses, and parasites can also led to immune-complex disorders. The list of the diseases of *autoaggression* caused by immune complexes is extensive. The type of disease does not depend only on the place where the immune complexes are fixed but also on the origin of the antigen.

There are many similar diseases elicited by the activation of the complement system. All of them are so-called *autoimmune diseases*. Until recently they were considered as incurable diseases, because they only could be influenced medically to a limited extent. Some clinical trials have helped to determine that certain enzymes help to interrupt the enzymatic cascade of the complement system. The interruption of the complement system cascade works to avoid tissue damage. *This is achieved by enzymatically diluting the pathogenic immune complexes and activating the macrophages.* This interrupts the vicious circle that leads to chronic degenerative diseases. Enzyme therapy can help to avoid the formation of autoantibodies, inhibit the production of immune complexes, and avoid the activation of complement. To some extent, virtually all diseases contain an immune system component. In conventional medicine, pathogenic immune complexes are eliminated through plasmapheresis, lymphopheresis, and cryoprecipitation. It is much easier, however, to remove the pathogenic immune complexes using enzymes that activate the "phagocytic macrophage system" or by breaking down the large complexes into smaller ones that can be eliminated far more efficiently.

In a few words, enzyme preparations accelerate the progress of the inflammation necessary for healing. They act in a similar way to a natural enzymatic cascade as a bodily alarm response. In autoimmune diseases, enzyme mixtures interrupt the autoaggressive complement cascade, enzymatic breakdown of pathogenic immune complexes, and essential activation of the macrophages. This way the vicious cycle is broken. Just as metabolic demand rises during many disease states, so can enzyme needs. Primary deficiencies may exist, or relative deficiencies may develop in relationship to ongoing illness. Therefore during certain circumstances, enzymatic requirements may be larger than the normal.

Enzymes have the ability to reduce the thick fibrin layer surrounding cancer growth, often 15 times thicker than normal. By reducing this fibrin layer, cancer cell adhesiveness is diminished, which may serve to reduce the risk of metastasis. Loss of this insulating fibrin layer also renders the cancer cell antigens more recognizable to the host's immunosurveillance.

These mechanisms of action justify the large number of indications for systemic enzyme therapy; it is therefore the basis of treatment in acute and chronic inflammatory conditions, autoimmune diseases such as polyarthritis, states of impaired resistance (viral and neoplastic diseases), and also for vascular conditions, in which the additional improvement in blood flow is of great importance. There also is increasing evidence for their prophylactic efficacy (prevention of tumor metastases).

Biologic Mechanism of Action

Enzymatic processes often occur in cascades, where one enzyme activates another in sequential fashion until the last enzyme completes the desired reaction. This process has two advantages. The first is for a saving of energy, as these small individual chemical steps require much less energy than an extensive transformation. The second is for security. The body must insure that these enzymatic cascades are not activated until necessary. An enzymatic cascade activated in the wrong place at the wrong time can cause dangerous or even lethal consequences.

Enzymes often travel throughout the circulatory and lymphatic systems in an inactive and innocuous form. Once needed, they are activated by changes in their structure. Their activation triggers the appropriate enzymatic cascade leading to the desired result. Enzymatic inhibitors are a second safety measure and can prevent the activation of the enzymes inappropriately. Some synthetic enzymatic inhibitors are antibiotics, such as penicillin, or anti-inflammatory medications, such as cortisone. Blocking an enzymatic cascade can prevent an unwanted result. Similarly, the deficiency of an enzyme can lead to chronic disease.

Rationale exists for the use of these substances in inflammatory conditions, autoimmune disease, and cancer.[6-9] Different enzymes have different optima of activity and different modes of action. For this reason, combinations are often more effective than single enzymes. The single substances described below (enzymes and rutosid) are these enzymes, which are well-investigated as monopreparations or are part of enzyme combination products.

Rutosid is a potent radical scavenger and some derivatives significantly reduce the permeability of normal and damaged capillaries.[10] The cysteine proteinase *bromelain*, extracted from pineapples,[11] has raised a longstanding interest in the clinical treatment of different conditions.[12] The antiinflammatory and serum fibrinolytic activity of bromelain after oral administration has been demonstrated in the older literature.[13,14] The serin endoproteases *trypsin* and *chymotrypsin* are obtained from porcine pancreas, the major source of this enzyme. Trypsin and chymotrypsin have been used as an oral supplement in inflammatory and autoimmune diseases and cancer.[15,16]

Papain is obtained by fractionated centrifugation and ultrafiltration of the milky juice [latex] from unripe fruits of the tropical papaya tree, *Carica papaya var. Linn.* Papain, like the other proteolytic enzymes reduces edema, cleaves antigen-antibody complexes, and modulates receptor structures on blood cells, endothelial lining, and cancer cells. Amylase and lipase are constituents of pancreatic extract. They are mainly used to broaden the spectrum of unspecific immune regulatory properties.

Demographics

Orally-administered proteolytic enzyme combinations are widely distributed throughout central and Eastern Europe, Latin America, and India. It is believed that Germany is the country that consumes most of the enzyme preparations. In the U.S. at the present time they are distributed as over-the-counter (OTC) products. In Europe, half of enzyme consumption occurs by self-medication and half is being prescribed by practitioners and hospitals. Patients using proteolytic enzyme combinations tend to be well-informed about their disease. In Mexico, Japan, and South America, systemic enzyme therapy is well-known and accepted by many mainstream physicians. This consists of medical enzyme preparations and food supplement enzyme preparations.

In the U.S. and many other countries, there are many enzymes that are used legally as an effective systemic treatment for a variety of medical conditions, which range from inflammations to cancer treatment. These enzymatic preparations are approved by the FDA to be used in the treatment of specific diseases. There are around 37 enzymatic preparations listed in the 1999 *Physician's Desk Reference*.

Because systemic enzyme therapy has a wide range of therapeutic effects, it is applicable to a wide variety of patients.

Forms of Therapy

Systemic enzyme therapy uses specific enzymes alone or in enzymatic mixtures. Enzymes can be administered orally, topically, rectally, and parenterally (intravenous, intramuscular, intraarterial, and intratumor). Many enzyme preparations are labeled as food supplements, so it easy to get them as such. When enzyme mixtures are administered some other way, such as parenterally, they are considered "orthodox drugs."

Indications and Reasons for Referral

There are the following four main indications for using proteolytic enzymes:

- Trauma
- Acute and chronic inflammation, fibrosis reactions, and autoimmune disease: Inflammations include those induced by sports-related overuse.
- Viral infections
- Cancer: Enzymes are used here for reduction of the side effects of chemotherapy and radiation, improvement of quality of life (QOL), reduction of the risk for infections, reduction of the potential for metastasis, and the prolonging of life.

Additional uses include applications in vascular diseases, such as thrombosis, phlebitis, and varicose veins, because enzymes inhibit the formation of thrombosis.

Office Applications

Because of the central role of the immune system in virtually all diseases and the ability of proteolytic enzymes to modulate the immune response, the magnitude of indications amenable for these enzymes is explainable. For further indications, please refer to the section "Efficacy."

Practical Applications

It is important to take oral proteolytic enzymes between meals with a minimum of 30 minutes before or 120 minutes after meals. Also, advise patients to take the enzymes together with a glass of water, which improves their activation in the upper intestinal tract.

Research Base

Evidence Based

Efficacy and safety of proteolytic enzymes was determined in placebo-controlled trials, in prospective reference-controlled studies, and in retrolective reference-controlled studies, in addition to studies of safety in healthy volunteers.

Basic Science

PROTEOLYTIC SERUM ACTIVITY: INTERACTION WITH α2-MACROGLOBULIN

Proteolytic serum activity is kept in balance by serum-proteinases and antiproteinases (α2-macroglobulin AMG, α1-anti-trypsin AAT). Enzymes retain their proteolytic activity after binding to AMG.[17] Physiologically protease-complexed (activated) AMG is important for the clearance and regulation of the turnover of cytokines in tissue.

INFLUENCE ON BLOOD VISCOSITY

Proteolytic enzymes have been shown to improve microcirculation, decrease blood viscosity, and reduce thrombotic events, which might help to prevent thromboembolic complications in malignant diseases.[18]

ANTIINFLAMMATORY EFFECTS

The anti-inflammatory and antiedemic efficacy of proteolytic enzymes administered through various routes, including peroral, has been assessed in classical animal models of acute and chronic inflammation.[19] Proteases have proven to have an influence on mediator substances, such as the reduction of bradykinin by bromelain.[20]

PAIN-REDUCING EFFECT

In a model of experimental hematoma in volunteers, the pain-reducing effect in the course of time by enzyme (Phlogenzym) treatment versus placebo could be demonstrated.[21,22]

IMMUNE REGULATORY EFFECTS

The basic immunologic modulatory capacity allows to explain the efficacy of oral enzymes in the treatment of inflammatory diseases as well as in cancer.

Regulation of the Cytokine Network   Cytokine effects are modulated by α2-macroglobulin-protease complexes.[23,24] Because α2-macroglobulin-protease complexes are formed at the sites of inflammation, the α2-macroglobulin-protease complexes contribute to the reduction of overexpressed cytokines, which are relevant for metastasis and chronic inflammation and fibrosis in vivo (see also "Antiinflammatory Effects").[25]

Modulation of Cell Adhesion Molecules (CAM)   A major mechanism for the metastatic spread of cancer is the attachment of tumor cells to the endothelial lining in blood vessels and body cavities through various adhesion molecules.[26,27] In inflammatory conditions, CAM also play a key role.[28] An alteration of CAM expression following in vivo and in vitro exposure to proteolytic enzymes has been described recently.[29,30] This might lead to a decreased metastatic process.

Fragmentation of Immune Complexes and Decreased Complement Activation   Circulating immunocomplexes (CIC) block immune competent cells and activated complement proteins, which causes edema and inflammation. High levels of CIC have been associated with an impaired immunity and prognosis in cancer patients.[31,32]

The efficacy of hydrolytic enzymes is partly based on their capability to modulate these molecules. Hydrolytic enzymes are able to restore the phagocytosis of macrophages.[33]

ANIMAL MODELS

Chronic Inflammation and Autoimmune Diseases   Investigations concerning the pathogenesis of autoimmune diseases focuses on the Th1-Th2 cytokine balance.[34] Disregulation of this balance leads to pathogenic effects. Among them, elevated levels of TGF-β have a disastrous role.[35] Enzyme therapy (Phlogenzym) has been demonstrated to support the clearance of TGF-β and restore the Th1-Th2 balance with improvement of clinical symptoms.[36-38]

Differentiation Induction, Cancer, and Metastasis Prevention Early and recent research showed effects of fed pancreatic extract and other proteolytic enzymes in reduction of tumor growth in different animal models.[39-41]

In patients suffering from burn injuries, oral trypsin and chymotrypsin reduced metalloproteinases.[42] This might be of interest in respect to metalloproteinases that are discussed to enhance metastasis and inflammatory processes.

Risk and Safety

OVERALL SAFETY EVALUATION Allergic reactions against single enzymes are possible and some comments can be found in the literature. The combination of enzymes does not increase the risks. Rather, the opposite is true: There is no report of serious allergic reactions in literature concerning the use of proteolytic enzymes. During many years there was no change in the pattern of listed adverse reactions, especially in severity, outcome, or target population.

Efficacy

There are many clinical studies on the efficacy of proteolytic enzymes in a wide variety of conditions. Clinical studies have proven proteolytic enzymes and enzyme combination to be effective in the following conditions:

TRAUMA, SURGERY, AND POSTOPERATIVE TREATMENT

Therapeutic efficacy of single enzymes and combinations has been studied in several placebo-controlled trials in postoperative treatment and following sport injuries (contusion, distortion).[43,44] The enzyme treatment lead to a pain reduction,[45] antiinflammatory effects, and shortened the period of immobility.[46]

ANGIOLOGY

In angiology, different enzyme combinations were proven effective in venous diseases,[47,48] postthrombotic syndrome,[49,50] reduction of thromboembolic complications,[51,52] and lymphatic edema following breast surgery.[53]

ACUTE AND CHRONIC INFLAMMATION

Clinical trials to examine the efficacy of enzyme and enzyme combinations were conducted in a variety of inflammatory conditions, such as acute and chronic sinusitis,[54] prostatitis,[55] cystitis and pyelonephritis,[56] adnexitis, and others. The enzyme treatment reduces the inflammatory process and rate of relapse. If necessary, the enzymes should be combined with anitbiotics. Papain as single enzyme successfully has been administered in the treatment of visceral infections.[57]

RHEUMATIC DISEASES

The different forms of rheumatic diseases, including rheumatism of the soft tissues, inflammatory episodes of degenerative joint diseases (osteoarthritis),[58,59] and spondylopathies and soft tissue rheumatism[60,61] benefit from the administration of proteolytic enzymes.[62] The rates of the inflammatory episodes are reduced. In the beginning of the treatment enzymes probably can be combined (for two days) with nsaids or analgesics for a faster pain reduction.

In general the patient should undergo basic immunotherapy, such as with methotrexate (MTX), combined with proteolytic enzymes. Newer research showed a better response, fewer side effects, and the possible reduction of the MTX dosage.

In the treatment of patients with juvenile chronic arthritis (JCA), Wobenzym (WE) has shown influence on both articular (tenderness, swelling, pain on motion, limitation of motion) and systemic signs (rash, lymphadenopathy).[63]

CANCER

Earlier clinical trials showed beneficial effects of the combination from proteolytic enzymes with chemotherapy and radiation therapy in cancer patients.[64] Proteolytic enzymes successfully have been administered for the treatment of lung cancer,[65] malignant pleural effusions,[66] pancreatic cancer,[67] and ovarian cancer.[68] In patients suffering from head and neck cancers undergoing radiotherapy a protective effect for proteolytic enzymes to prevent the mucositis was shown.[69] The bleomycin-induced pneumotoxicity in the treatment of advanced epithelial cancers of the head and neck could be prevented.[70]

Long-term results of treating patients with multiple myeloma with proteolytic enzymes in combination with chemotherapy have been published previously.[71,72] The results of a study with 330 patients[73] demonstrated a 3-year median survival benefit for the group of patients receiving proteolytic enzymes in addition to chemotherapy. These results recently initiated an orphan drug status for proteolytic enzymes for this indication at the FDA in the U.S.

HERPES ZOSTER AND VIRALLY MEDIATED DISEASES

The efficacy and safety of WOBE-MUGOS in the treatment of herpes zoster was assessed in prospective, randomized double-blind controlled studies against acyclovir. The proteolytic enzymes were as effective as acyclovir in achieving pain control and healing.[74,75]

Another study investigated the oral administration of proteolytic enzymes as adjuvant treatment in recurrent laryngeal papillomatosis.[76] Patients with chronic hepatitis C also have been shown to benefit from the administration of proteolytic enzymes.[77]

INNOVATIVE INDICATIONS

Further research is focusing on atherosklerosis,[78,80] multiple sclerosis,[81] diabetes type I, Cogan syndrome,[82] nephrosclerosis, and fibrosis (see "Animal Models").

Future Research Opportunities and Priorities

The combination of standard treatment regimens like chemotherapy and radiation in cancer or antibiotic drugs and basic therapy in inflammatory disorders are an attractive area of further research. The Enzyme Research Institute reports more than 150 scientific and clinical studies presently in progress at different medical centers in the world. In addition, Sociedad Médica de Invetigaciones Enzimáticas, A.C. in Mexico performs some research and teaching activities.

Druglike Information

Actions and Pharmacokinetics

In the bloodstream, enzymes consequently are bound to various transport molecules in the blood (for example, α1-antitrypsin or α2-macroglobulin). The carrier molecules suitable for transport lead to a "coating" of the antigenic determinants without causing a substantial change in the activity of hydrolases.

BIOAVAILABILITY

Interestingly, trypsin could be shown to recirculate in the gut following oral administration,[1] and both bromelain and trypsin exhibit a dose-related bioavailability following repeated oral administration[83,84]

DOSE-RESPONSE RELATIONSHIP

The dose-response effect of proteolytic enzymes was determined using an experimental hematoma model[22,75] comparing the recommended regular therapeutical dose (2 tablets three times per day by mouth) with a high-dose regimen (4 tablets three times per day by mouth), and a low-dose (2 tablets before bedtime by mouth), and a placebo in a randomized double-blind study. After a single oral dose of proteolytic enzymes a dose-dependent increase of serum-activity was observed in healthy volunteers. Its maximum is reached after approximately 3 to 4 hours. The results in this model demonstrated that the dose of 2 tablets three times per day was the optimal dose. Higher doses can be administered without risk.

Pharmacokinetics

The pharmacologic principle of systemic enzyme therapy depends on the absorption of enzymes as intact molecules after oral administration. Thus their biologic effects are fully preserved. The tablets or coated tablets must resist gastric secretion to prevent destruction by the acid milieu of the stomach. Once in the small bowel the large enzyme molecules, like all macromolecules, may be absorbed in two ways, as follows:

1. They may bind to specific receptors in a particular area of the intestinal mucosa and be transported through the gut's epithelium (pinocytosis); or
2. They may be taken up by lymphocytes "roaming" in the lumen of the bowel and be released again after passage through the gut wall.

   In this way a small percentage of the administered dose may find its way into the circulation and lymph system still in an active form. As already pointed out, it is important that the structure responsible for enzymatic activity remains largely intact so that the enzyme retains its activity.

ABSORPTION

The absorption data can be taken also from a recent study by Castell et al.[2,3] Data suggest that the absorption rate of different enzymes is not influenced when applied in the combination. About 1% to 3% of the enzymes and less than 1% of rutosid metabolites could be recovered in plasma. The limited bioavailability of pharmaceuticals does not necessarily mean limited systemic activity.[85]

DISTRIBUTION

In animal models the high amount of constituents of proteolytic enzymes found in the kidney after administration suggests a renal route of elimination.

METABOLISM

Proteolytic Enzymes: After absorption, most of the absorbed proteolytic enzymes do not exist in a free form but are bound to a carrier, such as the antiproteinase α2-macroglobulin. This protects the enzyme from interactions with other molecules and neutralizes potentially allergenic properties of these proteases. In spite of this carrier binding the enzyme remains active.

Rutosid: Rutosid is hydrolyzed to its constituent aglycone and sugars in the bowel by microorganisms.[86] The sum of the metabolites exhibited a half-life of 11 hours. Although clear-cut dose dependency could not be shown for rutosid metabolites, concentrations were elevated above baseline values.

ELIMINATION

Proteolytic Enzymes: In human volunteers the elimination half-life of peroral trypsin was estimated to be within the range of 9 to12 hours.[83]

Rutosid: After oral administration of rutosid, only metabolites could be detected in the urine.[87,88] The half-life was 2.4 ± 0.2 hours after intravenous administration. Recovery in feces of the oral dose was $53 \pm 5\%$, suggesting extensive degradation by intestinal microorganisms.

Warnings, Contraindications, and Precautions

Enzymes should not be used in the event of a known susceptibility to allergic reaction. The fibrinolytic action of proteolytic enzymes must be taken into consideration during diseases or surgical interventions associated with an increased risk of hemorrhage. In general, enzymatic mixtures should not be taken shortly before or after surgery involving a high risk of bleeding. Enzyme preparations are contraindicated in hemophiliacs and in persons with any disease state that inteferes with coagulation enough to create an abnormal danger of bleeding.

SPECIAL POPULATIONS

There is no evidence available that would preclude the use of proteolytic enzymes in the elderly or in children, although specific clinical data pertaining to these special populations is lacking. According to the "guideline on the excipients in the label and package leaflet" of the European Commission, lactose present as an excipient in proteolytic enzymes may be harmful for people with lactase insufficiency, galactosemia, or glucose or galactose malabsorption syndrome.

OVERDOSE

None are known. An acute median lethal dose has not yet been determined for the oral administration in different animal species.

Drug or Other Interactions

Because of the possible fibrinolytic effects, interactions with such drugs as the coumarins or heparin may occur. Patients undergoing anticoagulation therapy should consult their physicians before taking proteolytic enzymes and their coagulation profile should be checked regularly. Other interactions have neither been investigated, nor are any known from the literature.

Adverse Reactions

Proteolytic enzymes were well tolerated when tested versus placebo.[89] About half of the people taking enzymes describe a harmless change in the color and odor of their stools. About 240 cases of side effects have been reported worldwide. Most of the complaints were because of increased gas formation in the bowels or slightly increased bleeding tendencies following surgery or injury. Very rarely a systemic intolerability of proteolytic enzymes may occur. Allergic reactions may be observed rarely following oral administration of proteolytic enzymes. Allergic reactions and side effects have been reported mainly for plant derived proteolytic enzymes, such as papain and bromelain.[90,91] Slight burning or itching of the skin has been reported after enemas containing enzymes.

Pregnancy and Lactation

Insufficient information is available on the administration of proteolytic enzymes during pregnancy and breast-feeding. Unless the benefits of their administration clearly outweigh the potential risks, they are not routinely recommended.

Trade Products, Administration, and Dosage

Multiple enzyme formulations are available commercially, many of which resemble a natural enzymatic cascade. The main enzymes include: bromelain; pancreatin; amylase; lipase; papain; trypsin; chymotrypsin; desoxyrribonuclease; and cocarboxylase. Most of the information in this discussion refers to the following three formulas with which most of the clinical trials were conducted. The choice of formulation depends upon the indication.

1. The combination of enzymes from the pancreas (pancreatin, trypsin and chymotrypsin), pineapple (bromelain), papaya (papain), plus the flavonoid rutosid. For conditions with chronic inflammations (wobenzym N).
2. The combination of enzymes from the pancreas (pancreatin, trypsin), pineapple (bromelain), plus the flavonoid rutosid. For acute inflammation, chronic inflammation, and trauma (phlogenzym).

3. The combination of enzymes from pancreas (trypsin and chymotrypsin) and papaya (papain). For severe illnesses, including oncologic and viral diseases (WOBE-MUGOS E).

Dosages vary depending on the medical condition and formulation. Generally speaking, for acute inflammatory conditions, five tablets of enzymes three times daily should be taken for 10 days. For chronic problems the enzyme preparations should be taken for at least 3 months. The products listed in this discussion have lower dosages, ranging from two tablets daily to four tablets three times a day. As previously mentioned, 2 tablets three times daily is the optimal dose. Higher doses can be administered without risk.

Many enzyme formulations are available from a variety of sources. For the enzyme formulations specifically referred to in this chapter, Oral Enzymes International has a source in North America:

Marlyn Health Care
14851 N. Scottsdale Rd.
Scottsdale, AZ 85254
Tel: (602) 991-0200
Fax: (602) 991-0551

Self-Help versus Professional

Enzymes are natural substances. They can be taken as food supplements in the case of mild problems; that is, they can be used as any other over-the-counter drug. In fact, enzyme preparations can be purchased in any health food store as food supplements for mild problems, such as to aid digestion. For serious medical conditions, they must be prescribed by a physician, especially when intramuscularly or intravenously administered. Similarly, any natural substance administered at a high dosage should be monitored by a qualified physician.

Credentialing

No formal credentialing exists specifically for enzyme therapy. However, most high dose or parenteral applications of enzyme therapy fall in the domain of medical management. In these cases, credentialing applies to those of a standard mainstream medical practitioner.

Training

The knowledge for the general use of systemic enzyme therapy can be easily obtained by attending a several-day seminar on the subject. However, for special intracorporeal administration of enzymatic preparations, it is necessary to receive specific training. In Mexico, Sociedad Médica de Investigaciones Enzimáticas, A.C. has held many seminars on systemic enzyme therapy. At Universidad de Guadalajara, update seminars are held regularly on Systemic Enzyme Therapy. Such review and update courses also are offered in various locations worldwide.

What to Look for in a Provider

Look for the provider's ability to explain the rationale of the therapy and teach the patient how to handle route and dosage of administration, as well as the provider's commitment to continuing evaluation and screening of clinical effects. Practitioners providing enzyme therapy should have at least a certificate indicating some formal training on the subject along with experience in its administration, in addition to their medical credentials.

Associations

In the United States:

Immunoenzymology Research Foundation
Evanston, IL 60201

In Mexico:

Sociedad Médica de Investigaciones Enzimáticas, A.C.
Los Alpes No. 1014
Col. Independencia
44340 Guadalajara, Jal.
Tel: (3) 637-7237, 651-5476
Fax: (3) 637-0030

In Germany:

Medical Association of Research on Enzymes
Gerestried, Germany

Internet Resources

www.mucos.de (German)
www.mucos.cz (German, English, Russian, Czech)
www.mucos.de/uk/index (English)

Suggested Reading

1. Wrba H, Pecher O, Solorzano HE: *Enzimas, sustancias del futuro,* Munich, 1996, Deutchland.
2. Ransberger K, Solorzno H: *Enzimoterapia,* Guadalajara, 1991, Dirección de Publicaciones de la Universidad de Guadalajara (Spanish only).

3. Klaschka F: *New perspectives in tumor therapy,* Gräfelfing, Germany, 1996, forum Medizin.

4. *Oral enzymes: basic brochure on enzyme combinations,* MUCOS Pharma, Germany, 1992.

5. Williams M et al: *Enzymes: fountain of life,* 1994, Neville Press.

6. Wolf M, Ransberger K: *Enzyme therapy,* New York, 1972, Biological Research Institute.

7. Wrba H, Pecher O: *A drug of the future,* Landsberg, Germany, 1996, Ecomed-verlag.

References

1. Lake-Bakaar G et al: Metabolism of 125I-labelled trypsin in man: evidence for recirculation, *Gut* 21:580, 1980.

2. Castell JV et al: Intestinal absorption of undegraded proteins in men: presence of bromelain in plasma after oral intake, *Am J Physiol* 273(1):G139-136, 1997.

3. Gardner MLG, Steffens KJ, editors: *Absorption of orally administered enzymes,* Berlin, 1995, Springer.

4. Wrba H et al, editors: *Systemisch enzymtherapie. Aktueller stand und fortschritte,* Munich, 1996, MMW Medizin Verlag München.

5. Bertelli A, Mizushima Y, Ziff M, editors; Abstracts of 7th Interscience World Conference on Inflammation, Antirheumatics, Analgesics, Immunomodulators, *Int J Tissue Reactions,* XIX, ½, 1997.

6. Lehmann PV: Immunomodulation by proteolytic enzymes, *Nephrol Dial Transplant* 11:953-955.

7. Nouza K: Systemic enzyme therapy in angiology, *Bratisl Lek Listy* 96:566-569, 1995.

8. Lehmann PV, Rovensky J: Immunologic aspects of systemic enzyme therapy, New York Academy of Sciences, May 22, 1996, Prague.

9. Sy MS et La: Potential of targeting cell surface CD44 proteins with proteinases in preventing tumor growth and metastatis, *Int J Immunother* 8(3-4), 1977.

10. Timeus C: Objektivierung der Wirkung von Venenpharmaka auf die menschliche Mikrozirkulation. Dargestellt am Beispiel der O-(beta-hydroxyethyl)-rutosid, *ETH Zurich,* 1983.

11. Harrach T et al: *J Protein Chem* 14:41, 1995.

12. Batkin S, Taussig SJ, Szekerezes J: Antimetastatic effect of bromelain with or without its proteolytic and anticoagulant activity, *J Cancer Res Clin Oncol* 114:507-508, 1988.

13. Pirotta F et al: Bromelain, a deeper pharmacological study, antiinflammatory and serum fibrinolytic activity after oral administration in the rat, *Drugs Under Exper Clin Res* 4:1-20, 1978.

14. Munzig E et al: *FEBS Letters* 351:215, 1994.

15. Ransberger K, Stauder G, Streichhan P: *Enzymkombinationspraeparate—Wobenzym N, Mulsal N und Phlogenzym—wiseenschaftliche Monographie zur Praeklinik,* Graefelfing, Germany, 1991, Forum Medizin Verlag.

16. Wolf M, Ransberger K: *Enzymtherapie,* Vienna, 1970, Maudrich Verlag.

17. James K, Taylor FB, Fudenberg HH: Trypsin stabilizers in human serum. The role of α_2-macroglobulin, *Clin Chem Acta* 83:359-368, 1966.

18. Alban S, Franz ME, Franz G: Influence of the therapeutically used enzymes bromelain, papain, and trypsin on the blood coagulation in vitro, *Pharm Pharmacol Lett* 7(2-3):59-62, 1997.

19. Wood Gr et al: Sequential effects of an oral enzyme combination with rutosid in different in vitro and in vivo models of inflammation, *Int J Immunother* 13(3-4):139-145, 1997.

20. Majama M et al: Effects of an orally active nonpeptide bradykinin B2 receptor antagonist, FR173657, on plasma exudation in rat carrageenin-induced pleurisy, *Br J Pharmacol* 121:723-730, 1997.

21. Waldvogel HH, editor: *Analgetika, antinotzeptiva*, Heidelberg, 1995, Springer Verlag.

22. Kleine MW: Evidence of the efficacy of an enzyme combination preparation using the method of artificial hematomas in combination with a pressure meter: a placebo-controlled, randomized, prospective, double blind study, *J Clin Res* 1:87-102, 1998.

23. LaMarre J et al: Cytokine binding and clearance properties of proteinase-activated α_2-macroglobulin, *Lab Invest* 65:3, 1991.

24. Heumann D, Vischer TL: Immunomodulation by alpha2-macroglobulin and alpha2-macroglobulin-poteinase complexes: the effect on the human T lymphocyte response, *Eur J Immunol* 18:755-760, 1988.

25. Feige JJ et al: Alpha 2-macroglobulin: a binding protein for transforming growth factor-beta and various cytokines, *Horm Res* 45(3-5):227-232, 1996.

26. Stauder R et al: Different CD44 splicing patterns define prognostic subgroups in multiple myeloma, *Blood* 88(8):3101-3108, 1996.

27. CAM: Litratur.

28. Springer TA: Traffic signals for lymphocyte recirculation and leukocyte emigration: the multistep paradigm, *Cell* 76(2):301-314, 1994.

29. Sargent NSE, Price JE, Tarin D: Effect of enzymatic removal of cell surface constituents on metastatic colonization potential of mouse mammary tumor cells, *Br J Cancer* 4(8):569-577, 1983.

30. Jutila MA, Kishimoto TK, Finken M: Low-dose chrymotrypsin treatment inhibits neutrophil migration into sites of inflammation in vivo: effects on mac-1 and MEL-14 adhesion protein expression and function, *Cell Immunol* 132:201-214, 1991.

31. Vlock DR et al: Clinical correlates of circulating immune complexes and antibody reactivity in squamous cell carcinoma of the head and neck, *J Clin Oncol* 11(12):2427-2433, 1993.

32. Nerurkar AV, Advani SH, Gothoskar BP: Circulating immune complexes in Hodgkin's disease. Reactivity of IgG isolated from circulating immune complexes, *Neoplasma* 40(2):87-91, 1993.

33. Keskovar P: Immuntherapie unter Einbeziehung von aktivierten Makrophagen: Richtiges timing kann fur den Erfolg ausschlaggebend sein, *Dtsch Zschr Onkol* 24(2):29-40.

34. Miossec P, van den Berg W: Th1/Th2 cytokine balance in arthritis, *Arthritis Rheum* 40:2105-2115, 1997.

35. Wu Sm, Patel DD, Pizzo S: Oxidized α_2-macroglobulin (α_2M) differentially regulates receptor binding by cytokines (growth factors: implications for tissue injury and repair mechanisms in inflammation, *J Immunol* 161:4356-4363, 1998.

36. Targoni O, Lehman PV: Modulation of the autoreactive T cells via systemic enzyme therapy with Phlogenzym, *Int J Tiss Reac* 19:87, 1997.

37. Targoni OS, Tary-Lehmann M, Lehmann P: Prevention of murine EAE by oral hydrolytic enzyme treatment, *J Autoimmunity*, 12(3):191-198, 1999.

38. Desser L et al: Concentrations of soluble tumor necrosis factor receptors and TNF in serum of mulitple myeloma patients after chemotherapy and after combined enzyme-chemotherapy, *Int J Immunother* 13(3-4):121-131, 1997.

39. Sargent NSE, Price JE, Tarin D: Effect of enzymatic removal of cell surface constitutents on metastatic colonization potential of mouse mammary tumor cells, *Br J Cancer* 4(8):569-577, 1983.

40. Wald M et al: Polyenzyme preparation Wobe-Mugos inhibits growth of solid tumors and development of experimental metastases in mice, *Life Sci* 62(3):43-48, 1998.

41. Wald M et al: Proteinases reduce metastatic dissemination and increase survival time in C57B16 mice with the lewis lung carcinoma, *Life Sci* 63(17):237-243, 1998.

42. Latha B et al: Serum enzymatic changes modulated using trypsin: chymotrypsin preparation during burn wounds in humans, *Burns* 32(7-8):560-564, 1997.

43. Vinzenz K: Odembehandlung bei zahnchirurgischen eingriffen mit hydrolytischen enzyme, *Die Quintessenz* 7:1053, 1991.

44. Kleine MW: Systemische enzymtherapie in der sportmedizin, *Dtsch Zeitschr f Sportmedizin* 41:126, 1990.

45. Hoernecke R, Doenicke A: Perioperative enzymtherapie. Eine sinnvolle erganzung zur postoperativen schmerztherapie? *Anasthesist* 42:856-861, 1993.

46. Rahn HD: *Twenty-fourth FMS World Congress of Sport Medicine: Symposium on Enzyme Therapy in Sports Injuries,* May 28, 1990, Amsterdam, 1990, Elsevier Science.

47. Koshkin Vm: Systemische enzymtherapie bei akuter thrombophlebitis der oberflachlichen venen an den unteren extremitaten, *Vasomed* 4:220-224, 1996.

48. Inderst R: Enzumtherapie bei Gefaberkankungen, *Allgemeinmedizin* 19:154, 1990.

49. Mahr H: Zur Enzymtherapie entzundlicher Venererkrankungen der tiefen Beinvenenthrombose und des postthrombotischen synroms, *Erfahrungsheilkunde* 117, 1983.

50. Morl H: Behandlung des postthrombotischen syndroms mit einem enzymgemisch, *Therapiewoche* 36:2443, 1986.

51. Ernst E, Matrei A: Orale therapie mit proteolytischen enzymen modifiziert die blutrheologie, *Klin Wschr* 65:994, 1987.

52. Sampaio CAM et al: Inactivation of kinins by chymotrypsin, *Biochem Pharmacol* 25:2391, 1976.

53. Scheef W, Pischnamazadeh M: Proteolytische Enzyme als einfache und sichere Methode zur Verhütung des Lymphödems nach Ablatio mammae, *Med Welt* 35:1032, 1984.

54. Rayn RE: A double-blind clinical evaluation of bromelains in the treatment of acute sinusitis, *Headache* 7:13, 1967.

55. Rugendorff EW, Burghele A, Schneider HJ: Behandlung der chronischen abakteriellen Prostatitis mit hydrolytischen Enzymen, *Der Kassenarzt* 14:43, 1986.

56. Barsom S, Sasse-Rollenhagen K, Betterman A: Zur Behandlung von Zystitiden und Zystopyelitiden mit hydrolytischen Enzymen, *Acta Medica Empirica* 32:125, 1983.

57. Rogenski NM et al: Use of papain in visceral infections, *Rev Bras Enferm* 48(2):140-143, 1995.

58. Gallachi G: Hydrolytische Enzyme bei aktivierten Polyarthrosen, *Rheuma* 8, 1988.

59. Singer F, Oberleitner H: Ein Beitrag zur medikamentösen Therapie der aktivierten Arthrose, *WMW* 3:55-58, 1996.

60. Klein G, Kullich W, Brugger A: Phlogenzym in der Behandlung der Periarthropathia humeroscapularis tendopathica simplex, *Arzt&Praxis* 51(781):879-885, 1988.

61. Uffelmann K, Vogler W, Fruth C: Der Einsatz hydrolytischer Enzyme beim extraartikulären Rheumatismus, *Allgemeinmedizin* 19:151, 1990.

62. Panijel M: Entzündlich-rheumatische Erkrankungen, *Zeitschr f Allgemeinmedizin* 61:1305, 1985.

63. Shaikov AV et al: Oral enzyme therapy in patients with juvenile chronic arthritis, *Tissue Reactions* 19(1), 1997.

64. Klaschka F: *New perspectives in tumor therapy*, Gräfelfing, Germany, 1996, Forum Medizin.

65. Kesztele V, Huerbe E, Wischin W: Erfahrungen mit proteolytischen Enzymen beim Bronchuskarzinom, *Wiener Med Wochenschr* 25:412-414, 1976.

66. Kokron O et al: Proteolytic enzymes in the treatment of malignant pleural effusions and solid metastases. In Hellmann K, Connors TA, editors: *Chemotherapy*, vol 8, 1976.

67. Hager ED et al: Multimodal treatment of patients with advanced pancreatic cancer in combination with locoregional hyperthermia, *South Med J* 89(10):145, 1996.

68. Lahousen M: Modification of liver parameters by adjuvant administration of proteolytic enzymes following chemotherapy in patients with ovarian carcinoma, *Wien Med Wochenschr* 145(24):663-668, 1995.

69. Vinzenz K, Stauder U: Die Therapie der radiogenen Mucositis mit Enzymen. In Vinzenz K, Waclawiczek H, editors: *Chirugische therapie von Kopf-Hals-Karzinomen*, Berlin, 1992, Springer Verlag.

70. Schedler M et al: Adjuvant therapy with hydrolytic enzymes in oncology—a hopeful effort to avoid bleomycin induced pneumotoxicity? *J Cancer Res Clin Oncol* 116(Suppl 1), 1990.

71. Sakalova A et al.: The results of a randomized study of the treatment of multiple myeloma, *Klinicka Onkologie (Praha)* 9(4):130-134, 1996.

72. Sakalova A et al.: Long-term survival with multiple myeloma, *Vnitrni Lekarstvi (Praha)* 40(2):98-103, 1994.

73. Sakalová A et al: Survival analysis of an adjuvant therapy with oral enzymes in multiple myeloma, *Br J Haematol* 102:353, 1998.

74. Kleine MW: Comparison between an oral hydrolytic enzyme combination and oral acyclovir in the teatment of acute herpes zoster: a double-blind, controlled multicenter trial, *J Eur Acad Dermatol Venerol* 2:296-307, 1993.

75. Kleine MW et al: The intestinal absorption of orally administered hydrolytic enzymes and their effects in the treatment of acute herpes zoster as compared with those of acyclovir therapy, *Phytomedicine* 2(1):7-15, 1995.

76. Mudrak J, Bobak L, Sebova I: Adjuvant therapy with hydrolytic enzymes in recurrent laryngeal papillomatosis, *Acta Otolaryngol Suppl* 527:128-130, 1997.

77. Kabil SM et al: Oral enzymes in the treatment of chronic HCV, *JHGID* 4:4,1-8, 1996.

78. Gaciong Z et al: Protease therapy alleviates allograft arteriosclerosis in rats, *Transplant Proc* 28(6):3439-3440, 1996.

79. Muller J et al: Weaning from mechanical cardiac support in patients with idiopathic dilated cardiomyopathy, *Circulation* 96:542-549, 1997.

80. Mertin J et al: Use of oral enzymes in multiple sclerosis patients, *Tiss Reac* 19(1/2), 1997.

81. Schedler MGJ, Bartylla M: Retroskeptive und prospektive Untersuchungen an Patienten mit Cogan-I-Syndrom, *Laryngo Rhin Otol* 73:662-666, 1994.

82. Mai I et al: Oral bioavailability of bromelain and trypsin after repeated oral administration of commercial polyenzyme preparation, *Euro J Clin Pharmacol* 50(6):548, 1996.

83. Colac C, Streichhan P, Lehr CM: Oral bioavailability of proteolytic enzymes, *Eur J Pharm Biopharm* 42(4):222-232, 1996.

84. Pedersen AK, FitzGerald GA: Dose-related kinetics of aspirin. Presystemic acetylation of platelet cyclooxygenase, *N Eng J Med* 311:1206-1211, 1984.

85. Sawai Y et al: Serum concentration of rutosid metabolites after oral administration of a rutosid formulation to humans, *Arzneim Forsch* 37:729-732, 1987.

86. Gugler R, Leschik M, Dengler HJ: Disposition of quercetin in man after single oral and intravenous doses, *Eur J Clin Pharmacol* 9:229-234, 1975.

87. *Periodic safety update reports on wobenzym, WOBE-MUGOS, phlogenzym, mucozym,* MUCOS Pharma GmbH, Geretsreid, Germany, 1999.

88. Davis M, Thomas LC, Guice KS: Esophagitis after papain, *J Clin Gastroenterol* 9(2):127-130, 1987.

89. Wuthrich B: Proteolytic enzymes: potential allergens for the skin and respiratory tract? *Hautarzt* 36(3):123-125, 1985.

Flower Essences

EILEEN NAUMAN

Origins and History

Flower essences were discovered by English homeopath Edward Bach, MD during the early 1900s. A number of books have been written about him and his use of 38 essences. As a homeopath, he saw that a homeopathic remedy could cause severe and uncomfortable, even painful aggravations for his patient. He eventually left homeopathy because of this and experimented with hundreds of flowers in England to find something that was milder and gentler but still healing in nature. He believed illness was caused by emotional imbalance. From this platform, he identified concern for others, fear, loneliness, oversensitivity, disinterest in life, and uncertainty as the underlying reasons for health disorders.

As a homeopath, Bach understood the mind-body connection and applied this understanding to flower essences. In a process of experimentation, Bach would sip the dew that was found on the leaf or petals of the flower. He noted that almost every flower possessed physical symptoms except for 38 of them. These 38 created only emotional and mental symptoms. Following homeopathic tradition, after proving them on himself to find out what symptoms each essence created in him, he was able to define through this systematic methodology what constellation of symptoms each essence would treat. The 38 flowers he worked with are made by Nelson Pharmaceuticals in England and do not address physical symptoms or complaints in a person, only emotional ones as qualified above.

Flower essences are used the world over and in the U.S. there are a number of companies that make and sell them. Since 1970 a trend has evolved to move beyond Bach's 38 original essences and to incorporate many other essences. Currently, flower essences are used to address spiritual, mental, and emotional, as well as physical problems. People who are sensitive to the effects of traditional medical drugs and homeopathic remedies do best on flower essences. If the person is sensitive the flower essence often will have just as profound a healing effect as a homeopathic remedy.

Individuals who are drawn to flower essences are basically the people who work with them. They are highly sensitized individuals, and generally speaking, highly intuitive. There are few schools teaching this information, although more are forming in the U.S. as interest in flower essences has grown. Individuals who have used flower and gem essences and gained relief from their symptoms have fueled this interest.

Dr. Bach's original 38 essences were derived from flower, tree, bush, and water sources. A trend exists to stretch beyond these 38 and "see what else is out there in the organic world." Nor do some advocates of flower essences accept Bach's tenet that all disease originates from the emotional plane. Symptoms also extend to physical complaints and spiritual crises. Bach's essences do not address physical complaints, although it has been proposed by Bach consultants that by working with the emotional problem the physical symptoms will disappear. Other flower and gem essences can and do address all four levels—spiritual crisis, mental, emotional, and physical symptoms—although few address all these levels in one plant or gemstone.

Today, essences have expanded enormously to include an exciting array of possibilities. Imponderables, such as star, moon, and comet energy, can be made by placing a glass bowl filled with living water next to the eyepiece of a telescope. Many other flowers, bushes, and trees are used to make essences from around the world.

Mechanism of Action According to Its Own Theory

Depending on the flower essence practitioner's belief system, this can be highly diverse. In a Native American cosmology, each plant, rock, tree, and stream, and so on, is believed to possess an intelligence, a spirit that is connected to us through the energy exchange. Each one has the capacity to heal us.

In a human being, this spirit is known as an *aura*, which is composed of 9 layers or fields. Each field has a specific purpose and design in keeping a person physically healthy. In the first field, the etheric field, *chakras* or energy centers are embedded. There are seven major chakras. Each chakra works with a specific color or energy frequency.

Through homeopathic proving research currently in progress, flower and gem essences are being asssessed for the symptoms they create in a healthy person. These symptoms then can be used and matched as closely as possible to the ill person's symptoms and the correct flower or gem essence used. Please see "Research" for more explanation of this method.

The posologic concept of the infinitesimally small dose is part of the nature of flower essences. Hormesis is the fairly new and popular scientific field that studies the effects of extremely small doses of otherwise toxic substances to promote growth or healing. This field is part is an outgrowth of the Ardnt-Schultz Law, which states that for every substance, small doses stimulate, moderate doses inhibit, and large doses kill.

Another theory about the mechanism of action of flower essences is the idea of smart water. The understanding here is that the solvent (usually water) can carry information that is formed as a vibratory imprint of its solute. Every substance leaves a different vibratory imprint and this imprint gets stronger and clearer as the remedy is more potentized. This theory has been experimentally substantiated by the work of Dr. Shui-Yin Lo with ice crystals. Because flower essences are placed in a bowl of water for a certain length of time, there is an energy interchange between the crude substance and the water.

Biologic Mechanism of Action

It remains unknown to this day as to how flower essences work on the cellular level. More research is clearly needed. The Arndt-Schultz Law with reference to biologic activity provides a logical starting point for the use of minute doses.

Forms of Therapy

There are two types of flower essences: single essence and combination essence. A *single essence* means only one substance is contained in the bottle. Some flower and gem essences must be taken for a long period of time to see improvement. How long they are used also depends on whether the condition is acute or chronic.

Combination essences, where multiple essences are mixed together, also are used. This can mean a gem essence and a flower essence, a tree essence with a bush essence, and so on, are mixed together in one bottle.

Demographics

Flower essences are made and used around the world in the U.S., Australia, and Europe.

Users of flower essences are both genders and all ages, including infants, children, and adults. "New Age" or spiritually inclined people are more likely to use flower and gem essences. Individuals who are sensitive to traditional medications, manifested by malaise or other adverse effects, or have tried homeopathy and done nothing but *prove* a remedy and are miserable, will try flower and gem essences because they are so mild and gentle in comparison.

Indications and Reasons for Referral

Flower essences are often considered when an individual has had a negative experience with conventional drugs or homeopathic medications. These essences also are of value when the patient wishes to manifest greater control over self-medical care.

Office Applications

A simple ranking of conditions responsive to this form of therapy is as follows. As with all alternative therapies, use of flower essences does not preclude the use of mainstream medical therapies in addition.

Top level: *A therapy ideally suited for these conditions*
Arthritis (rheumatoid or osteoarthritis); backache; back pain; cataracts; chronic pain; emotional disorders; macular degeneration; night blindness; vision disorders; and whiplash

Second level: *One of the better therapies for these conditions*

Accidents; addictions; allergies; anger (uncontrolled); anxiety; attention deficit disorder; breathing disorders; bursitis; circulation disorders; connective tissue disorders; depression; fears; foot injuries; headaches; lower back disorders and injury; lymph gland disorders; lymph gland swelling; mental health; migraines; nerve disorders; osteoarthritis; osteoporosis; psychologic problems; psychotic behavior; rheumatoid arthritis; rheumatism; shortness of breath (dyspnea); sinus disorders (acute and chronic); sinusitis (acute and chronic); spinal injury; and violent behavior

Third level: *A valuable adjunctive therapy for these conditions*

Asthma; bone disorders; bronchitis; bruises; carpal tunnel syndrome; central nervous system diseases; children's health; colds; congestive heart failure; conjunctivitis; cornea disorders; detached retina; emphysema; eye diseases; fibromyalgia; floaters; fractures; hay fever; headaches (migraine and tension); hypoglycemia; influenza; insomnia; iritis; knee disorders and injuries; lung disorders; manic depressive illness; menopause; muscle or neck injuries; neuralgia; panic attack; posttraumatic stress disorder; premenstrual syndrome; Raynaud's syndrome; respiratory disorders; retinitis; retinal degeneration; sciatica; scoliosis; shoulder dislocation; sleep disorders; sports injuries; tinnitus; viral and bacterial infections; and women's health

Practical Applications

Because flower and gem essences rarely compete with any other form of traditional or alternative medicine the physician may feel confident in using them as an adjunct to ongoing treatment. In some cases they may reduce the drug of choice and this change in the patient's drug dosage must be monitored by a physician.

Physicians may consult the author of a book written on the topic or search the Internet under such headings as *flower essences*, *gem essence*, or *natural essences* to find a practitioner or information about a specific essence in question. Companies who sell flower and gem essences usually are very helpful and guiding when asked about a certain product, dosage, and administration. Attending workshops and seminars on this topic will help the physician know when to use this form of alternative medicine.

Research Base

Research in the formal sense does not exist for flower essences. Some nontraditional methods of data gathering do exist, as described in the following section.

Evidence Based

Depending on the company involved, evidence may vary in format. Some use "psychic intuiting" and consider this to be adequate evidence. The person uses intuition to discern what the essence might treat (and this can mean errors in such postulation). For others, it is deriving information anecdotally by feedback from their customers on what an essence did or did not address in their cases.

A far more scientific method is a *proving*. This method incorporates the use of 10 to 20 healthy male and female volunteers from around the world. A proving is the taking of a unknown (to the prover) substance over a period of time until it creates symptoms in the healthy persons. They do not know what essences they are proving. The prover then writes down these symptoms in painstaking detail. This can be a symptom that can come on emotionally, mentally, physically, or spiritually. The symptoms then are collected over a 14-day period in a diary or log and sent to the manager of the proving. The manager then gleans all the symptom information from all the provers' logs. A picture emerges of specific symptoms and in that way we know what a specific flower or gem essence will address in a person.

With this method, the correct essence can be confidently given because it is based on proving information and has been matched against the collected symptoms of the patient.

Risk and Safety

Little information is known for risks and safety. However, in provings, it has been observed that crested prickle poppy and datura essences can cause a loss of concentration, which could interfere with the driving of a car or a person's work.

Efficacy

Infants, children, and adults who have sensitivity to conventional drugs will do best on flower and gem essence treatment. Effectiveness is estimated by the author as 75%.

Future Research Opportunities and Priorities

Provings are ongoing regarding opal, emerald, and amethyst within one company beginning in Winter 1998. Eleven more flower and gem essences were proven in 1999.

A useful study would be on the effects of ocotillo essence in cases of chronic back pain.

Druglike Information

Preparing a Flower Essence

There are many ways to make a flower essence. The one presented here is the Bach method.

In this method the person avoids touching the flowering head of the plant with fingers, scissors or knife. The flowers then are placed in a clear glass bowl filled with distilled water. The bowl then is placed next to the plant in direct sunlight for 1 hour.

Making a gemstone essence depends on the size of the stone in question. For instance, in one method to create an amethyst essence, six tumbled amethysts (about the size of a dime) are chosen and placed in the water for 1 hour in direct sunlight. The water acts as a host that imprints and holds the memory of this plant, its color, and its uniqueness. The amethysts are strained off and the remaining water is mixed with 50% brandy to create what is known as a *mother essence* or ME. Fresh mother essences are created every year or two, depending upon the company's policy.

A stock bottle (usually varying from 2 dram size to 1-ounce eye dropper size) would, by FDA law in the U.S., have 5% alcohol in the base. Distilled or *living* (well or aquifer) water and a certain number of mother essence drops are placed into the bottle.

Warnings, Contraindications, and Precautions

Based on provings' information on essences, a warning exists for crested prickle poppy and datura. It should be used only once per day for 20 minutes before the person goes to bed. It is not to be used during the day because it causes poor concentration and inattentiveness to a job or driving a car. Datura is a known hallucinogen. Neither of these essences should be used in patients currently taking psychotropic medications.

When using coreopsis as an appetite suppressant the health practitioner should continue to follow the patient's progress. In some provings the subject did not want to eat for days at a time. Monitor the patient to insure that the patient eats daily. The normal dosage is four drops four times daily. If excessive anorexia occurs, reduce the amount of the essence accordingly. Similarly, when coreopsis is used for *hypoglycemia* the patient needs to be warned that this essence may suppress the appetite for much longer than 5 hours. Warn the patient to eat every 3 to 5 hours while on the essence. Over time, the Coreopsis will address this ailment so the person will not experience symptoms near the 4 to 5-hour mark.

If chaparral is used as an appetite stimulant in anorexic individuals the health practitioner must follow the patient's progress in the consumption of food. In cases of dehydration, chaparral encourages the person to drink more fluids, but its use does not eliminate the need for intravenous fluid and electrolyte replacement, if indicated.

Drug or Other Interactions

Flower and gem essences work with conventional drugs. They are not *antidoted* (neutralized) by drugs as homeopathic remedies may sometimes be. Flower and gem essences may be used in conjunction with homeopathic treatment, herbs, energy tools (Reiki, polarity therapy, hands-on healing), and traditional drugs without any problems, except as noted as follows:

Arizona poppy, blanket flower, chaparral, or cottonwood tree may potentiate the effects of anticoagulants.

When almond blossom, black tourmaline, century plant, chaparral, colvilles, columbine, cottonwood tree, foxglove, goldenrod, owls clover, pear blossom, shasta daisy, sunflower, yellow yarrow, or yellow evening primrose is used for depression the health practitioner may need to reduce any antidepressant medications the patient is currently using while taking a specific essence.

The use of bear grass, bellis perennis, blanket flower, chaparral, or red bromeliad requires close monitoring and adjustment of oxygen needs in patients with chronic obstructive pulmonary disease.

Dosage for methylphenidate HCL for hyperactivity, attention deficit disorder (ADD), or attention deficit hyperactivity disorder (ADHD) symptoms may need to be reduced incrementally when crimson columbine is used. In some cases the essence can dramatically cure or ease ADD or ADHD symptoms. Such reductions are often needed within 2 weeks of using the essence.

Adverse Reactions

Sometimes an individual will experience a brief *healing crisis*, felt as an aggravation in current symptoms for a few minutes or hours after taking a specific essence.

Trade Products, Administration, and Dosage

Some sources for flower essences are as follows. Many more equally credible suppliers exist.

Alaska Flower Essence Project
PO Box 1369
Homer, AK 99603
Tel: (907) 235-2188
Fax: (907) 235-2777
E-mail: afep@alaska.net

Blue Turtle Flower and Gem Essences
PO Box 2513
Cottonwood, AZ 86326
Tel: (520) 634-9298
Orders: (800) 815-1624
Fax: (520) 634-9298
E-mail: docbones@sedona.net
www.medicinegarden.com

Flower Essence Society
PO Box 459
Nevada City, CA 95959
Tel: (520) 634-9298
Orders: (800) 548-0075
Fax: (916) 265-6467

Perelandra
PO Box 3606
Warrenton, VA 20188
Tel: (540) 937-2123
Orders (USA and Canada): (800) 960-8806
Fax: (540) 937-3360
www.perelandra-ltd.com

Dosage

The FDA demands that dosage and the Latin name of the essence be listed on the product. The FDA does not dictate the dosage. Each company has its own regimen. In general, essences are often taken three times per day.

Self-Help versus Professional

Many health food stores carry flower and gem essences. This therapy can be self-applied but people without adequate training or backgrounds may not choose the correct essence. There are a few self-help books available to help casual users of flower and gem essences. Their training comes from the books and their applied knowledge. Or they go on the Internet; at our site we post the actual provers' symptoms with the essence so that people are assured of precise symptoms and a match with their own.

People who want to self-prescribe for acute conditions may do so successfully. Chronic conditions should be seen by a flower essence consultant.

Visiting a Professional

There are many ways to take a flower essence case. The following is one form. For an acute or chronic case a medical past and present history form is sent to the patient before seeing the essence consultant. The acute case is straightforward: a matching of the person's symptoms with flower and gem essence proving symptoms. The one that most closely matches is chosen. A constitutional case-taking may take longer, depending on the patient's medical history and chief complaints and how long it takes the essence consultant to discern the core imbalance to the patient's vital force. The person, after receiving the essence, is asked to check back in with the consultant. Usually, the person is seen every 4 weeks, although the person may call the consultant at any time with a question or concern. This process is ongoing until the patient no longer has any symptoms of the chief complaint remaining.

Credentialing

No formal standardized credentialing exists for this form of therapy.

Training

Some companies do provide training in flower essences. These include Bach, Flower Essence Society (FES), Perelandra, and Blue Turtle Flower and Gem Essences.*

FES conducts workshops and seminars on flower essences. Blue Turtle Flower and Gem Essence offers a 3-year training program.

Flower Essence Society
PO Box 459
Nevada City, CA 95959
Tel: (916) 265-9163
Fax: (916) 265-6467

---

*This company is owned by the author.

The Dr. Edward Bach Centre
Mount Vernon, Bakers Lane
Sotwell, Oxon, OX100PZ, UK
Tel: +44 (0) 1491 834678
Fax: +44 (0) 1491 825022
www.bachcentre.com

Blue Turtle Flower and Gem Essence
PO Box 2513
Cottonwood, AZ 86326
Tel/Fax: (520) 634-9298
E-mail: docbones@sedona.net
www.medicinegarden.com

The Internet also is another resource where advertisements for workshops or seminars will occasionally appear.

What to Look for in a Provider

The person or health practitioner should inquire of the consultant's training and degree of experience. Years working as a consultant are preferable. Some degree of medical training is recommended so that the consultant can differentiate between emergency and non-emergency medical conditions.

Barriers and Key Issues

The major barrier in flower essences is the lack of available research. Published information is forthcoming on cured cases using flower or gem essences. Visibility in mainstream medicine could be improved by the introduction of proving information into medical journals. Owners of flower essence companies are willing to speak to and give workshops to acquaint health practitioners with their area of expertise.

Associations

Manufacturers of flower essences and their respective practitioners are divided as to their belief systems. There is no one governing body or board to provide such information, nor is there a single composite directory that can give such information. Places to search include the following:

1. Health food stores
2. Internet search engines (type in *flower, gem,* or *natural essence*)
3. Direct contact with a flower and gem essence company
4. New Age newspapers, such as *Sage,* or New Age magazines, such as *Yoga Magazine*

The author suggests the following Internet resources as a starting point for further information (listed in alphabetic order):

1. Australian Bush Flower Essences
   http://www.ausflowers.com.au/essences/43.html
2. The Alchemy of the Desert
   http://www.desert-alchemy.com/txt/pub-AOD.html
3. Flower and Gem Essences
   http://www.medicinegarden.com/NE/Index.html
4. Perelandra, Ltd.
   http://www.perelandra-ltd.com/

Suggested Reading

1. Chancellor PM: *Bach flower remedies*, New Canaan, Conn, 1971, Keats.
   An excellent overview of the Bach remedies.
2. Devi L: *The essential flower essence handbook*, Nevada City, Calif, 1996, Masters Flower Essences Publishing.
   This author used a biofeedback experiment to gain information on the essences she tested.
3. Kaminski P, Katz R: *Flower essence repertory*, Nevada City, Calif, 1994, The Flower Essence Society.
   A repertory of flowers and the conditions they address.
4. Kramer D: *New Bach flower therapies*, Rochester, Vt, Healing Arts Press.
   New, additional material created by a Bach consultant.
5. Nauman E: *Crested prickle poppy*, Cottonwood, Ariz, 1994, Blue Turtle Publishing.
   A 14-day proving on an essence to find out what detailed symptoms it will address.
6. Wright M: *Flower essences*, Warrenton, Va, 1988, Perelandra, Ltd.
   A useful resource guide to flower essences that the author has worked with over the years.

Bibliography

Cook TM: *Homeopathic medicine today: a modern course of study*, New Canaan, Conn, 1989, Keats.

Lo SY: Anomalous states of ice, *Modern Physics Letters B* 10(19):909-919, 1996.

Schiff M: *The memory of water: homeopathy and the battle of ideas in the new science*, London, 1998, Thorsons.

Murphy R: *Lotus materia medica, lotus star medica,* ed 2, Pagosa Springs, Co, 1996 Lotus Star Academy.

Nauman E: *Crested prickle poppy flower essence proving*, Cottonwood, Ariz, 1996, Blue Turtle.

Nauman E: *NE quick guide, internet,* Cottonwood, Ariz, 1998, Blue Turtle.

Nauman E: *Natural essence materia medica and repertory,* vol 1, 1998, unpublished manuscript.

Tompkins P, Bird CO: *The secret life of plants,* New York, 1989, Harper Collins.

Herbal Medicine

MARY L. CHAVEZ

PEDRO I. CHAVEZ

Origins and History

Herbal medicine is defined by the European Union as "medicinal products containing as active ingredients exclusively plant material and/or vegetable drug preparations."[1-3] From a historical perspective, herbal medicines have been used since the dawn of humanity. There is evidence that plants were used for healing during the Neanderthal period before 60,000 BCE. Eight species of plants surrounded the body of a Neanderthal man discovered in a cave in northern Iraq, seven of which are still commonly used as herbal medicines.[3,4]

Herbal treatment was developed through experimentation, cultural and family tradition, and anecdotal accounts. Before the advent of writing, medicine men and women verbally handed down information about use. The first books to focus on herbals were written by the Chinese more than 5000 years ago. These books were written on silk and included such plants as the opium poppy and ephedra. The first written records of using herbals to treat illness were found on ancient Mesopotamian clay tablets and Egyptian papyrus written around 2000 BCE. These early pharmaceutic writings were designated as *materia medicas*. In the first century CE the Greek pharmacobotanist Pedanios Dioscorides wrote the most famous materia medica entitled *De Materia Medica Libri Cinque*.[5,6] This treatise contained more than 600 herbal drugs and remained the authoritative reference for almost 15 centuries.

Worldwide, many traditional medicine systems relied heavily on herbal therapies. Such systems included traditional Chinese medicine, Ayurvedic medicine of India, and Unanic medicine of the Middle East. Other indigenous medical systems also relied on herbal medicines, including South, Central, and North American Indian and African cultures. Many important drugs originated from these traditional medicine practices, including cocaine, ipecac, podophyllotoxin, physostigmine, quinine, and tubocurarine.[2]

Most of the folkloric use of herbals in the United States was based on uses established by Native Americans.[3] Early European settlers exchanged information on the use of herbals with the Native Americans. Almost 170 herbal drugs that have been officially listed in the U.S. *Pharmacopoeia and National Formulary* were used by American Indians and 50 more were used by indigenous peoples of the West Indies, Mexico, and Central and South America.[2] Thus, until the beginning of this century, physicians commonly used herbal preparations to treat various illnesses.

Gradually with time the use of herbals in medical practice declined in the U.S. However, the World Health Organization estimated that 4 billion people, or 80% of the world population, still relies on herbal medicines for some aspect of primary health care.[7] For these people it is a matter of economics because most cannot afford modern pharmaceuticals. Other reasons include living in rural areas where drugs are inaccessible or in areas with a shortage of physicians.[8]

The use of *phytomedicines* is markedly different in Western Europe. Physicians and pharmacists receive significant education and training on the use of phytomedicines (herbal medicine). The use of herbal medicines is strongly integrated with conventional medicine.[1]

In the last two decades, several changes in attitudes in the U.S. have occurred which have altered the opinions of the public and medical community toward use of herbal medicines. The public has become dissatisfied with the effectiveness and cost of modern medicine and is searching for alternative and less expensive methods of treatment. In addition, many people have learned to appreciate things that are "natural" and "organic." The "green" revolution has produced an appreciation for classical plant drugs.

Biologic Mechanism of Action

As early civilizations developed, it was a common belief that plants had been signed by the "creator" with a clue to their therapeutic effect. This belief assumed that the plant or plant part would resemble the human site of its clinical application. This notion has been called the *Doctrine of Signatures*. Thus, kidney beans should cure kidney disorders and cerebral malfunction should be treatable with walnuts.[9]

During the time of Dioscorides, use of herbals was based on the classical Galen classification.[10] Galen's system taught that health and the four bodily humors—black bile, blood, phlegm, and yellow bile—determined disease. The humors were associated with the elemental principals of antiquity, which were air, earth, fire, and water. The elements were thought to be combined with the four bodily humors (in various ratios and proportions) to produce the qualities of cold, dry, moist, or warmth. As a result diseases were classified as being moist, warm, or dry. Treatment involved administration of herbals having the opposite property.[5,6] The herbals were classified according to their property and graded on a four-point scale as to whether they were "imperceptible," "perceptible," "powerful," or "very powerful." To illustrate, opium was categorized as grade 4/cold, and pepper was categorized as grade 4/dry and warming.[5] The goal of treatment was to balance the humors by removing the excess or increasing what was deficient. This medical system became the dominant system throughout Europe through the medieval era.[2]

During the early nineteenth century with the development of the sciences and the scientific methods, herbal medicines began to be the object of scientific analysis. The first time that chemical and analytic methods were used to extract the active principal from a herbal involved the isolation of morphine from opium in 1803 to 1806.[9] Additional applications of chemical and analytic efforts resulted in enhancing the desired therapeutic properties by reducing adverse effects of various substances isolated from plants. As an example, acetylsalicylic acid was formed from salicin found in willow bark. During the later part of the nineteenth century, chemists began to synthesize large numbers of organic compounds with sophisticated chemical complexity. With the advent of synthetic medicines, the transition from herbal remedies to modern pharmaceutics began. However, regulations and economics were a major cause of the decline in the use of herbal remedies rather than lack of therapeutic efficacy.

Mechanisms of Action

Herbal remedies are phytomedicines that contain plant material with pharmacologically active constituents and often contain inert constituents such as starch, coloring matter, and other substances that have no defined pharmacologic activity. For most herbals the specific active compounds that produces the pharmacologic activity is unknown. The dried herbal or whole plant extract is considered the active ingredient.[9] Thus, herbal remedies may contain single chemical substances or complex mixtures of compounds that can produce a wide range of pharmacologic effects. The active constituents are mostly secondary metabolites that are present in small concentrations in the plant. It is hypothesized that the plant produces these secondary compounds as protection against insects and parasites. The amount of chemical constituents varies because of many factors, including type of soil, sunlight, rain, time of season of collection, temperature, maturity of the plant, associated flora, and storage conditions. Many herbals contain chemical compounds that are structurally related and can produce similar pharmacologic activity. Thus the therapeutic effect is likely the result of combined or synergistic action rather than one single compound. The active constituents are present in lower concentrations than in purified, single-compound synthetic pharmaceutics. Overall the risks associated with crude herbal remedies are much fewer than with conventional drugs, when administered in appropriate doses.

Forms of Therapy

Herbal medicines are preparations made from plants or plant parts or whole extracts or concentrates of active plant constituents.[5,6] The preparations are available as fresh plant products and as solid or liquid dosage forms. Fresh plant products are usually prepared as an infusion (tea) by pouring boiling water over the herb and letting it steep. A decoction is prepared by directly boiling the herb in water, then straining to remove excess plant material. The liquid forms include medicinal oils, medicinal spirits, plant juices, syrups and tinctures, glycerites, and related products. Solid dosage forms are available as powdered plant material, powdered extracts, and concentrates. Solid preparations include granules, uncoated tablets, coated tablets, capsules, and lozenges. Herbal medicines also are available as herbal combination products. Many herbal medicines also are available in standardized form. These products are standardized for pharmacologic activity or marker chemical constituents.

A survey of herbal sales by natural food stores in 1997 was conducted by *Whole Foods* magazine.[12] The ranking of the top 20 selling herbal supplements is presented in the corresponding table.

Ranking of Top-Selling Herbal Supplements by Natural Food Stores in 1997		
Ranking	**Herbal Medicine**	**% of Sales**
1	Echinacea	11.93%
2	Garlic	8.52%
3	Ginkgo	6.80%
4	Goldenseal	5.95%
5	Saw palmetto	4.87%
6 (tie)	Aloe	4.76%
7 (tie)	Ginseng	4.76%
8	Cat's claw	3.49%
9	Astragalus	3.07%
10	Cayenne	2.83%
11	Siberian ginseng	2.70%
12	Bilberry	2.61%
13	Cranberry	2.47%
14	Dong quai	2.13%
15	Grape seed extract	2.07%
16	Cascara sagrada	1.92%
17	St. John's wort	1.87%
18	Valerian	1.73%
19	Ginger	1.69%
20	Feverfew	1.59%

Demographics

Sales of herbal remedies in the U.S. are experiencing unprecedented growth. Although there is no collaborated effort by trade group to compile statistics, herbal medicinal sales for 1997 increased by 59%. An estimated 60 million adult Americans spent $3.24 billion on herbal medicines in 1997.[1] In a follow-up of their landmark national survey, Eisenberg et al[10] determined that 12.1% of adult Americans used herbal medicine in 1997. In a similar study conducted by Landmark Healthcare, 17% of the 1500 adults randomly surveyed used herbal therapy in 1997.

The follow-up national survey documented the prevalence and cost of alternative therapies in the U.S.[10] The researchers reported that use of alternative therapy (including herbal medicine) was more common among women (48.9%) than men (37.8%) ($p = 0.001$) and less common among African Americans (33.1%) compared to other racial groups (41.8%) ($p = 0.004$). Higher rates of use were found in people aged 35 to 49 years of age (50.1%) than in either older (39.1%) ($p = 0.001$) or younger persons (41.8%) ($p = 0.003$). Use was higher in those surveyed who had some college education (50.6%) compared to no college education (36.4%) ($p = 0.03$) and in people with an annual income above $50,000 (48.1%) compared with lower incomes (42.6%) ($p = 0.004$). In addition, use was higher among those who lived in the West (50.1%) compared to elsewhere in the U.S. (42.1%) ($p = 0.004$). A total of 62% of those who used alternative therapies did not inform their health care provider (including physicians and pharmacists) about their use.

Indications and Reasons for Referral

Herbal remedies should not be used for emergency and acute-care situations. They are mainly used as self-medications for chronic medical conditions or mild illnesses. In Germany, herbal medicines commonly are prescribed by physicians. The most common specific indications include respiratory tract disorders, central nervous system disorders, urinary tract remedies, cardiovascular disorders, gastrointestinal disorders, dermatologic and external antiinflammatory agents, immunostimulants, and gynecologic remedies. They also are used for treatment of rheumatoid disorders and other inflammatory conditions.

In 1997 a survey was conducted by *Prevention Magazine* to determine what sources most people used to learn about herbal remedies.[13] According to the results of the survey, 41% of American who used herbals learned about the remedies from friends or family; 37%, from magazines; 35%, from books; 13%, from health food stores; and 5%, from television. Only 9% of adults obtained their information from physicians, and pharmacists were the lowest source; only 4% of those surveyed obtained information from pharmacists.

The survey also explored attitudes toward used of herbal remedies and found that the majority of users thought herbal remedies were "just as good as or better than nonherbal remedies" in the areas of efficacy (53%), safety (65%) and cost (58%). A total of 42% of those surveyed felt that herbal remedies are effective for the treatment of serious illness, such as cancer.

Research Base

In general, scientific studies evaluating the therapeutic and pharmacologic effects of herbal remedies are lacking. There usually are no or very limited pharmacokinetic data for herbals since these medicines are of complex chemical composition. The active constituents usually are not known and thus it is impossible to determine the exact mechanism of action. The evaluation of the effectiveness of herbal remedies usually is through empiric observation in human patients treated with the herbal remedy. Herbal medicines cannot be patented in the U.S. and thus the pharmaceutic companies cannot recover research costs.

Evidence Based

For conventional pharmaceutics to be marketed, federal regulation requires documentation of therapeutic efficacy and safety of the drug to be evaluated before marketing. The scientific documentation requires toxicologic, pharmacologic, and clinical studies. At the present time the U.S. does not have a method to approve therapeutic claims for herbal medicines. Only a few herbals, such as cascara, psyllium, and senna, are approved as over-the-counter drugs.[6,14,19] Attempts are being made to apply the gold standard of randomized double-blind placebo-controlled studies to evaluate the efficacy and safety of herbal medications. Most of the scientific research has been conducted in Europe, particularly in Germany. The recent interest in alternative therapies in the U.S. has contributed to the formation of the National Center for Complementary and Alternative Medicine (formerly the Office of Alternative Medicine).[7] The Center currently is funding clinical trials evaluating alternative therapies including herbal therapies. The pharmaceutic industry and herbal manufacturers are beginning to conduct clinical trials involving herbal medicines.

Basic Science

Several basic scientific measures should be conducted to assure the safety, potency, and purity of herbal preparations, and some reputable herbal manufacturers conduct these quality assurance tests. Raw plant material should be authenticated by a qualified botanist. Common methods of identification include comparing a plant sample with an "herbarium sample," conducting macroscopic and microscopic examination of the plant material, and performing "organoleptic" testing (smelling, feeling, tasting).[15] Herbal preparations should be chemically analyzed to identify and quantitate active constituents and impurities. The analysis should include physicochemical analysis such as thin layer, gas, or high pressure liquid chromatography, which produces a "chromatographic fingerprint." This chromatographic fingerprint should be compared to a standard. Screening tests should be conducted to detect impurities.

Risk and Safety

It must be acknowledged that the therapeutic efficacy of conventional pharmaceutics is generally better than herbal medicines. The advantage of herbals is the patients that have a greater trust in these remedies based on their expectations of safety and efficacy. However, the claim of lower side effects has not been proven by modern statistical standards.[5] Clinical trials that evaluated the efficacy of herbal supplements are usually of short duration. The long-term adverse effects usually are not known.

There is a misconception among consumers that because herbal medicines are "natural" they are harmless. Side effects and toxic reactions have been reported with the use of herbal remedies. In some cases the adverse effects resulted from misidentification, mislabeling, and the patient's own self-selection. In addition there may be idiosyncratic reactions, including allergenic reactions.

Health professionals have many questions concerning the efficacy, potency, purity, safety, and consistency in dosage of herbal medicines. Under the current FDA regulations of herbal medicines, there is no guarantee that the product is pure or that potency is consistent. A large amount of variability can exist between herbal manufacturers and even within a single manufacturer's own lots, and batch-to-batch variation can occur. Product adulteration, mislabeling, and misidentification of herbs has occurred. Herbal preparations have been found to be adulterated with heavy metals (including arsenic, mercury, lead, and cadmium), nondeclared drugs (such as aminopyrine, diazepam, phenylbutazone, prednisone, and testosterone), pathogenic microorganisms such as *Salmonella* and *Aspergiullus*, pesticides, fumigants, and radioactive substances.[8]

Another concern is whether to use the whole plant or an extract of the plant. The extract may not contain the "active" constituent, or the whole plant preparation may not have sufficient quantity of the active constituents. A through literature review should be conducted to determine if a clinical trial has evaluated the efficacy and safety of the herbal medicine. Preparations with proven clinical evidence only should be recommended. Products should contain the complete labeling, including plant name with genus and species, batch number, standardized chemical constituents, amount of active ingredient per dose, and expiration date.

Patients with serious medical conditions such as cardiovascular disease, kidney disease, liver failure, depression, cancer, and HIV or AIDS should not use herbal medicines unless they are under the care of a qualified health professional. Very little information is available on use of herbal medicine during pregnancy, during lactation and in children, and therefore these products should not be used except with the advice of a qualified health care professional.

Herbal medicines should be stopped immediately if any adverse effects occur. Adverse reactions should be reported to the FDA Med-Watch monitoring system at (800) FDA-1088. Patients should be advised to consult their health care provider before using herbal medicine in combination with over-the-counter and prescription drugs. Herbal medicines can interact with each other and with conventional prescription and over-the-counter drugs. The table on page 555 lists herbal medicines that are considered unsafe and should not be recommended.

Efficacy

The table "Commonly Used Herbal Medicines" summarizes the available information. For several of the herbal medicine, some research studies have been conducted that supports the use, but for many herbals there is limited information.

Barriers and Key Issues

In 1994 the Dietary Supplement and Health and Education Act (DSHEA) separated "dietary supplements" from foods and drugs.[2,15] The Act broadly defined dietary supplements as herbals and other "natural medicines" including vitamins, minerals, and amino acids as dietary supplements. Most products manufactured as dietary are used as drugs, but the manufacturer does not need FDA approval or evaluation for safety before manufacturing. The proof of safety and adulteration rests with the FDA. A product can be removed from the market by the FDA if it poses an imminent health treat.

The Act does not allow therapeutic claims to be printed on the label but allows claims regarding the effect of the herbal on "structure and function" of the body. Herbal manufacturers must be able to substantiate the claims. The label must include the wording that "this statement has not intended to diagnose, treat, cure or prevent any disease." In addition, the label must include the term "dietary supplement."

Section 5 of the Act allows the use of scientific and other literature that promotes the sale of herbal medicines as long as the literature is not false or misleading and presents a balanced view. The literature cannot promote a specific brand, must be physically separated from the product container, and must be free of appended information. Previously such literature was considered as an extension of the label and was grounds for judging the product "mislabeled" and removed from the market.

Suggested Reading

There are numerous books, magazines, websites, and other reference material available. Much of the literature extols the benefits of herbs but very few provide scientific support. The following provides a listing of suggested readings:

Books

1. Bisset NG, editor: *Herbal drugs and phytopharmaceuticals*, Boca Raton, Fla, 1994, CRC Press.
   Includes 181 herbal monographs with information on sources, synonyms, chemical constituents, indications, adverse effects, preparation of tea, regulatory status, and macroscopic, microscopic, and chromatographic techniques for authentication.

2. Blumenthal M: *The complete German commission E monographs. Therapeutic guide to herbal medicines*, Newton, Mass, 1999, Integrative Medicine Communications.
   Includes 380 herbal monographs, 190 monographs of herbs, and fixed combinations. The monographs are arranged as tables with information of taxonomic cross-references, chemical constituents, pharmacology, indications, adverse effects, precautions, interactions, dosage, and administration.

3. Fetrow C, editor: *The professional's handbook of complementary and alternative medicines*, Springhouse, Pa, 1999, Springhouse Corp.
   Includes monographs of approximately 300 commonly used herbal and dietary supplements. The monographs includes generic names, synonyms, trade names, common forms, sources, chemical constituents, actions, uses, dosage, adverse effects, interactions, contraindication and precautions, special considerations, conclusion, and references.

4. Foster S, Tyler VE: *Tyler's honest herbal: a sensible guide to the use of herbs and related remedies*, New York, 1999, Haworth Herbal Press.
   Includes information of the folkloric and therapeutic use of more than 100 herbals.

5. Robbers JE, Speedie MK, Tyler VE: *Pharmacognosy and pharmacobiotechnology*. Baltimore, 1996, Williams & Wilkins.
   A textbook on pharmacognosy (the science of drugs from natural sources). Includes information of biotechnology-derived pharmaceutics, antibiotics, and herbal drugs.

6. Robbers JE, Tyler VE: *Tyler's herbs of choice: the therapeutic use of phytomedicinals*, New York, 1999, Haworth Herbal Press.
   Includes updated information on the regulation of herbals and monographs of commonly used herbals with clinical use, bioactive constituents, pharmacology, clinical efficacy, precautions, and adverse effects.

7. Schulz V, Hansel R, Tyler VE: *Rational phytotherapy: a physicians' guide to herbal medicine*, ed 3, New York, 1998, Haworth Herbal Press.
   Includes information on the extraction and standardization of phytomedicinals and the use of herbals for central nervous, cardiovascular, respiratory, digestive, gynecologic, skin, and connective tissue disorders, as well as to increase natural resistance.

Periodicals

1. *HerbalGram*, Boulder, Colo, Herbal Research Foundation; Austin, American Botanical Council.

   Includes feature-length articles, research reviews, conference reports, and book reviews.

2. *Pharmaceutical Biology* (formerly *International Journal of Crude Drug Research*), Ca Lisse, The Netherlands, Swets and Zeitlinger.

   Includes articles on biologically active chemicals and other substances, including drugs and pharmaceutic products used in traditional medicine.

3. *Journal of Natural Products*, Glendale, Ariz, American Chemical Society and American Society of Pharmacognosy, College of Pharmacy-Glendale.

   Includes articles on screening methods, isolation techniques, spectroscopy, structure elucidation, synthesis and biosynthesis, chematoxonomy, and pharmacology of natural products.

4. *The Herb Quarterly*, San Anselmo, Calif, SparrowHawk Press.

   Includes articles on gardening, healthy lifestyles, culinary use of herbs, and medicinal herbs.

5. *The Review of Natural Products*, St Louis, Facts and Comparison.

   Monographs of hundreds of natural products. Each monograph includes information about the products: scientific names, common names, botany, history, chemistry, pharmacology, toxicology, patient information, summary, and references. Updated monthly.

Retrieval Services

1. Internet GratefulMed or PubMed. www.igm.nlm.nih.gov

   Searchable bibliographic databases that include MEDLINE, PREMEDLINE, AIDSLINE, and other databases.

2. NAPRALERT (Natural Products ALERT), Program for Collaborative Research in the Pharmaceutical Sciences, College of Pharmacy, University of Illinois at Chicago.

   www.pmmp.uic.edu/mcp/nap1

   Contains bibliographic information on natural products and includes pharmacology, biologic activity, chemistry, taxonomic distribution, and ethnologic use. The file contains more than 100,000 records from over 150,000 citations.

3. National Center for Complementary and Alternative Medicine, Information Resources.

   www.altmed.od.nih.gov/nccam/resources

   Searchable index of over 90,000 bibliographic citations that the Center of Alternative Medicine obtained from MEDLINE.

4. Office of Dietary Supplements: International Bibliographic Information on Dietary Supplements (IBIDS).

   www.odp.nih.gov/ods/databases.ibids

   Searchable database on dietary supplements including vitamins, minerals, and botanicals produced by the Office of Dietary Supplements (ODS); contains more than 250,000 citations and abstracts.

5. The University of Texas Center for Alternative Medicine Research.

   www.sph.uth.tmc.edu:8052/utcam

   Provides information on the effectiveness of alternative and complementary therapies, including herbal for cancer prevention and control.

6. U.S. Food and Drug Administration Center for Food Safety and Applied Nutrition, Office of Special Nutritionals.
www.vm.cfsan.fda.gov/~dms/aens
Searchable database of the adverse reactions of nutritionals, including herbals from the Special Nutritionals Adverse Event Monitoring System (SN/AEMS) Web Report. The sources of information are obtained from a variety of sources, including the FDA's Med-Watch program and others.

References

1. Blumenthal M: *The complete German commission E monographs. Therapeutic guide to herbal medicines*, Newton, Mass, 1999, Integrative Medicine Communications.
2. Gillespie SG: Herbal drugs and phytomedicinal agents, *Pharm Times* 63(12):53-61, 1997.
3. Althoff S et al: *Consumer guide to alternative medicine*, Lincolnwood, Ill, 1997, Publications International.
4. Winslow LC, Kroll DJ: Herbs as medicines, *Arch Intern Med* 1998; 158(9):2192-2199, 1998.
5. Schulz V, Hansel R, Tyler VE: *Rational phytotherapy: a physicians' guide to herbal medicine*, ed 3, New York, 1998, Springer.
6. Robbers JE, Speedie MK, Tyler VE: *Pharmacognosy and pharmacobiotechnology*, Baltimore: 1996, Williams & Wilkins.
7. U.S. National Institutes of Health, Office of Alternative Medicine. Website: www.altmed.od.nih.gov.
8. Borins M: The dangers of using herbs. What your patients need to know, *Postgrad Med* 104(1):91-100, 1998.
9. Tyler VE: *Herbs of choice: the therapeutic use of phytomedicinals*, New York, 1994, Pharmaceutical Products Press.
10. Eisenberg DM: Trends in alternative medicine use in the United States, 1990-1997. Results of a follow-up national survey, *JAMA* 280(18):1569-1570, 1998.
11. The Landmark Report on Public Perceptions of Alternative Care. Website: www.landmarkhealthcare.com/constudy.
12. Richman A, Witkowski JP: Echinacea #1 in natural food trade, *HerbalGram* 41(Fall):53, 1997.
13. Johnston BA: One-third of nation's adults use herbal remedies. Market estimated at $3.24 billion, *HerbalGram* 40(Summer):49, 1997.
14. Tyler VE: *Honest herbal. A sensible guide to the use of herbs and related remedies*, ed 3, New York, 1993, Pharmaceutical Product Press.
15. Chavez ML: Natural products, *Rx Consult* 7(8):1-8, 1998.
16. Foster S: *An illustrated guide. 101 medicinal herbs*, Loveland, Colo, 1999, Interweave Press.
17. Bisset NG, editor: *Herbal drugs and phytopharmaceuticals*, Boca Raton, Fla, 1994, CRC Press.
18. *Review of natural products*, Facts and Comparison, St Louis.

Commonly Used Herbals with Documented or Suspected Risks[1,5,8,14]

Herbal	Plant Source	Common Use	Comments
Aconite (Monkshood)	*Aconitum napellus*	Analgesic, antipyretic, wound healing	Side effects include cardiac arrhythmia and respiratory paralysis.
Aloe (internally)	*Aloe barbadenis, Aloe vera,* various Aloe species	Constipation, general tonic, wound healing	Side effects include gastrointestinal (GI) cramping, diarrhea, nephritis, hypokalemia, albuminuria, and andhematuria with chronic use.
Borage	*Borago officinalis*	Antidiarrheal, diuretic	Contains low levels of pyrrolizidine alkaloids (lycosamine, amabiline, thesinine) that are potentially hepatotoxic and carcinogenic.
Calamus	*Acorus calamus*	Antipyretic, digestive aid	Some calamus species contain beta asarone, which may be carcinogenic.
Chaparral	*Larrea tridentata*	Anticancer	Case reports of liver toxicity have been associated with use.
Coltsfoot	*Tussilago farfara*	Antitussive, demulcent	Contains pyrrolizidine alkaloids that are potentially hepatotoxic and carcinogenic.
Comfrey	*Symphytum officinale,* various Smphytum species	Bruises, sprains, wound healing	Contains pyrrolizidine alkaloids that are potentially hepatotoxic and carcinogenic.
Ephedra (Ma-huang)	*Ephedra sinica,* various Ephedra species	Appetite suppressant, bronchodilator, athletic performance enhancement (often combined with caffeine-containing herbals)	Side effects include insomnia, irritability, GI disturbances, urinary retention, and tachycardia. Misuse can lead to hypertension and arrhythmias.
Germander	*Teucrium chamaedrys*	Appetite suppressant	Contains diterpneoid derivatives that are potentially hepatotoxic.
Licorice	*Glycyrrhiza glabra*	Antiulcer, expectorant	Should only be used in small doses for short duration (< 4 weeks). With high doses, hypertension, hypokalemia, and sodium and water retention may occur.
Life root	*Senecio aureus*	Emmenagogue	Contains pyrrolizidine alkaloids that are potentially hepatotoxic and carcinogenic.
Pokeroot	*Phytolacca americana*	Anticancer, antirheumatic	Contains a saponin mixture, phytolaccatoxin, and PWM (a proteinaceous mitogen), which can cause gastroenteris, hypotension, and diminished respiration.
Sassafras	*Sassafras albidum*	Antirheumatic, antispasmodic, stimulant	Contains the volatile oil safrole, which is potentially carcinogenic.
Yohimbe	*Pausinystalia yohimbe*	Impotence	Side effects include anxiety, nervousness, nausea, vomiting, and tachycardia.

Commonly Used Herbal Medicines[1,14-18]

Herbal Medicine	Scientific Name	Common Use	Potential Interactions	Potential Adverse Effects	Contraindications
Aloe vera (External only)	Aloe barbendenis, Aloe vera, various Aloe species.	External: first degree burns, cuts, abrasions	None known	Contact dermatitis	May delay healing of deep vertical (surgical) wounds
Arnica (External only)	Arnica montana	External: wound healing, inflammation	None known	Contact dermatitis; can damage skin with prolonged use	None unknown
Astragalus (or Tragacanth)	Astragalus membranaceus	Colds, flu, minor infections; hyperlipidemia, hyperglycemia (unproven)	None known	None known	None known
Bearberry	Arctostaphylos uva-ursi	Urinary tract inflammation	Any substance that acidifies the urine	Nausea and vomiting	Pregnancy, lactation, children under 12 years
Bilberry	Vaccinium myrtillus	Atherosclerosis, bruising, diarrhea, local inflammation of mucous membranes	Anticoagulants and antiplatelet drugs (possible)	Excessive consumption of berries constipation	None known
Black cohosh	Cimicifuga racemosa	Dysmenorrhea, menopausal symptoms, premenstrual syndrome	None known	Gastric discomfort, dizziness, nervous system and visual disturbances, hypotension, bradycardia, increased perspiration	Pregnancy, lactation
Blessed thistle	Centaurea enedictus	Appetite stimulant, dyspepsia	None known	Allergies	Allergies to blessed thistle

Common name	Scientific name	Uses	Drug interactions	Side effects	Contraindications/Warnings
Blue Cohosh	Caulophyllum thalictroides	Menstrual difficulties uterine stimulant	None known	Hypertension, respiratory stimulation, stimulation of intestinal motility	Should not be used without medical supervison; pregnancy, lactation, in children
Calendula	Calendula officinalis	External: wound healing	None known	None known	None known
Cascara sagrada	Rhamnus purshiana	Constipation	With chronic use due to potassium loss: cardiac glycoside, thiazide diuretics, corticosteroids, licorice root	Abdominal cramps	Intestinal obstruction, acute intestinal inflammation
Cat's claw	Unicaria tomentosa, U. guianensis	Cancer (anecdotal)	None known	None known	None known
Cayenne (Capsicum)	Capsicum frutescens	External: muscle spasms, chronic pain associated with herpes zoster, trigeminal neuralgia, surgical trauma	None known	Local burning sensation, hypersensitivity reaction	Injured skin, allergy
Chamomile	Matricaria recutita (formerly M. chamomile, Chamomile recutita)	External: skin and mucous membrane inflammation; internal: GI spasm and GI inflammatory disease	May delay concomitant drug absorption from the gut.	Allergies (rare)	Allergies to chamomile (and other herbs of the daisy family); avoid in pregnancy
Cranberry	Vaccinium macrocarpon	Prevention of urinary tract infection	None known	Overuse: diarrhea	None known
Dandelion	Tanaxacum officinale	Appetite stimulant, dyspepsia	None known	Contact dermatitis, gastric discomfort	None known

Continued

Commonly Used Herbal Medicines[1,14-18]—cont'd

Herbal Medicine	Scientific Name	Common Use	Potential Interactions	Potential Adverse Effects	Contraindications
Devil's claw	*Arpagophytum procumbens*	Appetite stimulant, supportive therapy for degenerative disorder of the locomotor system	None known	None known	Gastric and duodenal ulcers; gallstone (use only after consultation with health care provider)
Dong-quai	*Angelica sinensis*	CNS stimulant, suppression of immune system, analgesia, uterus stimulant (effective is controversial)	Contains courmarin derivatives, monitor with warfarin; possible synergism with calcium channel blockers	Photosensitivity; lowers blood pressure, possible CNS stimulation; possible carcinogenic (contains safrole)	Pregnancy
Echinacea	*Echinacea angustifolia, E. pallida, E. purpurea*	Supportive therapy for colds and flu	None known	Local tingling and numbing sensation with fresh juice	Long-term use not recommended; progressive systemic illness such as tuberculosis, leucosis, collagenosis, multiple sclerosis, AIDS and HIV infection, and other autoimmune diseases; allergy to plants in the daisy family
Eleuthero	*Eleuterococcus senticosus*	Improvement in well-being	Digitalis glycosides	High doses: irritability, insomnia, anxiety; skin eruptions, headache, diarrhea, hypertension, pericardial pain in rheumatic heart disease	Similar to ginseng
Evening primrose	*Oenothera biennis*	Hyperlipidemia, atopic eczema	None known	Nausea, GI disturbances, headache	None known

Eyebright	*Euphrasia officinalis*	Topical: conjunctivitis, eye irritations	None known	None known; cannot be recommended due to risk of potential contamination with homemade nonsterile preparations	See potential adverse effects
Fenugreek	*Trigonella foenum-graecum*	External: inflammation; internal: appetite stimulant	None known	Skin reactions with repeated external application	None known
Feverfew	*Tanacetum parthenium*	Migraine prophylaxis	Anticoagulants, antiplatelet drugs thrombolytics	Mouth ulceration with chewing leaves, oral irritation, GI disturbances, increase in heart rate	Allergy to feverfew and other plants in the daisy family; pregnancy
Fo-ti	*Polygonum multiforum*	Rejuvenation, decreased liver and kidney function, insomnia, hyperlipidemia, immunosuppression, antimicrobial	None known	None known	Pregnancy
Garlic	*Allium sativum*	Hyperlipidemia; other uses: antibacterial, anticancer, antifungal, antihypertensive, antiinflammatory agent, hypoglycemic,	Anticoagulants, antiplatelet drugs	GI disturbances, garlic odor; may increase insulin level producing decrease in blood glucose; high dose: anemia	Pregnancy and lactation
Ginger	*Zingiber officinale*	Dyspepsia, prevention of motion sickness	Anticoagulants, antiplatelet drugs; calcium channel blocker (possible)	None; GI irritation and discomfort with high dose	Gallstones (use only after consultation with health care provider); pregnancy (controversial)

Continued

Commonly Used Herbal Medicines[1,14-18] —cont'd

Herbal Medicine	Scientific Name	Common Use	Potential Interactions	Potential Adverse Effects	Contraindications
Ginkgo	*Ginkgo biloba*	Symptomatic treatment of age-related organic brain syndrome, peripheral arterial occlusive disease (Stage II of Fontaine), SSRI-induced sexual dysfunction, tinnitus, vertigo	Anticoagulants, antiplatelet drugs, thrombolytics	GI upset, headache, allergic skin reaction; cases of spontaneous bleeding have been reported	None known
Ginseng	*Panax ginseng, P quinquefolia*	Improvement in well-being	Anticoagulants, antiplatelet drugs, thrombolytics; may potentiate MOAIs; stimulants (including caffeine), antipsychotic drugs, hormone therapy	High dose: breast tenderness, nervousness, excitation; estrogenic effects in women, hypotension, hypertension	Chronic use (should use 2 weeks on and 2 weeks off); acute illnesses, any form of hemorrhage; pregnancy and lactation
Goldenseal	*Hydrastis canadensi*	Inflammation of mucous membranes (unproven); does not mask illegal drugs in urine drug screens	May interfere with the ability of colon to manufacture B vitamins and may decrease their absorption; heparin (possible)	Hypoglycemia	Pregnancy and lactation
Gotu kola	*Centella asiatica* (formerly *Hydrocotyle asiatica*)	External: wound healing	None known	Hypersensitivity	None known
Grape seed	*Vitis vinifera*	Antioxidant	None known	None known	None known

Common Name	Latin Name	Indication	Interactions	High dose	Pregnancy, lactation
Hawthorn	*Crataegus spp.*	Congestive heart failure Stage II of NYHA	Cardiotonic drugs, antihypertensive drugs	High dose: hypotension and sedation; nausea, fatigue, sweating, rash; none	Pregnancy, lactation
Horse chestnut	*Aeculus hippocastanum*	Chronic venous insufficiency	None known	GI disturbances, nausea, pruritus	None known
Hyssop	*Hyssopus officinalis*	Pharyngitis, expectorant	None known	None known	None known
Kava-kava	*Piper methysticum*	Anxiety, restlessness, sleep induction	Potentiation of CNS depressants and alcohol	Chronic use: kavaism with dry, flaking, discolored skin and reddened eyes; numbness of mouth with chewing, CNS depression	Pregnancy, nursing, endogenous depression
Licorice	*Glycyrrhiza glabra*	Gastric/duodenal ulcers	Due to potassium loss; digitalis glycosides, thiazide diuretics, corticosteroids, licorice	With prolonged use and with high doses: mineralocorticoid effects including sodium and water retention, hypokalemia, myoglobinuria	Gall bladder disease, kidney disease, pheochromocytoma and other adrenal tumors, diseases that cause low serum potassium livers, fasting, anorexia, bulimia, untreated hypothyroidism
Marshmallow	*Althaea officinalis*	Ingestion, irritation of oral and pharyngeal mucosa	May delay absorption of other drugs taken simultaneously	None known	None known
Milkthistle	*Silbum marianum*	Dyspepsia, supportive therapy for toxic liver damage	None known	Mild diarrhea	None known

Continued

Commonly Used Herbal Medicines[1,14-18] —cont'd

Herbal Medicine	Scientific Name	Common Use	Potential Interactions	Potential Adverse Effects	Contraindications
Passion flower	*Passiflora incarnata*	Anxiety, insomnia (unproven)	None known	None known; may have MAOI activity	None known
Pau d'arco	*Tabebuia impetiginosa*	Cancer	Vitamin K	Chronic use: anemia	Bleeding disorders
Peppermint	*Mentha X piperita*	External: myalgia and neuralgia; internal: GI spasms, nausea, inflammation of oral mucosa	External: irritation of mucous membranes; overuse: heartburn, relaxation of esophageal sphincter	External: contact dermatitis; internal: mouth irritation, muscle tremor, hypersensitivity reaction, heartburn, bradycardia	Obstruction of bile ducts, gallbladder inflammation, severe liver damage, pregnancy
Plantain	*Plantago major*	External: inflammation of skin; internal: cough, oral and pharyngeal mucosa inflammation	None known	None known	None known
Pygeum	*Pygeum africanum*	Benign prostatic hyperplasia	None known	GI disturbance	None known
Saw palmetto	*Serenoa repens*	Benign prostatic hyperplasia, stages I and II	Hormone therapy	GI disturbance	Pregnancy, lactation, children, breast cancer

Slippery elm	*Scutellaria lateriflora*	Pharyngitis, GI inflammatory disorders	None known	Contact dermatitis	None known
St. John's wort	*Hypericum perforatum*	External: oil preparation mild wounds and burns; internal: mild to moderate depression	Monoamine oxidase inhibitors; serotonin selective reuptake inhibitors and other antidepressants, sympathomimetics	Possible photosensitization, GI disturbance	Pregnancy and lactation
Stinging nettle	*Urtica dionica*	Benign prostatic hyperplasia	None known	Allergy	Pregnancy; cardiac and renal dysfunction
Tea tree	*Melaleuca alternifolia*	External: bacteriostatic	None known	Allergic contact dermatitis	None known
Tumeric	*Curuma longa*	Dyspepsia	None known	None known	Obstruction of bile passages
Valerian	*Valeriana officinalis*	Restlessness, sleeping disorders	Possible with CNS depressants and alcohol	Strong disagreeable odor, headache, excitability, cardiac disturbances, rare morning drowsiness	None known
Vitex (or Chaste Tree Berry)	*Vitex agnus-castus*	Menstrual disorders	May interfere with dopamine-receptor antagonists	GI disturbances, itching, urticaria	None known

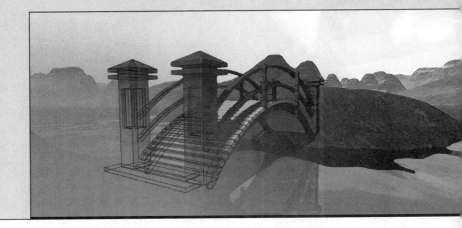

Diet and Nutrition in the Prevention and Treatment of Disease

Macronutrients, 566

Micronutrients, 576

Oxidative Stress, 595

Orthomolecular Medicine, 606

Nutritional Oncology and Integrative
  Cancer Care, 618

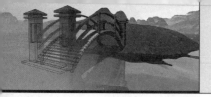

Macronutrients

MITCHELL J. GHEN

NANCY A. CORSO

Origins and History

Food is the basic resource of vitamins, minerals, and other nutrients that allow our body to do its daily performance. Our ability to eat foods and then extract the proper nutrients is what allows us to gain both energy and the building blocks for our immune system and other bodily functions. To understand human nutrition we must begin with the basics, that is, the building blocks and the chemical structure of food. Some reeducation is useful to help realize that many of the foods that we buy in food stores, fast food chains, and in health food stores may not actually be healthy for the human body. No longer may we overlook terms such as *complex carbohydrates*, *simple carbohydrates*, *processed foods*, *refined grains*, *caffeine ingestion*, *alcohol consumption*, and *refined oils*. Food intake and type have a profound effect on individual health. Although the ingestion of foods may not cause any acute deleterious effects on the health for humans, the long-term effects have been clearly documented in the literature.

As we cross the line into the new millennium, physicians and other health care providers need to consider how to effect change in our patients with less emphasis on the use of synthetic drugs and other chemical concoctions. Nutritional literature supports a growing realization that food could have a significant contributory factor in many of our chronic ailments of today, including cancer, collagen vascular diseases, arthritis, and even progressive aging. Our patients are spending billions of dollars on diets like high protein, low carbohydrate, low fat, low protein, Paleolithic, blood typing, zone, starvation, food pyramid, allergic disorder, caloric restriction, and juicing diets. Unfortunately, none of these specialized protocols is universally ideal. Individualized treatment and prescription of the appropriate diet is essential for the improvement for a patient's nutritional status.

Mechanism of Action According to Its Own Theory

The process of digestion is to allow nutrients, vitamins, and minerals to be extracted from the foods that we eat. By eating the proper foods and having a normal working digestive tract, we are assured of good cellular nutrition.

Biologic Mechanism of Action

Simple carbohydrates are empty calories that offer little to overall nutrition. The simple carbohydrates are sugars that include sucrose, dextrose, fructose, lactose, white sugars, maltose, honey, turbinado sugar, and corn syrup.

Grains, fruits, and vegetables are considered *complex carbohydrates*, which supply the nutrients our bodies need. More than half of calories should come from complex carbohydrates. However, when these foods are refined or processed the resultant is a product that now acts like a simple carbohydrate. White flour and white rice are examples of refining that removes at least 36 nutrients and then the "enrichment" process then adds back only four. Processed foods do not provide for adequate nutrition. Starches are just sugar molecules attached together and affect the body and immune cells in the same manner as simple sugars.[1]

There are three types of fiber. First, *insoluble fibers* are lignins, hemicellulose, and cellulose. These fibers make you feel full, help ease constipation, and subsequently can play a role in colorectal cancer reduction and diverticular disease. Second are the *soluble fibers*, which are pectin (which slows the absorption of food), gum mucilage (which helps reduce cholesterol), and glucomannan. Examples of soluble fibers are apples, pears, wheat bran, and vegetables. The third and new type of fiber is chitosan. It is from aquatic crustaceans (this fiber has been shown to bind fat). Diets high in fiber also help to control blood sugar and blood pressure.

Meat, fish, eggs, fowl, nuts, seeds, beans, milk, and legumes are examples of *proteins*. Proteins can be defined as any substance that is made up of amino acids in a peptide linkage and provide functions that are essential for life. Amino acids are involved in all the biochemical structure of hormones, enzymes, nutrient carriers, and antibodies. "Peptides are digested proteins, many of which are absorbed directly into the bloodstream after eating. Protein makes up ¾ of the dry weight of most body cells. There are considerable problems in determining a minimum protein requirement, it seems to be on the order of 0.3 to 0.4 gram of protein per kilo (2.2 pounds) of body weight per day or about 30 to 40 grams for the average adult male. This assumes a majority of the protein consumed is high-quality protein and contains most of the essential amino acids.

The current recommended dietary allowance (RDA) is 44 to 56 grams per day. In America even vegetarian diets contain 80 to 100 grams of protein per day. Every second the bone marrow makes 2.5 million red cells. White cells are usually replaced in 10 days. A person has the equivalent of new skin in 24 days and bone collagen in 30 years. All this maintenance and repair work requires amino acids. Determination of the ideal intake of these amino acids is more difficult than determination of the minimum daily requirement."[2]

Fats provide more energy per gram than any of the other macronutrients. Fat protects body organs, provides for fat-soluble vitamins, becomes the precursor for many hormones, and performs many other crucial body functions.

Essential fatty acids (EFAs) must be provided by food we eat or by supplementation. The two essential fatty acids are linolenic acid (an Omega-3 fat) and linoleic acid (an Omega-6 fat). Both are vital to the health of our immune system. Our diet ordinarily provides more Omega-6 than Omega-3 fatty acids. These substances are used by the body to make prostaglandins. "A lack can contribute to heart and skin disorders, bruising, flaking skin, dandruff, sun sensitivity, arthritis, allergies, obesity, behavior problems, digestive and immune system disorders, premenstrual syndrome, toxemia of pregnancy and many other problems."[1]

"Saturated fatty acids (SFA) or 'bad' fats are found in commercially-processed fat products, saturated animal fats and rancid or old fat should be avoided. They have undergone chemical changes so that even if their original sources provided essential fatty acids, they no longer do. Eating these fats interferes with the ability of essential fatty acids to function properly on the body. They are found mainly in animal foods like meat, whole milk and cheeses. It raises the blood cholesterol levels, and its impact is more profound than any other dietary substance. It should be limited to 10% of total calories."[3]

Cholesterol is an organic chemical compound that is a member of the family of alcohols. It looks and feels like soft wax. Cholesterol enters the body from food sources, and it is manufactured by the body in the liver. Cholesterol plays a vital role in the production of hormones and metabolic products. It is just one of a larger group of compounds in the body known as *sterols,* all of which are essential to life. Cholesterol has often been seen as an "enemy" to our bodies and as a culprit in many diseases. Too much cholesterol has been implicated as one of the risk factors in the genesis of heart disease. Although the lowering of cholesterol levels is advisable, the final role of cholesterol in vascular disease is still being delineated.

In addition to the macronutients, enzymes must be present to breakdown the food in a timely fashion. *Digestive enzymes* are proteins that allow chemical reactions to take place between other proteins, which may not occur at all without their presence. It has been suggested that enzymes will continue to work even after the organism's demise. "A single human liver cell contains at least 1000 different enzyme systems. Enzymes work by reducing the energy required for individual reactions to take place. They make it easier for two proteins to react together and they are not altered by the reactions they stimulate. Hundreds of thousands of reactions take place at any given second in your body and all of these functions involve numerous enzymes. The best way to make certain our bodies have adequate enzyme activity is to provide our bodies with the building blocks needed to make those enzymes which are components of the foods we eat: amino acids, carbohydrates, vitamins and minerals. Three basic kinds of digestive enzymes break down the proteins, starches and fats in the foods we eat and when ingested (encapsulated) with foods they may contribute to the digestion of those foods."[2] These include amylase for starches, lipase for fats, cellulase for cellulose, and protease for proteins. Consider that young cells contain 1000% or 10 times more enzymes than older cells, making digestion even more difficult in an older adult population.

From the moment food enters the mouth until it becomes waste material, there is a fine order of events that occurs, which allows for the proper extraction of the nutrients necessary for good health. Assuming that a patient has a normal digestive tract, the moment the food enters the mouth, ptyalin begins acting on the carbohydrates for its immediate breakdown into simple sugars. Unfortunately there is a narrow range of pH that allows this enzyme to work well. In the event that the saliva pH is greater than 7, then ptyalin is not produced and the first step of carbohydrate digestion ceases. Food then enters into the stomach where hydrochloric acid plays two roles: it sterilizes the foods that we are eating; and it slows or stops the reflex removal of foods too rapidly from the stomach. Enzymes, including intrinsic factor, help to absorb some vitamins, particularly B12. Too little acid in the stomach will let food and undigested protein exit the stomach too quickly. This has been implicated in several allergic conditions. Hyperchlorhydria or excess production of hydrochloric acid may cause marked delayed emptying of the stomach for as much as 6 to 8 hours. Commonly prescribed H2 blockers (antacids) can have a profound effect on this mechanism. Parietal cells produce hydrochloric acid, which mixes with the food. Once the food becomes saturated with the acid the food movement slows down. This lag time allows for the next step, which is the pressure of the stomach contents with the rising pH that will now allow the pyloris to relax and let the food enter the duodenum. Pancreatic exocrine juices, such as sodium bicarbonate and potassium bicarbonate in a ratio of 2:1, as well as liver bile, aid the transit of food into the small intestine. It is important to note that there are optimal pHs for the conversion of proteins to their building blocks, amino acids, as well as the conversion of starches to their common sugars.[4]

Demographics

Practitioners of nutrition can be found in almost every area of the country. The great difficulty becomes in finding one who is adept in suitable applications while considering the uniqueness of each patient. Nutritional information is taught to many individuals throughout their schooling, including herbalists (Western and Eastern), chiropractors, naturopaths, physicians, and academic degrees in nutrition. The authors believe that it is safe and befitting that each patient, regardless of age, should have a competent nutritional survey followed by a relevant treatment plan to help obtain optimal health.

Forms of Therapy

There is an endless amount of food combinations, diets, and food preparations available.

Indications and Reasons for Referral

Almost every acute and chronic disease can be improved to some degree by proper nutrition. Improper eating is partly responsible for coronary artery disease, peripheral vascular disease, food allergies, and cancer.

A simple ranking of conditions responsive to this form of therapy is as follows. As with all alternative therapies, careful use of macronutrients does not preclude the use of mainstream medical therapies in addition.

Top level: *A therapy ideally suited for these conditions*

Arthritis; cancer; child behavior disorders; colds and flu; constipation; diabetes; diarrhea; fibrocystic disease; food allergies; gastrointestinal disorders; heart disease; irritable bowel syndrome; and obesity

Second level: *One of the better therapies for these conditions*
Chronic fatigue syndrome, chronic pain, and depression

Third level: *A valuable adjunctive therapy for these conditions*
Migraine headaches, asthma, collagen vascular disease, and multiple sclerosis

Practical Applications

Sound nutritional applications require a scientific approach to determine the patient's individual needs. There are several instruments which will help the physician determine whether food is being adequately used for worthy nutrition.

We are a country that is overfed and undernourished. Our diets are fast, faddish, and nutritionally unfulfilling. They have animal proteins, chemically processed foods, saturated fats, and loads of sugar. Undernutrition without malnutrition is an important health and longevity secret. Overeating, regardless of the type of food, will cause chronic ailments and shorten life. According to Dr. Clive McCay of Cornell University, "The life span of rats doubled when food intake was halved." According to Professor Huxley, "Research has also shown undereating increases the life span in many animal life forms, including fruit flies, water fleas, trout, and worms by a factor of 19%." Luigi Corrao stated, "Sobriety, the art of eating in moderation, can be reduced to two simple guidelines: first, to avoid eating more than our system can easily digest and assimilate; and second, to avoid food and drink which disagree with the stomach. Sobriety means to pay intelligent attention to a quantity and quality of foods we eat." An old proverb states, "What we leave after taking a hearty meal does us more good than what we have eaten." "We must consume exactly what is necessary to assimilate the energy and biomolecular structures required to maintain our body as a mature human crystal. The right diet prepares and maintains the physical body as a superconductor."[5]

Druglike Information

Food is and can act like a drug. Foods when broken down into parts are nothing more than a group or combination of different chemicals. An apple alone has more than 280 different chemical entities. "When these chemicals get to certain areas of the brain, they stimulate 'neurotransmitters' that act as chemical messengers between brain neurons. For example food can cause excess epinephrine to be produced, creating extra energy. Individuals can have a physical reaction to the food/drug."[6] The cascade theory of reward explains how neurotransmitters stimulate and inhibit as they work in parallel or sequence in a spreading pattern that looks like a cascade ending with dopamine release.[7] "Deficiencies or an imbalance of dopamine release distorts this cascade and feelings of well-being may be displaced by craving for a substance, including food, to relieve the 'bad' feeling. Careful need in distinguishing between genetic, other anomalies and environmental stress/or drugs is important."[8] Compared to most drugs, food has a long breadth of effect. Jeffrey

Friedman of the University of Rockerfeller studied obese rats and found a gene that controls eating (OB Gene), which is homologous with the human gene. "The gene which controls the enzyme tyrosine hydroxylase which is involved in synthesis of dopamine and norepinephrine, when not present may cause eating disorders including overeating, anorexia and bulimia."[6]

"Peptides, which are digested proteins, are broken down into amino acids and work as neurotransmitters (chemical languages). There are about 50 such languages. They are also natural pain-relieving substances in the brain. It is no wonder it is not unusual for people after a meal to say they 'feel' much better. They can also control depression or produce sleep."[2]

Safety

Xenobiotics are foreign substances or toxins that enter the body. Food itself can act like a toxin. An individual's physiology and biochemistry, along with the quantity of food, food additives, environmental conditions, and the overall general health of the individual, can play a role in safety issues.

Seven hundred chemical pollutants have been identified in public water supplies. Most of these are carcinogenic and can cause birth defects. Many scientific studies have documented a consistent link between consumption of trace organic chemical contaminants in drinking water and elevated cancer mortality rates. Our foods often have hormones, pesticides, herbicides, and fungicides that compromise its safe consumption.

Not enough water can also decrease our margin for food safety. We should drink daily our weight in pounds divided by 2 and that resultant number converted to ounces is our minimum daily drinking requirement of pure water. For example a 150 pound male should drink 75 ounces of water a day (150 /2 = 75).

Actions and Pharmacokinetics

The mechanism of food digestion has been discussed. There are so many disorders that impair appropriate food assimilation that it is impossible to enumerate them all in this chapter. Aging and simple changes in the diet have a significant effect. For example, drinking a glass of water with a meal could increase the pH of the stomach before the normal physiologic increase has occurred. This would cause a too rapid emptying of the stomach contents. Many food interactions, such as caffeine, can increase the amount of acid in the stomach and hasten transit time.

Warnings, Contraindications, and Precautions

"When a person does finally succeed in selecting a well balanced and healthful diet they often do not take into consideration the harmful effects of pollution, pesticides, and soil depletion. Even when we are told most chemicals added to foods are safe they are really not. The food industry is a big business with annual sales well over $200 billion with $500 million of chemicals added to the foods. Literally thousands of chemicals are added to food. Few have been adequately tested and none have been tested in combination with others.

Many even banned are still used by producers anyway or by the time the ban is obtained dozens of similar chemicals replace the ones banned, some being worse than the previous. Agribusiness encourages a way of eating that disrupts our physical health. Fast-foods enter the community and home with deleterious effects. Industrialized foods are dependent on salt, sugar and chemicals to taste 'good'. Most additives are not there to prevent spoilage or increase the shelf life of the food but to make it 'look good', taste, feel and nourish like the real thing."[9]

Our representative food supply provides a shortage of essential fatty acids. "Food manufacturers process vegetable oils so they will not become rancid so easily. Refining and hydrogenating oils do extend the shelf life of these products but they also destroy the essential fatty acids (vital to health) present in the food source of the oil. A second reason for our lack of EFA's is that when whole grains are refined, essential fatty acids as well as many other nutrients are removed. Refined grains produce products with a longer shelf life than products made of whole grains since its the essential fatty acids in the whole grains that turn rancid. Finally, commercially grown beef, poultry eggs and dairy products do not provide the essential fatty acids that free range products do."[1] Processed foods have nitrate and nitrite preservatives that have constantly been shown to convert in the stomach to a potent carcinogen.

"A study comparing diets of Chinese and American people in 1991 showed that Chinese consumed 20% more calories but Americans ate 25% more fats."[10] "More Americans are overweight now than ever and the number is climbing! Many of our major health problems and weight problems are indeed nutritional, from eating the refined, processed and revitalized off of the modern world. The health-problem foods that are waiting to ambush you are sugar, sweeteners, hydrogenated oils, white flour, margarine and soda pop. If one is overweight they are already subjecting themselves to blood sugar and insulin problems as well as a risk for heart disease, fatigue, irritability, diabetes."[11] (Atkins, 1994)

Adverse Reactions

Any food at any time can cause an adverse reaction either in combinations with other foods as an allergen or as a toxin itself. There are also several conditions that would in effect cause more adverse reactions to certain types of foods. Organ insufficiencies, such as kidney, liver, and pancreas conditions, may all affect the way foods are processed and handled.

Pregnancy and Lactation

Pregnant women should not use fad diets and should be cautious about their sodium intake.

Self-Help versus Professional

The complexity of nutritional science is such that education and expertise only can be realized through academic affiliation and graduate program attendance.

Visiting a Professional

A good nutritional counselor will spend at least 1.5 hours to listen and discover your eating habits and with that information develop a treatment plan.

Credentialing

Credentialed individuals such as MDs, DCs, DOs, NDs, Registered Dietitians, and Nutritionists are all credentialed under their separate licensure (depending on the state) to deliver nutritional advice to their patients.

Training

Training can be obtained from most of the health care professional organizations. Contact your individual association for programs available. If time permits, investigate colleges or universities for programs leading to a master's degree or a PhD in nutrition.

Barriers and Key Issues

There is much confusion over which type of food diet a practitioner should choose for a patient. We can tell by watching or listening to different forms of media that we are constantly bombarded with many diet choices. Television, radio, Internet sites, health food store personnel, magazines, news reports, and book clubs give us a variety of diets to select. It is quite difficult to discriminate which are reliable, scientifically-based, or safe. Often they are misleading. Even the nutritional "experts" disagree among themselves. Hundreds of books on diet and nutrition by a myriad of authors also leads to the confusion among the general public as well as professionals. Until recently, intrinsic diet and nutritional information was sparse in the professional literature. Each organization gives nutritional information that can be very different from the next organization. The mainstream medical community presently is inclined to listen to and consider the plethora of information now dispensed on food science.

Many "dieters" are on an endless search for the "perfect" diet that will finally help them lose those fat inches and look better or feel more energetic. They gravitate to diets based on what friends or strangers convince them are facts or truths. Many diets are based on testimonials alone and may ultimately jeopardize health.

Fresh foods provide vitality, sunlight energy, nutrition, flavor and aliveness, which they permit to those who eat them, like taking a fresh bite of sunshine!

"Overall, the diet which will ultimately work best is one which can reduce your appetite by a natural body function, produces steady weight loss, sets no limits on the amount of certain foods you can eat, excludes hunger from the dieting experience, includes rich and luxurious foods, gives a metabolic edge or boost, consistently produces improvements in overall health and is adaptable to use as a lifetime diet where the lost weight will not come back." (Atkins, 1994)

Associations

American Chiropractic Association
PO Box 902
Falls Church, VA 22040
Tel: (800) 986-4636

The American College for Advancement in Medicine (ACAM)
23121 Verdugo Dr., Suite 4
Laguna Hills, CA 92653
Tel: (800) 532-3688
E-mail: acam@acam.org
www.acam.org

Great Lakes College of Clinical Medicine
1407-B N. Wells St.
Chicago, IL 60610
Tel: (800) 286-6013
E-mail: info@glccm.org
www.glccm.org

International College of Advanced Longevity Medicine (ICALM)
1407-B N. Wells St.
Chicago, IL 60610
Tel: (800) 286-6013
E-mail: drgary@netzone.com
www.incalm.com

Suggested Reading

1. Loiselle B: *The healing power of whole foods*, Nicholasville, Ky, 1993, Healthways Nutrition.
   An easy-to-understand minicourse on nutrition.
2. Braverman E: *The healing nutrients within*, New Canaan, Conn, 1997, Keats.
   A basic description of carbohydrates, proteins, and fats.
3. Galland L: *Superimmunity for kids*, New York, 1989, Delacourte.
   An overview of ways to maintain good health using foods in children.
4. Cousens G: *Spiritual nutrition and the rainbow diet*, San Rafael, Calif, 1986, Cassandra Press.
   A thought-provoking book that helps you connect mind to food.
5. Null G: *Guide to sensible eating*, New York, 1992, Golden Health.
   A good explanation of agribusiness and what it means to you and your family.

Bibliography

Heinerman J: *Heinerman's new encyclopedia of fruits and vegetables*, New York, 1995, Parker.

Heinerman J: *Heinerman's encyclopedia of nuts, berries, and seeds*, New York, 1995, Parker.

Kowalski R: *The eight week cholesterol cure*, New York, 1987, Harper & Row.

Sears B: *Enter the zone*, New York, 1995, HarperCollins.

Seibold R: *Cereal grass. What's in it for you!* Lawrence, Kan, 1990, Wilderness Community Education Foundation.

References

1. Loiselle B: *The healing power of whole foods*, Nicholasville, Ky, 1993, Healthways Nutrition.
2. Braverman E: *The healing nutrients within*, New Canaan, Conn, 1997, Keats.
3. Sonberg L: *The health nutrient bible*, Upper Saddle River, N.J., 1995, Simon & Schuster.
4. Haywood C: *Heidelberg pH capsule system*, Heidelberg, 1995, Heidelberg International.
5. Cousens G: *Spiritual nutrition and the rainbow diet*, San Rafael, Calif, 1986, Cassandra Press.
6. Blum K, Trachtenberg D: *Alcoholic gene*, 1993, Neurogenesis.
7. Lowinson J, Ruiz P, Millman R: *Substance abuse. A comprehensive textbook*, Baltimore, 1992, Williams & Wilkins.
8. Holder J, Blum K: *The addictive brain, perspective on brain functioning*, New York, 1991, MacMillan.
9. Null G: *Guide to sensible eating*, New York, 1993, Four Walls Eight Windows.
10. Null G, Null S: *The joy of juicing*, New York, 1992, Golden Health.
11. Atkins R, Gare F: *Dr. Atkins' new diet cookbook*, New York, 1995, M. Evans.

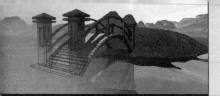

Micronutrients

MELVYN R. WERBACH

MITCHELL J. GHEN

Origins and History

The Recommended Dietary Allowances represent the best currently available assessment of safe and adequate intakes. . . . There are no demonstrated benefits of self-supplementation beyond these allowances.

American Dietetic Association
American Institute of Nutrition
American Society for Clinical Nutrition
National Council Against Health Fraud

The "popular concept" that vitamin supplementation for the American population is medically unnecessary is not supported by . . . biochemical and clinical data. Vitamin supplementation is needed for the "best health"—"optimal health." [1]

Karl Folkers, PhD
Institute for Biomedical Research
The University of Texas at Austin

The value of micronutrients has been cited numerous times in history, with an acceleration through the past 3 centuries. The discovery of relationships between B vitamins and pellegra, vitamin C and scurvy, and iodine and thyroid goiter are but a few of the indications that deficiencies in particular essential nutrients lead to disease states.

The concept of *nutritional medicine* involves the evaluation and treatment of dietary and specific nutritional factors that may promote the illness, including the following:

- Macronutrient deficiencies and imbalances
- Marginal nutrient deficiencies
- Factors interfering with nutrient digestion and absorption
- Food sensitivities

In recent decades, advances in the discovery, isolation, and synthesis of vitamins, minerals, amino acids, fatty acids, and other nutrients have resulted in the availability of numerous substances provided in various formulations designed to supplement the diet to improve health, prevent illness, and promote healing. Such supplementations include the administration of pharmacologic (supraphysiologic) dosages of nutrients and products of intermediary metabolism and administration of *probiotics* (microorganisms with antagonistic activity toward pathogens in vivo).

When should these supplements be recommended to patients? The answer to the question is highly controversial in the light of blanket statements against the use of nutritional supplements that have been made by major mainstream professional organizations. Yet the use of supplements applied in a thoughtful and methodic manner can have a beneficial influence on health and healing.

Biologic Mechanism of Action

By definition, *micronutrients* are vitamins and minerals. They are unlike the macronutrients, carbohydrates, proteins, and fats in that they themselves they do not provide the cells with energy. Vitamins are organic compounds that act as catalysts to allow chemical reactions to occur quickly that would otherwise proceed extremely slowly or not at all. Minerals are inorganic elements that also allow for appropriate cellular activity. In addition to vitamins' role as coenzymes, they also perform other actions. For example, vitamin E is an antioxidant and vitamin D can function as a hormone.

Vitamins are classified as either fat-soluble (vitamins A, D, E, K, and F [essential fatty acids]) or water-soluble (vitamins C and B complex). Minerals are broken down into *macrominerals* (calcium, chloride, magnesium, phosphorous, potassium, silicon, sodium, and sulfur), *trace minerals* (chromium, cobalt, copper, iodine, iron, manganese, molybdenum, selenium, zinc, boron, fluoride, germanium, lithium, nickel, rubidium, strontium, tin, and vanadium) and *heavy metals* (aluminum, arsenic, cadmium, lead, mercury, antimony, barium, beryllium, bismuth, bromine, thallium, and germanium). Heavy metals do not have specific physiologic functions and often are present in the body as contaminants.

Both vitamins and minerals play a part in the function of all cells in our body. Conventional medicine used to view vitamin therapy for only frank nutritional deficiencies. Mineral replacement was considered only where medicines tended to cause deficiencies (such as diuretics) and an occasional disorder like the use of calcium replacement for osteoporosis. Today, however, thousands of articles and excellent research has led us to recognize that *subclinical* deficiencies of a micronutrient will eventually cause a less than optimal situation for an individual's health.

The biologic mechanisms of micronutrients are numerous. However, it is easy to learn the common nutritional deficiencies. These include B-complex, vitamin D, calcium, copper, iron, zinc, chromium, folic acid, iodine, magnesium, potassium, selenium, vitamin E, and vitamin C. Each of these play an integral part in human nutrition. For example, marginal deficiencies of zinc, copper, vitamin C, and selenium all have been implicated in immune disorders. Low calcium and magnesium levels often have been found in hypertensive patients. Cardiac dysrhythmias have been associated with low copper and potassium levels. Congestive heart failure patients often have low selenium levels and often are seen with low folic acid, copper, iron, and vitamin C levels. Even hypothyroidism has been associated with low iodine levels. It is important to recognize that vitamins and minerals also play an integral part with proper functioning of the brain and they have an important role in the adjunctive treatment of mental illness.

Impressive results for inpatients with virtually all chronic diseases have been seen with vitamin and mineral repletion. These micronutrients have been shown to improve fatigue, increase energy levels, improve muscular strength, coordination, decrease fatigue, increase energy, improve sleep patterns, decrease pain, and improve mental well-being, hormone levels, digestion, cardiovascular function, and immune status.

Marginal Deficiencies

Analyses of the adequacy of the diet for health usually use the Recommended Dietary Allowances (RDAs) as a measure of nutrient adequacy. These standards have been developed by the Food and Nutrition Board of the National Research Council (U.S.) as "the levels of intake of essential nutrients that, on the basis of scientific knowledge, are judged by the Food and Nutrition Board to be adequate to meet the known nutrient needs of practically all healthy persons."[2]

RDA levels are intentionally set high to provide a large margin of safety above the level of nutrient intake at which the earliest evidence of a deficiency begins to appear. For this reason, an intake of less than 70% of the RDA is often used as a measure below which a person is considered to be at risk of developing a deficiency of that nutrient.

When this measure is used as a cutoff point to analyze the data collected by the large surveys of food consumption by Americans, the results suggest that micronutrient deficiency may be common.[3] For example, analysis of data from the U.S.D.A. Nationwide Food Consumption Survey, conducted between 1977 and 1978, showed that up to 50% of all individuals surveyed may be at least marginally deficient in vitamin B6, almost one-third may be at least marginally deficient in vitamin A, and one-fourth may be at least marginally deficient in vitamin C.[4] These data, although suggestive, should not be taken as proof of widespread micronutrient deficiencies. The actual prevalence of micronutrient deficiencies in the survey populations was not studied and the methodology used in large dietary surveys tends to have many flaws.[5]

Micronutrient deficiencies are likely to be particularly common for several subgroups of the population that repeatedly have been shown to be at greater risk of becoming nutritionally deficient either because of increased needs or reduced intake.[6] In addition to the poor, these subgroups include the following: adolescents; moderate to heavy consumers of alcohol; cigarette smokers; drug users; diabetics; women who are pregnant, lactating, or on oral contraceptives; dieters; vegans; the chronically ill; and older adults.[7]

For example, analysis of data from the First Health and Nutrition Examination Survey conducted by the National Center for Health between 1971 and 1972 showed that 40% of older adults failed to consume two-thirds of the RDA for vitamin C; 28%, for calcium; 26%, for vitamin A; and 24%, for iron.[8] Examination and testing of people taken from these subpopulations has tended to confirm the suggestion of nutritional surveys that deficiencies are indeed common. As an example, in the U.S., roughly 5% to 10% of people over 60 years of age have clinical findings associated with vitamin deficiency.[9]

Gross malnutrition, advanced disease, and genetic factors may foster the development of severe nutrient deficiencies (see the table, "Stages of Micronutrient Deficiency"). These deficiencies take the form of numerous signs and symptoms, many of which are traceable to structural lesions and even organ failure. Frequently, however, nutrient deficiencies are only marginal; in this case, there may be no evidence of organic pathology, yet the deficiencies may adversely affect the body's ability to maintain health in the face of biologic and psychologic stressors.[1,6]

Stages of Micronutrient Deficiency

Degree of Deficiency	Stage	Presentation
Marginal (subclinical)	Preliminary	Normal (gradual depletion of micronutrient stores)
	Biochemical	Low energy (impaired biochemistry)
	Physiologic	Nonspecific symptoms
Definite (classical)	Clinical	Classical deficiency disease
	Anatomic	Fatal illness if untreated

Modified from Brin and Myron, *JAMA* 187:762-766, 1964.

Most of the evidence for the adverse effects of marginal nutrient deficiencies has come from studies of vitamins.[10] Numerous biologic changes now are known to be associated with marginal deficiencies, including fetal abnormalities, interference with the production or composition of breast milk, growth retardation, increased susceptibility to infection, altered response to dietary constituents, and the promotion of degenerative tissue changes.[11] Neuropsychologic symptoms such as lethargy, irritability, insomnia, and difficulty concentrating may develop (marginal vitamin deficiency), which, on testing, are associated with objective deficits in cognitive performance; moreover, these deficits can be correlated with electroencephalographic indices of neuropsychologic function (see the table, "Marginal Vitamin Deficiencies").[12]

Marginal Vitamin Deficiencies

Biologic Effects

Fetal abnormalities
Reduced breast milk production, adverse changes in breast milk composition
Growth retardation
Increased susceptibility to infection
Altered response to dietary constituents
Promotion of degenerative tissue changes
Neuropsychologic effects
Lethargy
Irritability
Insomnia
Difficulty concentrating

Iron is an example of a mineral that may have adverse health effects when only marginally deficient. Both fatigue[3] and cold intolerance[13] have been shown to be associated with a deficiency of iron that is too slight to produce iron-deficiency anemia.[14]

With aging, the need for certain nutrients increases, yet the ability to absorb these nutrients unfortunately decreases. This phenomenon contributes to the decline into many chronic diseases. The problem is compounded by several additional factors. First, the ingestion of empty calories in the form of refined starches, oils, and simple sugars increases requirements for certain micronutrients. Second, dieting often can create further deficiencies. Finally, soils in this country may be deficient in important nutrients making the task of obtaining the appropriate levels of micronutrients without supplementation nearly impossible. Without proper levels of micronutrients, metabolism is compromised, making healthy weight control difficult at best.

Although there are unique considerations concerning the therapeutic indications for each nutrient, there are certain general issues that need to be addressed before health practitioners can make informed decisions. The field of nutritional medicine generally can be divided into two parts: nutrient repletion and nutrient pharmacotherapy.

NUTRIENT REPLETION

Nutrient repletion consists of identifying nutritional deficiencies, prescribing appropriate foods and dietary supplements to attempt to correct those deficiencies, and monitoring progress. Although, in general, nutrient repletion is quite safe, there is the danger that repletion of a micronutrient may worsen a deficiency of another that is not being supplemented. The competitive interaction of copper and zinc is one of the most studied. Just a modest increase in dietary zinc can reduce copper absorption[1] and occasionally even produce a copper-deficiency anemia.[14] Zinc also interferes with the intestinal absorption of iron, and zinc supplementation can result in impaired iron nutriture.[15]

As long as nutrient repletion is accomplished by improving the diet, such negative interactions would not be expected to be a problem. A varied diet rich in any nutrients found to be deficient is likely to contain sufficient quantities of micronutrients whose adequacy may be threatened by negative interactions.

Sometimes, however, a recommendation for improving the diet, even with detailed instructions, is not sufficient to result in adequate nutrient repletion. Patients may fail to follow the recommendation over the long-term because of inadequate motivation to make what for them may be a major lifestyle change. Also, a healthy diet, although adequate to prevent nutritional deficiencies in most of the general population, may still prove to be inadequate to fully replete their deficiencies.

When dietary recommendations are not adequate to correct nutritional deficiencies, repletion may require nutrient supplementation. Because supplementation is focused on a limited list of nutrients, some nutrient deficiencies may not be identified and thus supplemented. Moreover, all nutrients that negatively interact with those supplemented may not be provided in adequate dosages to prevent their further depletion. These risks easily can be minimized, however, by the careful choice of nutrients for supplementation. Given the obvious benefits of nutrient repletion, they appear to be only a minor consideration.

NUTRIENT PHARMACOTHERAPY

Nutrient pharmacotherapy refers to the use of nutrients, often at dosages well in excess of the recommended dietary allowances, for the purpose of preventing or treating illnesses that are not caused by nutrient deficiencies.

The risks of nutrient pharmacotherapy generally are much greater than those risks of nutrient repletion. Nutrient pharmacotherapy shares with nutrient repletion the risk of negative interactions with other nutrients. However, because of the relatively larger dosages that are provided, the risk of creating deficiencies is substantially greater in nutrient pharmacotherapy.

LABORATORY TESTING

Studies of a group of people whose intake of a nutrient is marginally deficient often find that the serum levels of that nutrient are significantly lower for that group than those of a normal control group; however, the serum level of that nutrient for an individual with a marginally deficient intake frequently is within the normal range. In other words, the correlation from individual to individual between nutrient intake and serum levels is poor. This does not mean that marginal nutrient intake is necessarily unrelated to serum levels, for if the study group is divided into quartiles, those in the lowest quartile are more likely than those in the highest quartile to have below-normal serum levels of that nutrient.[16]

Because a patient with a marginal deficiency still may have a normal serum level of that nutrient, a procedure that tests the *functional adequacy* of the nutrient, when it is available, may be the best laboratory method of objectively proving the existence of a marginal nutrient deficiency that then may require dietary changes or possibly dietary supplementation.

A functional test specifically for vitamins compares the in vitro activity of an enzyme that requires a vitamin as coenzyme with versus without an additional supply of the vitamin in its active form. For example, erythrocyte glutamate-pyruvate transaminase activity is measured both with and without added pyridoxal phosphate (the active form of vitamin B_6).

Microbiologic assays are another type of functional vitamin assay. Microorganisms are given all the vitamins they need for growth except for the one being tested and the subject's blood is added to their dish. Later the proliferation of the organisms is quantified and compared to norms to provide a measure of the functional adequacy of that vitamin.

Loading tests are a type of functional testing that are applicable to a number of different nutrients. With this form of testing, the subject receives a fairly large dosage of the nutrient that is being tested, and the subsequent excretion of that nutrient is then measured. The greater the deficiency, the lower the percentage of the nutrient that the body will be able to excrete.

CLINICAL FINDINGS

Significant nutrient deficiencies can reflect in a variety of physical findings. One example of these physical findings include changes in nails, as seen in the corresponding table, "Nail Abnormality and Nutritional Deficiency."

Nail Abnormality and Nutritional Deficiency

Nail Abnormality	Nutritional Deficiency
Brittle	Calcium ↓ Essential fatty acids ↓ Iron ↓ Selenium ↑, (also thickened) Vitamin A ↑ Zinc ↓
Hyperpigmentation (subungual)	Vitamin B_{12} ↓ (brown, reticular)
Koilonychia (spooning)	Chromium ↓ Iron ↓ with ridging, brittleness, thinness, and lack of luster Vitamin C ↓ (scurvy), with other ungual alterations
Leukonychia (white spots on nails)	Zinc ↓
Splinter hemorrhages	Vitamin C ↓ (scurvy) (rare) (extensive hemorrhages in a semicircular lattice)

Forms of Therapy

Micronutrient therapy can be given through the use of several routes. The most common route for therapy is oral ingestion of the vitamin or minerals to be administered. Intravenous replacement also is used by physicians, particularly when the patient is unable to absorb oral nutrients. Other mechanisms, such as transcutaneous, intranasal, buccal, and sublingual routes and methods, also have been used to deliver these nutrients.

Demographics

Practitioners who are using micronutrients as part of medical care or part of the healing arts are homogenously spread throughout the United States and across the world. Individuals of all ages, ranging from infants to older adults, use micronutrients, which are often taken in the form of vitamin supplements. Although there seems to be no cultural or sex prevalence for users of micronutrients or micronutrient therapy, it is usually the female head of household who buys the majority of all foods and supplements for use by the entire family.

Practical Applications

Nutritional Evaluation

Although medical evaluation often is unnecessary before starting nutritional supplements, a full medical evaluation often is helpful in identifying problems that may benefit from supplementation. Ideally, every general medical evaluation should include a careful nutritional assessment. Not only does a nutritional evaluation extend the findings of the general medical evaluation, but the results of the general medical evaluation will suggest possible nutritional interventions, whether through diet or the use of supplementation.

History

Identify the major complaints that convinced the patient to seek professional help and then ask for the history of these complaints from inception until the present. Clues often can be found by asking what factors seem to influence these complaints, such as stress, particular foods, or the phase of the menstrual cycle. Ask yourself if any of these symptoms or a combination of them could be the result of a nutritional deficiency. For example, a history of diminished taste and smell should cause you to suspect a zinc deficiency. The history of any other illnesses, including allergies, should be included. A history of illnesses in the immediate family may bring out the possibility of a common genetic factor that would increase the chances of the patient having the same illness as previously diagnosed in a biologic relative.

Information on the current diet, as well as a dietary history, are essential. Include the use of alcoholic and caffeinated beverages. Ask about food cravings, a symptom that may suggest food sensitivities. Bloating after meals is particularly suspicious of a deficiency of hydrochloric acid. Is there a history of abdominal cramping or abnormal bowel movements? This may suggest the possibility of abnormal gut microecology, which could be responsible for nutritional deficiencies.

Record all use of nutritional supplements and ask if ingestion of any of these supplements has had a noticeable effect. All drugs, including illegal drugs and tobacco, should be listed and their interactions with nutrients should be investigated.

Physical Examination

Every physical examination should include evaluation for gross malnutrition, something that most practicing physicians fail to do.

Between 25% and 50% of patients admitted to an acute medical service are malnourished. Physicians are often unaware which patients are admitted at nutritional risk and make no attempt to arrest further nutritional decline until a dramatic deterioration has occurred.

We studied all patients admitted to an acute medical ward before and after their physicians were taught to recognize nutritional deficiency early and to intervene appropriately. During the initial period, the house staff correctly identified two (12.5%) of 16 patients as being malnourished. During the posteducation period, physicians correctly identified all 14 patients admitted at nutritional risk (100%).[17]

Malnourished patients may appear to be obviously wasted, with muscle atrophy, flaccid subcutaneous tissue, and pallor. Most, however, will not seem to be overtly malnourished.[18] Two objective measures of malnourishment include: 1) lean body mass (skeletal muscle mass), in which the nondominant midarm circumference is subtracted from the triceps skinfold thickness, multiplied by 0.314, and then expressed as the percent deviation from published norms; and 2) body fat stores, in which three consecutive measurements of the skinfold thickness of the nondominant midarm triceps skinfold are measured with a Lange caliper, averaged, and compared to published norms.

Also look for signs of deficiencies of micronutrients. For example, a swollen, magenta-colored tongue suggests a niacin or a riboflavin deficiency, while dry skin suggests a deficiency of essential fatty acids.

Laboratory Testing

As in many areas of medicine, there has been a explosion of laboratory tests relevant to nutritional medicine. It always is tempting to do some testing because the additional information makes the clinical picture more comprehensive. However, because of the additional charges, practitioners should ask themselves which tests, if any, are necessary to make appropriate treatment decisions. This question is best answered after the history and physical examination have been completed. Often, at that point, enough information already has been gleaned so that testing is unlikely to affect current treatment.

A common situation that may require testing is in the evaluation of a patient with nonspecific symptoms and an inconclusive physical exam. The question then becomes one of choosing which tests are most needed to clarify the clinical picture. Sometimes testing is not needed initially but becomes important to find new diagnostic clues later on, when the initial treatment has failed.

Some types of laboratory testing that can be particularly helpful include the following:

1. General medical evaluation
   a. Hematologic parameters
   b. Measures of endocrine function
   c. Measures of immune function
   d. Measures of kidney function
   e. Measures of liver function
2. Measures of digestive function
   a. Gastric acidity
   b. Intestinal permeability
   c. Stool analysis
3. Nutritional evaluation
   a. Protein-energy malnutrition
   b. Vitamins
   c. Minerals
   d. Amino acids
   e. Fatty acids

Prescribing Nutritional Supplements

Nutritional medicines have been claimed to be beneficial for thousands of applications, although scientific proof of their efficacy often has not been well-established. A practical approach applies to the use of nutritional supplements as much as it does to prescription medications. A trial of a nutrient at a pharmacologic dosage for an unproved application is inadvisable unless the risk of adverse effects is fairly well-established. If, however, the risk is known, then treatment may be considered with that nutrient, based on its relative advantages and disadvantages to the patient when compared to competing treatments.

The following suggestions that apply specifically to choosing nutritional supplements:

1. Start with improving the diet.
2. Consider drug-nutrient, disease-nutrient, and nutrient-nutrient interactions.
3. Investigate the supplement's bioavailability.
4. If your patient may be sensitive to foods or food additives, recommend supplements that are not derived from the inciting foods and minimize the use of excipients (colorings, binders, and others).[19]

Research Base

Evidence Based

There are literally thousands of articles supporting the use of micronutrients, often targeted at specific effects of excess or deficiency for the various vitamins and minerals in normal and disease states. Standard texts on the subject are listed in "Suggested Reading."

Clinical Trials

Whatever the appeal of a specific nutritional supplement, remember that supplements are designed to *supplement* nutrients found in the diet. Whole foods are complex mixtures of numerous chemical substances, many of which have been poorly researched. Our knowledge of the relationship of these substances to health and healing is fragmentary and largely rudimentary. We know even less about the nutritional importance of the ratios that exist between the quantities of these substances within a food, as well as the ratios that exist between foods.

In repeated instances, our conclusions regarding therapeutic diets have been refuted long after they have become standard clinical practice. Examples are sugar avoidance in diabetic diets (refuted when the actual glycemic responses of individual carbohydrates were measured) and the milk-based diet for the treatment of peptic ulcer (refuted when it was found that milk produces an acid rebound).

We also suffer from limited knowledge about individual differences in nutrient needs, including differences in absorption, metabolism, use, and excretion. In addition to differences in baseline nutrient intake, these differences are due to numerous factors, including genetics, gender, age, illness, physical exercise, psychologic stress, exposure to toxins, and others.

The decision to add a specific quantity of a nutrient as a supplement to the diet of a particular person is therefore not an entirely rational one, even when there is an extensive body of scientific literature documenting the efficacy of that nutrient for a proposed clinical application. Therefore until we better understand the underlying mechanisms by which diet affects health, nutritional supplements should be viewed as adjunctive to the best possible diet.

Basic Science

See "Suggested Reading."

Risk and Safety

In large doses, micronutrients can have adverse reactions. These are mainly gastrointestinal in nature. Pain, diarrhea, and nausea have been noted. In addition, rashes, headaches, and allergic complications also have been noted.

In the case of organ dysfunction, other problems may occur. For example, liver disorders may affect how beta-carotene is absorbed and used. The same difficulty could occur with other fat-soluble vitamins. Minerals in large doses can be toxic to the liver, kidney, heart, and digestive tract. High doses of fat-soluble vitamins cannot be effectively excreted and can lead to toxicity. Sufficiently large doses of certain minerals could prove fatal. For example, in patients with kidney failure, foods rich in potassium may lead to hyperkalemia and potentially fatal cardiac arrhythmias.

Efficacy

A massive volume of data suggests that nutrients provided above their RDA level can reduce the risk of illness, although in most cases the efficacy of preventive nutrient supplementation in greater than RDA dosages has yet to be proven by long-term, randomized, double-blind studies.

As a recent example of the growing epidemiologic evidence, 11,348 noninstitutionalized adults were followed for a median of 10 years and mortality was related to their total vitamin C intake. The relationship between the standardized mortality ratio for all causes of death and increasing vitamin C intake was found to be strongly inverse for men and weakly inverse for women. When men with a daily vitamin C intake in the 300 to 400 mg range were compared to those who consume less than 50 mg per day, their death rate was 35% lower, while the death rate for women was 10% lower. Even after adjustment for the usual confounding variables, the relationship between vitamin C intake and mortality remained for the men.[20]

In regard to the treatment of established illness, controlled studies demonstrating the efficacy of high-dose nutrient supplementation continue to appear in the literature although most of the evidence supporting the thousands of applications of nutrient pharmacotherapy is only preliminary in nature.[21] Some of the better proven applications include niacin supplementation to reduce elevated cholesterol levels, pyridoxine to reduce infantile seizures and premenstrual symptoms, folic acid in early pregnancy to prevent neural tube defects, and magnesium in acute coronary insufficiency to reduce the risk of myocardial infarction, cardiac arrhythmias, and death.

Future Research Opportunities and Priorities

Constant disease-oriented research with micronutrients is occurring. The literature is replete with new studies monthly.

Druglike Information

Safety

When providing micronutrients for patients, we must always consider the possibility that we will create potential imbalances or relative deficiencies in other phytonutrients that have not been extracted or artificially produced in a tablet or capsule. The good news is that vitamin toxicity is extremely rare and fatalities are almost unheard of. Minerals, on the other hand, have a narrow range of "normal" within our systems. Too much or too little can have serious consequences. A thorough understanding of physiology and anatomy is required for safe application of pharmacologic doses of micronutrients. Recognize that there are nutrient-nutrient as well as drug-nutrient interactions. These interactions may either potentiate or reduce the effectiveness of one or the other substances.

Actions and Pharmacokinetics

Most micronutrients are metabolized by the liver and excreted by the kidney or gastrointestinal tract. If any of these systems are impaired, so will be the use of the vitamin or mineral. Dosages must be adjusted accordingly.

Warnings, Contraindications, and Precautions

As long as nutrient repletion is accomplished by improving the diet, such negative interactions would not be expected to be a problem. A varied diet rich in the nutrients found to be deficient is likely to contain sufficient quantities of micronutrients whose adequacy may be threatened by negative interactions, including those that are marginally deficient but may not have been identified as such.

Sometimes, however, a recommendation for improving the diet, even with detailed instructions, is not sufficient to result in adequate nutrient repletion. Patients may fail to follow the recommendation over the long term because of inadequate motivation to make what for them may be a major lifestyle change. Also, a healthy diet, although adequate to prevent nutritional deficiencies in most of the general population, still may prove inadequate to fully replete their deficiencies. The failure may be a result of poor nutrient absorption or nutrient dependency; that is, a requirement for an unusually large amount of a nutrient to achieve an adequate state of nutriture to satisfy metabolic needs.

For example, some people have an inborn deficiency of the enzyme cystathionine beta-synthase. This enzyme is quite important because it metabolizes homocysteine, a toxic amino acid that contributes to the development of atherosclerosis. For about 50% of the people with cystathionine beta-synthase deficiency, high supplementary doses of vitamin

B_6 will push the reaction forward, markedly reducing or even eliminating the biochemical abnormalities.[22] In other words, this subgroup is dependent on doses of vitamin B_6 well in excess of the RDA if they wish to prevent their genetic abnormality from promoting the development of atherosclerotic changes.

When dietary recommendations are not adequate to correct nutritional deficiencies, repletion may require nutrient supplementation. Because supplementation is focused on a limited list of nutrients, some nutrient deficiencies may not be identified and thus supplemented. Moreover, all nutrients that negatively interact with the ones being supplemented may not be provided in adequate dosages to prevent their further depletion. These risks can easily be minimized, however, by the careful choice of nutrients for supplementation. Given the obvious benefits of nutrient repletion, they appear to be only a minor consideration.

Adverse Reactions

Four risk factors are shared by drugs and nutritional medicines. First, adverse effects can be the result of exaggerated responses to either the desired or undesired pharmacologic effects. These reactions are believed to be the most common cause of untoward effects and often can be treated by adjustment of the dosage. Second, impurities formed during the manufacturing process may cause untoward reactions. Eosinophilia-myalgia syndrome, for example, has been largely traced to a contaminant formed during the manufacture of L-tryptophan.[23] Third, the active substance may be formulated with other ingredients to facilitate its administration and increase its bioavailability. These preservatives, vehicles and excipients, although considered therapeutically inactive, occasionally may be the cause of adverse reactions.[6] Fourth, there may be unpredictable "allergic" reactions, such as occurs extremely rarely with injections of thiamine at pharmacologic dosages.

There also is the risk of adverse effects from nutrient toxicity, a risk that is not encountered in nutrient repletion. Fortunately, the body has a number of mechanisms unique to nutrients for preventing high doses from becoming toxic. For example, as the oral dose of some of the vitamins, major minerals, trace elements, amino acids, and glucose increases beyond a threshold, the percentage of absorption from the gut is reduced. Similarly, the percentage of the dosage excreted tends to increase as the dosage of a nutrient is increased beyond a threshold. These mechanisms can become overwhelmed, however, if the dosages are too high. Other factors, such as the storage of fat-soluble vitamins in body tissues, also contribute to the danger of toxicity from high dosages of nutrients.

The relationship between effective pharmacologic doses of nutrients and nutrient toxicity is highly variable. A number of nutrients, such as vitamin B_{12}, have no known toxicity at any dose. Most, such as calcium, only are administered at doses well below their minimum toxic dose, while a few, such as vitamin A, are sometimes used at doses at the low end of their toxic range.

The table "Poison Exposures: Outcomes" is excerpted from the 1988 annual report by the American Association of Poison Control Centers Data Collection System.[24] It supports the hypothesis that nutritional supplements in general are considerably less toxic than drugs.

Poison Exposures: Outcomes			
	Vitamins	**Minerals**	**Drugs**
Totals	23,870	8416	298,284
No effect	81.0%	69.0%	61.0%
Minor effect	18.0%	27.0%	32.0%
Moderate effect	1.3%	3.2%	6.1%
Major effect	0.03%	0.25%	1.21%
Death	0.004%	0.05%	0.15%

Few nutrients at appropriate pharmacologic doses are as dangerous as easily available over-the-counter medications, such as aspirin. Some (such as folacin, pantothenic acid, riboflavin, and vitamin B_{12}) fail to show evidence of toxicity even at dosages of 100 times their RDAs. As long as the dosage of a nutrient is below its minimum toxic dose, it is doubtful that it is as dangerous as aspirin. If its therapeutic dosage reaches into the toxic range, however, the risk of toxicity must be weighed against its potential benefits.

For example, vitamin A, the most potentially toxic of the vitamins, is an example of a nutrient with therapeutic applications at dosages that are sometimes above its minimum toxic dosage of approximately 25,000 IU daily. Its pharmacologic benefits usually can be obtained at doses of 100,000 IU daily or less, especially if it is combined with vitamin E, with which it has a synergistic effect.[25] Because toxicity is uncommon at doses below 100,000 IU[26] and because adverse effects not due to toxicity are rare, its safety profile at pharmacologic doses compares reasonably well with that of many prescription drugs. Iron, by contrast, even though it is an essential trace mineral, should not be supplemented other than to prevent or replete a deficiency; otherwise there are no known benefits and considerable risks of overdose, particularly in infants and small children.

As is the case for drugs, the level of nutrient supplementation that results in toxicity, as well as the length of time that it takes before toxicity develops, varies enormously between individuals. Therefore if the risk-benefit ratio is sufficiently low, it still may be appropriate to use a dosage of a nutrient that is known to be above its minimum toxic dosage, but only as long as the patient is monitored for the earliest signs of toxicity. If toxicity starts to develop, discontinuing the supplement then will be considered.

Drug or Other Interactions

If a person is taking a medication, nutrient-drug interactions are of concern. Examples are folic acid supplements, which decrease the anticonvulsant action of phenytoin, and calcium supplements, which practically nullify the efficacy of tetracycline if the two are taken together. (Many of these interactions can be avoided by instructing patients to take their supplements 1 hour before or at least 2 hours after taking medication.)

Negative interactions are a danger that is not limited to nutrients. Just as nutrient supplementation carries the risk of negative interactions with other nutrients, drugs often have potentially dangerous interactions with other drugs, a factor that contributes substantially to adverse drug reactions in people taking multiple drugs—as is often the case with cancer patients. Moreover, many drugs also have negative interactions with nutrients, potentially causing nutrient deficiencies that are unhealthy. A well-known example is impairment of gastrointestinal absorption and increased urinary excretion of sodium and potassium caused by thiazide diuretics, an interaction that may result in an inadequate supply of these two essential minerals, manifested by muscle weakness and other adverse effects. In the field of cancer chemotherapy an example of a drug-nutrient interaction would be methotrexate causing inhibition of the dihydrofolate reductase enzyme and possibly leading to manifestations of a folate deficiency.

Pregnancy and Lactation

Pregnant and lactating women must be cautious as to their ingestion of the fat-soluble vitamins. The only mineral whose requirement doubles in pregnancy is calcium, and the only vitamin requirement that doubles is folic acid.

Trade Products, Administration, and Dosage

Dosages vary from condition to condition. There are many companies that make micronutrients. We prefer the professional lines whose standards seem to be better. The FDA does not regulate micronutrients except as part of a food. Therefore the potencies on the bottles can vary significantly from company to company. We suggest you find a product you are comfortable with and that will allow you to titrate the dosage as needed.

Consider bioavailability issues when choosing a particular supplement for your patient. Fillers, capsules, sprays, tablets, and patches all may affect the absorption potential. Minerals are best absorbed if in a chelated or Kreb's Cycle formulation.

Self-Help versus Professional

Many individuals read popular books on nutrition and begin a supplement program. This often leads to supplement polypharmacy, as the individual keeps adding supplements to the regimen, one at a time. For basic supplementation of a vitamin or mineral tablet, self-prescribing is fine. But for the use of micronutrient supplements to assist with managing illness, professional help for individual needs is imperative.

Visiting a Professional

A first visit usually is long enough to assess nutritional status and may include a complete history and physical examination. Discussion on all aspects of the patient's medical history includes a detailed evaluation of current diet and micronutrient intake. Further studies would be discussed and a future appointment should be made to go over all results and set an individualized treatment plan. Some of the thought process involved in the evaluation is detailed in "Practical Applications."

Credentialing

Two certifying examinations do exist for nutritional therapy. Licensing varies greatly from state to state. The two certifying boards are the Certification Board for Nutrition Specialists and the Clinical Nutrition Board.

Certification Board for Nutrition Specialists
Hospital for Joint Diseases
301 E. 17th St.
New York, NY 10003
Tel: (212) 777-1037
Fax: (212) 777-1103

Clinical Nutrition Certification Board
5200 Keller Springs Rd., Suite 410
Dallas, TX 75248
Tel: (972) 250-2829
Fax: (972) 250-0333

The Certification Board for Nutrition Specialists provides Certification as a Certified Nutrition Specialist (CNS). Eligibility requires an advanced degree (masters or doctoral level) from a regionally accredited university program in the field of nutrition, nutritional sciences, or a field allied to nutrition and relevant to the practice of nutrition in a professional setting. Licensed physicians also are eligible. Please contact the board for more detailed information on eligibility.

The Clinical Nutrition Board provides the title of Certified Clinical Nutritionist (CCN). Eligibility requires a bachelor's degree or equivalent, plus a 900 hour clinical nutrition internship.

Training

Advanced training in nutrition is available at many universities.

What to Look for in a Provider

Experience is paramount. The practitioner who is prescribing for you should have significant training. Good examples are terminal degrees such as a master's degree or PhD in Nutrition, or naturopathic physicians or medical physicians (DOs or MDs) with significant amounts of postgraduate course work in nutrition.

Barriers and Key Issues

In regard to treating nutrient deficiencies, the risks of nutrient repletion are small, while the benefits are compelling. The lack of sufficient randomized and controlled intervention trials makes it more difficult to make generalizations concerning the risk-benefit ratio of nutrient pharmacotherapy. In general, nutritional medicines appear to be far safer than drugs, but more evidence is needed to confirm this impression.

As more articles appear in the conventional literature, interest and acceptance is developing for vitamin and mineral replacement. Pharmaceutic companies, which often are responsible in large part for physician training in a particular drug use, now are beginning to produce vitamins and minerals. It no longer is unusual for a cardiologist to suggest that a patient take vitamin E, a family physician to prescribe vitamin C or a general multivitamin, or an internist to suggest B-complex to improve a patient's energy. Patients now expect their physician to have a working knowledge of nutrition and supplements. Failure to have this knowledge is an open invitation for the patient to seek counsel elsewhere, and often from potentially less reliable sources.

Associations

The American College for Advancement in Medicine (ACAM)
23121 Verdugo Dr., Suite 4
Laguna Hills, CA 92653
Tel: (800) 532-3688
E-mail: acam@acam.org
www.acam.org

Great Lakes College of Clinical Medicine
1407-B N. Wells St.
Chicago, IL 60610
Tel: (800) 286-6013
E-mail: info@glccm.org
www.glccm.org

International College of Advanced Longevity Medicine (ICALM)
1407-B N. Wells St.
Chicago, IL 60610
Tel: (800) 286-6013
E-mail: drgary@netzone.com
www.incalm.com

Suggested Reading

1. Werbach M: *Nutritional influences on illness,* ed 2, Tarzana, Calif, 1993, Third Line Press.
2. Werbach M: *Nutritional influences on mental illness,* ed 2, Tarzana, Calif, 1999, Third Line Press.
   A text categorized by disease that allows the user to see possible micronutrient usage. There are hundreds of scientific studies cited.
3. Werbach M, Moss J: *Textbook of nutritional medicine,* Tarzana, Calif, 1999, Third Line Press.
   The first true textbook in the field.

4. Werbach M: *Foundations of nutritional medicine*.
   An excellent reference text that discusses common nutritional deficiencies, nutrient interactions, and bioavailability.

5. Hamilton K: *Clinical pearls*, Sacramento, ITServices.
   There are several years of these texts to choose from. They are a compilation of thousands of articles in the literature about micronutrients and their application to the treatment of disease. For more information, e-mail at office@clinicalpearls.com.

Bibliography

American Medical News, October 5, 1992, p. 32.

Belongia EA et al: An investigation of the cause of the eosinophilia-myalgia syndrome associated with tryptophan use, *N Engl J Med* 323(6):357-365, 1990.

Crayhon R: *Nutrition made simple*, New York, 1994, M. Evans.

Dean C: *Complementary natural prescriptions for common ailments*, New Canaan, Conn, 1994, Keats.

Drug Evaluations Subscription, Chicago, 1990, American Medical Association, 1:22-26.

Forbes RM, Erdman JW Jr: Bioavailability of trace mineral elements, *Annu Rev Nutr* 3:213-221, 1983.

Jick H: Drugs—remarkably nontoxic, *N Engl J Med* 291(16):824-828, 1974.

Kaldor JM et al: Leukemia following chemotherapy for ovarian cancer, *N Engl J Med* 322:1-6, 1990.

Kaldor JM et al: Leukemia following Hodgkin's disease, *N Engl J Med* 322:7-13, 1990.

Lieberman S, Bruning N: *The real vitamin and mineral book*, York, 1997, Avery.

Marginal vitamin deficiency: the "gray area" of nutrition, *Vitamin issues* 2(2), 1980.

Melmon KL: Preventable drug reactions: causes and cures, *N Engl J Med* 284(24):1361-1368, 1971.

Murray M, Pizzorno J: *Encyclopedia of natural medicine*, Rocklin, Calif, 1991, Prima.

Schneider-Helmert D, Spinweber CL: *Evaluation of L-tryptophan for treatment of insomnia: a review*, Naval Health Res Center, Naval Med Res Develop Com, Rep 84(4), Jan 1984.

Sears B: *The zone*, New York, 1995, Regan Books.

Stewart ML et al: Vitamin/mineral supplement use: a telephone survey of adults in the United States, *J Am Diet Assoc* 85:1585-1590, 1985.

Werbach M: *Foundations of nutritional medicine*, Tarzana, Calif, 1997, Third Line Press.

Werbach M: *Nutritional influences on illness*, ed 2, Tarzana, Calif, 1993, Third Line Press.

Werbach M: *Nutritional influences on mental illness*, ed 2, Tarzana, Calif, 1999, Third Line Press.

References

1. Folkers K: Renaissance in biomedical and clinical research on vitamins and coenzymes, *J Optimal Nutr* 1(1):11-15, 1992.

2. *Recommended dietary allowances*, Washington, DC, 1989, National Academy Press.

3. Beutler E et al: Iron therapy in chronically fatigued nonanemic women: a double-blind study, *Ann Intern Med* 52:378, 1960.

4. Pao EM, Mickle SJ: Problem nutrients in the United States, *Food Technol* 35:58-79, 1981.

5. National Research Council: *Nutrient adequacy: assessment using food consumption surveys,* Washington, D.C., 1986, National Academy Press.

6. Brin M: Erythrocyte as a biopsy tissue in the functional evaluation of thiamin status, *JAMA* 187:762-766, 1964.

7. Enstrom JE, Kanim LE, Klein MA: Vitamin C intake and mortality among a sample of the United States population, *Epidemiol* 3(3):194-202, 1992.

8. Norton L, Wozny MC: Residential location and nutritional adequacy among elderly adults, *J Gerontol* 39(5):592-595, 1984.

9. Bowman BB, Rosenberg IH: Assessment of the nutritional status of the elderly, *Am J Clin Nutr* 35(5 Suppl):1142-1151, 1982.

10. Forbes RM, Erdman JW Jr: *Annu Rev Nutr* 3:213, 1983.

11. Thurnham DI: Red cell enzyme tests of vitamin status: do marginal deficiencies have any physiological significance? *Proc Nutr Soc* 40:155-163, 1981.

12. Tucker DM et al: Nutrition status and brain function in aging, *Am J Clin Nutr* 52:93-102, 1990.

13. Kirn TF: Do low levels of iron affect body's ability to regulate temperature, experience cold? News, *JAMA* 260(5):607, 1988.

14. Gordon DJ, Levander OA, editors: *Nutrition '87,* Washington, DC, 1987, American Institute of Nutrition.

15. Yadrick MK et al: Iron, copper, and zinc status: response to supplementation with zinc or zinc and iron in adult females, *Am J Clin Nutr* 49:145-150, 1989.

16. Smith JL: Dietary status of Americans. In *Vitamin supplementation: a factual perspective,* Nutley, N.J., 1983, Hoffman-La Roche.

17. Roubenoff R et al: Malnutrition among hospitalized patients. A problem of physician awareness, *Arch Intern Med* 147(8):1462-1465, 1987.

18. Wright RA: Commentary: nutritional assessment, *JAMA* 244(6):559-560, 1980.

19. Napke E, Stevens DG: Excipients and additives: hidden hazards in drug products and in product substitution, *Can Med Assoc J* 131(12):1449-1452, 1984.

20. Enstrom JE, Kanim LE, Klein MA: Vitamin C intake and mortality among a sample of the United States population, *Epidemiol* 3(3):194-202, 1992.

21. National Research Council: *Nutrient adequacy: assessment using food consumption surveys,* Washington, DC, 1986, National Academy Press.

22. Mudd SH: Homocystinuria. In Wyngaarden JB, Smith LH Jr, editors: *Cecil: textbook of medicine,* ed 18, Philadelphia, 1988, W.B. Saunders.

23. Belongia EA et al: An investigation of the cause of the eosinophilia-myalgia syndrome associated with tryptophan use, *N Engl J Med* 323(6):357-365, 1990.

24. Lotovitz TL, Schmitz BF, Holm KC: 1988 annual report of the American Association of Poison Control Centers National Data Collection System, *Am J Emerg Med* 7(5):495, 1989.

25. Ayres S, Mihan R, Scribner MD: Synergism of vitamins A and E with dermatologic applications, *Cutis* 23:600-603, 689-690, 1979.

26. Bauernfeind JC: *The safe use of vitamin A: a report of the International Vitamin A Consultative Group,* Washington, DC, 1980, The Nutrition Foundation.

Oxidative Stress

JEFFREY S. BLAND

Origins and History

In a landmark paper published in 1957, Denham Harman, MD, PhD, speculated that aging in all living systems might be related to free radical chemistry and the damaging effects of free radicals on cellular constituents.[1] Harman pointed out that free radicals increased with increasing metabolic activity and their production is related to alterations in biologic oxidation-reduction reactions. He suggested that aging and degenerative diseases may be caused by side effects of free radicals and that antioxidants may help protect against free radical oxidative damage.

During the early 1970s, Irwin Fridovich, MD, pointed out that one of the most important oxidants in cellular systems could be superoxide, created as a consequence of the univalent reduction of molecular oxygen to a free radical-like species.[2] It was Linus Pauling, PhD, who first proposed in the 1920s that oxygen could be converted to superoxide and could be important in physiology.[3] Fridovich suggested that superoxide might have significant relevance to biology and medicine through its ability to increase free radical activity in cellular systems. Superoxide, in turn, may be interrelated with other reactive oxygen species, such as hydrogen peroxide, lipid peroxides, single oxygen, and hydroxyl radical.

William Pryor, PhD, was one of the first scientists to study free radical reactions in biochemical systems, using kinetic measurements.[4] A *free radical* is a molecule with an unpaired electron, which as an electrophile is in search of high electron density. The electron-deficient species, such as hydroxyl radical or lipid peroxy radical that has been derived from the oxidative damage of unsaturated fatty acids, will seek out sites of high electron density within biologic systems, such as membrane lipids, nucleic acids, and the amino acid residues within proteins and enzymes. Pryor pointed out that free radicals can be produced within biologic systems by exposure to ionizing radiation, enzyme activity, activation of the oxidative burst within phagocytic cells in the immune system, exposure to dietary free radical catalysts, transition metal-catalyzed oxidative reactions (as from excessive free iron, copper or other transition metals), and airborne prooxidants that can be exchanged across the lung-blood barrier (such as those derived from cigarette smoke).

More recently, Helmut Sies, PhD, described the physiologic state associated with increased production of reactive oxygen species (ROS) as "oxidative stress."[5] In 1985 he defined oxidative stress as a disturbance in the prooxidant-antioxidant balance in favor of the

595

prooxidant state. In this situation the organism is under increased exposure to ROS, which participate in free radical-induced alteration of cellular components through an exponential chain radical-carrying mechanism.

Protection against the pathology induced by these oxidant species is provided by a broad class of agents called *antioxidants*, represented by both small molecules such as tocopherol and ascorbate, and enzymes like superoxide dismutase.

Increased risk of oxidative stress and the adverse effects of ROS on cellular species can result from many factors, including exposure to alcohol, medications, trauma, cold, toxins, or radiation, as indicated in the figure below.

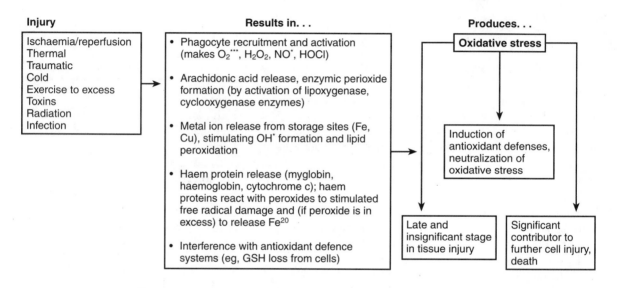

Protection against all of these processes depends upon the adequacy of various antioxident substances derived either directly or indirectly from diet, as shown in the corresponding table.

Oxidative stress also can result from exposure of the liver to xenobiotic substances that induce oxidative reactions by upregulating cytochrome P-450 mixed-function oxidase. This process can deplete specific cellular antioxidants, such as glutathione, vitamin C, or vitamin E.[6] Recently, ROS have been associated with the pathology of a number of liver diseases, and antioxidants have been found to provide important protection.[7] Our own research found that an antioxidant-enriched diet is capable of supporting liver detoxification function in "apparently healthy" humans, helping to defend against oxidative stress.[8]

Oxygen-Induced Pathology

Over millennia of natural selection, aerobic organisms have developed a sophisticated antioxidant protection system to defend against oxidative stress and ROS. As a result of breathing atmospheric gases that are 21% oxygen, oxygen-breathing organisms have developed antioxidant systems that are perfectly adapted to this level of oxygen but not to levels exceeding 21%.

Antioxidants from the Diet	
Constituent	**Action**
Known to be important Vitamin E (fat-soluble)	General name for group of compounds, of which α-tocopherol is most important, that inhibit lipid peroxidation. Important in protection against cardiovascular disease.
Widely thought to be an important antioxidant Vitamin C (ascorbic acid)	Essential for several metabolic roles, for example, in collagen synthesis and hormone production. Inhibits nitrosamine carcinogenesis by direct reduction of these compounds. Probably assists α-tocopherol in inhibition of lipid peroxidation by recycling the tocopherol radical: $T^{\bullet}$ + ascorbate → TH + ascorbate. Good scavenger of many free radicals and may help to detoxify inhaled oxidizing air pollutants (ozone, $NO_2^{\bullet}$, free radicals in cigarette smoke) in the respiratory tract. In animals, high concentrations of ascorbate partly compensate for low levels of GSH. However, mixtures of ascorbate with iron or copper ions can accelerate oxidative damage in vitro; this often is dismissed as irrelevant in vivo because such ions usually are safely protein-bound. However, "free" iron or copper ions can be released at sites of tissue injury and there is increasing evidence to link high body-stores of iron or copper to human disease.
Probably important, but not necessarily as antioxidants β-carotene, other carotenoids, related plant pigments	Increasing epidemiologic evidence exists that high intake of such molecules is associated with diminished risk of cancer and cardiovascular disease, especially in smokers. Often simplistically grouped with vitamins E and C as antioxidants. Many carotenoids exert antioxidant effects in vitro under certain conditions.
Possibly important Flavonoids, other plant phenolics	Plants contain phenolic compounds that inhibit lipid peroxidation and lipoxygenases in vitro (such as flavonoids), although (similar to ascorbate) they can sometimes be prooxidant if mixed with iron ions in vitro. The bioavailability of these plant-derived substances from the diet is not yet well understood, and therefore their full impact on the antioxidant potential of the individual is unclear.

Organisms exposed to greater oxygen concentrations for an extended period of time may risk increased oxidative damage. For example, Halliwell pointed out that exposure of adults to pure oxygen at one atmosphere for as little as 6 hours causes chest soreness, cough, and sore throat in some subjects, and longer periods of exposure leads to oxidative damage to the alveoli.[9] Exposure of premature infants to the oxygen-enriched environment of the incubator has been shown to increase the risk of ocular damage and the condition known as *retrolental fibroplasia* (RF), which is the formation of fibrous tissue behind the lens of the eye. Administration of higher doses of vitamin E to these children significantly decreases the incidence of RF, indicating the important role of an enhanced level of antioxidants in protecting against oxidative stress.[10]

There is strong evidence that damage to DNA, proteins and enzymes, lipids, and small molecules such as uric acid occurs as a consequence of increased production of ROS within cellular systems. Many years ago it was shown that animals exposed to oxidative stress in the absence of adequate antioxidants had enhanced production of "age pigments" called *lipofuscin* and *ceroid*.[11] The accumulation of cellular debris as a consequence of exposure to ROS is associated with a number of disorders ascribed to premature biologic aging. Control of free radicals and ROS in biologic systems may therefore be very important in defending against disease processes that contribute to age-related disorders.

Oxidants, Antioxidants, and Atherosclerosis

Accumulating evidence indicates that oxidative stress also contributes to damage to lipoproteins that may relate to the origin of atherosclerosis. For several years, considerable attention has been placed on hypercholesterolemia as a major risk factor for heart disease, but the oxidation hypothesis of atherogenesis has recently emerged, suggesting that factors other than cholesterol can contribute to the incidence of heart disease.[12] Oxidative modification of LDL is a prerequisite for macrophage uptake and cellular accumulation of cholesterol. Earl Benditt, MD, advanced the monoclonal theory of atherosclerosis more than 10 years ago. Benditt proposed that certain mutagenic insults may have transformed the cells within the arterial wall into a state of monoclonal hyperplasia that results in the atheroma.[13] This model suggests that agents like ROS, which could cause alteration in the replication rate of cells within the arterial wall, could initiate an atheroma. It now is felt that reactive oxygen species result not only in the oxidative modification of cells in the arterial wall and plasma lipoproteins, but also in cholesterol itself, producing cholesterol oxides, all of which may be mutagenic and induce monoclonal hyperplasia.

Antioxidants may help prevent oxidation of LDL and may play a role in protecting against atherogenesis. LDL is very rich in antioxidants like vitamin E, which appear to be critical for its protection.[14] It may be possible to reduce prooxidant activity by enhancing the antioxidant content of cells, such as enriching them with ascorbate, tocopherol, or beta-carotene.

A genetic propensity toward oxidation of LDL may account for certain family-related risk factors for heart disease. Drs. Iris Rajman, Martin Kendall, and Robert Cramb at Queen Elizabeth Hospital in Birmingham, England, recently proposed that antioxidant therapy to prevent atherosclerosis might be most effective in patients who have genetically-determined small LDL particles, which are more susceptible to oxidative stress.[15]

In a recent retrospective study, Walter Willett, PhD, and his colleagues found that nurses who consumed higher amounts of vitamin E on a routine basis had a 41% lower incidence of heart disease than nurses who consumed the lowest level of vitamin E from their diet and supplements.[16]

Oxidants, Antioxidants, and Cellular Physiology

According to Peter Cerutti, MD, from the Swiss Institute of Experimental Cancer Research, ROS also are involved in alterations in cellular communication related to cancer. Carcinogen-induced tumor initiation is related to the carcinogen's ability to cause structural damage in DNA as base-pair mutations, deletions, insertions, rearrangements, and sequence amplification and to alter nuclear signal transduction pathways. All of these processes may be initiated by exposure of DNA to ROS.[17]

Epidemiologic studies by Marilyn Menkes, MD, and her colleagues and William Blot, PhD, and his colleagues evaluating serum antioxidants and dietary antioxidants suggest that an increased level of vitamin E and carotene is associated with a significant reduction of mortality from cancer in both the lung and colon.[18,19] Myron Brin, PhD, was the first to show prospectively that those with the highest serum levels of vitamins E and C had the lowest incidence of heart disease and cancer.[20] These epidemiologic studies, although not proof of the antioxidant hypothesis, are highly suggestive of the relationship between antioxidant intake and the prevention of both heart disease and cancer.

Reactive oxygen species and oxidative stress also are related to pulmonary and respiratory tract disorders.[21] Because of its very large surface area, the respiratory tract is a major target for potential oxidative injury from inhaled radicals like nitrogen dioxide, cigarette smoke, aerosol toxic minerals like cadmium and lead, nonradicals like ozone, and products of inflammatory cells that release reactive oxygen species and nitric oxide. The significant amounts of antioxidants in fluids lining the respiratory tract help provide initial defense against reactive oxygen species exposure. In either a large or long-term oxidative challenge, these defenses can be depleted, resulting in injury to the pulmonary system.[22]

One oxidant species that recently has been studied in pulmonary disorders is nitric oxide. Nitric oxide synthase (NOS) is reasonably active in most lung cells. The predominance of the inducible NOS in "activated" pulmonary macrophages indicates nitric oxide may play a role in lung inflammation and lung oxidant stress. As a modulator of cellular function, nitric oxide can be either a defensive agent or, when produced in excess quantities, a prooxidant, inducing oxidative stress.

Under normal conditions, nitric oxide interacts with superoxide anion to protect lungs against superoxide, but when nitric oxide and superoxide both are produced in very high quantities they react rapidly to form the very powerful oxidant peroxynitrite, which may contribute to lung injury. The relationship between pulmonary toxicity as a consequence of exposure to reactive oxygen species is shown in the box "Lung Conditions in Which Oxidative Stress May Be Involved."

LUNG CONDITIONS IN WHICH OXIDATIVE STRESS MAY BE INVOLVED

Oxygen toxicity

Cigarette smoke effects

Lung cancer

Ischemia-reperfusion injury (as in lung transplantation)

Air-pollutant exposure (O_2, NO_2, SO_2)

Mineral-dust pneumoconiosis

Bleomycin or paraquat toxicity

Idiopathic pulmonary fibrosis

Infant respiratory distress syndrome

Bronchopulmonary dysplasia

Adult respiratory distress syndrome

Cystic fibrosis

Immune-complex-mediated lung injury

HIV-associated lung disease

Asthma

Acid aspiration

Lung transplantation

Protection against reactive oxygen species in the lung depends on the activity of glutathione, mucins that line the lung, vitamin E, and vitamin C. Lung cells under sustained oxidative stress have increased activity of copper, zinc, and manganese superoxide dismutase, as well as catalase and glutathione peroxidase upregulation.[23] This is an example of the body's trying to protect itself against increased oxidative stress that, if sustained at a high level, ultimately overrides the antioxidant protection systems and induces free radical damage.

Assessment of Oxidant Stress and Antioxidant Need

Analysis of oxidative stress and its relationship to antioxidant need has been approached by two different strategies. The first is to measure the results of oxidative stress and free radical damage. The second is to examine the antioxidant reserve through what might be called *oxidative stress resistance*. The former of these two strategies focuses on the presence of oxidative stress-induced molecular pathology. The latter focuses on functional redox dynamics and oxidative stress resistance.

One of the primary methods that has been used to examine the result of oxidative stress and free radical-induced damage to DNA is the analysis in the blood of the oxidatively damaged nucleotide 8-hydroxy-2' deoxyguanosine, which is considered to be a biomarker of in vivo oxidative damage.[24]

According to a recent report, a number of oxidized DNA bases are found in the sera of patients suffering from a variety of inflammatory diseases (including systemic lupus erythematosis and other autoimmune disorders) thought to be related to oxidant stress.[25] The analysis of oxidized DNA bases in sera by high-pressure lipid chromatography or electrochemical methods may therefore prove to be clinically valuable in assessing pathologic processes related to oxidative stress.

Another method that has been used to evaluate the degree of oxidative stress-induced damage is the exhalation of breath ethane and pentane that occurs as a consequence of the oxidative cleavage of unsaturated lipids found in membranes and other cellular organelles. These hydrocarbon molecules are a consequence of the oxidative cleavage of the unsaturated tails of omega-3 and omega-6 fatty acids, respectively. The measurement of these volatile hydrocarbons in the breath therefore has been suggested as a useful assessment tool for defining the presence of oxidative stress in vivo.[26] Investigators have used breath ethane generation during total body irradiation as a marker of in vivo oxygen free radical-mediated lipid peroxidation. Although not a standard procedure in all clinical reference laboratories, the mass spectrometric analysis of breath pentane and ethane after suitable collection may provide a useful screening tool for measuring lipid peroxidation as a consequence of oxidative stress, and it may help define needs for antioxidants.[27] A number of investigators have shown that in situations in which an increase in oxidative stress is not compensated for by adequate antioxidant protection there is either an increase in the blood levels of malondialdehyde (MDA) or the conjugation of the double bonds in linoleic acid. Both of these conditions can be readily measured by laboratory test and represent presumptive screening methods for assessing oxidative stress.

To evaluate oxidative stress resistance and antioxidant potential, a challenge procedure either in vitro or in vivo must be employed. The oxygen radical absorbency capacity developed recently by Richard Cutler, PhD, and his colleagues at the National Institutes on Aging represents such an in vitro method. In this assay, a patient's serum is challenged in vitro with a defined oxidative stress, and chemoluminescent products generated as a consequence of free radical oxidative reactions are measured. The higher the level of antioxidant reserve of the patient, the lower the level of chemoluminescent products produced after exposure to the defined oxidants. This challenge test may be able to measure aspects of antioxidant reserve in the body using whole serum as the biologic fluid for evaluation.[28] This test evaluates the reserve of protection through the oxidant challenge procedure. It may be that using two tests (one that measures antioxidant reserve and another that measures the presence of free radical oxidant-induced damage) together as a panel provides the best indication for overall redox balance in the patient.

The salicylate challenge test represents an example of an in vivo challenge method to evaluate the oxidative stress resistance. Salicylate is administered orally to the patient in a standard dose graded to body weight, and the urinary metabolites are analyzed.

In patients who are experiencing high degrees of oxidative stress due to hydroxyl radical-mediated reactions, there is a greater production of the salicylate metabolite 2,3-dihydroxybenzoic acid and catechol than in control patients who were not undergoing oxidative stress.[29]

Challenge studies with vitamin C also have been used to evaluate the presence of oxidative stress. Vitamin C in the presence of oxidants is converted into ascorbyl radical, which has been identified as an indicator of oxidative stress.[30] Electron spin resonance spectroscopy or other instrumental techniques can be used to evaluate the presence of ascorbyl radical in sera after a patient has taken a challenge dose of ascorbic acid. The higher the levels of electron spin resonance signal for ascorbyl radical after the vitamin C challenge, the more in vivo oxidative stress is present. This test indicates that if an individual is under high oxidative stress, administration of high doses of ascorbic acid actually may result in an increased level of a secondary free radical species, ascorbyl radical, which could be harmful in its own right.[31] Ascorbyl radical is quenched by tocopherol (vitamin E), which subsequently is regenerated through the activity of glutathione. This demonstrates that the antioxidant family of nutrients works together as a team in providing proper redox protection. Giving one antioxidant nutrient at high levels without the others may produce an inappropriate oxidation-reduction system that may further amplify specific free radical reactions. Balz Frei, PhD, has demonstrated that antioxidants are depleted from the blood at different rates upon exposure to oxidative stress, with ascorbate being depleted first, followed by active sulfhydryl antioxidants, bilirubin, ureate, and α-tocopherol.[32]

Oxidants, Antioxidants, and Diseases of Aging

All of this later research lends credibility to Dr. Denham Harman's proposal, some 40 years ago, that oxidant stress plays a role in aging and antioxidants may help defend against certain aspects of biologic aging. Recently, Bruce Ames, PhD, pointed out that metabolism, like life itself, involves tradeoffs. We must have oxygen to support aerobic metabolism, which gives mammals a competitive advantage over nonoxygen-requiring organisms. This dependence on oxygen, however, puts us at risk to reactive oxygen species and oxygen radical-induced tissue pathology. The longer we live, the more reactive oxygen species we are exposed to and the more potential damage there is to critical cellular organelles and biomolecules. This damage to cells leads to sequential reduction in function, which finds ultimate expression in degenerative diseases of aging.[33] Ames pointed out that antioxidant defense systems help protect against oxidant-induced degenerative diseases of aging, such as cancer, cardiovascular disease and immune system declines, brain dysfunction, and cataracts. We now recognize that the principal sources of dietary antioxidants are fruits, vegetables, and whole grains, which in our present diets may be inadequate to meet our needs for fulfilling the expectation of health for seven, eight, or nine decades.

As our expectations for good health and longevity have increased, our need for antioxidants to defend function throughout the aging process has increased as well. The Recommended Dietary Allowance (RDA) levels for antioxidants were not established with the amounts of those nutrients required to protect function over many decades of life for individuals exposed to reactive oxygen species. Edward Schneider, MD, has suggested reformulating the RDAs for older adults to acknowledge the role nutrients play in defending against biochemical processes associated with decline of function and aging.[34] We now recognize that activities of antioxidant enzyme systems (for example, glutathione peroxidase, catalase, and superoxide dismutase), along with sufficient intercellular levels of antioxidant nutrients (for example, ascorbate, tocopherol, glutathione, carotenoids, and flavonoids), help protect against oxidative processes and encourage improved cell survival and the potential of enhanced function and health throughout the aging process.[35,36]

Strong evidence from studies of aging humans indicates that healthy older adults have much higher levels of glutathione than their peers who evince signs of premature biologic aging and disease and that glutathione levels in the body may be one of the best predictors of biologic aging and health.[37,38] Levels of glutathione in the body reflect both diet and health-related factors.[39] Other extracellular antioxidants also may help protect against oxidative stress. Knowledge about these antioxidants, combined with an understanding of tocopherols, ascorbate, carotenoids, flavonoids, and glutathione status, increases the understanding of risk of diseases associated with premature biologic aging.

According to Mohsen Meydani, PhD, only in recent years have "antioxidant vitamins" made their way into the vocabulary of health practitioners. There is a rapid increase in our understanding of the importance of free radicals in biologic disorders and the potential role of antioxidants in protecting against free radical effects and preventing disease. Our diet contains many antioxidants other than those that traditionally have been studied, such as members of the flavonol, polyphenol, flavonoid, and quinoid families (such as vitamin K-related nutrients).[40] Many antioxidant investigators have pointed out that vitamin E (tocopherol) may play an important role in protection against heart disease, problems related to excessive platelet aggregation, certain forms of cancer, disorders of the immune system, and the pathologic consequences of diabetes, all of which are age-related health disorders. There appears to be increasing evidence that intake of vitamin E beyond the RDA may provide a benefit in reducing the risk of these age-related diseases. In the context of the broader research in the antioxidant field, however, we should not limit our clinical attention to any one antioxidant but instead examine the full complement of redox agents that help protect against oxygen radical-induced injury.

Clinical Conclusions

A tremendous amount of research remains to be done before we can fully understand both the preventive and therapeutic application of antioxidants in clinical medicine. However, what can be derived from our state of understanding today is that oxidant stress and reactive oxygen species play a significant role in the modulation of diseases we associate with aging.

In addition, cellular-specific antioxidants help defend against the adverse effects in the mitochondria of imbalanced cellular redox potential. In the 1970s, Linus Pauling, PhD, discussed the use of therapeutic doses of vitamin C to prevent and treat viral infections.[41] Following his suggestions, Robert Cathcart, MD, reported in numerous clinical instances therapeutic benefit of using "bowel tolerance" doses of vitamin C (in other words, the oral dose that will initiate diarrhea) for the treatment of many virally related disorders.[42] His rationale is that vitamin C given at these doses has an entirely different physiologic effect on redox potential and mitochondrial function from lower therapeutic doses. Although this theory has not been proven through detailed mechanistic studies, many clinicians have anecdotally reported benefits in their patients using this therapeutic approach. Clinical observations over the past 25 years point out the need for more research on the nutritional pharmacology and physiochemistry of vitamin C and potentially other antioxidants applied to disease states related to altered mitochondrial oxidative phosphorylation and its relationship to oxidative stress.

Individual antioxidants may not have as broad clinical benefit as the intake of balanced antioxidants that incorporate all the dietary redox-active substances we have consumed for millennia. Specific antioxidants include the well-researched ascorbate, carotenoids, and tocopherols, but they also extend into other phytonutrients, such as phenols, flavonoids, and quinoids. The list of beneficial nutrients includes coenzyme Q10, lipoic acid, N-acetylcarnitine, catechins (from green tea), quercetin from onions and garlic, ginkgolides from *Ginkgo biloba*, silymarins from milk thistle, and curcumin from the spice turmeric.

We now recognize that complex plant formulations containing many redox-active substances may play a different role in modulating physiologic function than the single nutrient agents like vitamin C or vitamin E.[43] There is acceptance among the scientific and medical communities that enhanced antioxidant intake in the diet and specific application of antioxidants in certain states of oxidative stress may provide both preventive and therapeutic advantage.[44] In 1977 G.L. Engel, MD, suggested that the challenge for biomedicine was to find a new model for understanding the origin of disease that is consistent with the increasing understanding of the pathophysiology of age-related disorders.[45] Assessment of oxidative stress susceptibility and antioxidant protection may play an important role in establishing the scientific foundation for biologic aspects of this risk of oxidant stress-induced disorders.

References

1. Harman D: Aging: a theory based on free radical and radiation chemistry, *Gerontol* 298-300, 1956.

2. Fridovich I: The chemistry and biology of superoxide (O2-): central concepts and residual problems. In *The molecular basis of oxidative damage by leukocytes*, Boca Raton, Fla, 1992, CRC Press.

3. Czapski G: The chemistry of superoxide anion, *Ann Rev Phys Chem* 22:171, 1971.

4. Pryor WA: Free radical reactions and their importance in biochemical systems, *Fed Proc* 32:1862-1868, 1973.

5. Sies H, editor: *Oxidative stress*, New York, 1981, Academic Press.

6. Cosmos G, Feher J, editors: *Free radicals and the liver*, Berlin, 1992, Springer-Verlag.

7. Aust SD et al: Free radicals in toxicology, *Toxicol Appl Pharmacol* 120:168-178, 1993.

8. Bland JS, Bralley AJ: Nutritional upregulation of hepatic detoxication enzymes, *J App Nutr* 44:2-15, 1992.

9. Halliwell B: Free radicals and antioxidants: a personal view, *Nutr Rev* 52:253-265, 1994.

10. Ehrenkranz RA: Vitamin E and retinopathy of prematurity: still controversial, *J Pediatr* 114:801-803, 1988.

11. Tappel AL: Free-radical lipid peroxidation damage and its inhibition by vitamin E and selenium, *Fed Proc* 24:73, 1965.

12. Witztum JL: The oxidation hypothesis of atherosclerosis, *Lancet* 344:793-795, 1994.

13. Benditt E: The origin of atherosclerosis, *Sci Am* 236:74-85, 1977.

14. Esterbauer H et al: The role of lipid peroxidation and antioxidants in oxidative modification of LDL, *Free Rad Biol Med* 13:341-390, 1992.

15. Rajman I, Kendall M, Cramb R: The oxidation hypothesis of atherosclerosis, *Lancet* 344:1363-1364, 1994.

16. Stampfer MJ et al: Postmenopausal estrogen therapy and cardiovascular disease, *N Engl J Med* 325:756-762, 1991.

17. Cerutti PA: Oxy-radicals and cancer, *Lancet* 344:862-863, 1994.

18. Menkes M et al: Serum B-carotene, vitamins A and E, selenium and the risk of lung cancer, *N Engl J Med* 315(20):1250-1254, 1986.

19. Blot W et al: Nutrition intervention trials in Linxian China: supplementation with specific vitamin/mineral combination, cancer incidence and disease-specific mortality in the general population, *J Natl Cancer Inst* 85:1483-1492, 1993.

20. Gey KF et al: Inverse correlation between plasma vitamin E and mortality from ischemic heart disease in cross-cultural epidemiology, *Am J Clin Nutr* 53:3265-3345, 1991.

21. Cross CE et al: Reactive oxygen species and the lung, *Lancet* 344:930-933, 1994.

22. Cross CE et al: Oxidants, antioxidants, and respiratory tract lining fluids, *Environ Health Perspect* 102:185-191, 1994.

23. Fridovich I: Superoxide dismutases, *Methods Enzymol* 58:61-97, 1986.

24. Shigenaga MK, Ames BN: Assays for 8-hydroxy-2'-deoxyguanosine: a biomarker of in vivo oxidative DNA damage, *Free Rad Biol Med* 10:211-216, 1991.

25. Frenkel K et al: Recognition of oxidized DNA bases by sera of patients with inflammatory diseases, *Free Rad Biol Med* 14:483-494, 1993.

26. Arterbery VE et al: Breath ethane generation during clinical total body irradiation as a marker of oxygen-free-radical-mediated lipid peroxidation: a case study, *Free Rad Biol Med* 17:569-576, 1994.

27. Kneepkens CM, Lepage G, Roy CC: The potential of the hydrocarbon breath test as a measure of lipid peroxidation, *Free Rad Biol Med* 17:127-160, 1994.

28. Cao G, Alessio HM, Cutler RG: Oxygen-radical absorbance capacity assay for antioxidants, *Free Rad Biol Med* 14:303-311, 1993.

29. Ghiselli A et al: Salicylate hydroxylation as an early marker of in vivo oxidative stress in diabetic patients, *Free Rad Biol Med* 13:621-626, 1992.

30. Roginsky VA, Stegmann HB: Ascorbyl radical as natural indicator of oxidative stress: quantitative regularities, *Free Rad Biol Med* 17:93-103, 1994.

31. Halliwell B: Vitamin C: the key to health or a slow-acting carcinogen? *Redox Report* 1:5-9, 1994.

32. Stocker R, Frei B: Endogenous antioxidant defenses in human blood plasma. In Sies H, editor: *Oxidative stress*, New York, 1985, Academic Press.

33. Ames BN, Shigenaga MK, Hagen TM: Oxidants, antioxidants, and the degenerative diseases of aging, *Proc Natl Acad Sci USA* 90:7915-7922, 1993.

34. Schneider EL et al: Recommended dietary allowances and the health of the elderly, *N Engl J Med* 314:157, 1986.

35. Michiels C et al: Importance of SE-glutathione peroxidase catalase, and CuZn-SOD for cell survival against oxidative stress, *Free Rad Biol Med* 17:235-248, 1994.

36. Warner HR: Superoxide dismutase, aging, and degenerative disease, *Free Rad Biol Med* 17:249-258, 1994.

37. Meskini N et al: Glutathione peroxidase activity and metabolism of arachidonic acid in peripheral blood mononuclear cells from elderly subjects, *Clin Sci* 85:203-211, 1993.

38. Lang CA et al: Low blood glutathione levels in healthy aging adults, *J Lab Clin Med* 120:720-775, 1992.

39. Lang CA et al: Low blood glutathione levels in healthy aging adults, *J Lab Clin Med* 120:720-725, 1992.

40. Meydani M: Vitamin E, *Lancet* 345:170-175, 1995.

41. Pauling L: Ascorbic acid and the common cold: evaluation of its efficacy and toxicity, *Med Trib* Mar 24, 1976:1-3. and *Med Trib* Apr 7, 1976:4-6.

42. Cathcart R: Vitamin C: the nontoxic, nonrate-limited, antioxidant free radical scavenger, *Med Hypoth* 1985;18:61-77, 1985.

43. Fishman RHB: Antioxidants and phytotherapy, *Lancet* 344:1356, 1994.

44. Marantz PR: Beta carotene, vitamin E, and lung cancer, *N Engl J Med* 331:611, 1994.

45. Engel GL: The need for a new medical model: a challenge for biomedicine, *Science* 196:129-136, 1977.

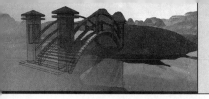

Orthomolecular Medicine

HECTOR E. SOLORZANO DEL RIO

Origins and History

Orthomolecular medicine involves the prevention and treatment of diseases using the optimal amounts of natural substances, such as vitamins, minerals, trace elements, amino acids, enzymes, and friendly bacteria. The term *orthomolecular* was first used by Linus Pauling in a paper he wrote in the journal *Science* in 1968. With remarkable insight, he described many of the theoretic scientific foundations of this form of complementary medicine. *Ortho* means "correct," and the physicians using this kind of therapy attempt to reestablish patients' health by prescribing nutrients in an amount sufficient to produce adequate levels of them.

Biochemical pathways of the body have significant genetic variability in terms of individual enzyme concentrations and transcriptional potential, receptor-ligand affinities, and protein transporter efficiency. Nutrition also is one of the many factors that plays an important role in the intensity and duration of disease states. By studying the complex interactions of genes with specific nutrients, variations in symptoms can be understood.

The premise behind orthomolecular therapy began around 1920 when nutrients were used to treat some clinical conditions. Magnesium, for example, was used for cardiac arrhythmias. Although some of these therapies were empirically effective, no relationship to nutritional deficiencies was seen at that time. Intentional consideration of deficiencies began around 1950, when Drs. Abram Hoffer and Humphrey Osmond began to treat schizophrenics with megadoses of vitamin B-3 (niacin).

Mechanism of Action According to Its Own Theory

Adequate nutrition is essential for good health. Nutrition provides our body with the raw material necessary to make tissues, blood, hormones, bones, and so on. Nutrients are essential for every biochemical pathway in our organism. Failure to meet the body's nutritional requirements results inevitably in illness. A deficiency in vitamin C results in scurvy. Deficiency syndromes exist for nearly every nutrient, including vitamins, minerals, amino acids, essential fatty acids, enzymes, and so on. Unfortunately, blood tests reflect the momentary level of nutrients, useful in extreme deficiencies but not necessarily tissue levels. Other, more functional studies can best detect more subtle deficiencies.

The main difference between mainstream and orthomolecular medicine is that ortho-dox medicine regularly prescribes *anti-drugs*. For example, we prescribe anti-cough drugs, antiinflamatory drugs, antipyretic drugs, antiacid drugs, antihypertensive drugs, and many others. All these medications serve only to inhibit the normal bodily mechanisms of reac-tion of our bodies. They do not address the cause of the clinical condition. In contrast, or-thomolecular medicine attempts to give the body the raw nutritional materials it needs to heal itself.

Biologic Mechanism of Action

Orthomolecular medicine is based on a very important principle called *biochemical individ-uality*. The late Roger Williams, PhD, of the University of Texas showed that in any group of 15 to 20 people there can be a range of nutritional requirements from person to person that varies by as much as 700%. So, if the official recommended dietary allowance (RDA) for vitamin B-1 is 1 mg daily, then any healthy individual can need up to 7 mg every day to keep the body functioning well.

An important term in orthomolecular medicine is *subclinical deficiency*. This means that the patient lacks a certain nutrient, but the deficiency has not reached a degree where we would expect to find the deficiency symptoms taught by the orthodox medical community.

There are many cases in Mexico diagnosed as noninsulin-dependent diabetes that, af-ter closer scrutiny, are only a severe deficiency of chromium. Chromium is necessary for carbohydrates metabolism.[1,2] Chromium is a key constituent of the glucose tolerance fac-tor. It works closely with insulin in facilitating the uptake of glucose into cells. Diabetes is a leading cause of death in adulthood. Potentially thousands of cases labeled as diabetes may only be chronic chromium deficiencies. Although somewhat controversial, a similar relationship exists between chronic zinc deficiency and benign prostatic hypertrophy.

Another important factor is the dosage. Nutrients act as such only at a certain amounts. But if the same nutrient is administered at a higher dosage, then the effect of the nutrient changes. In essence, all nutrients become a drug when administered at a high dosage. This is why they can be used as remedies to treat many diseases. For example, the RDA for vi-tamin A is 5000 IU. Administering 50,000 IU instead can act as an immunostimulant. Caution must be used, however, to avoid toxicity.

Forms of Therapy

In orthomolecular medicine the practitioner must do a nutritional assessment along with laboratory studies. Some of the laboratory testing is conventional and some is not. Ac-cording to the results, the treatment will be given in a very specific way to address the (of-ten subclinical) nutritional deficiencies. There are no set protocols for each disease as in the conventional medicine. There are theoretically as many treatments as patients.

As an example, treatment of heart disease may involve supplementation with coenzyme Q-10. Elevated homocysteine levels, an emerging risk factor in heart disease, often reflect a subclinical deficiency of pyridoxine (vitamin B-6) and folic acid. Modifying cardiac risk using an orthomolecular approach therefore involves supplementation with coenzyme Q-10, vitamin B-6, and folic acid, rather than focusing on cholesterol levels.

Treatment may also involve changing the biologic environment. For example, if the orthomolecular doctor finds through a mineral hair analysis that the patient has a chronic heavy metal intoxication, then the doctor will know that most likely there is a corresponding deficiency because of a pharmacologic antagonism. A high level of mercury released from dental fillings can produce a chronic deficiency of magnesium or zinc. So, in this case, it not only is necessary to supplement with magnesium or zinc, but it also is important to reduce the origin of the problem: the releasing of mercury from the dental fillings.

Demographics

There are many practitioners of orthomolecular medicine worldwide. In Mexico the use of this nutritional therapy has been spread since 1985 through the courses offered by Universidad de Guadalajara. In the United States, the followers of Dr. Linus Pauling are abundant. The largest density of this type of practitioners is in California. Canada also has many practitioners of this kind of nutritional therapy.

The patients who tend to use this therapy are from all ages, genders, and cultures. Regrettably, most patients who turn to orthomolecular medicine do not do so until they are told or feel that orthodox medicine does not have anything more to offer for their condition.

Indications and Reasons for Referral

Virtually any illness can benefit from nutritional therapy, either as primary or adjunctive therapy. Historically, certain illnesses are treated more often with orthomolecular medicine than others, as listed in the following section.

Office Applications

A simple ranking of conditions responsive to this form of therapy is as follows. As with all alternative therapies, use of orthomolecular medicine does not preclude the use of mainstream medical therapies in addition. The listings here are the best uses of supplements for therapy of the illnesses described. The nutritional supplements are prescribed according to the nutritional imbalance of each person, depending on the biochemical individuality.

Top level: *A therapy ideally suited for these conditions*
Arthritis, asthma, colds, and flu

Second level: *One of the better therapies for these conditions*
Fever, premenstrual syndrome, sleep disorders, and vision disorders

Third level: *A valuable adjunctive therapy for these conditions*
Genital warts, hay fever, gastritis, and parasitic infections

Additional indications include autism, benign prostatic hypertrophy, cancer, diabetes, heart disease, hypertension, mental health, and yeast infections.

Practical Applications

Any patient needs nutritional support. Remember the words of Hippocrates: "Let your medicine be your food and your food be your medicine." Nutrients are most readily available in nonprocessed foods.

As an example of application, consider the management of a postmenopausal patient with osteoporosis. From an orthodox medical perspective, treatment includes hormone replacement therapy, calcium supplementation, and in some cases, potent modifiers of osteoclastic and osteoblastic activity. From an orthomolecular medicine perspective, the treatment focus would be on several nutritional imbalances. These would include the following:

- A subclinical deficiency of vitamin C, which is necessary for the production of collagen
- A deficiency of vitamin D, which is needed for healthy bones
- A subclinical deficiency of vitamin E, which is a precursor of many hormones, including estrogens
- A deficiency of Boron, which is necessary not only for healthy bones but also the production of female hormones. Serum estrogen levels in women who are taking boron sometimes rise to levels that are similar to those levels of estrogen replacement therapy.
- A subclinical deficiency of vitamin B-6, which is necessary for the production of female hormones
- A subclinical deficiency of vitamin K, which is required to form the hormone osteocalcin
- In some cases, a deficiency of "friendly microflora" in the intestines may hinder the conjugation of estrogens.
- A subclinical deficiency of silicon, which is essential for the metabolism of connective and bone tissue
- A subclinical deficiency of magnesium, which is a powerful agent in the fixation of calcium

These deficiencies would be specifically supplemented.
Some lesser-known applications of supplementation are as follows:

- Vitamin B-6 (pyridoxine) may have value in the adjunctive therapy of carpal tunnel syndrome by supplementing the patient with vitamin B-6, between 50 mg to 200 mg daily for 30 to 90 days.

- Folic acid deficiency correlates with a higher incidence of cervical dysplasia.[3] Its value in treating preexisting dysplasia is controversial.[4]
- L-tryptophan has applications in the management of seasonal affective disorder,[5] premenstrual dysphoria,[6] and mild depression.[7]

Evidence is accumulating for the use of supplemental vitamin E in the treatment of Alzheimer's disease.[8] Serum aluminum levels may be involved with the development of patients with dementia, including Alzheimer's disease.[9] Aluminum intoxication is not rare. It can be seen in heavy users of aluminum hydroxide or users of aluminum kitchen tools.

Several studies have demonstrated value in the administration of dehydroepiandrosterone (DHEA) in patients with lupus.[10-12]

Taurine deficiency is described in patients with epilepsy, suggesting the value of taurine supplementation as adjunctive therapy of seizure disorders.[13] In clinical studies in Guadalajara, we have seen that taurine has a powerful, lasting anticonvulsant effect. Patients who did not respond to orthodox therapy responded to this nutritional treatment.

Research Base

Evidence Based

There are literally thousands of studies that demonstrate the impact of nutrition on health. In a randomized, placebo-controlled, serial angiographic clinical trial, Vitamin E supplementation was found to slow the progression of coronary artery atherosclerosis.[11] In another study, dietary selenium in an amount of 200 micrograms daily was shown to reduce the risk of skin cancer by as much as 52%.[15] A keyword search in the standard literature on almost any vitamin or mineral will yield an ample return of studies on the subject.

Risk and Safety

All nutrients are naturally occurring substances. If we use only the amount required by each patient according to biochemical individuality, then there no risks. In addition, genetic errors make some people physiologically require more amounts of certain nutrients. Toxicity can occur, particularly with fat-soluble vitamins. Dosing needs to be based on available literature regarding toxicity of the supplements to be administered.

Efficacy

If there is a deficiency, then the best medicine for that patient will be exactly the nutrient that is being missed. The main difference between the paradigms used in orthodox and orthomolecular medicine is that mainstream health care practitioners were only taught the symptoms of an extreme nutritional deficiency. For example, beri beri results from a B-1 deficiency, and scurvy results from an extreme vitamin C deficiency. However, in ortho-molecular medicine, we have seen that there are subclinical deficiencies. This means that a patient can have a specific nutritional deficiency but not an extreme deficiency. This can elicit symptoms but not to the same extent as an extreme deficiency. The reasons for this are the length of time (usually chronic diseases) and the extent of the deficiency.

Other

Many clinical trials are in progress worldwide. Since natural substances cannot be patented, they are not profitable. This is changing as larger pharmaceutic firms enter the business of nutritional supplements.

Druglike Information

Safety

Orthomolecular medicine is not only safe; it is essential for continued good health. Headaches are not a deficiency of aspirin. Nutrients are not strange substances to our bod-ies. If dosages are administered according to the biochemical individuality of the patient, there seldom will be a problem. Toxicity can occur with improper dosing of many nutri-ents. For example, more than 100,000 IU of vitamin A, when taken for several months, can produce toxic effects.

Actions and Pharmacokinetics

As previously mentioned, the deficiency of any given nutrient will result in a group of symp-toms, depending on the extent and duration of the deficiency. Nutrients can interact with any medication or food. Knowledge of these interactions is a necessity for any practitioner of this therapy. Nutrients are necessary for genetic expression. For many genetic errors, the composition and quantity of the food that is consumed can modify the phenotypic ex-pression of the genotype. Ideally, a diet design should potentiates the expression of the in-dividual's genes for normal growth, development, and longevity while suppressing the ex-pression of genes associated with disease.[16]

Warnings, Contraindications, and Precautions

In sufficient doses, contraindications do exist. For example, Vitamin E sometimes can in-terfere with platelet aggregation and should be used with caution in patients on warfarin or other platelet antagonists. In addition, there are some precautions that are related to the proper nutritional imbalance of a specific patient in a given moment. Caution also must be exercised if patients have an allergy or intolerance to a particular nutrient. There are certain reactions that nutrients can produce. Tolerance dose is not the same for everyone. Vitamin C, for example, can produce diarrhea at dosages of 6 grams or more.

Drug or Other Interactions

More than 3000 food-drug interactions currently exist. Knowledge of these interactions is an integral part of any approach to nutritional medicine. For example, vitamin B-6 (pyridoxine) is contraindicated in patients that receiving levadopa for the treatment of Parkinson's disease.

Adverse Reactions

The only possible direct reaction to a nutrient could be an allergy. A patient who is allergic to a particular food will be allergic to any food supplement containing that food. In well-prescribed orthomolecular medicine, adverse reactions are few or seldom occur. If adverse effects do occur, they often indicate that the dosage is inappropriate for that patient. The incidence of supplement-related adverse effects is considerably lower than that of prescription medications.

Pregnancy and Lactation

Nutrients are essential during pregnancy and lactation. For example, l-taurine is an amino acid required for both the baby and mother. It is essential for brain development of the baby as well as the production of milk by the mother. During pregnancy, many women may have a deficiency of magnesium or vitamin B-6. So the specific treatment for preeclampsia is their supplementation. There are no contraindications during pregnancy and lactation for orthomolecular medicine when scientifically administered. As in all uses of supplements, a knowledge of their safe dosing potential and potential toxicity is a requirement for the prescriber.

Trade Products, Administration, and Dosage

There are literally hundreds of food supplements or nutrients sold everywhere. Most of them are sold as food supplements.

There are nutrients that are used in orthodox medicine; for example, the amino acid l-carnitine now is widely used for heart problems such as myocardial infarction, especially in intensive care units.[17,18]

Self-Help versus Professional

For mild problems and conditions, self-supplementation is appropriate. For example, many clinical studies have demonstrated that the taking of zinc lozenges can shorten the duration of a common cold and also minimize symptoms. Many publications for lay audience exist that can provide information on the use of nutrients to treat some clinical conditions.

It is not recommended to use food supplements for a major medical problem without the supervision of a physician, preferably one trained in orthomolecular medicine.

Visiting a Professional

Besides the history and physical examination that is commonly performed by orthodox physicians, orthomolecular physicians perform a nutritional assessment to determine the specific nutritional deficiencies and needs of an individual patient. Sometimes it is necessary to have the results of a mineral hair analysis or intracellular vitamin analysis, or other laboratory studies that are not regularly requested by the conventional medical community. Some of the tests that are commonly requested by orthomolecular physicians include the following:

- Heidelberg test (to measure stomach pH)
- Biologic terrain assessment (to measure pH, resistivity, and redox index of samples of blood, saliva, and urine)
- Intraerythrocitic magnesium levels
- Electroacupuncture of Voll (EAV) medication testing
- Measures of blood levels of amino acids, blood levels of enzymes, and blood levels of vitamins

After the assessment is completed, the orthomolecular physician not only will prescribe certain food supplements, but the orthomolecular physician also will advise on lifestyle habits and changes and a specific diet that the patient should follow, according to the results of the assessment.

Credentialing

In some countries, it is necessary to be a medical doctor to prescribe high dosages of nutrients. Credentialing depends on local laws.

Training

There are seminars on orthomolecular medicine worldwide. There is a center in Canada, the International Society of Orthomolecular Medicine. In Mexico, the Universidad de Guadalajara also holds many seminars. More information can be acquired by searching for country-specific associations on the International Society for Orthomolecular Medicine website at www.orthomed.org.

What to Look for in a Provider

In general, the practitioner of orthomolecular medicine often is a physician whose practice style shows an awareness that environment and lifestyle are as important as the eating habits of the patient.

Barriers and Key Issues

Because natural substances cannot be patented the multinational pharmaceutic companies historically have not been interested in them and do not heavily promote the use of supplements. Multinational pharmaceutic companies seldom produce any natural products, although this is changing in response to current public demand. In general, pharmaceutic firms promote their prescription medications and their few natural products. If a company paid for a research study of a nutrient, then any other company could promote the same nutrient using claims based on the other company's research. It is more profitable if a company has a copyright on a certain molecule that does not exist spontaneously in nature. In this way, only that company will get profits from this research for the duration of the patent.

As the production and marketing of vitamins, supplements, and herbals becomes cost-effective, pharmaceutic firms will join in as sources. A benefit of this economic evolution is a likely outpouring of supplement-related research.

Associations

International Society for Orthomolecular Medicine
16 Florence Ave.
Toronto, Ontario, Canada M2N 1E9
Tel: (416) 733-2117
Fax: (416) 733-2352
E-mail: centre@orthomed.org
www.orthomed.org

SIAMO
Los Alpes No. 962
44280 Guadalajara, Jal. Mexico
Fax: 3 637 0030

Suggested Reading

1. Hoffer A, Walker M, Pauling L: *Putting it all together: the new orthomolecular nutrition*, New Canaan, Conn, 1989, Keats.

    In this book the authors discuss the definition of orthomolecular and how it treats the diseases. It contains case histories and also explains the functions of major nutrients.

2. Hoffer A: *Orthomolecular medicine for physicians*, New Canaan, Conn, 1989, Keats.

    The author explains that orthomolecular medicine is simply the treatment and prevention of diseases by adjusting the chemical constituents of our body. To do this, we manage nutrition. He suggests a simple trial; just ask any patient to follow a sugar-free diet and prescribe one or two vitamins. Any doctor will be amazed with the results.

Bibliography

Arsenian MA, New PS, Cafasso CM: Safety, tolerability, and efficacy of a glucose-insulin-potassium-magnesium-carnitine solution in acute myocardial infarction, *Am J Cardiol* 78(4):477-479, 1996.

Clark LC et al: Effects of selenium supplementation for cancer prevention in patients with carcinoma of the skin. A randomized controlled trial, Nutritional Prevention of Cancer Study Group, *JAMA* 276(24):1957-1963, 1957. Published erratum appears in *JAMA* 277(19):1520, 1997.

Slate EH et al: (1979), *Dr. Mandell's 5-day allergy relief system*, New York, 1979, Thomas Y. Crowell.

Mednick SA et al: Genetic influences in criminal convictions: Evidence from an adoption cohort, *Science* 224:891-894, 1984.

Nichols P: *Minimal brain dysfunction*, 1981, Lawrence Erlbaum Association.

Paterson ET: Towards the orthomolecular environment, *J Ortho Psychol* 10:269-283, 1981.

Pauling, L. (1968), Orthomolecular psychiatry, *Science* 160:265-271.

Pauling L: *How to live longer and feel better*, New York, 1986, W. H. Freeman.

Prinz, RJ et al: Dietary correlation of hyperactive behavior in children, *J Consult Clin Psychol* 48:760-769, 1980.

Reed B: *Food, teens, and behavior*, Manitowoc, Wis, 1983, Natural Press.

Rimland B: Risks and benefits in the treatment of autistic children, *J Autism Childhood Schiz* 8:100-104, 1978.

Rimland B: The Feingold diet: An assessment of the reviews by Mattes, Kavale, and Fomess and others, *J Learn Disabil* 16:331-333, 1983.

Rimland B, Larson GE: Nutritional and ecological approaches to the reduction of criminality, delinquency and violence, *J Applied Nutr* 33:116-137, 1981.

Rippere V: *The allergy problem*, Wellingborough, England, 1983, Thorsons.

Rippere V: Food additives and hyperactive children: a critique of Connors, *Br J Clin Psychol* 22:19-32, 1983.

Rippere V: (1983), Nutritional approaches to behavior modification, Progress in Behavioral Modification 14:299-354.

Ross H: *Fighting depression*, New York, 1975, Larchmont Books.

Rudin DO, Felix C: *Omega 3 oils to improve mental health, fight degenerative diseases, and extend your life*, New York, 1996, Avery.

Schauss A: Differential outcomes among probationers comparing orthomolecular approaches to conventional casework counseling, *J Ortho Psych* 8:158-168, 1979.

Schauss A: *Diet, crime, and delinquency*, Berkeley, Calif, 1980, Parker House.

Schauss AG, Simonsen CE: A critical analysis of the diets of chronic juvenile offenders, *I Ortho Psychol* 8:149-157, 1979.

Siegler M, Osmond H: (1966), Models of madness, *Br J Psychol* 112:1193-1203, 1966.

Siegler M, Osmond H: *Models of madness, models of medicine*, New York, 1974, Macmillan.

Silverman LJ, Metz AS: Minimal brain dysfunction. 3. Epidemiology. Numbers of pupils with specific learning disabilities in local public schools in the United States: spring 1970, *Ann NY Acad Sci* 205:146-157, 1973.

Singh RB et al: A randomized, double-blind, placebo-controlled trial of L-carnitine in suspected acute myocardial infarction, *Postgrad Med J* 72(843):45-50, 1996.

Smith LH: *Improving your child's behavior chemistry*. Englewood Cliffs, NJ, 1976, Prentice-Hall.

Smith RF: A five-year field trial of massive nicotine acid therapy of alcoholics in Michigan, *I Ortho Psych* 3:327-331, 1974.

Stewart MA: Hyperactive children, *Sci Am* 222:94-98, 1970.

Stewart M et al: The hyperactive child syndrome, *Am J Orthopsychiatry* 36:861-867, 1966.

Stone I: The natural history of ascorbic acid in the evolution of the mammals and primates and its significance for present-day man, *J Ortho Psychiatry* 1:82-89, 1972.

Stone I: *The healing factor: vitamin C against disease*, New York, 1972, Grosset and Dunlap.

Von Hillsheimer G: *How to live with your special child*, Washington, D.C., 1970, Acropolic Books.

Williams RJ: *Biochemical individuality*, New York, 1956, John Wiley.

Williams RJ: *The wonderful world within you*, New York, 1977, Bantam Books.

References

1. Anderson RA: Chromium, glucose intolerance, and diabetes, *J Am Coll Nutr* 17(6):548-555, 1998.

2. Fox GN, Sabovic Z: Chromium picolinate supplementation for diabetes mellitus, *J Fam Pract* 46(1):83-86, 1998.

3. Kwasniewska A, Tukendorf A, Semczuk M: Folate deficiency and cervical intraepithelial neoplasia, *Eur J Gynecol Oncol* 18(6):526-530, 1997.

4. Butterworth CE Jr et al: Oral folic acid supplementation for cervical dysplasia: a clinical trial, *Am J Obstet Gynecol* 166(3):803-809, 1992.

5. Ghadirian AM, Murphy BE, Gendron MJ: Efficacy of light versus tryptophan therapy in seasonal affective disorder, *J Affect Disord* 50(1):23-27, 1998.

6. Steinberg S et al: A placebo-controlled clinical trial of L-tryptophan in premenstrual dysphoria, *Biol Psychiatry* 45(3):313-320, 1999.

7. Riemann D, Vorderholzer U: Treatment of depression and sleep disorders. Significance of serotonin and L-tryptophan in pathophysiology and therapy (in German), *Fortschr Med* 116(32):40-42, 1998.

8. Pitchumoni SS, Doraiswamy PM: Current status of antioxidant therapy for Alzheimer's Disease, *J Am Geriatr Soc* 46(12):1566-1572, 1998.

9. Roberts NB et al: Increased absorption of aluminum from a normal dietary intake in dementia, *J Inorg Biochem* 69(3):171-176, 1998.

10. Barry NN, McGuire JL, van Vollenhoven RF: Dehydroepiandrosterone in systemic lupus erythematous: relationship between dosage, serum levels, and clinical response, *J Rheumatol* 25(12):2352-2356, 1998.

11. Hodis HN, Mack WJ, LaBree L: Serial coronary angiographic evidence that antioxidant vitamin intake reduces progression of coronary artery atherosclerosis, *JAMA* 273(23):1849-1854, 1995.

12. van Vollenhoven RF et al: Treatment of systemic lupus erythematosus with dehydroepiandrosterone: 50 patients treated up to 12 months, *J Rheumatol* 25(2):285-289, 1998.

13. Goodman Ho, Shihabi Z, Oles KS: Antiepileptic drugs and plasma and platelet taurine in epilepsy, *Epilepsia* 30(2):201-207, 1989.

14. Hodis HN, Mack WJ, LaBree L: Serial coronary angiographic evidence that antioxidant vitamin intake reduces progression of coronary artery artherosclerosis, JAMA 273(23):1848-1854, 1995.

15. Clark LC et al: Effects of selenium supplementation for cancer prevention in patients with carcinoma of the skin. A randomized controlled trial. Nutritional Prevention of Cancer Study Group, JAMA 276(24):1957-1963, 1996.

16. Berdanier CD, Wolinsky I, editors: *Nutrients and gene expression: clinical aspects, modern nutrition,* Boca Raton, Fla, 1996, CRC Press.

17. Singh RB et al: A randomized, double-blind, placebo-controlled trial of L-carnitine in suspected acute myocardial infarction, *Postgrad Med J* 72(843):45-50, 1996.

18. Arsenian MA, New PS, Cafasso CM: Safety, tolerability, and efficacy of a glucose-insulin-potassium-magnesium-carnitine solution in acute myocardial infarction, *Am J Cardiol* 78(4):477-479, 1996.

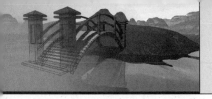

Nutritional Oncology and Integrative Cancer Care

A Rational, Mechanism-Based Approach

KEITH I. BLOCK

CANCER REMAINS one of the most formidable biologic enigmas suffered by modern humanity. Although patients and clinicians alike tend to think of cancer as a distinct morphologic entity, it is perhaps better understood as a *multistep process* in which numerous factors—many of them within our control—can determine its malignant behavior. Additionally, the multifactorial etiology of each cancer varies from one type to the next, as well as from one patient to the next. It therefore stands to reason that comprehensive therapy for this complex disorder necessitates a multifaceted and pluralistic strategy tailored to the disease, the patients' particular biochemistry, and the biopsychosocial uniqueness of each potential survivor. The essential components of integrative cancer care comprise the primary focus of this chapter.

With very few facilities offering integrative care in the field of oncology, we have taken liberty in this chapter to refer to our center as a model for future interest. For the past two decades, this author's clinical work at the Block Medical Center and research through the Institute for Integrative Cancer Care, both located in Evanston, Illinois, have focused on modulating the biochemical milieu toward actively inhibiting oncogenesis. Ongoing integration of information derived from clinical observation and literature research is coordinated through the Institute. Along with colleagues at the University of Illinois, this author's research staff has been investigating the following five areas of integrative cancer management: (1) toxicity mitigation for chemotherapy and radiotherapy; (2) adjuvant nutrition for standard oncologic care; (3) physical care, stress reduction, and support groups; (4) safety and efficacy of phytochemical and botanic agents as adjuncts to standard anticancer therapy; and (5) remission consolidation, which involves secondary, tertiary, and quarternary prevention strategies.[1]

There still is considerable room for improvement concerning standard therapy and long-range management for most cancers. Despite some indications that clinical outcomes for certain cancers are improving, overall efficacy of many chemotherapy agents now has reached a plateau, at least as they are currently implemented in the oncologic setting.[2] Even with several limited additions of new chemotherapy agents, improvements in clinical outcome in general have been modest. Cancer mortality rates remain unacceptably high, and survival rates for most cancers have improved only marginally in recent years, if at all. Since 1971, when Nixon proclaimed "war on cancer," 5-year survival and mortality rates have declined only marginally for most types of solid tumors.[3]

It is the aim of integrative cancer care to improve patient care and patient outcome by transforming the landscape of mainstream cancer medicine. A wealth of both clinical and laboratory data indicate that specific nutrients and other natural agents can block and even reverse the processes that underlie tumor growth and metastasis. Many of these agents can augment the effectiveness of standard medical treatments, all of which play an integral role in our approach. Some have proved highly useful in the mitigation of treatment-related toxicities resulting primarily from the use of chemotherapy and radiation treatments. We believe that the optimal approach to cancer biotherapy involves tailoring the selection of these natural agents to the specific disease, treatment, individual biochemistry, and individual psychologic orientation.

In addition to this biologic focus, however, our approach makes extensive use of psychotherapeutic and biobehavioral strategies for controlling cancer. In our view, achieving a "cure" or prolonged survival is only one important goal in the battle against cancer. In this regard, conceptualizing and treating neoplastic disease as a chronic illness that can be managed for an extensive time is gaining favor. No less important is the physician's unremitting attention to the patient's personal needs, energy levels, and other quality-of-life concerns. To live longer is no more important than feeling vital and at peace with the condition, connected to family or extended family, and in harmony with surroundings. Finding meaning and purpose in life and experiencing a renewed sense of vitality—these more intangible outcomes are linked inextricably to the healing experience, as well as survivorship per se.[4] Thus, our approach extends beyond the classical patient-physician relationship.

For physicians who endorse a truly integrative approach, it is important to exploit the full range of biologically based strategies aimed at halting the progression of cancer. Our Evanston experience suggests that practitioners should consider enlisting the support of ancillary caregivers, including dietitians, fitness trainers, acupuncturists, massage therapists, psychologists, and behavioral medicine specialists with expertise in techniques like imagery, meditation, biofeedback, and relaxation.

Modulating the Malignant Terrain

To better understand the rationale behind an individually tailored approach to cancer treatment, it is first necessary to explore the dynamic relationship between neoplastic disease and the host environment. We refer to this biochemical milieu, which can either support or restrain the development and progression of cancer, as the *terrain*. The clinical behavior of malignant cells reflects interactions between the intrinsic aggressive potential of these cells on the one hand and the tumor- and metastasis-retarding influences of the host on the other hand.[5] Biologically comprehensive cancer therapy is designed to alter the terrain in which the malignant "seed" of cancer takes root.

Let us take a closer look at how the host environment can influence the course of this disease. The transformation from normal cells to cancer cells is thought to result from successive and cumulative genetic defects. Moreover, cancer cells themselves are genetically unstable, and various defective aspects of malignant DNA metabolism, such as those involving telomere maintenance and DNA repair mechanisms, contribute to tumor growth and progression.[6] Cancer cells produce numerous immune-suppressive factors that enable tumors to evade immune recognition, thus allowing effective invasion and eventual spreading of the malignancy. Within the disease process, defective genes clearly do not exist in isolation. Such genetic instability can be increased under the intracellular influence of free radicals derived from diets high in fat[7,8] and low in antioxidants.[9,10] High-fat diets also may increase a tumor's metastatic potential, possibly through a mechanism involving alterations in cholesterol metabolism.[11] In breast tumors and other cancers, higher concentrations of DNA lesions have been found in cancerous tissues compared to cancer-free surrounding tissues,[12] and the pattern of these lesions changes as a tumor's metastatic potential increases.[13] These higher levels of DNA lesions suggest that free radical reactions may help determine the malignant character of these cells. In breast cancer patients, high-fat intakes correlate with adverse prognostic factors, such as high circulating estradiol levels[14,15] and an aneuploid DNA pattern.[16]

A great deal of recent evidence has demonstrated that in most, if not all cancers, tumor cell biology can be altered biochemically. The tumor terrain or biochemical milieu can vary tremendously from one patient to the next depending on dietary habits, genetic makeup, body composition, psychologic stress, and exercise patterns. The tumor-growth regulatory influence of the biochemical terrain can be modulated by a low-fat, high-vegetable diet and nutritional pharmacology, which includes supplemental agents such as nutrients, phytochemicals, and botanicals. Other factors aimed at blocking the terrain's ability to enhance tumor growth and invasiveness include mind-body techniques and therapeutic exercise. Accordingly, such noninvasive interventions are integral to the treatment and long-term management of cancer.

The idea that the host environment may be essential to tumor progression is illustrated by a 1992 report in which breast cancer growth characteristics were associated with a wide range of host factors in 91 postmenopausal women with breast cancer.[17] The researchers reported that high consumption of saturated and monounsaturated fat correlated significantly with increased tumor growth; conversely, consumption of fiber, vitamins, vegetables, and fruits was associated with a significant decrease in tumor-growth characteristics. Perhaps because so little attention is focused on adjusting and fine-tuning the terrain, dietary fat and lack of antioxidant compounds may be a stronger contributor to advanced cancer than is currently realized. Instead, virtually all medical attention is aimed at eradicating the tumor, often at the expense of host-defense mechanisms. Chemotherapy and radiation treatments figure prominently in this endeavor, and though they continue to reap substantial clinical rewards, the need for improved outcomes warrants a broader approach.

The Seven-Part Approach of Block Integrative Cancer Care

Based on clinical experience and observations at the Institute for Integrative Cancer Care, seven major components of clinical care have been identified. These components of the Block Integrative Cancer Care (BICCTM) program are not listed in order of importance, although it is true that much of the initial emphasis is placed on the first aspect, which pertains to the healing persona of the patient. Nutrition may be considered a primary mediating factor in treatment and thus will be addressed in greater detail in this chapter. Each component is intended to work in tandem to alleviate the side effects of cytotoxic treatments and enhance the prospects for recovery from cancer. To provide a limited treatment approach focusing on only one dimension of care is to forsake the profound healing potential afforded by mind-body interactions and somatic care strategies.

1. Attitudes and Beliefs

The clinician's consideration of the impact of attitudes and beliefs comprises the first of our seven components. In all clinical interactions the patient can and should be viewed as a whole person, not simply as a case or disease. Our team of health professionals strives to recognize each individual's aspirations and agendas (including those that predate the illness), as well as reactions to the diagnosis, specific type of illness, fears of treatment, and concerns regarding prognosis. In some cases, for example, the cancer may have occurred previously in the family and therefore carries a strong emotional charge. The powerful impact of beliefs has been demonstrated through studies of the placebo effect in which people who adhered to the placebo had better therapeutic outcomes than those who did not.[18,19]

Additionally, we strive to help patients cultivate a life-affirming philosophy and willingness to actively participate in their healing process. Thus, our physicians and other caregivers are encouraged to evince an enthusiastic, hope-oriented, caring, and supportive attitude in all clinical proceedings. We value hope as a positive healing force, something to be promoted and reinforced. Some clinicians may feel concerned that what it being offered here is a kind of "false hope." In this author's view, however, far more worrisome than false hope is any insensitive incitement of hopelessness, a reckless stealing of hope that characterizes some aspects of conventional oncologic practice today.

Feelings often are suppressed around the time of diagnosis, usually in response to the diagnosis itself.[20,21] The tendency to suppress feelings has consistently shown associations with the decline of the body's anticancer defenses.[22,23] Thus, the undermining of hope by insensitive communications from the caregiver (even when well-intentioned) can have a profoundly adverse effect on survival (also known as the "nocebo effect," in contradistinction with that of the placebo).[24] Hope connotes a positive, adaptive mode of engaging with life, which recognizes that connecting with and expressing feelings is beneficial. Physicians therefore should encourage their patients to ask questions and assert their needs while also providing the space and time for the expression of feelings. Also core to our clinical approach is assisting the patient in lifestyle and personal introspection to influence self-care, personal well-being, and overall life experience.

2. Medical Care

Our next major component, medical care, is of course an integral part of all cancer management decisions. The development of a comprehensive therapeutic plan must be based on a thorough understanding of the effects of treatment on both the tumor *and* the host (patient). For example, because chemotherapy drugs tend to be immunosuppressive, immune augmentation strategies may be employed to minimize this side effect. Studies in nutritional and medicinal chemistry have uncovered numerous ways to integrate cytotoxic therapies with natural or semisynthetic bioactive agents (also referred to here as *biologic response modifiers*) capable of mitigating treatment-related toxicities while also augmenting the immunologic attack on malignant cells. For example, the glutathione precursor N-acetyl cysteine is not only synergistic with doxorubicin[25] but also happens to protect the heart against the drug's toxic effects without reducing its antitumor activity.[26,27] Other natural agents that have shown promise in preventing or limiting the cardiotoxicity produced by doxorubicin include selenium compounds,[28] niacin and isocitrate,[29] and coenzyme Q10[30,31] or a combined regimen of coenzyme Q10, dextran sulfate, and reduced glutathione.[32] Thus, the BICC approach includes relatively low-cost forms of immunotherapy that serve not only as therapy per se but as adjuvant strategies for restoring optimal immunocompetence during and after periods of chemotherapy or radiotherapy. Full medical and diagnostic workups are performed on each patient. Conventional anticancer treatments and reasonable options for the specific disorders, including the potential for treatment-related complications, are covered in detail. Although not all patients are willing to follow our recommendations for conventional therapy, we continue to work with them with regard to responsible use of alternative, experimental, and complementary therapies (discussed in the following section). Thus, for example, our clinic provides full oncology services in which each patient's protocol is adjusted on both an inpatient and outpatient basis to provide the options of treatment modalities most consistent with state-of-the-art science, while recognizing the important broader needs of each patient.

Our course of medical treatment follows a graduated scheme where appropriate, depending on tumor type and disease stage, moving from a less invasive strategy to a more invasive one, as the need calls for and as the informed patient chooses. We often advise the administering of chemotherapy in fractionated doses as a continuous infusion to attempt to reduce adverse side effects and increase treatment efficacy (for example, the potential for immune enhancement using 5-FU).[33] For the treatment of testicular carcinoma or advanced-stage lymphoma, a more aggressive approach to cytotoxic therapy is commonly recommended. However, intensive chemotherapy and radiation treatments are followed up with an equally intensive program of immune enhancement, detoxification, tissue repair, and systemic rebuilding.

In some cases, the scheduling of treatment regimens is aligned with circadian variations in drug metabolism and tissue sensitivity to drugs. Administering drugs at selective times of the day, an innovative strategy known as *cancer chronotherapy*, has demonstrated the capacity to potentiate the drugs' activity and diminish toxicity.[34,35,36] This innovative approach has shown considerable promise in the cytotoxic treatment of gastrointestinal cancers,[37] as well as, to a lesser degree, in treating cancers of the lung[38] and breast.[39] Supplementary agents, acupuncture, hypnotherapy, biofeedback training, and practices such as Qi Gong also are provided to decrease side effects of chemotherapy and radiotherapy. The goal of these strategies is to minimize untoward effects while maximizing therapeutic efficacy, as documented earlier.

3. Therapeutic Nutrition

Our approach to nutritional biotherapy entails personally tailored use of diet and nutrition to modulate host-tumor relationships and treatment effects.[40-42] Dietary modification involves changes in food selection and preparation of foods and diets that are aimed at modulating specific anticancer mechanisms to reinforce treatment effects or mitigate adverse side effects.[43] In the majority of cases, this refers to adoption of a diet low in fat, moderate in protein, and high in complex carbohydrates and fiber. Additionally, however, certain foods and food combinations may be highlighted for individual consumption depending on biochemical individuality and disease-related factors.

In agreement with the more up-to-date scientific literature on adjuvant nutrition for cancer treatment, the basic dietary approach is low in fat (15% to 18% in most cases), moderate in protein (chiefly from vegetarian sources), and high in vegetables, fruits, and whole grain cereals, breads, and pastas. Fish and egg whites are acceptable alternate sources of protein, particularly if a patient desires animal products or would benefit clinically from such concentrated protein sources (for example, in the case of cachexia or during therapies that result in increased catabolism). With the complex nature of malignant disease and treatments, optimal care warrants a personalized and tailored regimen for each patient. Along with adjusting for body composition, we perform a variety of tests to determine macronutrient and micronutrient needs, adjusting these according to other individual factors as well, such as appetite decline and lean-tissue wasting, hormonal levels, lipid peroxidation, antioxidant levels, and immunosuppression.

Specific dietary components can be emphasized to increase the intake of phytochemicals with known anticancer and detoxification properties. Regular consumption of soy products, for instance, is recommended for most patients, in part based on the high genistein content. Investigations of soy isoflavones have demonstrated antiestrogenic activity, inhibition of topoisomerases and protein tyrosine kinases, regulation of cell cycle progression and apoptosis, and inhibition of both angiogenesis and cell proliferation.[44-46] Several reports have suggested that dietary supplementation with soybean products deters the growth of primary tumors (breast, colon, liver, and prostate tumors), as well as the development of metastatic secondary tumors.[47-50] Numerous other properties make soy products a potentially valuable adjunctive strategy for breast cancer patients, although more research is needed to evaluate this possibility. Dietary modulation of hormonal balances that influence tumor biology has intriguing therapeutic potential. At the molecular level, dietary lipids can induce specific changes in oncogenes and the metabolism of both estrogens and androgens.[51-53] Low-fat, high-fiber dietary patterns are generally associated with lower blood concentrations of estrogens and androgens. For instance, plasma testosterone and estradiol levels in Seventh-Day Adventist men were both significantly lower among lactovegetarians compared to omnivores when fat intakes were comparable; notably, the sex hormone levels within these subpopulations were inversely correlated with dietary fiber.[54] Among the Japanese, mortality rates for cancers of the breast and prostate are significantly lower than they are among North Americans diagnosed with these cancers. Japanese men and women have lower androgen and estrogen levels compared to their U.S. counterparts, and this may reflect lower body mass as well as the high-fiber, low-fat dietary pattern that has become the traditional trademark of Asian populations.[55]

Indeed, from the epidemiologic perspective, a low-fat, plant-based diet seems to be critically important in moderating sex hormone levels in men and women alike. Lowering the intake of total fat from 40% to 25% of total calories and increasing the ratio of dietary polyunsaturated to saturated fatty acids has been associated with significant decreases in total serum testosterone and nonprotein-bound testosterone.[56] A low-fat, plant-based diet tends to moderate circulating estrogen levels, as reflected in the substantial differences in patterns of estrogen metabolism between vegan and omnivorous women.[57-60] The intestinal flora of vegans excrete more byproducts of estrogen metabolism and reabsorb the least compared to the flora of lactovegetarians or meat-eaters.[61]

Within the area of dietary modification, recommendations are formulated as exchange lists ("trade-off groups") to quantify a regimen to meet individual needs. Patients receive personalized dietary counseling and training to guide them in proper food selection. Caloric needs are calculated based on body size, severity of illness, and treatment plan, and numbers of each exchange in the daily diet then are outlined and discussed with the patient and other caregivers who may attend the consultation. The BINTTM program was developed through extensive research in the early 1980s to provide a system of optimal food choices, quantifiably tailored to the needs of each patient. The program also specifies foods that are less advantageous and thus reduced or avoided. Among these are meats (with the exception of fish), dairy products, sugar and refined flour products, and caffeine and other stimulants.

4. Supplementation

The fourth component uses biologically active agents in supplement form. Our nutritional biotherapy program is individually tailored to the unique biochemistry of each individual as well as the treatments and disease itself (type and stage of cancer, relative aggressiveness, and so on). These supplements, which include macro and micronutrients, phytochemicals, and botanicals, including some select biochemical agents, enhance the therapeutic effects of the diet. Examples include the antitumor role of vitamin E, which may block oncogenesis by downregulating protein kinase C,[62] as well as tumorigenic cytokines (while also upregulating cytokines associated with enhanced immunologic function).[63,64] By inhibiting the aggregation of platelets,[65] vitamin E potentially may restrain the metastatic process.

Immune modulation is another important avenue through which nutritional pharmacology may prove useful. Vitamin A compounds (retinoids), along with the vitamin A precursor beta-carotene, enhances a number of anticancer defense mechanisms, including the cytotoxic activity of natural killer (NK) cells,[66-68] T-lymphocytes,[69,70] and tumoricidal macrophages,[71-73] which may be involved in the removal of chemoresistant residual cancer cells. Vitamin E supplements have been shown to prevent age-related immune dysfunction[74] and may reduce muscular atrophy during immobilization (hospitalization).[75] Vitamin E invariably is used in conjunction with eicosapentaenoic acid (EPA), the highly unsaturated omega-3 fatty acid within fish oil. EPA has been shown to inhibit tumor growth and block metastasis through a variety of mechanisms.[76-79] EPA and other omega-3 fatty acids may also reverse immune suppression,[80] radioresistance,[81] and the cachectic state often associated with advanced malignancy.[82] Some studies have focused on EPA's ability to downregulate the production of inflammatory cytokines and eicosanoids, thus helping to impede tumor progression.

Although such a mechanism-based perspective on nutritional oncology is helpful in illuminating potential avenues for effective treatment, the efficacy of these treatment possibilities must be substantiated through an evidence-based assessment of treatment efficacy and clinical outcomes. Evidence-based medicine* has been defined as "the conscientious, explicit, and judicious use of current best evidence in making decisions about the care of individual patients."[83] With regard to treatment, for example, adjuvant nutrition has demonstrated efficacy in treating cancers of the lung,[84,85] breast,[86,87] bladder,[88,89] and pancreas.[90,91] However, because of insufficient funding for conducting randomized clinical trials of adjuvant nutrition, nutritional oncology relies heavily on findings from nonrandomized studies and the experiences or anecdotal reports of the relatively few clinicians who are working in this still incipient field. With limited time for keeping abreast of this fast-growing body of literature, physicians must make special efforts to identify and meet their ongoing learning needs and apply their knowledge appropriately and consistently in the nutritional oncologic setting.

Besides scientific evaluation, one of the areas that distinguishes our approach to nutritional oncology from those that have been introduced in the past (primarily through lay books and journal articles) is our emphasis on individual tailoring rather than a shotgun or "everything and the kitchen sink" approach. The need for tailoring is highlighted by the adverse effects of certain drug-nutrient interactions, nutrient-nutrient interactions, and nutrient-disease interactions. Within breast cancer, for example, the following deficiencies are not uncommon: 1) the vitamin-like substance, coenzyme Q10 (CoQ10) and one of its precursors, pyridoxine;[92,93] 2) vitamin D and magnesium as a consequence of cisplatin treatment;[94,95] 3) zinc, selenium, and vitamins A and E, resulting from doxorubicin treatment;[96,97] and 4) vitamins C and B1 (thiamin), due to treatment with fluorouracil (5FU), one of the chemotherapy agents often used for treatment of metastatic breast cancer.[98,99] Whether such nutritional problems are caused by the disease or treatment or both, in each instance there are grounds for nutritional modulation to restore the patient's functional status and to enhance overall treatment efficacy.[100,101]

The BICC approach to supplementation, along with the diagnostic testing used to assist in the design of the therapeutic plan, is beyond the scope of this discussion. However, the box "Sample Tests of the BINTTM Nutrition Screening Panel" briefly summarizes three important tests that we have found useful for tailoring our biotherapeutic approach to the individual cancer patient.

One of the areas that has become of special interest to proponents of cancer biotherapy is the inhibition of angiogenesis, the formation of new blood vessels by which growing tumors obtain their nourishment. Recent research indicates that antiangiogenic agents may synergistically enhance the effectiveness of chemotherapy treatments.[102-106] Moreover, the

---

*The process that characterizes evidence-based medicine includes problem formulation, study location and retrieval, critical appraisal of evidence, application to patient management, and self-evaluation. Findings from clinical trials can be used to answer a host of health-related questions regarding symptomology, diagnostic signs, prognostic indicators, treatment, and even cost effectiveness.

combination of the antiangiogenic agent with minocycline (an antibiotic) potentiated the lethal effects of fractionated radiotherapy.[107] Based on a more recent series of animal experiments, Teicher and colleagues conclude "that a broad range of antiangiogenic therapies can interact in a positive manner with cytotoxic therapies."[108] Among the angiogenic inhibitors that may work well in combination with cytotoxic agents are suramin, TNP-470, minocycline, linomide, and interferon-delta-4.[109] In the absence of controlled clinical trials, however, the long-range safety and efficacy of these agents remains questionable.

For a variety of reasons, antiangiogenic therapy appears to require implementation over a period of months or even years, without a break in therapy. This approach is aimed at stabilizing the residual primary tumor and to extend "dormancy" of micrometastases. Thus the goal is improved control of tumor growth rather than outright tumor eradication. Because of this, we recommend the broad-spectrum, daily use of natural agents capable of inhibiting angiogenesis, as these agents generally have low toxicity. The following candidates appear to have some promise based on laboratory research: soy genistein, the dominant isoflavone found in legumes;[110,111] thiol compounds such as glutathione, acetyl-cysteine, and other sulfur-containing compounds from *Allium sativum*, or garlic;[112] the bioflavonoids apigenin and luteolin;[113] omega-3 fatty acids from fish oil;[114] cartilage products;[115,116] vitamin A and its analogues;[117] vitamin D and analogues;[118] vitamin E;[119] alpha-interferon combined with 13-cis-retinoic acid;[120] and various natural agents such as chitin (a polysaccharide derived from insect exoskeletons) and extracts of magnolia (*Magnolia liliflora*).[121] Research on animal models to date suggests some combination of these agents could be effective in blocking angiogenesis, thus aiding in the prevention of metastasis. The selection of nutrients and other bioactive agents for each biomodulation regimen is planned with the help of information obtained from testing as described in the box. Biochemical test results are carefully assessed to design an appropriate supplementation regimen. A few of the categories we consider when developing personalized programs include the following: 1) protein, calorie, and fiber food supplements; b) vitamin and mineral supplements; and 3) botanic agents. These may be described as follows:

1. Protein, calorie, and fiber food supplements: We recommend the use of either a soy-based or rice protein-based supplement to minimize allergic reactions. These supplements contain natural sweeteners derived from brown rice rather than the refined carbohydrates found in conventional protein and calorie food supplements. The plant-based formula includes fiber supplements and food sources containing both soluble and insoluble fiber types.

2. Vitamin and mineral supplements: A variety of vitamin and mineral supplements are used to increase the patient's intake of antioxidants and other critical elements to achieve supraphysiologic levels. In many patients, micronutrients may be deficient because of the biochemical assaults posed by chemotherapy, surgery, radiation, or disease-related cachexia or anorexia.

3. Botanic agents and fatty-acid based supplements: European and Chinese botanic agents are examples commonly used in our clinics. These include combined formulations designed for specific needs with items such as borage oil, fish oil, astragalus, saw palmetto, garlic, and other substances that have shown potential as anticancer agents or can be used in specifically tailored situations to reduce side effects or enhance efficacy of conventional therapy.

5. Physical Care

Physical care, the fifth component of integrative care, includes both therapeutic exercise and physical or somatic treatments. Most cancer patients are assigned exercise programs according to personal preference as well as physical abilities and limitations. We employ specialists in bodywork of different types (orthobionomy, shiatsu, and deep-tissue massage), as well as acupressure and electrical stimulation for pain care. These treatments appear to be of particular benefit in work with patients who require pain reduction. Asian yoga practices, Qi Gong, and a series of Tai Chi-like exercises (slow, gentle, rhythmic movements aimed at relaxation and raising energy levels) are used for strengthening and rebuilding. In a study of 122 cancer patients in China, physicians reported that the longer Qi Gong was practiced, the greater was the inhibition of tumor growth and reduction in pain.[122] In another study of Qi Gong practitioners, immune cell counts remained stable and relatively few patients experienced the adverse side effects typically seen with chemotherapy, such as poor appetite and vomiting; also, whereas only 8% of Qi Gong cases showed no response to the chemotherapy, 39% of the control cases (no Qi Gong) were nonresponders.[123] It should be noted that these relaxing yet rejuvenating exercises also are specially tailored for bedridden or extremely weak patients with cancer.

6. Stress Care

Our sixth component, stress care, pertains to the psychologic well-being of patients with cancer. Data from several psychooncology studies of cancer survivorship[124-126] have indicated significant clinical benefits resulting from psychosocial support and stress management in patients with cancer. Comprehensive approaches to the patient include stress care provided on an individualized basis, respecting personal preference or inclination. Specialists in our clinics provide guidance in cognitive restructuring, imaging and visualization, support group programs, use of prayer, logotherapy, biofeedback, meditation, journals, drawing (a creative, imagery projection exercise), and a variety of other stress reduction techniques and interventions uniquely suited to the patient. Individuals will tend to vary in the benefits they can derive from different stress reduction techniques. The therapeutic value is even more impressive when stress care is not focused solely on mitigating stress but also on augmenting the patient's inner resources for active healing.

7. Reasonable and Responsible Use of Alternative and Experimental Therapies

Responsible use of selected experimental and alternative treatment options is encouraged for patients who seek such options when a reasonable therapeutic situation arises. These options may be recommended or at least supported for patients, either when options for conventional therapy have been exhausted or when patients desire their inclusion along with orthodox medical treatments. Reasonable and responsible alternative or experimental treatments may be recommended when the patient is unwilling to consider conventional strategies; however, these treatments should be chosen with consideration for the following: 1) the type and stage of disease; 2) age and condition of the patient; 3) a poor benefit-risk ratio for conventional treatment; and 4) a reasonable rationale or meaningful evidence exists to support the usefulness of the therapy. For example, some patients may choose echinacea along with their standard regimen, hoping to benefit from its immune-potentiating effects. An arabinogalactan in echinacea has been shown to stimulate the tumor-killing activity of macrophages.[127] In a study of patients with inoperable liver cancer, the cytotoxic activity of their natural killer cells increased by 90% with the addition of echinacea to thymostimulin.[128] Thus, where clinical data may be sparse, agents such as echinacea may be used safely and reasonably from a mechanism-based perspective.

Conclusion

Many innovative technologies and gene therapies will help revolutionize oncology in the coming years. Our clinical experience over the past two decades confirms an emergent consensus provided by clinical and laboratory data. This rapidly growing body of evidence suggests that substantial advances in cancer care will continue to develop by combining nutrition and other biomodulation strategies with established treatment modalities, including surgery, radiotherapy, chemotherapy, and hyperthermia. The benefits of psychotherapy and psychosocial support for patients with cancer can be further augmented by interweaving these modalities with complementary therapies. Quality of life, which subsumes performance status, is an independent predictor of survival duration for several types of cancer, and thus any improvement in this aspect of survivorship may be considered a valid if not essential goal of optimal cancer care.[129] The basic goal of our integrated, multifaceted approach is to exploit the full range of the patient's self-healing resources.[130] Future intervention trials will help provide the substantiation required to make more definitive statements regarding the efficacy of specific protocols.

Oncologic care strategies must be extended beyond achieving disease stabilization or remission to encompass long-range management or what we refer to as "remission consolidation." With respect to colorectal cancer, for example, the initial prevention is termed *primary prevention*. Following diagnosis and treatment, however, the prevention of a recurrence of colorectal cancer is termed *secondary prevention*. Calcium supplementation has been shown to inhibit the formation of adenomatous polyps after polypectomy and after colorectal surgery.[131] Supplementation with omega-3 fatty acids (notably fish oils)[132] and antioxidants such as vitamin C[133,134] and N-acetyl cysteine[135] may provide additional long-range protection against colorectal cancer for both men and women. Admittedly the weight of evidence for secondary prevention is considerably lighter than for primary prevention. However, findings from studies of primary prevention may be used to inform efforts at secondary prevention: the likelihood of successful remission consolidation is enhanced by implementing and *intensifying* the primary prevention strategies. Remission consolidation strategies must in general be more rigorous than primary prevention strategies because cancer patients represent a high-risk group (for recurrence and relapse) compared to the general population.

Metastasis continues to be the nemesis of oncologic care. To improve treatments and outcomes for those suffering from neoplastic dissemination, it will be necessary to go beyond the standard approaches embraced in major treatment centers. By including nutritional biotherapy, physical care, and psychotherapeutic support as integral components of cancer care, this new treatment paradigm which this author refers to as *biopsychooncology*[136] makes it possible to discuss managing cancers much as chronic illnesses such as diabetes, arthritis, and cardiovascular disorders. Thus, instead of limiting care to an aggressive, kill-and-cure paradigm that has prevailed for several generations of oncological care, where this is not a successful reality, a more control-oriented approach to treatment should be embraced.[137,138] The question at this point is not whether such control is possible, but which combinations of biomodulation strategies are most appropriate for any given clinical situation. With new innovations in the emerging field of integrative cancer care, the hope of controlling oncogenesis now is coming within reach.

In closing, let us keep in mind that treatment of advanced cancer is *not* a straightforward medical problem. Tumor growth and metastasis involve a highly complex set of processes, all of which may be subject to nutritional modulation.[139] Most, if not all, nutrition-related malignant processes depend on the intricate interplay of intracellular signaling, growth factor regulation, immune and hormonal modulation, detoxification pathways, and host defense systems. As stated at the outset, malignant cells are genetically unstable, and cancer cell function can be further disrupted by the biochemical milieu, which is in constant flux and may greatly vary from one patient to the next. Our research at the Institute for Integrative Cancer Care suggests that further research into the ability to more precisely tailor regimens to each patient's disease, treatments, biochemistry, psychoemotional profile, and personal preferences will continue to improve treatment outcomes.

SAMPLE TESTS OF THE BINT™ NUTRITION SCREENING PANEL*

Vitamin A, E, and carotenoids: This micronutrient assessment tool measures the concentrations of selected vitamins and carotenoids in the blood. Low or suboptimal levels of these micronutrients have been correlated with tumor progression, suggesting that the body uses them to combat neoplastic disease. Analysis of carotenoids reflects overall intake of vegetables and thus serves as a barometer for healthy eating patterns. Concentrations of each vitamin and carotenoid are recorded separately, providing important information for tailoring the supplementation regimen for each patient.

Oxidative Stress Index: This clinical assessment tool indicates the patient's degree of free radical damage. Oxidative stress as measured by the blood level of oxidized low-density lipoproteins, lipid peroxide levels, and total oxidative protection (TOPI index) is correlated with tumor growth and metastasis. Once the level of oxidative stress is established the physician can select appropriate supplemental antioxidants and dietary modifications, all tailored to individual needs.

Essential Fatty Acids: This clinical assessment tool measures the concentrations of fatty acids in blood. Omega-3 fatty acids have been shown to cause a substantial reduction in inflammatory processes and both tumor growth and metastasis. The Block Integrative Nutrition Treatment (BINT) program was in part formulated to raise the level of omega-3 fatty acids relative to omega-6 fatty acids and to increase monounsaturates while decreasing saturated fatty acids. Adjusting the nutritional biotherapy strategy toward optimal ratios may result in numerous anticancer benefits.

---

*Additional assessments include measures of immunocompetence, detoxification pathways, and cancer markers, among other standard tests.

SAMPLE BICCTM ASSESSMENT CHECKLIST

ASSESSMENT
General panels
Oxidative stress index
Antioxidant status
Immune function index
Inflammatory markers
Coagulation index
General stress index
Metabolic profile
Detox capacity
Hormone panels
Nutrition status
Fitness index

References

1. Adjuvant nutrition.
2. Hollander S, Gordon M: The plateau in cytotoxic cancer drug discovery, *J Med* 21(3-4):143-163, 1990.
3. Taylor PR: Personal communication, 1995.
4. Block KI: The role of self in healthy cancer survivorship, *Advances* 13(1):6-26, 1997.
5. NCAB Subcommittee to Evaluate the National Cancer Program: *Cancer at a crossroads: a report to Congress for the nation*, Bethesda, Md, 1994, National Cancer Advisory Board.
6. Miyagawa K: Genetic instability and cancer, *Int J Hermatol* 67(1):3-14, 1998.
7. Djuric Z et al: Dietary modulation of oxidative DNA damage, *Adv Exper Med Biol* 354:71-83, 1994.
8. Yang MH, Schaich KM: Factors affecting DNA damage caused by lipid hydroperoxides and aldehydes, *Free Radical Biol Med* 20(2):225-236, 1996.
9. Jacob RA, Burri BJ: Oxidative damage and defense, *Am J Clin Nutr* 63(6):985S-990S, 1996.
10. Anderson D: Antioxidant defenses against reactive oxygen species causing genetic and other damage, *Mut Res* 350(1):103-108, 1996.
11. Mehta N et al: Cellular effects of hypercholesterolemia in modulation of cancer growth and metastasis: a review of the evidence, *Surg Oncol* 6(3):179-185, 1997.
12. Malins DC et al: The etiology and prediction of breast cancer. Fourier transform-infrared spectroscopy reveals progressive alterations in breast DNA leading to a cancer-like phenotype in a high proportion of normal women, *Cancer* 75(2):503-517, 1995.
13. Malins DC, Polissar NL, Gunselman SJ: Tumor progression to the metastatic state involves structural modifications in DNA markedly different from those associated with primary tumor formation, *Proceedings of the National Academy of Sciences of the United States of America* 93(24):14047-14052, 1996.

14. Stoll BA: Diet and exercise regimens to improve breast carcinoma prognosis, *Cancer* 78(12):2465-2470, 1996.

15. Kuller LH: Dietary fat and chronic diseases: epidemiologic overview, *JADA* 97(7):S9-S15, 1997.

16. Furst CJ et al: DNA pattern and dietary habits in patients with breast cancer, *Eur J Cancer* 29A(9):1285-1288, 1993.

17. Ingram DM, Roberts A, Nottage EM: Host factors and breast cancer growth characteristics, *Eur J Cancer* 28A(6-7):1153-1161, 1992.

18. Horwitz RI et al: Treatment adherence and risk of death after a myocardial infarction, *Lancet* 336:542-546, 1990.

19. Brown W: Harnessing the placebo effect, *Hosp Prac* 107-116, 1998.

20. Kreitler S et al: Repressiveness: cause or result of cancer? *Psychooncol* 2:43-54, 1993.

21. Greer S, Morris T: Psychological attributes of women who develop breast cancer: a controlled study, *J Psychosom Res* 19:147-153, 1975.

22. Chiappelli F et al: Differential effect of beta-endorphin on three human cytotoxic cell populations, *Int J Immunopharmacol* 13:291-297, 1991.

23. Aarstead JH et al: The effect of stress in vivo on the function of mouse macrophages in vitro, *Scan J Immunol* 33:673-681, 1991.

24. Spiegel H: Nocebo: the power of suggestibility, *Prevent Med* 26(5):616-621, 1997.

25. De Flora SD et al: Synergism between N-acetylcysteine and doxorubicin in the prevention of tumorigenicity and metastasis in murine models, *Int J Cancer* 67(6):842-848, 1996.

26. Doroshow JH et al: Prevention of doxorubicin cardiac toxicity in the mouse by N-acetylcysteine, *J Clin Invest* 68(4):1053-1064, 1981.

27. Wagdi P et al: Cardioprotection in patients undergoing chemo- and/or radiotherapy for neoplastic disease. A pilot study, *Japan Heart J* 37(3):353-359, 1996.

28. Pritsos CA, Sokoloff M, Gustafson DL: PZ-51 (ebselen) in vivo protection against adriamycin-induced mouse cardiac and hepatic lipid peroxidation and toxicity, *Biochem Pharmacol* 44(4):839-841, 1992.

29. Schmitt-Graff A, Scheulen ME: Prevention of adriamycin cardiotoxicity by niacin, isocitrate or N-acetyl-cysteine in mice. A morphological study, *Pathol Res Prac* 181(2):168-174, 1986.

30. Sugiyama S et al: Approaches that mitigate doxorubicin-induced delayed adverse effects on mitochondrial function in rat hearts; liposome-encapsulated doxorubicin or combination therapy with antioxidant, *Biochem Molec Biol Int* 36(5):1001-1007, 1995.

31. Shinozawa S, Gomita Y, Araki Y: Protective effects of various drugs on adriamycin (doxorubicin)-induced toxicity and microsomal lipid peroxidation in mice and rats, *Biol Pharm Bull* 16(11):1114-1117, 1993.

32. Shinozawa S, Kawasaki H, Gomita Y: Effect of biological membrane stabilizing drugs (coenzyme Q10, dextran sulfate and reduced glutathione) on adriamycin (doxorubicin)-induced toxicity and microsomal lipid peroxidation in mice, *Japan J Cancer Chemother* 23(1):93-98, 1996.

33. Daemen T et al: The effect of liver macrophages on in vitro cytolytic activity of 5FU and FUdR on colon carcinoma cells: evidence of macrophage activation, *Int J Immunopharmacol* 14(5):857-864, 1992.

34. Hrushesky WJ: Circadian pharmacodynamics of anticancer therapies, *Clin Chem* 39(11):2413-2418, 1993.

35. Hrushesky WJ, Bjarnason GA: Circadian cancer therapy, *J Clin Oncol* 11(7):1403-1417, 1993.

36. Hrushesky WJ: Cancer chronotherapy: is there a right time in the day to treat? *J Infus Chemother* 5(1):38-43, 1995.

37. Levi F: Chronotherapy for gastrointestinal cancers, *Current Op Oncol* 8(4):334-341, 1996.

38. Yamamoto N et al: Chronopharmacology of etoposide given by low dose prolonged infusion in lung cancer patients, *Anticancer Res* 17(1B):669-672, 1997.

39. Canal P et al: Chronopharmacokinetics of doxorubicin in patients with breast cancer, *Eur J Clin Pharmacol* 40(3):287-291, 1991.

40. Oldham RK: Cancer biotherapy: general principles. In Oldham RK, editor: *Principles of cancer biotherapy*, ed 2, New York, 1991, Marcel Dekker.

41. DeVita VT, Hellman S. Rosenberg SA: *Biologic therapy of cancer*, ed 2, Hagerstown, Md, 1995, Lippincott-Raven.

42. Tuttle-Newhall JE, Blackburn GL: Cancer and nutrition: a challenge to the nutritional specialist. In Quillin P, Williams RM, editors: *Adjuvant nutrition in cancer treatment*, Arlington Heights, Ill, 1993, Cancer Treatment Research Foundation/American College of Nutrition.

43. Block KI: Dietary impact on quality and quantity of life in cancer patients. In Quillin P, Williams RM, editors: *Adjuvant nutrition in cancer treatment*, Arlington Heights, Ill, 1993, Cancer Treatment Research Foundation/American College of Nutrition.

44. Messina MJ et al: Soy intake and cancer risk: a review of the in vitro and in vivo data, *Nutr Cancer* 21(2):113-131, 1994.

45. Barnes S: Effect of genistein on in vitro and in vivo models of cancer, *J Nutr* 125(3 Suppl):777S-783S, 1995.

46. Fotsis T et al: Genistein, a dietary ingested isoflavonoid, inhibits cell proliferation and in vitro angiogenesis, *J Nutr* 125(3 Suppl):790S-797S, 1995.

47. Messina MJ et al: Soy intake and cancer risk: a review of the in vitro and in vivo data, *Nutr Cancer* 21(2):113-131, 1994.

48. Barnes S, Peterson TG: Biochemical targets of the isoflavone genistein in tumor cell lines, *Proc Soc Exp Biol Med* 208:103-108, 1995.

49. Naik HR, Lehr JE, Pienta KJ: An in vitro and in vivo study of antitumor effects of genistein on hormone refractory prostate cancer, *Anticancer Res* 14(6B):2617-2619, 1994.

50. Stoll BA: Eating to beat breast cancer: potential role for soy supplements, *Ann Oncol* 8(3):223-225, 1997.

51. Kaput J et al: Diet-disease interactions at the molecular level: an experimental paradigm, *J Nutr* 124(8 Suppl):1296S-1305S, 1994.

52. DeWille JW et al: Dietary fat promotes mammary tumorigenesis in MMTV/v-Ha-ras transgenic mice, *Cancer Letters* 69(1):59-66, 1993.

53. Lanson M, Besson P, Bougnoux P: Supplementation of MCF-7 cells with essential fatty acids induces the activation of protein kinase C in response to IGF-1, *J Lipid Mediat Cell Signal* 16(3):189-197, 1997.

54. Howie BJ, Shultz TD: Dietary and hormonal interrelationships among vegetarian and Seventh-Day Adventists and nonvegetarian men, *Am J Clin Nutr* 42:127-134, 1985.

55. Wynder EL, Cohen LA, Winters BL: The challenges of assessing fat intake in cancer research investigations, *JADA* 97(7 Suppl):S5-8, 1997.

56. Hamalaine E et al: Diet and serum sex hormones in healthy men, *J Steroid Biochem* 20:459-464, 1984.

57. Goldin BR et al: Estrogen excretion patterns and plasma levels in vegetarian and omnivorous women, *New Engl J Med* 307:1542, 1982.

58. Gorbach SL, Goldin BR: Diet and the excretion and enterohepatic cycling of estrogens, *Prevent Med* 16(4):525-531, 1987.

59. Adlercreutz H et al: Urinary estrogen profile determination in young Finnish vegetarian and omnivorous women, *J Steroid Biochem* 24:289, 1986.

60. Hill PB et al: Gonadotrophin release and meat consumption in vegetarian women, *Am J Clin Nutr* 43:37, 1986.

61. Gorbach SL: Estrogens, breast cancer, and intestinal flora, *Rev Infect Dis* 6(Suppl 1):S85, 1984.

62. Azzi A et al: Vitamin E: a sensor and an information transducer of the cell oxidation state, *Am J Clin Nutr* 62(6 Suppl):1337S-1346S, 1995.

63. Wang Y, Watson RR: Vitamin E supplementation at various levels alters cytokine production by thymocytes during retrovirus infection causing murine AIDS, *Thymus* 22(3):153-165, 1994.

64. McCarty MF: Promotion of interleukin-2 activity as a strategy for "rejuvenating" geriatric immune function, *Med Hypoth* 48(1):47-54, 1997.

65. Bruckner G: Microcirculation, vitamin E and omega 3 fatty acids: an overview, *Adv Exper Med Biol* 415:195-208, 1997.

66. Zhao Z et al: Effects of N-(4-hydroxyphenyl)-retinamide on the number and cytotoxicity of natural killer cells in vitamin-A-sufficient and -deficient rats, *Nat Immun* 13(5):280-288, 1994.

67. Santoni A et al: Modulation of natural killer activity in mice by prolonged administration of various doses of dietary retinoids, *Nat Immun Cell Growth Reg* 5(5):259-266, 1986.

68. Gergely P et al: Effect of vitamin A treatment on cellular immune reactivity in patients with CLL, *Acta Medica Hungarica* 45(3-4):307-311, 1988.

69. Garbe A, Buck J, Hammerling U: Retinoids are important cofactors in T cell activation, *J Exper Med* 176(1):109-117, 1992.

70. Watson RR et al: Effect of beta-carotene on lymphocyte subpopulations in elderly humans: evidence for a dose-response relationship, *Am J Clin Nutr* 53(1):90-94, 1991.

71. Watson RR, Moriguchi S, Gensler HL: Effects of dietary retinyl palmitate and selenium on tumoricidal capacity of macrophages in mice undergoing tumor promotion, *Cancer Letters* 36(2):181-187, 1987.

72. Tachibana K et al: Stimulatory effect of vitamin A on tumoricidal activity of rat alveolar macrophages, *Brit J Cancer* 49(3):343-348, 1984.

73. Kishino Y, Moriguchi S: Nutritional factors and cellular immune responses, *Nutr Health* 8(2-3):133-141, 1992.

74. Losonczy KG, Harris TB, Havlik RJ: Vitamin E and vitamin C supplement use and risk of all-cause and coronary heart disease mortality in older persons: the established populations for epidemiologic studies of the elderly, *Am J Clin Nutr* 64(2):190-196, 1996.

75. Appell HJ, Duarte JA, Soares JM: Supplementation of vitamin E may attenuate skeletal muscle immobilization atrophy, *Int J Sports Med* 18(3):157-160, 1997.

76. Cave WT Jr: Omega 3 fatty acid diet effects on tumorigenesis in experimental animals, *World Rev Nutr Diet* 66:462-476, 1991.

77. Rose DP, Connolly JM: Effects of dietary omega-3 fatty acids on human breast cancer growth and metastases in nude mice, *J N Cancer Inst* 85(21):1743-1747, 1993.

78. Karmali RA, Adams L, Trout JR: Plant and marine n-3 fatty acids inhibit experimental metastasis of rat mammary adenocarcinoma cells, *Prostagland Leukotr Essen Fat Acid* 48(4):309-314, 1993.

79. Karmali R: n-3 fatty acids: biochemical actions in cancer, *J Nutr Sci Vitaminol* special edition:148-152, 1992.

80. Gogos CA et al: The effect of dietary omega-3 polyunsaturated fatty acids on T-lymphocyte subsets of patients with solid tumors, *Cancer Detect Prevent* 19(5):415-417, 1995.

81. Baronzio G et al: Omega-3 fatty acids can improve radioresponse modifying tumor interstitial pressure, blood rheology, and membrane peroxidability, *Anticancer Res* 14(3A):1145-1154, 1994.

82. Tisdale MJ: Mechanism of lipid mobilization associated with cancer cachexia: interaction between the polyunsaturated acid, eicosapentaenoic acid, and inhibitory nucleotide-regulatory protein, *Prostaglan Leukotr Essen Fat Acid* 48(1):105-109, 1993.

83. Sackett DL et al: Evidence-based medicine: what it is and what it isn't, *BMJ* 312:71-72, 1996.

84. Pastorino U et al: Adjuvant treatment of stage I lung cancer with high-dose vitamin, *Am J Clin Oncol* 11:1216-1222, 1993.

85. Jaakkola K et al: Treatment with antioxidant and other nutrients in combination with chemotherapy and irradiation in patients with small-cell lung cancer, *Anticancer Res* 12:599-606, 1992.

86. Lockwood K et al: Apparent partial remission of breast cancer in 'high risk' patients supplemented with nutritional antioxidants, essential fatty acids and coenzyme Q10, *Mol Aspect Med* 15 Suppl:231-240, 1994.

87. Lockwood K et al: Progress on therapy of breast cancer with vitamin Q10 and the regression of metastases, *Biochem Biophys Res Commun* 212(1):172-177, 1995.

88. Yoshida O et al: Prophylactic effect of etretinate on the recurrence of superficial bladder tumors—results of a randomized control study, *Hinyokika Kiyo* 32:1349-1358, 1986.

89. Lamm DL et al: Megadose vitamins in bladder cancer: a double-blind clinical trial, *J Urol* 151:21-26, 1994.

90. Carter JP et al: Dietary management may improve survival from nutritionally linked cancers based on analysis of representative cases, *J Am Coll Nutr* 12:209-226, 1993.

91. Recchia F et al: Advanced carcinoma of the pancreas: phase II study of combined chemotherapy, beta-interferon, and retinoids, *Am J Clin Oncol* 21:275-278, 1998.

92. Folkers K et al: Activities of vitamin Q10 in animal models and a serious deficiency in patients with cancer, *Biochem Biophys Res Commun* 1997;234:296-299.

93. Folkers K: Relevance of the biosynthesis of coenzyme Q10 and of the four bases of DNA as a rationale for the molecular causes of cancer and a therapy, *Biochem Biophys Res Commun* 1996;224:358-361, 1996.

94. Gao Y et al: The effects of chemotherapy including cisplatin on vitamin D metabolism, *Endocr J* 40:737-742, 1993.

95. Evans TR et al: A randomised study to determine whether routine intravenous magnesium supplements are necessary in patients receiving cisplatin chemotherapy with continuous infusion 5-fluorouracil, *Eur J Cancer* 31A:174-178, 1995.

96. Faure H et al: 5-Hydroxymethyluracil excretion, plasma TBARS and plasma antioxidant vitamins in adriamycin-treated patients, *Free Radic Biol Med* 20:979-983, 1996.

97. Faber M et al: Lipid peroxidation products, and vitamin and trace element status in patients with cancer before and after chemotherapy, including adriamycin. A preliminary study, *Biol Trace Elem Res* 47:117-123, 1995.

98. Dickerson JW: Nutrition and breast cancer, *J Hum Nutr* 33:17-23, 1979.

99. Heier MS, Dornish JM: Effect of the fluoropyrimidines 5-fluorouracil and doxifluridine on cellular uptake of thiamin, *Anticancer Res* 9:1073-1077, 1989.

100. Simone CB: Use of therapeutic levels of nutrients to augment oncology care. In Quillin P, Williams RM, editors: *Adjuvant nutrition in cancer treatment*, Arlington Heights, Ill, 1993, Cancer Treatment Research Foundation/American College of Nutrition.

101. Prasad KN: Vitamin E induces differentiation, growth inhibiton, and enhances the efficacy of therapeutic agents on cancer cells. In Quillin P, Williams RM, editors: *Adjuvant nutrition in cancer treatment*, Arlington Heights, Ill, 1993, Cancer Treatment Research Foundation/American College of Nutrition.

102. Teicher BA et al: Response of the Fsall fibrosarcoma to antiangiogenic modulators plus cytotoxic agents, *Anticancer Res* 13:2101-2106, 1993.

103. Teicher BA et al: Potentiation of cytotoxic cancer therapies by TNP-470 alone and with other antiangiogenic agents, *Int J Cancer* 57(6):920-925, 1994.

104. Teicher BA et al: Potentiation of cytotoxic therapies by TNP-470 and minocycline in mice bearing EMT-6 mammary carcinoma, *Breast Cancer Res Treat* 36(2):227-236, 1995.

105. Teicher BA et al: Antiangiogenic treatment (TNP-470/minocycline) increases tissue levels of anticancer drugs in mice bearing Lewis lung carcinoma, *Oncol Res* 7(5):237-243, 1995.

106. Teicher BA et al: Comparison of several antiangiogenic regimens alone and with cytotoxic therapies in the Lewis lung carcinoma, *Cancer Chemother Pharmacol* 38(2):169-177, 1996.

107. Teicher BA et al: Potentiation of cytotoxic therapies by TNP-470 and minocycline in mice bearing EMT-6 mammary carcinoma, *Breast Cancer Res Treat* 36(2):227-236, 1995.

108. Teicher BA et al: Comparison of several antiangiogenic regimens alone and with cytotoxic therapies in the Lewis lung carcinoma, *Cancer Chemother Pharmacol* 38(2):169-177, 1996.

109. Teicher BA et al: Comparison of several antiangiogenic regimens alone and with cytotoxic therapies in the Lewis lung carcinoma, *Cancer Chemother Pharmacol* 38(2):169-177, 1996.

110. Fotsis T et al: Flavonoids, dietary-derived inhibitors of cell proliferation and in vitro angiogenesis, *Cancer Res* 57(14):2916-2921, 1997.

111. Fotsis T et al: Genistein, a dietary ingested isoflavonoid, inhibits cell proliferation and in vitro angiogenesis, *J Nutr* 125(3 Suppl):790S-797S, 1995.

112. Koch AE et al: Inhibition of production of monocyte/macrophage-derived angiogenic activity by oxygen free-radical scavengers, *Cell Biol Int Rep* 16(5):415-425, 1992.

113. Fotsis T et al: Flavonoids, dietary-derived inhibitors of cell proliferation and in vitro angiogenesis, *Cancer Res* 57(14):2916-2921, 1997.

114. McCarty MF: Fish oil may impede tumor angiogenesis and invasiveness by down-regulating protein kinase C and modulating eicosanoid production, *Med Hypo* 46(2):107-115, 1996.

115. Moses MA, Sudhalter J, Langer R: Identification of an inhibitor of neovascularization from cartilage, *Science* 248(4961):1408-1410, 1990.

116. Hunt TJ, Connelly JF: Shark cartilage for cancer treatment, *Am J Health-Sys Pharm* 52(16):1756-1760, 1995.

117. Oikawa T et al: A highly potent antiangiogenic activity of retinoids, *Cancer Let* 48(2):157-162, 1989.

118. Majewski S et al: Retinoids, interferon alpha, 1,25-dihydroxyvitamin D3 and their combination inhibit angiogenesis induced by non-HPV-harboring tumor cell lines. RAR alpha mediates the antiangiogenic effect of retinoids, *Cancer Let* 89(1):117-124, 1995.

119. Shklar G, Schwartz JL: Vitamin E inhibits experimental carcinogenesis and tumour angiogenesis, *Eur J Cancer* 32B(2):114-119, 1996.

120. Marshall JL, Hawkins MJ: The clinical experience with antiangiogenic agents, *Breast Cancer Res Treat* 36:253-261, 1995.

121. Boik J: Natural agents that inhibit angiogenesis. In *Cancer and natural medicine*, Princeton, Minn, 1996, Oregon Medical Press.

122. Hongmei A, Jingnan B: Curative effect analysis of 122 tumor patients treated by the intelligence Qi Gong, Second World Conference on Academic Exchange of Medical Qigong, September 15, 1993.

123. Shouzhang W et al: A clinical study of the routine treatment of cancer coordinated by Qigong, Second World Conference on Academic Exchange of Medical Qigong, September 15, 1993.

124. Greer S, Morris T, Pettingale KW: Psychological response to breast cancer: effect on outcome, *Lancet* 2(8146):785-787, 1979.

125. Kogon MM et al: Effects of medical and psychotherapeutic treatment on the survival of women with metastatic breast carcinoma, *Cancer* 80(2):225-230, 1997.

126. Fawzy FI et al: Malignant melanoma. Effects of an early structured psychiatric intervention, coping, and affective state on recurrence and survival 6 years later, *Arch Gen Psychiatry* 50(9):681-689, 1993.

127. Luettig B et al: Macrophage activation by the polysaccharide arabinogalactan isolated from plant cell cultures of Echinacea purpurea, *J Natl Cancer Inst* 81(9): 669-675, 1989.

128. Lersch C et al: Stimulation of the immune response in outpatients with hepatocellular carcinomas by low doses of cyclophopsphamide (LDCY), echinacea purpurea extracts (Echinacin) and thymostimulin, *Arch Geschhwulstforsch* [German] 60(5):379-383, 1990.

129. Ruckdeschel JC, Piantodosi S: Quality of life assessment in lung surgery for bronchogenic carcinoma, *Theoret Surg* 6:201-205, 1991.

130. Block KI: The role of self in healthy cancer survivorship, *Advances* 13(1):6-26, 1997.

131. Duris I et al: Calcium chemoprevention in colorectal cancer, *Hepato Gastroenterol* 43(7):152-154, 1996.

132. Caygill CP, Charlett A, Hill MJ: Fat, fish, fish oil, and cancer, *Br J Cancer* 74(1):159-164, 1996.

133. Pappalardo G et al: Antioxidant agents and colorectal carcinogenesis: role of beta-carotene, vitamin E, and vitamin C, *Tumori* 82(1):6-11, 1996.

134. Ferraroni M et al: Selected micronutrient intake and the risk of colorectal cancer, *Br J Cancer* 70(6):1150-1155, 1994.

135. Roncucci L et al: Antioxidant vitamins or lactulose for the prevention of the recurrence of colorectal adenomas. Colorectal Cancer Study Group of the University of Modena and the Health Care District 16, *Dis Col Rect* 36(3):227-234, 1993.

136. Block KI: The role of self in healthy cancer survivorship, *Advances* 13(1):6-26, 1997.

137. Oldham RK: Cancer and diabetes: are there similarities, *Cancer Biother Radiopharm* 2(1):1-3, 1997.

138. Schipper H, Goh CR, Wang TL: Shifting the cancer paradigm: must we kill to cure? *J Clin Oncol* 13(4):801-807, 1995.

139. Anonymous: Diet and cancer: molecular mechanisms of interaction. Conference proceedings. Washington, D.C., September 1-2, 1994, *Adv Exper Med Biol* 375:1-222, 1995.

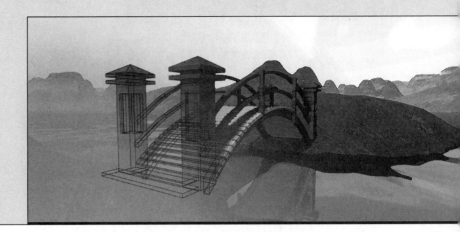

Unclassified Diagnostic and Treatment Methods

Applied Kinesiology,   **638**

Aromatherapy,   **651**

Biologic Dentistry,   **667**

Colon Hydrotherapy,   **679**

Color Therapy,   **690**

Detoxification Therapy,   **702**

Environmental Medicine,   **716**

Fasting,   **728**

Juice Therapy,   **741**

Iridology,   **756**

Quartz Crystal Therapy,   **770**

Reflexology,   **779**

Applied Kinesiology

PHILIP MAFFETONE

Origins and History

Applied kinesiology (AK) combines many existing complementary medicine therapies into one system, much like traditional Chinese medicine. AK focuses on the predisease, subclinical, or dysfunctional condition rather than disease. In AK the terms *functional* and *dysfunctional* refers to subclinical structural, chemical, and mental states, rather than the traditional medical definition in which functional means emotionally-based or psychosomatic.

The use of manual muscle testing as a means of assessing the patient's subclinical or functional state is a key component in AK. After assessments are made, the therapies applied may include acupressure, manipulation and other touch-based therapies, diet and nutrition, and lifestyle issues such as exercise and stress control. AK is used worldwide by chiropractors, medical doctors, osteopaths, and other practitioners.

A unique feature of AK is its use of manual muscle testing as part of an interactive neurologic assessment process that helps the practitioner determine areas of structural, chemical, and mental dysfunction. Through the use of muscle testing, combined with other methods of assessment such as a complete history and physical exam, the practitioner seeks to find the therapies that best match the patient's specific needs. This process is done each and every time the practitioner and patient meet. For example, in a patient with low back pain, abdominal muscle function may be impaired. The use of a particular therapy may prove effective if and when it results in normalization of the abdominal muscle dysfunction.

Applied kinesiologists theorize that structural, chemical, and mental dysfunction is associated with secondary muscle imbalance; specifically muscle inhibition (usually followed by overfacilitation or tightness of an opposing muscle). Applying the proper therapy results in normalization of the inhibited muscle. This allows the practitioner to immediately assess the efficacy of certain therapies.

Applied kinesiology was developed by George Goodheart, DC, beginning in 1964. Goodheart found that significant and immediate improvements in posture and function and reductions in pain could be made by applying pressure in an inhibited muscle's attachments. The inhibited muscle initially was detected using manual muscle testing. He theorized that the improvements were the result of an effect on the muscle's neurologic components: Golgi tendon organs and spindle cells.

Gradually a variety of existing modalities, including acupressure, osteopathic techniques, nutrition, and others, also were found to improve muscle function. By using muscle testing as a guide, the efficacy of the therapy could be determined immediately. Improvements in posture and gait and reductions in pain and disability (such as range of motion) also were immediately improved.

Goodheart later observed that specific muscles sometimes were inhibited by dysfunction in other areas, including organs or glands, acupuncture meridian imbalance, and nutrition needs. For example, following the Chinese model, if a meridian was low in Qi, a specific muscle was often found inhibited, and the corresponding meridian with too much Qi was associated with an overfacilitated or tight muscle.

Applied kinesiology also incorporates manipulation of the cranium, spine, and extravertebral joints as described by the chiropractic and osteopathic professions. In addition, many other techniques have been borrowed, refined, and incorporated into AK, including those directed at the nervous system, temporomandibular joint, diaphragm muscle, and a system of nutritional assessment.

Mechanism of Action According to Its Own Theory

An important concept in AK is the association of muscle dysfunction secondary to dysfunction in other areas of the body. This includes local muscle trauma, joint dysfunction, neurologic stress, cranial faults, temporomandibular joint dysfunction, and others. Chemical causes of muscle dysfunction may include nutritional imbalance, drug interactions, hormonal dysfunction, and others. Mental and emotional stress factors also can affect muscle function.

In addition to muscles becoming abnormally inhibited as a result of stress, specific muscles are thought to be associated with specific areas of the body. For example, applied kinesiologists have observed organ-muscle and glandular-muscle relationships. Dysfunction of a specific gland, for example, may result in a specific muscle inhibition. This typically will change posture and gait and also may cause secondary symptoms, such as knee pain. Adrenal dysfunction causing secondary sartorius muscle inhibition is one such example. In this case, increased adrenal stress often is associated with increased cortisol levels[1,2] followed by reduced dehydroepiandrosterone (DHEA).[3] This can be measured easily and accurately using salivary samples.[4,5] Treatment of adrenal dysfunction using acupuncture or other modalities, for example, may be monitored by testing the related muscle function (the sartorius muscle). Restoration of normal muscle function may indicate successful therapy. Applied kinesiologists have observed that when hormone levels return to normal, as in the example given here, sartorius muscle function also normalizes.

Biologic Mechanism of Action

The relationship of one body system affecting another has been previously observed. For example, Newsholme[6] discussed a relationship between muscles and the immune system; Parry-Billings et al[7] describes a similar relationship between the muscles, immune system, and brain; Weidner et al[8] demonstrated secondary gait changes in athletes who had colds; and Boda et al[9] showed gait abnormalities in patients with chronic fatigue syndrome. Essentially, any change in a patient's physiologic state will be ultimately reflected in the cortex, cerebellum, brain stem, and spinal cord, and it is postulated that these changes can be monitored at the level of the anterior horn motor neurons in the spinal cord through manual muscle testing.

Manual muscle testing is used in AK to help the practitioner distinguish between normal and abnormal function. Abnormal facilitation and inhibition are described as the contraction and lack of contraction, respectively, of skeletal muscles. Although it is understood that even though the central state of the alpha motor neuron is a reflection of multiple facilitory and inhibitory effects, the final outcome is either facilitation or inhibition. (*Excitation* occurs when facilitation reaches the threshold for depolarization, where the "all or none" phenomenon takes place.)

In AK, facilitated muscles have sometimes been referred to as "strong" and inhibited muscles as "weak."[10] However, these terms may not be the best available to describe muscle function. Skeletal muscles can be normally facilitated or inhibited; they also can be abnormally facilitated or inhibited. So the terms *normal or abnormal facilitation* or *normal or abnormal inhibition* are preferred.

Normal muscle facilitation and inhibition occurs constantly in the human body. For example, the normal gait consists of muscles that are normally facilitated or inhibited. Facilitation occurs at the neuromuscular junction with an action potential traveling the length of the muscle fiber and resulting in contraction. Inhibition of the motor neuron occurs postsynaptically (and presynaptically on some neurons) and results in the decreased likelihood of contraction of the muscle. When muscle function is not normal, imbalance results.

Muscular imbalance is described as a deviation from the expected normal facilitated or inhibited muscle and is discussed in the works of Janda,[11] Jull and Janda,[12] and Sahrmann.[13] This imbalance often begins as a muscle inhibition resulting from some physical, chemical, or mental stress and may cause further secondary muscle overfacilitation, followed by dysfunction in the related joints. The outcome of this series of imbalances, which may take weeks, months, or years to develop, may be pain, disability, or some other dysfunction.

Physical causes of muscle inhibition are the result of an imbalance between the external demand and functional capacity of the muscle. This may include too much or too little activity and macro or micro trauma. Muscle inhibition also may occur secondary to joint dysfunction and was described as early as 1965 by DeAndrade et al[14] and more recently by others.[15,16]

Originally, manual muscle testing was used in traditional medicine for the evaluation of poliomyelitis patients, with graded tests ranging from no muscle contraction to normal strength. Today, general muscle tests may be part of a standard neurologic exam to rule out pathology.

Manual muscle testing as described by Kendall et al[17] and Walther[18] is a clinical tool used to determine the function of the specific muscle. The works of Leisman et al,[10,19] Perot et al,[20] and Lawson and Calderon[21] have begun to demonstrate the scientific merits of muscle testing as used in AK to be a reproducible, effective clinical tool. Like other aspects of clinical practice, manual muscle testing is both an art and science. Proficiency comes with experience and an understanding of biomechanics.

It should be noted that in this type of manual muscle testing, function is being evaluated rather than strength or power. Muscular strength is the maximum force generated by the muscle. A more clinical definition is that strength is the maximum weight a person can lift one time. Power is defined with a time component. It is the combination of strength and speed of the movement.

Forms of Therapy

In addition to AK, many other different versions of manual muscle testing are used, and under many different names. Most often, the word *kinesiology* is part of this name. These versions include clinical kinesiology, where different types of muscle testing are used; behavioral kinesiology, which focuses on the mental or emotional and psychologic aspects of the patient; and the O-ring technique used in Japan, which only tests the hand muscles as an assessment.

Not only are various kinesiology methods used by clinicians, but many lay groups use various forms of kinesiology throughout the world as well. The Touch for Health association may be the largest, with many similar but differentiated groups using more simple muscle tests to guide various conservative self-help therapies.

Demographics

AK is used throughout the world by chiropractors, medical doctors, osteopaths, dentists, podiatrists, and other practitioners. It mostly is used in conjunction with modalities such as acupuncture, cranial-sacral therapy, and other alternative approaches, although some medical practitioners incorporate it into their modern medical approach.

Applied kinesiologists treat patients of all ages and genders for functional problems. In many cases, there also is a complementary approach, where one patient is under the care of a medical specialist for a specific disease and also is seen by an AK doctor. In this case, it is best that both practitioners communicate with each other to best serve the needs of the patient.

Indications and Reasons for Referral

Perhaps the most common reason to refer a patient to an applied kinesiologist is for assessment and treatment of functional (subclinical) structural, chemical, or mental and emotional problems. This may be the case following an exhaustive assessment that finds no disease or other serious condition, but the patient still has complaints. For example, a patient complaining of low back pain may have negative radiographs and other necessary evaluations, but the pain and disability persists. An AK doctor would consider a functional problem (see the previous definition), especially in the muscles that support or influence the low back.

Office Applications

It is important to note that AK doctors do not have predetermined therapies for given named conditions. The conditions listed as follows can serve as a general guide.

Allergies and hypersensitivities: When necessary, food and environmental allergy blood tests may be performed as part of the assessment process. Treatment may include dietary adjustment, nutrition, and other natural remedies.

Arthritis: As a complementary approach the AK doctor may work with a specialist in matching the best diet, nutrition, and exercise program.

Asthma: This may be accompanied by autonomic imbalance, which the AK practitioner can assess. Treatment may include diet and nutrition.

Children's health: AK practitioners usually have pediatric patients, often in conjunction with regular pediatrician care. They are assessed and treated like other patients.

Chronic fatigue syndrome: Dietary, nutritional, and other lifestyle factors may be applicable in these patients.

Colds, flu, and other infections: The AK practitioner would consider the best dietary and nutritional factors that match the patient's needs to improve immunity, including evaluation of lifestyle stress.

Constipation, diarrhea, and other nondisease gastrointestinal problems: This is another example of a subclinical (functional) problem that is commonly treated by an AK practitioner.

Diabetes: The AK doctor would complement the approach with a specialist.

Heart disease: The AK doctor could complement the specialists and consider dietary, nutritional, and lifestyle factors, including exercise needs.

Hemorrhoids: Treatment may be through the use of diet, nutrition, and herbal remedies.

Hypertension: The AK doctor could complement the specialists and consider dietary, nutritional, and lifestyle factors.

Insomnia and other sleeping disorders: The AK doctor could complement the specialists and consider dietary, nutritional, and lifestyle factors.

Intestinal disease: Treatment would be complementary with a specialist.

Menstrual and menopausal symptoms: AK practitioners can perform hormonal evaluations as part of the assessment process. Treatment may include diet, nutrition, and exercise.

Musculoskeletal problems (back, neck, other joint and muscle pain, including chronic pain, and headache): This often is a functional (nonpathologic and subclinical) problem easily assessed and treated with hands-on therapies, such as manipulation, acupressure, and muscle therapy.

Obesity and weight management: The AK doctor could consider dietary, nutritional, and lifestyle factors.

Restless leg syndrome: This may be the result of a minor neuromuscular imbalance. Treatment may include hands-on therapy, such as manipulation, acupressure, and muscle therapy.

Sports injuries: This is a specific therapy best treated by an AK doctor except in cases that require surgery or first aid.

Stress: AK practitioners can evaluate adrenal function, as well as other issues that are related to stress.

A simple ranking of conditions responsive to this form of therapy is as follows. As with all alternative therapies, use of AK does not preclude the use of mainstream medical therapies in addition.

Top level: *A therapy ideally suited for these conditions*

Allergies; amenorrhea; restless leg syndrome; back pain; chronic fatigue syndrome; colds and flu; constipation; diarrhea; hay fever; headaches; insomnia; irritable bowel syndrome; joint pain; obesity and weight management; osteoporosis; premenstrual syndrome; sinusitis; sports injuries; stomachache; and stress

Second level: *One of the better therapies for these conditions*

None

Third level: *A valuable adjunctive therapy for these conditions*

Arthritis; asthma; bronchitis; children's health; chronic pain; colic; colitis and Crohn's disease; diabetes; diverticulosis and diverticulitis; ear infections; emphysema; endometriosis; female health; fever; gastrointestinal disorders; general ear pain; gout; heart disease; hemorrhoids; hyperactivity; hypertension; male health; menstrual cramps; osteoarthritis; sleep apnea; and sleep disorders

Practical Applications

AK is used in the normal office setting. Patients are evaluated in an examination room with a standard table. During this time, more traditional tests are performed, such as blood pressure, along with specific tests, such as muscle testing.

AK often involves the following process: 1) assessment for functional imbalances; 2) treatment procedures; and 3) reassessment. This process may continue for 20 minutes to 45 minutes. Depending on the condition, the patient typically may return for the same assessment-treatment-reassessment process in 1 or 2 weeks, or the patient may not return for 1 or 2 months.

In some cases, such as in the health care of athletes, the AK practitioner may assess and then treat patients in their setting, such as a football field or on a college campus. In many athletic cases, assessment and treatment are provided directly on the field.

Research Base

Evidence Based

Peterson[22] studied muscle testing and phobia. This preliminary inquiry demonstrates the need for musculoskeletal, attentional, and presensitized subject variables to be controlled to ascertain if muscle testing can be reliably used as a tool to identify emotional arousal.

Froehle[23] did a retrospective study on ear infections. This retrospective study had several limitations but demonstrated a successful complementary approach of treating children with ear infections.

Hsieh and Phillips[24] discussed reproducibility. This study investigated the reliability of manual dynamometry using two different types of muscle testing. The authors found that patient-initiated muscle testing was reproducible, but the doctor-initiated method was not reproducible.

Efficacy

Perot et al compared mechanical and electromyographic parameters and showed that muscle testing is mostly dependent on satisfactory subject-examiner coordination, which also is necessary in standard clinical manual muscle testing.

In addition to those studies previously cited (Leisman et al,[10,19] Perot et al,[20] and Lawson and Calderon[21]), peer-reviewed, indexed papers that further discuss the efficacy or use of applied kinesiology include those authored by Motyka and Yanuck[25] and Schmitt and Yanuck.[26] Other references can be found in the textbooks that are listed in this discussion in "Suggested Reading."

Future Research Opportunities and Priorities

A number of areas of research have yet to be evaluated in AK. These include the basic technique of manually inducing facilitation and inhibition in an abnormal muscle (referred to as "origin and insertion technique"), the muscle organ-gland relationships, and aerobic or anaerobic muscle testing.

Other

Gin and Green[27] discussed the history of AK. References to the individual therapies that are used by applied kinesiologists can be further studied in their respective discussions in this text.

Druglike Information

For information about an individual AK therapy, please refer to its discussion in this text. There is no such information for AK muscle testing itself.

Self-Help versus Professional

Licensed practitioners who use AK are more able than the patient to objectively evaluate the patient. Self-application of AK may be limited to the use of diet and nutrition, for example, as discussed elsewhere in this text.

Visiting a Professional

A visit to an AK practitioner typically begins with the completion of various forms, which inventory the patient's symptoms. This includes questions about past personal and family medical history, current nutritional supplements and drugs, exercise habits, and stress. A separate dietary analysis also is frequently used by many practitioners.

This is usually followed by a history taking process, one-on-one with the doctor. If the doctor decides to accept the patient for care, this is followed by a physical examination. This process may begin with some standard evaluations, including vital signs. The examination continues with a routine heart and lung examination, as well as other systems as necessary, along with neurologic and sometimes orthopedic tests based on the particular patient's needs.

Postural blood pressure measurements often are performed to rule out the possibility of orthostatic hypotension or its functional counterpart. Such postural changes, as theorized in AK, may be associated with adrenal dysfunction. Vital capacity often is included in testing, as it is directly associated with overall health.[28] It commonly is used by many AK practitioners to compare general therapeutic efficacy (pretreatment and posttreatment or over longer time periods).

This is followed by a postural analysis, sometimes with the use of a standard plum line. Some practitioners also use other evaluations, such as treadmill or ergometer tests to measure blood pressure, pulse changes, and gait. Next, various manual muscle tests are performed. The patient is tested in both prone and supine positions and often sitting and standing as well. The practitioner also may evaluate how the muscles react to other factors, including mental stimulus (asking the patient to think of a stressful situation), nutrient or food (by asking the patient to taste it), or pushing on certain joints or muscles.

Certain laboratory evaluations may also be ordered by the AK doctor. These include radiographs, standard blood and urine tests, and sometimes more specialized tests, such as salivary hormone tests.

Only after extensive evaluations is the patient treated. This may include the use of a variety of therapies, including finger pressure applied to an acupuncture point (some may use needles if within their scope of practice) or specific areas on muscles, or mild manipulation to the cranium, spine, pelvis or extravertebral joints. This process is followed by a reevaluation: Did the rendered therapy change any abnormal findings observed during the initial assessment? For example, is the postural distortion improved, muscle dysfunction normalized, or pain reduced? This process may take 90 minutes for a typical patient.

This process also may result in the doctor recommending specific nutritional supplements, if necessary. In addition, certain dietary recommendations also may be discussed with the patient on the next visit. Most of these recommendations follow the results of the dietary analysis, where both patient and practitioner can see which nutrients, if any, are below recommended dietary allowance (RDA) levels, balance of various dietary fats (such as omega-3 and -6), macronutrient balance, and others.

This process also may result in the doctor making lifestyle recommendations, such as beginning a walking program or modifying an existing program that is interfering with the patient's condition. In addition, stress may be a subject that is discussed. Some of this may be postponed until the second visit.

Patients usually are scheduled for the next visit based on their current condition, and their response to therapy during the first session. This timeframe varies. In the author's opinion, scheduling the patient for 1 or 2 weeks later is typical. On this second visit a very similar approach is taken, other than repeating much of the history and examination process. Some tests are performed again as necessary (such as those that were not within normal parameters), and many muscles are tested.

A similar treatment process follows, with the patient scheduled for another visit if necessary. In some cases, very few treatments are necessary. However, in patients with chronic problems, more long-term care may be necessary. Typically the patient may have treatment sessions scheduled monthly or as necessary. These sessions may last 20 to 30 minutes or as long as 1 hour.

Credentialing

There is no specific degree for AK; rather, it is practiced by those already possessing a doctorate degree (such as DC, DO, MD, and others) and a license to diagnose. Courses and certifications are given by the International College of Applied Kinesiology (ICAK), which has chapters throughout the world.

Specific practitioners either practice as an applied kinesiologist (within the scope of their particular license) or use AK as an adjunct to their particular specialty. For example, chiropractors, medical doctors, or osteopaths may practice predominantly their specialty but use AK assessment and treatment methods as an adjunct. This blend is applicable because AK is an open system based on sound physiologic principles, and many therapeutic approaches can be incorporated as per the doctor's expertise and interests.

Training

The ICAK provides various levels of certification for physicians. To receive proper certification, approved courses must be taken from certified teachers approved by the Board of Certified Teachers. These include the following:

1. The Basic Applied Kinesiology 100-hour course is the essential basic program.
2. A separate certification is given for those successfully passing a Proficiency Exam or Test of Clinical Competence following the 100-hour course.

3. ICAK Diplomate status is granted by the International Board of Examiners following successful completion of 300 hours of instruction by at least two diplomates and successful completion of a written and practical exam.
4. A Certified Teacher must be an ICAK Diplomate, complete various teaching requirements, and maintain regular recertification.

Barriers and Key Issues

AK has not been widely accepted, which most likely results from the misunderstanding of this approach. Much of this may come from the small "fringe" groups that use muscle testing, with many observers seeing all muscle-testing clinicians performing the same therapy. In fact, AK is not part of most approaches that use muscle testing. The status statement of the International College of Applied Kinesiology clearly defines the approach and role of the AK doctor:

Applied Kinesiology *is*:

- A diagnostic system using muscle testing to augment normal examination procedures. It was founded and developed by Dr. George Goodheart, Jr., a chiropractor. Further advances have been made by members of the International College of Applied Kinesiology.
- A diagnostic tool that uses the neuromuscular system and other measurable parameters to aid in evaluating what is wrong and what to do for a patient.
- An expanding body of knowledge that covers in depth the structural and chemical imbalances that are at the base of most patient's problems.

In addition:

- An applied kinesiology examination depends on knowledge of functional neurology, anatomy, physiology, biomechanics, and biochemistry and is combined with standard physical examination procedures, laboratory findings, radiographs, and history taking.
- The different procedures developed by Dr. Goodheart and others in the International College of Applied Kinesiology are derived from many disciplines, including chiropractic, osteopathy, medicine, dentistry, acupuncture, biochemistry, and others and are currently being used by doctors of chiropractic, osteopathy, homeopathy, dentistry, and medicine.

Applied Kinesiology is *not*:

- A simple yes or no, radionics, or pendulum type of testing system.
- Testing bottles in the hand or pills on the skin.
- Testing using mental telepathy.
- Using crystals or magnets as treatment modalities.

- Touch for Health or any other form of evaluation using muscle testing as a simple yes or no answer system.
- A simplistic, "cookie cutter" approach to treatment.

Most professionals and patients are unaware of the current published research that shows AK to be a useful, effective, and logical approach. However, much more research is still necessary.

AK does not always fit into the current model of health care; for example, treatment X for condition Y. This also may have an adverse effect on acceptance, especially when third-party reimbursement is considered.

Associations

The International College of Applied Kinesiology
6405 Metcalf Ave., Suite 503
Shawnee Mission, KS 66202
Tel: (913) 384-5336
Fax: (913) 384-5112
E-mail: icakusa@usa.net
www.icakusa.com

Local chapter contacts in their respective countries can be received from the ICAK headquarters.

The Touch for Health Kinesiology Association
11262 Washington Blvd.
Culver City, CA 90230
Tel: (800) 466-8342
Fax: (310) 313-9319
E-mail: admin@tfh.org
www.tfh.org

Suggested Reading

The following referenced textbooks may be helpful in the understanding and use of applied kinesiology:

1. Walther D: *Applied kinesiology synopsis*, Pueblo, Colo, 1988, Systems DC.
   This is a standard text for those who practice AK.
2. Maffetone P: *Complementary sports medicine*, Champaign, Ill, 1999, Human Kinetics.
   This is a text on AK focused more on exercise, diet, and nutrition along with presenting the reader with an introduction to applied kinesiology and other aspects of complementary sports medicine.
3. Kendall FP, McCreary EK, Provance PG: *Muscles, testing, and function*, ed 4, Baltimore, 1993, Williams & Wilkins.
   This is a standard text on manual muscle testing. It does not discuss applied kinesiology.

The following general audience books reflect the approach used by an applied kinesiologist:

1. Maffetone P: *In fitness and in health*, Stamford, N.Y., 1997, Barmore Productions.
   This book includes a chapter on applied kinesiology to help patients understand the concepts, a chapter on complementary medicine, and discusses nutrition, diet, and exercise.
2. Thie J: *Touch for health*, Marina Del Ray, Calif, 1996, DeVorss & Co.
   This is a book for lay people (and may serve as an introduction for professionals) on some very basic techniques of using kinesiology.

References

1. Henry JP: Biological basis of the stress response, *Integr Physiol Behav Sci* 27(1):66-83, 1992.
2. Pollard TM: Physiological consequences of everyday psychosocial stress, *Coll Antropol* 21(1):17-28, 1997.
3. Parker LN, Levin ER, Lifrak ET: Evidence for adrenocortical adaptation to severe illness, *J Clin Endocrinol Metab* 60:947-952, 1985.
4. Peters JR et al: Salivary cortisol assays for assessing pituitary-adrenal reserve, *Clin Endocrinol Oxf* 17(6):583-592, 1982.
5. Kahn J et al: Salivary cortisol: a practical method for evaluation of adrenal function, *Biol Psychiatry* 23:335-349, 1988.
6. Newsholme EA: Biochemical mechanisms to explain immunosuppression in well-trained and overtrained athletes, *Int J Sports Med* 15:142-147, 1994.
7. Parry-Billings M et al: A communicational link between skeletal muscle, brain, and cells of the immune system, *Int J Sports Med* 11(Suppl 2):S122-S128, 1990.
8. Weidner TG et al: Effects of viral upper respiratory illness on running gait, *J Athl Train* 32(4):309-314, 1997.
9. Boda WL et al: Gait abnormalities in chronic fatigue syndrome, *J Neurol Sci* 131(2):156-161, 1995.
10. Leisman G, Shambaugh P, Ferentz A: Somatosensory evoked potential changes during muscle testing, *Int J Neurosci* 45:143-151, 1989.
11. Janda V: Some aspects of extracranial causes of facial pain, *J Prosthet Dent* 56:484, 1986.
12. Jull G, Janda V: (1987). Muscles and motor control in low back pain. In Twomey LT, Taylor JR, editors: *Physical therapy for the low back; clinics in physical therapy*, New York, 1987, Churchill Livingstone.
13. Sahrmann S: Posture and muscle imbalance: faulty lumbar pelvic alignments, *Phys Ther* 67:1840, 1987.
14. DeAndrade JR, Grant C, Dixon ASJ: Joint distention and reflex muscle inhibition in the knee [Abstract], *J Bone Joint Surg* 47:313, 1965.
15. Fisher NM et al: Muscle function and gait in patients with knee osteoarthritis before and after muscle rehabilitation, *Disabil Rehabil* 19(2):47-55, 1997.
16. Spencer JD, Hayes KC, Alexander IJ: Knee joint effusion and quadriceps reflex inhibition in man, *Arch Phys Med Rehabil* 65:171, 1984.
17. Kendall FP, McCreary EK, Provance PG: *Muscles, testing, and function*, ed 4, Baltimore, 1993, Williams & Wilkins.

18. Walther D: *Applied kinesiology synopsis*, Pueblo, Colo, 1988, Systems DC.

19. Leisman G et al: Electromyographic effects of fatigue and task repetition on the validity of strong and weak muscle estimates in applied kinesiology muscle testing procedures, *Percep Motor Skills* 80:963-977, 1995.

20. Perot C, Meldener R, Goubel F: Objective measurement of proprioceptive technique consequences on muscular maximal voluntary contraction during manual muscle testing [Abstract], *Agressologie* (French): 32(10):471-474, 1991.

21. Lawson A, Calderon L: Interexaminer reliability of applied kinesiology manual muscle testing, *Percep Motor Skills* 84:539-546, 1997.

22. Peterson KB: A preliminary inquiry into manual muscle testing response in phobic and control subjects exposed to threatening stimuli, *J Manip Physiol Ther* 19(5):310-316, 1996.

23. Froehle RM: Ear infection: a retrospective study examining improvement from chiropractic care and analyzing for influencing factors, *J Manip Physiol Ther* 19(3):169-177, 1996.

24. Hsieh CY, Phillips RB: Reliability of manual muscle testing with a computerized dynamometer, *J Manip Physiol Ther* 13(2):72-82, 1990.

25. Motyka T, Yanuck S: Expanding the neurological examination using functional neurologic assessment. Part I: methodological considerations, *Int J Neurosci* 97:61-76, 1999.

26. Schmitt W, Yanuck S: Expanding the neurological examination using functional neurologic assessment. Part II: neurologic basis of applied kinesiology, *Int J Neurosci* 97:77-108, 1999.

27. Gin RH, Green BN: George Goodheart, Jr, DC, and a history of applied kinesiology, *J Manip Physiol Ther* 20(5):331-337, 1997.

28. Benfante R, Reed D, Brody J: Biological and social predictors of health in an aging cohort, *J Chronic Dis* 38(5):385-395, 1985.

Aromatherapy

JANE BUCKLE

Origins and History

Aromatherapy, with its roots in herbal medicine, is perhaps one of the oldest therapies, dating back 6000 years to its use in India, China, North and South America, Greece, the Middle East, and Europe.

The renaissance of modern aromatherapy occurred in France just before World War II. Medical doctor Jean Valnet, chemist Maurice Gattefosse, and surgical assistant Marguerite Maury were key figures and used aromatherapy clinically to help wounds heal, fight infection, and improve skin texture. An example is thymol, the antiseptic discovered by Lister, and one of the components of thyme essential oil. In France, more than 1500 trained physicians use essential oils as an alternative to antibiotics. The use of synthetic scents, which only has appeared in the last few decades, has nothing to do with aromatherapy.

Aromatherapy uses essential oils. True essential oils are steam-distilled (or expressed from the peel of citrus plants) from aromatic plants; many of them have familiar smells, such as lavender, rose, and rosemary. However, there can be many different species of the same genus. For example, the genus of thyme is *Thymus* but there are more than 60 different species or varieties of thyme, each with a different chemistry and therefore different therapeutic effects. There are three different species of lavender and 600 different species of eucalyptus. Although suppliers of essential oils do not carry all species of a genus, many do supply several different species that may have very different therapeutic effects. For this reason, it is very important to identify an essential oil with its full botanic name. Please see the table "Essential Oils Mentioned in This Discussion."

Mechanism of Action According to Its Own Theory

The term *aromatherapy* refers to the therapeutic use of essential oils, which are the volatile organic constituents of plants. Essential oils are common ingredients in the pharmaceutic, perfume, and food industries and as such are experienced by most of the population on a daily basis.

Aromatherapy is thought to work at psychologic, physiologic, and cellular levels. The effects of aroma can be rapid—sometimes just thinking about a smell can be as powerful as

651

Essential Oils Mentioned in this Discussion	
Essential Oil	**Botanic Name**
Aniseed	*Pimpinella anisum*
Basil	*Ocimum basilicum*
Chamomile german	*Matricaria recutita*
Chamomile roman	*Chamomelum nobile*
Clary sage	*Salvia sclarea*
Coriander seed	*Coriandrum sativum*
Eucalyptus	*Eucalyptus globulus*
Fennel	*Foeniculum vulgare*
Geranium	*Pelargonium graveolens*
Ginger	*Zingeber officinale*
Hyssop	*Hyssopus officinalis*
Lavender true	*Lavandula officinalis*
Lemongrass	*Cymbopogon citruatus*
Neroli	*Citrus aurantium var amara*
Palmarosa	*Cymbopogon martinii*
Parlsey	*Petroselinum sativum*
Pennyroyal	*Mentha pulegium*
Peppermint	*Mentha piperita*
Rose	*Rosa damascena*
Rosewood	*Aniba rosaeodora*
Sage	*Salvia officinalis*
Sandalwood	*Santalum album*
Tarragon	*Artemesia dracunculus*
Wintergreen	*Gaultheria procumbens*
Ylang ylang	*Cananga orodata*

the actual smell itself. These effects can be relaxing or stimulating depending on the previous experiences of the individual as well as the chemistry of the essential oils used.

Biologic Mechanism of Action

Olfaction

Essential oils are composed of many different chemical components or molecules. These olfactory stimulants travel through the nose to the olfactory bulb and from there, nerve impulses travel on to the limbic system of the brain, an inner complex ring of brain structures below the cerebral cortex that is arranged into 53 regions and 35 associated tracts. Of these regions the amygdala and the hippocampus are of particular importance in the processing of aromas.

The amygdala governs our emotional response. Diazepam (valium) is thought to reduce the effect of external emotional stimuli by increasing gamma aminobutyric acid (GABA)-containing inhibitory neurons in the amygdala. Lavandula angustifolia (true lavender) is thought to have a similar effect on the amygdala, producing a sedative effect similar to diazepam. The hippocampus is involved in the formation and retrieval of explicit memories. This is where chemicals in an aroma trigger learned memory. Smell is very important in our lives, beginning with the newborn's identification of its mother and continuing into old age where studies have shown the depression of residential older adults was reduced with the aromas of fruit and flowers.

The effect of odors on the brain has been mapped using computer-generated topographics. These Brain Electrical Activity Maps (BEAM) indicate how a subject, linked to an electroencephalogram (EEG), psychometrically rated odors presented to them. Smells can have a psychologic effect even when the aroma is below the level of human awareness.

Dermal

Essential oils are absorbed through the skin through diffusion, with the dermis and fat layer acting as a reservoir before the components within the essential oils reach the dermis and then the bloodstream. There is some evidence that massage or hot water enhances the absorption of at least some of the essential oil's components.

Forms of Therapy

There are the following four basic types of aromatherapy:

1. Esthetic: the aromas are used purely for pleasure, such as candles and soaps;
2. Holistic: aromatherapy is used for general *stress*;
3. Environmental fragrancing: aromas are used to manipulate mood or enhance sales; and
4. Clinical: where essential oils are used for specific outcomes that are measurable

Demographics

Aromatherapy is commonly practiced in the UK, France, Germany, Switzerland, Sweden, Australia, New Zealand, and Japan. Many nurses and other health professionals train in aromatherapy to enhance their care. In France, medical doctors and pharmacists use aromatherapy as part of conventional medicine, often for the control of infection.

Indications and Reasons for Referral

CAUTION: Aromatherapy should not be used as a replacement therapy. It is an adjunctive rather than alternative therapy and can be very useful alongside orthodox medicine. Aromatherapy is particularly effective in mind-body illnesses. Please refer to the table "Indications and Methods of Application."

Indications and Methods of Application

Category	Condition	Method	Essential Oils
Psychologic	Insomnia	I, T	Lavender, ylang ylang, clary sage, frankincense, and neroli
	Depression	I, T	Bergamot, basil, lavender, geranium, neroli, angelica, rose, and melissa
	Stress and anxiety	I, T	Lavender, frankincense, Roman chamomile, mandarin, angelica, and rose (especially with touch)
	Anorexia	I, T	Rose, neroli, lemon, and fennel
	Substance abuse	T	Helichrysum and angelica
Pain relief	Migraine	T	Peppermint and lavender
	Osteoarthritis	T	Eucalyptus, black pepper, ginger, Spike lavender, Roman chamomile, rosemary, and myrrh
	Rheumatoid	T	German chamomile, lavender, peppermint, and frankincense
	Low back pain	T	Lemongrass, rosemary, lavender, and sweet marjoram
	Cramps	T	Roman chamomile, clary sage, lavender, and sweet marjoram
	General aches and pains		Rosemary, lavender, lemongrass, clary sage, black pepper, lemon eucalyptus, and spike lavender
Gynecologic	Menopausal	I, T	Clary sage, sage, fennel, aniseed, geranium, rose, and cypress
	Menstrual cramping	T	Roman chamomile, lavender, and clary sage
	Premenstural syndrome	T	Clary sage, sage, fennel, aniseed, geranium, and rose
	Idiopathic infertility	T	Clary sage, sage, fennel, aniseed, geranium, and rose
Cardiovascular	Borderline HTN		Ylang ylang and lavender
	Antidepressant induced orthostasis		Rosemary and spike lavender
Urinary	Cystitis	T	Teatree, palma rosa, and especially sitz bath
	Water retention	T	Juniper, cypress, and fennel
Gastrointestinal	Irritable bowel		Roman chamomile, clary sage, mandarin, cardomon, peppermint, mandarin, fennel, and lavender
	Constipation	T	Fennel and black pepper
	Indigestion	I	Peppermint and ginger
Infection	Staph including MRSA	I, T	Teatree
	Bacterial, nonspecific	I, T	Eucalyptus, naiouli, sweet marjoram, oregano, tarragon, savroy, German chamomile, thyme, and manuka
	Viral	I, T	Ravansara, palma rosa, lemon, Eucalyptus smithii, melissa, rose, and bergamot
	Fungal	T	Lemongrass, black pepper, holy basil, clove, cajuput, caraway geranium, and teatree (particularly good for toenail; apply QD to nailbed)

Office Applications

Aromatherapy has been useful in treating the following areas, starting with conditions most likely to respond and progressing to those less likely to respond.

Chronic pain: Aromatherapy is used with touch particularly to enhance strong analgesics such as morphine passive cutaneous anaphylaxis (PCA), as well as pain relief (spiritual, physical, and emotional).

Indications and Methods of Application—cont'd

Category	Condition	Method	Essential Oils
Pediatrics	Behavioral problems	I, T	Mandarin, lavender, Roman chamomile, and rose
	Colic	T	Rating 2: Roman chamomile and mandarin
	Diaper rash		Lavender
	Sleep problems		Lavender, rose, and mandarin
	Autism		Rose; can help children with multiple disabilities to interact socially
Respiratory	Bronchitis	I	Ravansara, eucalyptus globlulus, eucalyptus smithi, teatree, and spike lavender
	Sinusitis	I	Eucalyptus globulus, lavender, Spike lavender, and rosemary
	Mild asthma	I	Lavender, clary sage, and Roman chamomile
Dermatology	Mild acne	T	Teatree, juniper, cypress, and naiouli
	Mild psoriasis	T	Lavender and German chamomile
	Diabetic ulcers	T	Lavender, frankincense, and myrrh
Chemotherapy side effects	Nausea	I	Peppermint, ginger, and mandarin
	Postradiation burns	T	Lavender, German chamomile, and Tamanu carrier oil
Muscular	Sports injuries	T	Spike lavender, rosemary, sweet marjoram, and black pepper
Geriatrics	Memory loss	I	Rosemary and rose
	Dry, flaky skin	T	Geranium, frankincense, and oil of evening primrose carrier oil
	Alzheimer's disease	I	Rating 4: rosemary, lavender, pine, and frankincense
Palliative care	Pain:		
	Spiritual	I, T	Rose, angelica, and frankincense
	Physical	I, T	Lavender, peppermint, lavender, lemongrass, and rosemary
	Emotional	I, T	Geranium, pine, and sandalwood
	Relaxation	I, T	Lavender, clary sage, mandarin, frankincense, and ylang ylang
	Bed sores	T	Lavender, teatree, and sweet marjoram
Care of the dying	Rites of passage	I	Choose selection of patient's favorite aromas or frankincense or rose
	Bereavement	I	Rose, sandalwood, patchouli, and angelica

I, inhalation; *T,* topical

Stress and anxiety: Aromatherapy facilitates the parasympathetic response as shown on heart-variation monitors and EEGs.

Chemotherapy side-effects: Aromatherapy is effective for nausea and postradiation burns.

Vaginal infections: Use vaginally 2 drops of tea tree in 5 ccs (1 teaspoon) of almond oil. Absorb mixture into tampon and insert into the vagina. Change tampon for new mixture daily. Leave in situ over night. (As tea tree oil varies in content and quality, be sure to obtain from a reliable source; see the listings presented here). Highly effective against Candida albicans, anaerobic infections, and chlamydia.

Premenstrual syndrome, menopausal symptoms, and menstrual problems: The mixture of estrogen-like essential oils, such as fennel, aniseed, sage, and clary-sage, with touch appears to help reduce symptoms. These can be used in conjunction with herbal medicine or orthodox hormone replacement therapy.

Borderline hypertension diastolic and transient hypotension caused by some antidepressants: Aromatherapy is a simple and effective way for patients to care for themselves in an enjoyable way.

Decubitus ulcers: Aromatherapy is effective for diabetic ulcers, herpes zoster, and simplex type 1 (some success with type 2), as well as loss of skin integrity in lymphoedema.

Insomnia: Place two drops of relaxing essential oil on cotton ball. Place under pillowcase. The effects of inhaled essential oils on insomnia have been shown in clinical studies.

Depression: Aromatherapy can empower patients and give pleasure. Essential oils can be used in tandem with conventional medication and to help wean patients off medication where appropriate.

Recurrent upper respiratory tract infections: Aromatherapy is effective in the treatment of bronchitis and sinusitis.

Resistant infections: Aromatherapy is effective in the treatment of bacterial (including methicillin-resistant and vancomycin-resistant staphylococcal aureus), viral, and fungal infections.

Sports injuries: Aromatherapy is effective in the treatment of sports injuries.

Bereavement: Aromatherapy is effective for bereavement.

Memory loss, dry flaky skin, Alzheimer's disease, dementia: Aromatherapy is effective in the treatment of these conditions (all rating 4).

Infertility with no physiologic cause: The hormonal balancing essential oils fennel, aniseed, sage, clary-sage, geranium, cypress, and the use of touch can accentuate the mind-body link. This takes several months to achieve.

Behavioral problems: Aromatherapy is effective in the treatment of colic, diaper rash, sleep problems, and autism; it can help children with multiple disabilities to interact socially. Aromatherapy uses the powerful nonverbal stimulus of smell and touch to communicate with a child at a basic level.

Practical Applications

Methods of Using Aromatherapy

Essential oils can be absorbed by the body in one of the following three ways:

1. Through the olfactory system: 1 to 5 drops, without touch, by direct and indirect inhalation

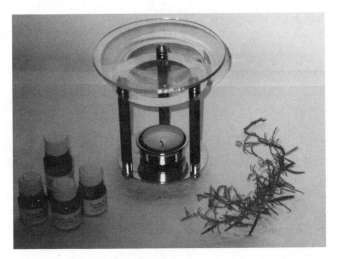

2. Through the skin in baths: 1 to 8 drops in compresses, massage, through touch
3. Through the mouth: 1 to 2 drops (this is accepted as aromatic *medicine* requiring the training of a primary care provider, MD, OD, or chiropractor)

INHALATION

Direct inhalation means that an essential oil is directly targeted to the patient through 1 to 5 drops on a tissue (or floated on hot water in a bowl) and inhaled for 5 to 10 minutes.

Indirect inhalation includes the use of burners, nebulizers, and vaporizers, which can be heat, battery, or electrically operated and may or may not include the use of water. Larger but portable aroma systems are available to control the release of essential oils on a commercial scale into rooms up to 1500 square feet. This is similar to environmental fragrancing (using synthetics), which is common practice in hotels and department stores, and it is useful for mood enhancement and stress reduction.

BATHS

Put 4 to 6 drops of essential oil into a teaspoon of milk, rubbing alcohol, or carrier oil (as essential oils do not dissolve in water and would float on the top, giving an uneven treatment) and add to the bath water. Agitate vigorously. Relax in bath for 10 minutes.

COMPRESSES

Add 4 to 6 drops of essential oil to warm water. Soak a soft cotton cloth in mixture, wring out, and apply to affected area (contusion or abrasion). Cover external surface with plastic wrap (as for food) to maintain moisture and cover with a towel. Keep in place for 4 hours.

TOUCH

Aromatherapy often is used in a gentle massage or the *m* technique. Use 1 to 5 drops of essential oils diluted in a teaspoonful (5 ccs) of cold-pressed vegetable oil, cream, or gel. Gentle friction and hot water enhance absorption of essential oils through the skin into the blood stream. The amount of essential oil absorbed from an aromatherapy massage will normally be 0.025 ccs to 0.1 ml, or approximately 0.5 to 2.0 drops.

Research Base

Evidence Based

Wilkinson[1] found Roman chamomile to be effective in altering perceptions of pain in palliative cancer care in a randomized study. Moate[2] used sandalwood and lavender in depression with psychiatric patients with positive effects in a descriptive study. Styles[3] used a mixture of lavender, Roman chamomile, neroli, mandarin, sandalwood, palmarosa, and geranium to reduce pain, stress and anxiety in HIV-positive hospitalized children in a descriptive study. Betts[4] reduced the severity of seizures and increased the period of time between seizures with ylang ylang. Gobel et al[5] found peppermint to be as effective as conventional medication for headaches in a randomized, double-blind cross-over study. Krall and Krause,[6] in an open, randomized study, found peppermint was effective for periarthritic pain. Woolfson[7] found lavender reduced pain by 50% in patients in a critical care unit. Buchbauer et al[8] showed measurable sedative effects from inhaling the essential oil of lavender. Stevensen[9] found neroli reduced anxiety and alleviated stress in a cardiac unit in a controlled study. Lemongrass was shown to have an analgesic effect and potentiate the effects of morphine in an animal study by Seth et al.[10] This findings were later explored and replicated by Lorenzetti et al.[11]

Komori[12] showed that citrus enhanced immune function and reduced depression in human studies. Manly[13] found that lemon, lemongrass, peppermint, and basil were psychologically stimulating and lavender and rose were relaxing in human studies. Schiffman[14] showed pleasant odors improved mood of women and men at midlife. Kichuri et al[15] showed several essential oils had a beneficial effect on insomnia.

Carson[16] showed that tea tree was effective against Staph aureus, MRSA, and VRSA in in vitro studies. A multicentered hospital study in the UK has shown similar effects in pilot human studies (results yet to be published). Larrondo showed lavender, melissa, and rosemary inhibited three species of pseudomonas by 75% in an in vitro study.[17] Benouda[18] showed the effect of eucalyptus globulus on staph aureus, strep C and D, proteum klebsiella, salmonella typhi, and haemophilus influenze was comparable to the action of antibiotics in an in vitro study. Deininger[19] presented the antiviral effects of numerous components, such as citronellol, citronellal, linalol, linalyl acetate, and eugenol, that are found in essential oils in an in vitro study. Wannisorm[20] showed that lemongrass was a powerful antifungal agent against many fungi, including ringworm, in an action comparable to clotrimzole, in an in vitro study.

Risk and Safety

Most essential oils have been tested by the food and drinks industry because many essential oils are used as flavorings. Other research has been carried out by the perfume industry.[21-23] Most of the commonly used essential oils in aromatherapy have been given GRAS (generally regarded as safe) status.

Efficacy

Aromatherapy works very well on insomnia, stress, and emotional problems, particularly if touch is involved. The author would put the success rate in this area as high as 75% based on published research, case studies, and personal clinical experience. In other areas, such as hormonal imbalance, aromatherapy is worth trying, although the effects of aromatherapy will not equate hormone replacement therapy. In other words, aromatherapy will ameliorate the symptoms but not remove the cause. For pain, aromatherapy works on pain perception and the ability of the patient to relax. Aromatherapy can be a useful ingredient of a multiple-disciplinary pain management team.

Future Research Opportunities and Priorities

Ongoing studies on hospital-acquired infection are in progress. This could move aromatherapy further into the clinical field. Essential oils are complicated and contain between 100 and 400 different components, which are divided into functional groups such as alcohols, aldehydes, phenols, esters and so on. The exact percentage of each component will vary with the batch of essential oil and is directly related to the climatic growing conditions, harvesting, and distillation process. Further studies on human subjects are needed in all areas previously listed.

Druglike Information

Safety

Aromatherapy is a very safe complementary therapy if it is used within the guidelines. Avoid use with patients with atopic eczema. Some essential oils have caused dermal sensitivity, mostly through impure extracts. Do not administer essential oils orally unless extensively trained; poisoning (and in some circumstances fatalities) have been documented. There is a list of banned or contraindicated essential oils to guide the novice (see the table "Essential Oils to Avoid"). Essential oils that are high in esters and alcohols tend to be gentle in their action and the safest to use. Essential oils that are high in phenols tend to be more aggressive and should not be used over long periods of time.

Actions and Pharmacokinetics

The pharmacologically active components in essential oils work at psychologic, physical, and cellular levels. Essential oils are absorbed rapidly through the skin, and some essential oils now are used to help the dermal penetration of orthodox medication. Essential oils are lipotrophic and excreted through respiration, kidneys, and insensate loss.

Essential Oils to Avoid

Common Name	Botanic Name	Constituent	Reason
Basil (exotic)	*Ocimum basilicum*	High % estragole	Carcinogenic
Birch	*Betula lenta*	90% methyl salicylate	Systemic toxicity
Boldo	*Peumus boldus*	Ascaridole	Toxic to humans
Buchu	*Agothosma betulina*	Pulegone	Liver toxicity and abortifacient
Cade	*Juniperus oxycedrus*	Benzoapyrene	Carcinogenic
Calamus	*Acorus clamus var angustatus*	Asarone	Genotoxic
Camphor (brown)	*Cinnamomum camphora*	Safrole	Carcinogenic
Camphor (yellow)	*Cinnamomum camphora*	Safrole	Carcinogenic
Cassia	*Cinnamomum cassia*	Cinnamaldehyde	Skin sensitizer
Cinnamon bark	*Cinnamomum zeylanicum*	Cinnamaldehyde	Skin sensitizer
Costus	*Saussurea costus*	Costuslactone	Skin sensitizer
Elecampane	*Inula helenium*	Alantolactone	Skin sensitizer
Horseradish	*Armoracia rusticana*	Allyl isothiocyanate	Irritating to skin
Melaleuca	*Melaleuca bracteata*	Methyleugenol	Carcinogenic
Mustard	*Brassica nigra*	Allyl isothiocyanate	Mucous membrane irritant
Pennyroyal	*Mentha pulegium*	Pulegone	Liver toxicity and abortifacient
Ravensara	*Ravensara anisata*	Estragole	Carcinogenic
Sage (dalmatian)	*Salvia officinalis*	Thujone	Convulsant
Sassafras	*Sassafras albidum*	Safrole	Carcinogenic
Tansy	*Tanacetum vulgare*	Thujone	Convulsant
Tarragon*	*Artemesia dracunculus*	Estragole and methyleugenol	Carcinogenic
Thuja	*Thuja occidentalis*	Thujone	Convulsant
Wintergree	*Gaultheria procumbens*	Methyl salicylate	Systemic toxicity
Wormseed	*Chenopodium ambrosiodes var*	Ascaridole	Toxic anthelminticum
Wormwood	*Artemesia absinthium*	Thujone	Convulsant

*Somewhat controversial. Thujone is in very small quantities. Many aromatherapists use tarragon.

Warnings, Contraindications, and Precautions

In general, use the following precautions:

1. Do not take essential oils by mouth, unless trained and a primary care provider.
2. Do not touch your eyes with essential oils. If essential oils get into your eyes, rinse with milk or carrier oil (essential oils do not dissolve in water) and then water.
3. Store essential oils away from fire or naked flame. Essential oils are highly volatile and flammable.
4. Store essential oils in a cool place out of sunlight and in colored glass (amber or blue). Store expensive essential oils in the refrigerator.
5. Many essential oils stain clothing. Beware!
6. Do not use essential oils undiluted on the skin.
7. Keep essential oils away from children and pets.
8. Only use essential oils from reputable supplier.
9. Always close the container immediately.

10. Avoid during early pregnancy.
11. Use extra care with patients receiving chemotherapy.
12. Be aware of which essential oils are photosensitive, such as bergamot.
13. Avoid with patients with severe asthma or multiple allergies.

Drug or Other Interactions

The following precautions are recommended:

1. Avoid with patients receiving homeopathy. Strong aromas like peppermint and eucalyptus can negate homeopathic remedies.
2. Avoid chamomile in patients who are allergic to ragweed.
3. Avoid peppermint in G6PD deficiency.
4. Eucalyptus globulus and Cananga odorata can effect the absorption of 5-fluorouracil.
5. 1,8 cineole (a component of some essential oils) was found to significantly decrease the narcotic effect of pentobarbitol.
6. Cymbopogon citratus (West Indian lemongrass) was found to potentiate the effects of morphine in studies in rats.
7. Peppermint can negate effects of quinidine in treatment of arrhythmias.
8. Lavender can potentiate barbiturates.
9. Tranquilizers, anticonvulsants, and antihistamines may be slightly potentiated by sedative essential oils.
10. Sage, clary-sage, fennel, and aniseed, which mimic the effect of estradiol, should be avoided in estrogen-dependent tumors.
11. Emmenogogic essential oils, such as hyssop, should be avoided in pregnancy.
12. Hypertensive essential oils, such as rosemary, should be avoided in patients with hypertension.
13. Hyssop should be avoided in patients prone to seizures.
14. Some essential oils, such as ylang ylang, and lavender potentiate the effects of some orthodox medications, such as barbiturates.
15. Some essential oils, such as eucalyptus, enhance the effect of some antibiotics.
16. Some essential oils, such as cinnamon, contain high levels of phenols which can cause dermal irritation.
17. Some essential oils, such as bergamot, contain furanocoumarins, which can cause dermal irritation or burns when in the presence of ultraviolet light.

Adverse Reactions

There is some evidence of adverse skin reactions caused by sensitivity in remote cases. The majority of cases were from extracts that contained topical preservatives, rather than essential oils, which do not contain preservatives. People with multiple allergies are more likely to be sensitive to aromas. Most of the information is available from *The Food and Cosmetics Toxicology Journals*. Tisserand and Balacs mention the following:

1. Undiluted peppermint on a recent scar caused necrosis and warranted further surgery.
2. Taking essential oils orally without specialized knowledge can be dangerous: 5 ccs of *Eucalyptus globulus* can kill a 5-year-old child.
3. Essential oils that contain furanocoumarins (all the citrus peel oils) can cause photosensitivity from erythema to full-thickness burns.

Pregnancy and Lactation

Essential oils should be avoided during the first trimester, and it is suggested that essential oils thought to have emmenogogic action should be avoided altogether. These include sage, pennyroyal, camphor, parsley, tarragon, wintergreen, juniper, hyssop, and basil. The following are thought to be safe in pregnancy: cardomon, chamomile (Roman and German), clary sage, coriander seed, geranium, ginger, lavender, neroli, palmarosa, patchouli, petitgrain, rose, rosewood, and sandalwood.

Tisserand and Balacs state there is "no evidence that they are abortifacient in the amounts used in aromatherapy" (see "Suggested Reading").

Trade Products, Administration, and Dosage

Recommended companies, according to the author, are listed as follows:
Essential Oils Distributors:

Scents and Scentsibility Ltd.
PO Box 8013
Bridgewater, NJ 08807
Tel: (732) 469-2757
www.scentsibility.com

Elizabeth Van Buren Aromatherapy Ltd.
303 Potrero St. #33
Santa Cruz, CA 95060
Tel: (408) 425-8218

Fragrant Earth Ltd and Oshadi Ltd.
Distributor: Quality of Life
15 Meadow Lane
Dedham, MA 02026
Tel: (800) 688-8343

Administration

Essential oils can be used topically or inhaled. Between one and five drops of essential oils are diluted in a 5 ccs (a teaspoon) cold-pressed vegetable oil, such as sweet almond oil, for topical application. Some French doctors who are trained in aromatic medicine give essential oils (diluted in carrier oil orally) in gelatin capsules to treat infections. For topically applications (for example, chronic pain), use every four hours. For inhalation (for example, insomnia, nausea, and depression), inhale for 10 minutes as necessary. Use touch methods such as massage or the *m technique*. This technique is becoming accepted as a method of using touch for aromatherapy where appropriate, especially with nurses or when the practitioner is not a licensed massage therapist. Simple stress management can be incorporated into everyday regime with the use of baths and foot soaks, vaporizers, and sprays.

Self-Help versus Professional

This therapy can be self-applied for stress-management, but for more clinical uses it is better to have some training and knowledge of the chemistry and extraction methods. Many essential oils are sold under their *common name*. Origanum marjorana (sweet marjoram) is an excellent essential oil for insomnia. However, Thymus mastichina (Spanish marjoram) is frequently sold as "marjoram," but it is not a marjoram and certainly will not help insomnia! Lavandula angustifolia and Lavandula latifolia both are sold as "lavender." Angustifolia has sedative and antispasmodic properties; latifolia is a stimulant and expectorant.

Visiting a Professional

The field of aromatherapy is vast. Patients need to be aware of what kind of aromatherapy they need. Do they need help with stress management, to make their home smell more welcoming, do they have clinical symptoms, or are they on medication?

If a patient wants clinical aromatherapy it is best to see a trained health professional who has taken a clinical course in aromatherapy to enhance practice, such as a licensed massage therapist, registered nurse, physical therapist, and so on. If patients want medical aromatherapy, they need a physician with extensive training in the internal use of essential oils. Treatment can include some touch, if appropriate. A typical session would be an extensive background history and symptomology, a discussion of what aromas are liked and disliked, a discussion of the appropriateness of the application, a discussion of expectancies, and either an inhalation, topical application, or aromatic capsules, if the practitioner is so qualified.

Credentialing

At the moment there is no recognized national certification examination. Obviously there will be different requirements depending on the type of aromatherapy being practiced. There is no governing body at present, but the steering committee for Educational Standards in Aromatherapy in the U.S. is currently setting up the Aromatherapy Registration Board, which as a nonprofit entity will be responsible for administering a national exam and providing the public with a list of registered practitioners. The largest professional body is the National Association of Holistic Aromatherapy (NAHA). At present there are no requirements to become certified or accredited. Trainings can range from 1 weekend to several years. Anyone can train in this therapy.

What to Look for in a Provider

This is difficult, particularly because the field is so diverse. There are many self-taught aromatherapists who have extensive knowledge, but there are others whose knowledge is very limited. For clinical aromatherapy, it would be wisest to choose a licensed health professional who has completed a course of at least 200 hours from a school or organization whose exam has been accepted by an external organization like NAHA or the ARB.

Barriers and Key Issues

Aromatherapy is misunderstood because it is so broad. However, it encompasses many facets, from pleasure to pain to infection, and it is not limited to scented candles and potpourri. Commercial use of the word *aromatherapy* to boost sales of products such as shampoos has further confused the public. In fact, few if any cosmetic or pharmaceutic products currently include essential oils; they use synthetic fragrances as they are much cheaper. More clinical studies need to be carried out for aromatherapy to be taken seriously by the medical profession in the U.S., as well as more dialogue with French physicians.

Associations

National Association for Holistic Aromatherapy
PO Box 17622
Boulder, CO 80308
Tel: (888) ASK-NAHA or (314) 963-2071
Fax: (314) 963-4454
E-mail: info@naha.org
www.naha.org

Suggested Reading

1. Tisserand R, Balacs T: *Essential oil safety*, London, 1995, Churchill Livingstone.
   Written by an internationally recognized aromatherapist and a molecular biologist, this excellent book outlines all the safety issues, metabolism of essential oils, toxicity, dangerous essential oils, contraindications, and much more. With 500 references.
2. Buckle J: *Clinical aromatherapy*, San Diego, 1997, Singular.
   Written by a critical care nurse with an MA in Clinical Aromatherapy, this book puts aro-

matherapy squarely into the clinical area, outlining specialist departments such as oncology and pediatrics. It has a comprehensive section on infection and outlines protocols and policies. With 700 references.

3. Valnet J: *The practice of aromatherapy: holistic health and the essential oils of flowers and herbs*, Vermont, 1990, Healing Arts Press.

   The classic text book for the novice written by a French MD and translated into English by Tisserand.

4. Ackerman D: *A natural history of the senses*, New York, 1990, Vintage Books.

   A fascinating look at all the senses, including touch and smell, which are basic components of aromatherapy. Beautifully written.

References

1. Wilkinson S: Aromatherapy in palliative care, *Int J Pall Nurs* 1(1):21-30, 1995.

2. Moate S: Anxiety and depression, *Int J Aromather*, 7(1):18-21, 1995.

3. Styles JL: The use of aromatherapy in hospitalized children with HIV disease, *Comp Ther* 2:16-21, 1997.

4. Betts T: The fragrant breeze: the role of aromatherapy in treating epilepsy, *Aromather Q* 51:25-27, 1996.

5. Gobel H, Schmidt G, Soyka D: Effect of peppermint and eucalyptus oil preparations on neurophysiologic and experimental algesimetric headache parameters, *Cephalalgia* 14:228-234, 1995.

6. Krall B, Krause W: Efficacy and tolerance of Mentha arvensis aetheroleum, *Programme Abstracts*, 24th International Symposium of Essential, Grasse, France, 1993.

7. Woolfson A, Hewitt D: Intensive aromacare, *Int J Aromather* 4(2):12-14, 1992.

8. Buchbauer G, Jirovetz L, Jager W: Aromatherapy: evidence for sedative effects of the essential oil of lavender after inhalation, *Z Naturforsch* 46:1067-1072, 1991.

9. Stevensen CJ: The psychophysiological effects of aromatherapy massage following cardiac surgery, *Comp Ther Med* 2(1):27-35, 1994.

10. Seth G, Kokate CK, Varma KC: Effect of essential oil of Cymbopogon citratus on the central nervous system, *India J Exper Biol* 14(3):370-371, 1976.

11. Lorenzetti B et al: Myrcene mimics the peripheral analgesic activity of lemongrass tea, *Ethnopharmacol* 34:43-48, 1991.

12. Komori T et al: Effects of citrus fragrance on immune function and depressive states, *Neuroimmunomodul* 2:174-180, 1995.

13. Manly CH: Psychophysiologic effects of odor, *Crit Rev Food Sci Nutr* 33(9):57-62, 1993.

14. Schiffman S: Pleasant odors improve mood of women and men at mid-life, *Compendium of Olfactory Research* pp. 97-103, 1995, Olfactory Research Fund.

15. Kichuri A: Effects of fragrance on insomniac tendency in health human beings. In Baser KHC, editor: *Conference proceedings: flavors, fragrances, and essential oils*, Istanbul, 1995, Anadolu University Press.

16. Carson CF et al: Susceptibility of methicillin resistant Staph aureus to the essential oil of Melaleuca alternifolia, *J Antimicrob Chemother* 35:421-424, 1995.

17. Larrondo JV, Agut M, Calvo-Torras MA: Antimicrobial activity of essences from libiates, *Microbios* 82:171-172, 1995.

18. Benouda A, Hassar M, Benjilali B: The antiseptic properties of essential oils in vitro tested against pathogenic germs found in hospitals, *Fitogerapia* 59(2):115-119, 1988.

19. Deininger R: The spectrum of activity of plant drugs containing essential oils—their antibacterial, antifungal, and antiviral activity, *Proceedings from Holistic Aromatherapy: a scientific conference on the therapeutic uses of essential oils* 406:15-43, 1995.

20. Wannisorm B, Jarikasem S, Soontormtanasart T: Antifungal activity of lemongrass oil and lemongrass oil cream, *Phytother Res* 10:551-554, 1996.

21. Heng MC: Local necrosis and interstitial nephritis due to topical methyl salicylate and menthol (re: wintergreen), *Cutis* 39(5):442-444, 1987.

22. Opdyke DLJ: Safety testing of fragrances: problems and implications, *Clin Toxicol* 19(1):61-67, 1977.

23. Millet Y: Toxicity of some essential plant oils: clinical and experimental study, *Clin Toxicol* 18(12):1485-1498, 1981.

Biologic Dentistry

PHILLIP P. SUKEL

Origins and History

Alternative or complementary dentistry also may be called *biologic, environmental, biocompatible,* or *holistic* dentistry. The biologic dentist is concerned about the effect dentistry may have on the overall health of an individual. Patients become "mercury-free" when amalgams are replaced with nonmercury restoratives, although they still have mercury deposited in body tissues (body burden). *Mercury-free* only means that the practitioner is not placing new mercury amalgams. Unlike the traditional dental paradigm, biologic dentists treat the mouth as part of the human body, and dental care, as well as dental health, cannot be separated from the body and its influence on systemic health.

As early as the seventh century the Chinese used a "silver paste" containing mercury (Hg) to fill decayed teeth.[1] With advancements in metallurgy, this pliable mass was a relatively inexpensive and very easy compound to put into teeth. The problem is the impact that mercury and other components have on an individual's systemic health.

In the last 20 years, research evidence confirms that every therapeutic medication or material we use *may* affect our patients depending on their individual characteristics. Other dental materials like base metals, fluoride, root canals, anesthetics and analgesics, the myriad of new restorative materials, and even the precious (gold) and nonprecious (nickel) alloys may have an adverse effect. The treatment goal of the biologic dentist is not to put anything back into the mouth that may have an adverse impact on health. This discussion primarily addresses the mercury amalgam issue.

Proper protection must be used for the patient, doctor, and staff before, during, and after the removal of mercury amalgam. Protection protocols are based on research evidence, some of which are funded, interpreted, and integrated into clinical applications by the International Academy of Oral Medicine and Toxicology (IAOMT). See "Associations."

Mechanism of Action According to Its Own Theory

There are four principle ways that dental materials may influence health, as follows:

1. *Toxic:* Research evidence shows that mercury is a poison.[2] There are two detoxification steps from a poison: get away from the source (mercury amalgams are removed from the

667

mouth), and eliminate the deposited body burden of toxins. Mercury detoxification is complex.[3] Therapies include diet, drugs (DMPS, DMSA), vitamins and minerals, homeopathy, exercise, sauna, hydrotherapy, herbs, and manual lymphatic drainage.

2. *Galvanism:* Almost all dental restorative materials contain metals that impart physical properties to make the material more color-stable, easier to use, less corrosive, wear longer, resist breakage, and expand or contract more like a tooth. Two or more metals in an environment with an electrolyte (saliva) result in corrosion.[4] Mercury amalgam is a semi-solid containing several metals: about 50% mercury, 30% silver, and the remaining 20% mainly copper, tin, and zinc.

3. *Immune system:* There is significant literature showing the immune sensitivity and allergy of dental materials, especially mercury. Dental materials in the mouth corrode. The corrosion byproducts react immunologically (Clifford Material Reactivity Test).

4. *Acupuncture:* Every tooth lies on an acupuncture meridian influencing the energy of that meridian. *Electrodermal screening* is a form of acupuncture using a computer to help assess the impact dental materials may have on specific meridians by way of specific acupuncture points (generally the hands).

Once all materials are properly removed from the mouth, the toxic, galvanic, immune, and acupuncture influences are eliminated as long as good professional judgement is used in placing new "clean" materials.

Biologic Mechanism of Action

Mercury is released from amalgams in at least 3 forms: elemental mercury vapor (Hg^0)[4], ionic mercury (Hg^{2+}) through electrogalvanism[5], and particulate mercury (in Hg complexes with metal alloys and salts). Mercury vapor is released continuously throughout the life of the filling. The release rate increases after chewing or tooth brushing.[6] This exposure takes up to 90 minutes to return to pre-chew levels.[7]

Elemental mercury vapor is 80% to 100% absorbed through the lungs, passing within seconds into tissue sites (sulfur binding). A Mercury Vapor Risk Factor Analysis (IAOMT Standard of Care) determines an individual's risk for toxicity from mercury vapor exposure, as follows:

1. *Psychologic disturbances (erethysm):* Irritability, nervousness, shyness or timidity, loss of memory, lack of attention, loss of self-confidence, decline of intellect, lack of self-control, fits of anger, depression, anxiety, drowsiness, or insomnia

2. *Oral cavity disorders:* Bleeding gums, alveolar bone loss, loosening of teeth, excessive salivation, foul breath, metallic taste, leukoplakia (white patches), gingivitis (inflammation of the gums), stomatitis (mouth inflammation), ulceration (gingiva, palate, tongue), burning sensation in the mouth or throat, or tissue pigmentation

3. *Gastrointestinal effects:* Abdominal cramps, constipation or diarrhea, or gastrointestinal problems including colitis

4. *Systemic effects*
   a. Cardiovascular: Irregular heartbeat (tachycardia, bradycardia), feeble and irregular pulse, alterations in blood pressure, or pain or pressure in the chest

b. Neurologic: Chronic or frequent headaches, dizziness, ringing or noises in the ears, or fine tremors (hands, feet, lips, eyelids, and tongue)

c. Respiratory: Persistent cough, emphysema, or shallow and irregular respiration

d. Immunologic: Allergies, asthma, rhinitis (inflammation of the nose), sinusitis, or lymphadenopathy (especially neck)

e. Endocrine: Subnormal temperature, cold, clammy skin (hands and feet), or excessive perspiration

f. Other: Muscle weakness, speech disorders, dim or double vision, fatigue, anemia, hypoxia (lack of oxygen), edema (swelling), loss of appetite (anorexia), loss of weight, or joint pains

5. *Severe cases:* Hallucinations or manic depression

Organic mercury exposure comes from dietary sources like seafood. Mercury from the fillings is transported through saliva to the gut where it is changed into organic forms (methyl mercury) by resident microorganisms. Some microorganisms become resistant to the toxic effects of mercury, and this exposure provokes antibiotic resistance.[8] The earliest symptoms include fatigue, headache, forgetfulness, inability to concentrate, apathy, depression, outburst on anger, and decline of intellect. Later findings include the following symptoms: numbness and tingling in the hands, feet, or lips; muscle weakness progressing to paralysis; dim or restricted vision; hearing difficulty; speech disorders; loss of memory; incoordination; emotional instability; dermatitis; renal damage; and general central nervous system dysfunction.[9]

Forms of Therapy

Biologic dentistry can take many forms depending on the training and expertise of the practitioner. It can range from simple mercury removal (mercury-free) to the practitioner that may use advanced diagnostic testing, protection protocols, and detoxification,[3] biocompatible replacement identification tests, root canal and jaw bone cavitation therapy, and physician-assisted support and detoxification.

Demographics

Trained biologic dentists are not common but can be found worldwide. Many dentists now consider themselves "mercury-free" in that they no longer place new amalgams, but the vast majority of these dentists are not biologic. See "Associations."

At present there are basically the following two groups of patients using biologic dentistry:

1. Those patients with health concerns (some very serious) who usually have exhausted conventional medical therapies with little or no results. Informed physicians, relatives, or friends refer these patients for this modality.[9-13]

2. Anyone who is health-centered and wants optimum health. These people use other alternative modalities as found in this publication. Biologic dentists believe and re-

search supports that individuals cannot avoid dental pollution, short of removal and replacement.[3,9,11-13]

Indications and Reasons for Referral

Dentists may not make a medical diagnosis or suggest amalgam removal as a medical treatment. A biologic dentist must work closely with an aware physician in caring for the patient. Everyone has the right to know the medical science and have access to it. Only then can they make an informed choice as to treatment. Clinical sign and symptoms resulting from Hg exposure are listed in "Biologic Mechanism of Action."

Research Base

Evidence Based

Animal and human experiments show that the uptake, distribution in tissues, and elimination of amalgam mercury is significant and amalgam mercury is the primary source of human mercury body burden.[14] Research on the pathophysiologic effects of mercury centers on the immune system, renal system, oral and intestinal bacteria, reproductive system, and central nervous system. Amalgam safety is not supported by research.[15]

Basic Science

There are three species of mercury. The main source of Hg^0 is vapor from dental amalgam tooth fillings (3 to 17μg/d). Organic Hg (Hg^+) is derived from fish and seafood (2.3μg/d). Inorganic Hg (Hg^{2+}) comes from other foods, water, and air (0.3μg/d). Hg^0 is absorbed across the lung and converted to Hg^{2+} intracellularly by catalase oxidation. The high lipid solubility of Hg^0 permits it to easily cross cell membranes, including the blood brain barrier, permitting easy entry to the brain. The kidney is the major site of Hg accumulation during compartmental redistribution after Hg^0 exposure. Some Hg^0 is dissolved in saliva and is swallowed and converted to Hg^{2+} by peroxidase oxidation. The majority is eliminated in the feces. Hg^{2+} is the toxic product responsible for the adverse effects of inhaled Hg^0.[15] Hg^+ and Hg^{2+} have retention half-lives in the body tissues ranging from days to years.[2,16-18]

Risk and Safety

Amalgam fillings are routinely removed and replaced. There are the following two elements to risk and safety:

1. The trauma from the removal process may lead to pulpitis (irritated nerve manifested by increased sensitivity to temperature) or even its death (treated by a root canal or removal).[12]

2. When an amalgam filling is removed for any reason, many conventional medical dentists choose to replace it with another mercury amalgam. This only continues the cycle of acute (removal process without protection) and chronic (long-term release of mercury vapor from a new mercury amalgam) exposure, thus perpetuating problems of risk and safety. Material safety data sheets (MSDS) from dental amalgam manufacturers now confirm that the dental industry is aware of the risk and the lack of safety of mercury amalgam filling. The first aid or emergency solution to chronic inhalation exposure to mercury vapor is to get away from the source of mercury and into fresh air immediately, which is impossible when amalgams are placed in the teeth.

Efficacy

Will replacing amalgam fillings improve an individual's health and reduce overall health care costs? Unfortunately, there have not been any large-scale scientific studies that would provide definitive answers to the question that are acceptable to the conventional medical establishment. However, there have been a number of small studies, which all indicate a positive health benefit accruing from the elimination of mercury-containing dental fillings. The vast majority of individuals who have undergone amalgam replacement and reduction of their mercury body burden have experienced improvements in health that have ranged from minor to startlingly dramatic. For example, the statistics listed in the table were compiled by the Foundation for Toxic Free Dentistry (FTFD) on 1569 patients from six different reports.[9]

Future Research Opportunities and Priorities

Research opportunities are limitless. There is a need for studies in mercury detoxification, protective protocols and replacement material identification, and pathophysiologic effects. Priority also must be placed on the clinical integration of the research and distribution of that information.

Druglike Information

Safety

Mercury vapor is continuously released from amalgam fillings and the levels increase immediately with chewing or toothbrushing.[6] The process of removal dramatically increases the acute exposure. Safe removal depends on a number of variables, such as health history problems, inadequate protection before, during, and after treatment, overly quick removal (in terms of number of fillings per visit), and the selection of replacement material that is incorrect or harmful. The biologic approach believes that it is safer to remove the mercury amalgams, risking a transient acute but protected exposure so that the body can begin the detoxification process, rather than risk continued chronic exposure.

Improvements in Health Resulting from Amalgam Replacements

% of Total	Symptom	Total Number of Patients	Number Improved	% of Cured
6%	Lack of energy	91	88	97%
17%	Metallic taste	260	247	95%
8%	Gum problems	129	121	94%
5%	Anxiety	86	80	93%
22%	Depression	347	317	91%
8%	Irritability	132	119	90%
14%	Allergy	221	196	89%
5%	Bad temper	81	68	89%
6%	Bloating	88	70	88%
22%	Dizziness	434	301	88%
5%	Chest pains	79	69	87%
34%	Headaches	531	460	87%
3%	Migraine headaches	45	39	87%
10%	Irregular heartbeat	159	139	87%
45%	Fatigue	705	603	86%
9%	Sore throat	149	128	86%
12%	Ulcers and sores (oral cavity)	189	162	86%
15%	Gastrointestinal problems	231	192	83%
8%	Muscle tremor	126	104	83%
10%	Nervousness	158	131	83%
8%	Numbness anywhere	118	97	82%
20%	Skin disturbances	310	251	81%
17%	Lack of concentration	270	216	80%
4%	Thyroid problems	56	44	79%
12%	Insomnia	187	146	78%
7%	Multiple sclerosis	113	86	76%
7%	Urinary tract problems	115	87	76%
17%	Memory loss	265	193	73%
6%	Tachycardia (rapid heart beat)	97	68	70%
29%	Vision problems	462	289	63%
6%	Blood pressure problems	99	53	54%

Warnings, Contraindications, and Precautions

There is great concern for those patients who have a compromised neurologic, immune, and central nervous systems, decreased kidney and liver function, and reproductive problems.[10,15] Although care must be exercised with everyone, a knowledgeable practitioner must more closely manage those patients with clinical manifestation of disease states related to mercury.[9] Using the health history and testing, a treatment plan for restorative replacement is developed according to the principles of biologic dentistry. The following is a short, very incomplete but helpful starter list of potential problem restorative materials, according to the principles of biologic dentistry:

> *Never use:* mercury amalgams; metal alloys (semi and nonprecious) that contain nickel, cobalt, chromium, and beryllium; fluoride; and gutta percha root canal filling

Use with caution: composite fillings and restoratives; materials that "out gas" formalde-
hyde; local anesthetics; nitrous oxide analgesic; metal alloys (precious); and Biocalex root canal filling

Adverse Reactions

Caution must be exercised before, during, and after removal of amalgams. Patients of highest risk for adverse reactions are those with allergies to the new materials or detoxification
limitations. Patients with neurologic and immunologic histories (especially environmental universal reactors) are at more risk to exposure and replacement materials. Care may be
necessary in how many amalgams are removed per visit and the use of anesthetics with
preservatives.[3,9,10,14] See "Efficacy."

Pregnancy and Lactation

Pregnant sheep received amalgam fillings containing radioactive tracer, demonstrating
the accumulation of amalgam mercury in both maternal and fetal tissues within several
days of placement. As gestation advanced, maternal-fetal transfer progressed and mercury also transferred to breast milk postpartum.[4] Human fetal-neonatal studies have since
demonstrated mercury concentrations in fetal kidney and liver and cerebral cortex of infants, which correlates significantly with the number of amalgam-filled teeth of their
mothers.[19]

The IAOMT has addressed this issue with a standard of care for "Optional Mercury Removal During Pregnancy and Lactation." Only emergency and absolutely necessary dental
mercury amalgam work should be done during these periods. If it is necessary to remove
mercury amalgams at this time, replace with biocompatible materials and follow IAOMT
protective protocols ("Reducing Mercury Vapor Exposure for the Patient During Amalgam
Removal").[11,20]

Self-Help versus Professional

The dental diagnosis, treatment planning, removal, and replacement of amalgams and other
dentistry must be done by a licensed dentist. Many other aspects of patient protection before and detoxification after can be self-taught with guidance by the dentist or physician.
Some protocols have been found to be more effective than others; for this reason, professional advice is helpful if not necessary, especially for the medically compromised patient.[3]

Visiting a Professional

There are two parts to visiting a biologic dentist, as follows:

1. *Interview, examination, and additional testing:* The initial examination would
   include all the usual information and data gathering as a nonbiologic dentist, such
   as the health history, necessary radiographs and documentation of the condition of

the hard and soft tissues, existing dentistry, periodontal (gum) health, and temporomandibular dysfunction. A biologic dentist would take much more time with patients on their health history (HH) to help them understand the relationship between their HH and current dentistry. Once the patient is comfortable with the issues and their goals are understood, a biocompatible treatment plan would be developed. Additional biologic tests include the following:

  a. Clifford material reactivity test: Antibody detection testing performed from blood serum to establish existing sensitivity to components of dental restorations and assist in selecting materials of lowest risk to the patient

  b. Oral potential test: A galvanic test to assess the electrical potential and current between restorations and from restorations to soft tissues

  c. Microscopic periodontal evaluation: To assess the possible presence of parasites, fungi, and other pathologic organisms in the gums tissues

  d. Dental kinesiology: To determine the compatibility of future restorative materials of lower risk

  e. Electroacupuncture assessment: A computerized assessment of the relationship of dental materials to acupuncture meridians to help with choosing replacement restorative materials

  f. Root canal and bone cavitation lesion assessment: Through radiographs, palpation, and anesthetic confirmation. Some practitioners use kinesiology or electroacupuncture evaluation. All should biopsy the removed tissues.

  g. Hair analysis: To determine heavy metal levels of the body, including mercury (synergistic effects)

  h. DMPS challenge test: Performed by a MD or DO to determine the tissue sequestering of mercury

  i. Other medical test deemed necessary by the attending physician

2. *Treatment plan and dentistry removal:* Once a treatment plan for the removal and biocompatible replacement is agreed on, the safe removal of the existing dentistry is of utmost importance to protect the patient and minimize the risk of additional mercury exposure before, during, and after the removal process.

  a. Patient protection before removal usually involves supplementation. For the average patient (complex patients need specific additional support), some of the common supplements include general multiple vitamins, vitamin C, chlorella, homeopathic lymphatic drainage remedies, cilantro, charcoal to bind heavy metals in the gastrointestinal tract, purified or spring water, and sulfur loading with supplements like selenium, N-Acetyl-L-Cysteine (NAC), glutathione, and methyl sulphonyl methane (MSM).[3,11]

  b. Patient protection during amalgam removal: The IAOMT has a specific protocol called "Reducing Mercury Vapor Exposure for the Patient During Amalgam Removal."

  c. Detoxification after amalgam removal generally is a continuation of the protection before with perhaps increases in chlorella, the addition of DMPS or DMSA, and more homeopathic remedies or preparations, depending on the specific needs of the patient.[3,11] The length of this phase usually is dictated by symptoms or, if possible, DMPS challenge.

Credentialing and Training

To practice dentistry in the U.S., individuals must have a license. There are a limited number of dental specialties. This modality is not a specialty, only an area of special interest. The International Academy of Oral Medicine and Toxicology offers levels of Accreditation (AIAOMT) and Fellowship (FIAOMT) attesting to a practitioner's level of biologic expertise and competence. See "Associations."

What to Look for in a Provider

Trained and practicing biologic dentists will have knowledge and experience in the following areas:

- Relating your health history to the medical research, *not leading you to believe* that the removal of amalgam fillings will cure or ameliorate your health concerns
- Understanding and being able to advise and protect you before, during, and after mercury removal. Removal can be done either with or without a rubber dam (both procedures are defined by the IAOMT *Standards of Care*). Also, there is no scientific support of the notion of "sequential removal."
- Recognizing the difference between allergy and toxicity, as well as the forms, advantages, and limitations of detoxification
- Knowing the potential problems and limitations of antibiotics, candida, parasites, root canals, fluoride, base metals, composites, and amalgam tattoos
- Understanding (if not performing) a mercury vapor risk factor analysis, oral galvanism screening, Clifford material reactivity test, jaw cavitation lesion palpation and anesthetic confirmation, dental kinesiology, electroacupuncture screening, and low speed drilling
- Using and being knowledgeable or at least familiar with homeopathy, nutrition, vitamin and mineral supplementation, herbal therapy, and Bach flower remedies
- Being familiar with other therapies not commonly practiced because of the need for additional training or dental licensure restrictions and concerns, including chiropractic, chelation, naturopathy, colonotherapy, sweat therapy, dark field microscopy, iridology, auricular therapy, manual lymphatic drainage, essential oils, magnets, cranial osteopathy, and neurotherapy

Some key questions to help find a biologic dentist include the following:

- Are you mercury-free? (If not, find someone else.) Are you a biologic dentist?
- What are your goals and do you have a mission statement?
- With my health history, should I be immediately concerned about removal of my amalgams?
- How do you protect me before, during, and after removal of the mercury amalgams? Do you use "Clean Up" (a device that attaches to the high-volume evacuation of

the dentist and fits around the tooth, removing the vast majority mercury and minimizing patient, doctor, and staff exposure during removal)?

- Do you use fluoride?
- Are you concerned about root canals? Are you using Biocalex?
- How do you decide on compatible replacement materials?
- Are you a member of the International Academy of Oral Medicine and Toxicology (IAOMT)? If so, are you accredited or a Fellow? (See "Associations.")

Barriers and Key Issues

As the key issue of the pathophysiologic effects of amalgam mercury becomes more widely recognized and accepted, the use of this restorative material eventually will fall into disfavor.[15] Much research is being done on all aspects of dental biocompatibility, bringing into question not only materials but also techniques and equipment to break down the barriers. When this medical research filters down to the clinical physicians, biologic dentistry must be included in the differential diagnosis.[10,13]

Associations

International Academy of Oral Medicine and Toxicology (IAOMT)
PO Box 608531
Orlando, FL 32860
Tel: (407) 298-2450
www.iaomt.org
Membership for professionals only, dedicated to research and education of professionals and a referral source for patients. IAOMT funds medical research, develops Standard of Care, and is the only organization with formal training and accreditation for professionals.

Foundation For Toxic Free Dentistry
PO Box 608010
Orlando, FL 32860
Send a self-addressed, stamped #10 envelope with $1.00 postage for a copy of the latest newsletter and a referral to a dentist closest to you.

The Holistic Dental Association
PO Box 5007
Durango, CO 81301
www.holisticdental.org

Clifford Consulting and Research
PO Box 17597
Colorado Springs, CO 80935
www.ccrlab.com

American Academy of Biologic Dentistry
PO Box 856
Carmel Valley, CA 93934
E-mail: aabd@thevortex.com
www.biologicdentistry.org

Suggested Reading:

1. Strong G: *Does mercury from dental amalgams influence systemic health? A referenced topical guide to the potential role of mercury from "silver" fillings in systemic pathology*, Billings, Mont, Strong Health Publications.
   Fully referenced topics include: Alzheimer's disease, cardiovascular disease, free radical pathology, immune system dysfunction, ion metabolism dysfunction, kidney dysfunction, neuropsychologic dysfunction, reproductive disorders, and useful summaries of mercury related information.

2. Ziff S, Ziff MF, Hanson M: *Dental mercury detox*, Orlando, Fla, 1995, Bioprobe.
   This edition has various protocols reflected in the scientific literature that may help reduce mercury body burden.

3. Ziff S, Ziff MF: *Dentistry without mercury*, Orlando, Fla, Bioprobe.
   Contains the latest scientific information on the mercury controversy and issues involved.

4. Walker G: *Fluoridation: poison on tap*, Mulgrove, Victoria, Australia, Magenta Press.
   A complete referenced guide on the influences of fluoride and fluoridated water on systemic health.

5. Ziff S, Ziff M: *Infertility and birth defects*, Orlando, Fla, Bioprobe.
   A major reference book that explains and documents the amazing facts about mercury and lead and why "silver" fillings may increase the risk of being infertile or bearing children who are mentally impaired. With 500 scientific references.

6. Kennedy D: *How to save your teeth*, Delaware, Ohio, Health Action Press.
   A fully referenced guide for the public and dentist seeking information on alternative preventive dentistry, including the dangers of mercury amalgams, root canals, and especially fluoride.

7. Hanson M: *Mercury bibliography update*, Orlando, Fla, Bioprobe.
   Includes 1404 citations and 610 abstracts covering 1991 to 1993.

8. Meinig GE: *Root canal cover-up*, Ojai, Calif, Bion.
   A referenced book that reveals how root canals can damage health, cripple the immune system, and affect the heart.

9. Ziff M, Ziff S: *The missing link? A persuasive look at heart disease as it relates to mercury*, Orlando, Fla, Bioprobe.
   A fully referenced book on the relationships of mercury, from "silver" amalgam dental fillings to heart disease.

10. Ziff S: *Silver dental fillings—the toxic time bomb*, Orlando, Fla, Bioprobe.
    This book covers the history of the amalgam controversy from 1819 to the present time.

References

1. Ring ME: *Dentistry: an illustrated history,* New York, 1985, M.H. Abrams.
2. Clarkson TW et al: Mercury. In Clarkston TW et al: *Biological monitoring of toxic metals,* New York, 1998, Plenum.
3. Ziff S, Ziff MF, Hanson M: *Dental mercury detox,* Orlando, Fla, 1995, Bioprobe.
4. Vimy MJ, Takahashi Y, Lorscheider FL: Maternal-fetal distribution of mercury (203-Hg) released from dental amalgam fillings, *Am J Physiol* 258:R939-R945, 1990.
5. Masi JV: Corrosion of amalgams in restorative materials: the problem and the promise. In Freiberg L, Schrauzer GN, editors: *Status quo and perspectives of amalgam and other dental materials,* Stuttgart, 1995, Theime-Verlag.
6. Patterson JE, Weissberg B, Dennison PJ: Mercury in human breath from dental amalgam, *Bull Environ Contam Toxicol* 34:459-468, 1985.
7. Vimy MJ, Lorscheider FL: Serial measurements of intraoral air mercury: estimation of daily dose from dental amalgam, *J Dent Res* 64:1072-1075, 1995.
8. Summers AO et al: Mercury released from dental "silver" fillings provokes an increase in mercury- and antibiotic-resistant bacteria in oral and intestinal floras of primates, *Antimicrob Agents Chemother* 37:825-834, 1993.
9. Ziff S, Ziff MF: *Dentistry without mercury,* Orlando, Fla, Bioprobe.
10. Strong G: *Does mercury from dental amalgams influence systemic health? A referenced topical guide to the potential role of mercury from "silver" fillings in systemic pathology,* Billings, Mt, Strong Health Publications.
11. Kennedy D: *How to save your teeth,* Delaware, Ohio, Health Action Press.
12. Meinig GE: *Root canal cover-up,* Ojai, Calif, Bion Publishing.
13. Ziff S: *Silver dental fillings: the toxic time bomb,* Orlando, Fla, Bioprobe.
14. Hanson M: *Mercury bibliography update,* Orlando, Fla, Bioprobe.
15. Lorscheider FL, Vimy MJ, Summers AO: Mercury exposure from "silver" tooth fillings: emerging evidence questions a traditional dental paradigm, *FASEB J* 9:504-508, 1995.
16. Klaassen CD: Heavy metals and heavy-metal antagonists. In Gilman AG et al, editors: *The pharmacological basis of therapeutics,* ed 8, New York, 1990, Pergamon Press.
17. Skare I, Engqvist A: Human exposure to mercury and silver released from dental amalgam restorations, *Arch Environ Health* 49:384-394, 1994.
18. Friberg L, editor: *World Health Organization: environmental health critieria no 118: inorganic mercury,* Geneva, 1991, World Health Organization.
19. Drasch G et al: Mercury burden of human fetal and infant tissues, *Eur J Pediatr* 153:607-610, 1994.
20. Ziff S, Ziff M: *Infertility and birth defects,* Orlando, Fla, Bioprobe.
21. Goering PL et al: Toxicity assessment of mercury vapor from dental amalgams, *Fundam Appl Toxicol* 19:319-328, 1992.

Colon Hydrotherapy

AUGUSTINE RICHARD HOENNINGER III

Origins and History

It is difficult to identify the exact time in history that colon hydrotherapy emerged, but many historians trace it back to the ancient Egyptians. The practice of colon hydrotherapy or in its most basic form, the enemas, was passed down from the gods to the Egyptians. Dr. Otto Bettman describes the occasion: "Thoth himself had revealed the enema one day to a few priest-physicians who were standing on the banks of the Nile. The god of medicine and science had landed on the water in the form of a sacred ibis. Filling his beak with water, he had injected it into his anus. The doctors took the hint, and the result was a great boon to humanity, the Devine Clyster."[1]

The ancient Egyptians appear to have made very frequent use of the enema or clyster. The *Ebers Papyrus* of the fourteenth century BCE, obtained in 1873 by George Ebers, and the *Edwin Smith Papyrus* (also Eighteenth Dynasty), one of the earliest surgical textbooks (circa 1700 BCE), also mentions enemas, gives directions for the use of the enema, and prescribes remedies for 20 stomach and intestinal complaints.

Enemas were not limited to just the Egyptians. The use of clysters are recorded as early as 600 BCE on the cuneiform inscriptions on Babylonian and Assyrian tablets[2] and in Hindu medical texts such as the *Susruta Samhita*, the work of Susruta, the father of Hindu surgery.[3] There also are depictions of clysters in the pre-Colombian Mayan art.[4] Hippocrates (fourth and fifth century BCE) recorded using enemas for fever therapy and disorders of the regime in his "On Regimen in Acute Disease."[5] Galen (second century CE) also was a proponent of the use of enemas. In fact, throughout history there is an abundance of writings and pictures of the varying procedures for the administering of enemas or clysters.[6]

The seventeenth century became known as the "age of the enema" or the "age of clysters." It was the fashion in Parisian society to enjoy as many as three or four enemas per day, the popular belief being that an internal washing or *lavement* was essential to well-being. During this period, Regnier de Graaf, who is credited with the first description of the Graafian follicle, described the proper method to use the clyster syringe in his treatise *De Clysteribus*, published in 1668.[7]

The clyster reached the true height of its fashion in the early years of the reign of Louis XIV (1638-1715). It is reported by William Lieberman that Louis XIV had more than 2000 enemas during his career, sometimes even receiving court functionaries and visitors during the procedure.[8]

By the middle of the eighteenth century the introduction of rubber made it possible to use this material for the enema apparatus. Pump systems were incorporated, allowing individuals to perform their own enemas.[9] Improvements in the quality and effectiveness of the equipment continued into the twentieth century. These improvements allowed a much greater cleansing of larger portions of the colon.

The therapy was brought to prominence in the United States by Dr. Kellogg, who reported in the 1917 *Journal of American Medicine* that in more than 40,000 cases, as a result of diet, exercise, and enema (colon hydrotherapy), "in all but twenty cases" he had used no surgery for the treatment of gastrointestinal disease in his patients.[10]

Colon hydrotherapy eventually gained the attention of James A. Wiltsie, MD, who contended that "our knowledge of the normal and abnormal physiology of the colon, its pathology and management, has not kept pace with that of other organs and systems of the body." He went on to say, "As long as we continue to assume that the colon will take care of itself, just that long will we remain in complete ignorance of perhaps the most important source of ill health in the whole body."[11]

By the early 1950s colon hydrotherapy was flourishing in the U.S. The prestigious Beverly Boulevard in California was then known as "Colonic Row." However, towards the mid-1960s the use of colon irrigations and colon hydrotherapy slowly dwindled until approximately 1972, when most colon hydrotherapy instruments were removed from the hospitals and nursing homes as the more favored medical procedure, the colostomy, and prescriptive laxatives became the vogue.

A few doctors, however, continued to recommend colon hydrotherapy. The profession continued to grow and the equipment continued to be improved.

The safety and effectiveness of the current, state-of-the-art colon hydrotherapy equipment has been strengthened by the enactment of the Medical Device Amendments of 1976, which revised and extended the device requirements of the 1938 Federal Food, Drug, and Cosmetic Act. This act was subsequently amended by the Safe Medical Devices Act of 1990 (SMDA) and the Medical Device Amendments of 1992. These amendments enhance premarket and postmarket controls and provide for additional regulatory authority over equipment manufactured for colon hydrotherapy.

Just as equipment has been greatly improved in the past 50 years, the training and professionalism of the colon hydrotherapist also has greatly improved. The formation of the International Association for Colon Hydrotherapy (I-ACT) (formerly the American Colon Therapy Association, founded in 1989), provides training and certification for colon hydrotherapist in the U.S. and around the world.

Today, with modern technologic advancements in colon hydrotherapy equipment, safety, and skilled therapists, colon hydrotherapy has become a valuable adjunctive modality to the physician in treating disease.

Mechanism of Action According to Its Own Theory

Colon hydrotherapy is an extended and more complete form of an enema. It is not a cure-all but an important complementary therapy in the overall health care of the patient. It is a safe, effective method of removing waste from the large intestine without the use of drugs.

The standard enema and colonotherapy treatment both use the infusion of aqueous substances into the rectum. A standard enema involves the injection of water (one way) into the colon, which is retained and evacuated by the patient. Colon hydrotherapy is an instrument-controlled continual bathing of the colon for cleansing and therapeutic purposes. There is no offensive odor or health risk to those in contact with the sick patients as with enemas and bed pans, and the dignity of the patient is maintained. The enema's cleansing ability is limited to the area of the rectosigmoid and for shorter periods of time because of the body's natural wish to expel material from the rectum. Colon hydrotherapy extends beyond the natural expulsion area to offer greater cleansing and therapeutic benefits.

During the session the patient's dignity is maintained at all times as most clothing may be kept on while draped, or a gown might be used to ensure the patient's modesty.

The procedure involves the patient inserting a small rectal tube or speculum into the rectum approximately 1 to 3 inches. This speculum or rectal tube allows for temperature and pressure-controlled, warm, filtered water to flow into the rectum and through the colon with the objective of cleansing and balancing the colon. This allows for the softening of fecal material, which assists the removal of fecal material in the large intestine. The colon hydrotherapist may gently manipulate the abdomen during the procedure to enhance the removal of waste material. The therapeutic effect of colon hydrotherapy is improved muscle tone, which facilitates peristaltic action and enhances the absorption of nutrients from the cecum and ascending colon while minimizing the absorption of toxic waste material. The cleansing effects of colon hydrotherapy reduce stagnation and subsequent bacterial proliferation in the colon and assists in maintaining harmony of the intestinal flora in promoting optimal health. The process of filling and releasing is repeated several times during a session.

Colon hydrotherapy best benefits the body when used in combination with adequate nutrient and fluid intake, as well as exercise.

Forms of Therapy

There only is one form of therapy for colon hydrotherapy when practiced according to the scope of practice of I-ACT; however, this therapy allows for variations in the duration of the session, temperature of the water, and pressure of the water. Therapists may vary their techniques as to the types of abdominal manipulation, lymphatic drainage, reflexology, or energy work applied to each patient based on the knowledge and techniques of the attending therapist.

The physician may prescribe the use of oxygen or other substances, such as bifidus, acidophilus, cell salts, and others, but these variations must be made only at the direction of a physician.

Demographics

The International Association for Colon Hydrotherapists (I-ACT) estimates there are more than 5000 colon hydrotherapists in the world, with more than 1500 colon hydrotherapists in the U.S. In the past 3 years I-ACT reported a 200% increase in the number of certified colon hydrotherapists in the U.S. alone. These colon hydrotherapists see patients from all walks of life.

Indications and Reasons for Referral

There are three primary reasons a physician may recommend colon hydrotherapy: 1) constipation or impaction; 2) preparation for diagnostic studies of the large intestine (barium enema, sigmoidoscopy, or colonoscopy); and 3) preparation for or after surgery (such as after a barium enema to cleanse the large intestine of the barium) as rapidly as possible.

Additionally, the physician may consider recommending colon hydrotherapy for diarrhea, bowel training (paraplegics or quadriplegics), arthritis, and suspected autointoxication or intestinal toxemia (toxins or microorganism absorption through damaged cells in the intestinal mucosa).

A simple ranking of applicable conditions is as follows:

Top level: *A therapy ideally suited for these conditions*
Constipation, diarrhea, and gastrointestinal disorders.

Second level: *One of the better therapies for these conditions*
Addictions; allergies; asthma; back pain; bladder infection; bronchitis; candidiasis; chronic fatigue syndrome; chronic pain; colds and flu; colitis and Crohn's disease; diverticulosis and diverticulitis; fever; gastritis; irritable bowel syndrome; osteoarthritis; rheumatoid arthritis; stomachache; stress; viral and bacterial infections; and yeast infections

Third level: *A valuable adjunctive therapy for these conditions*
AIDS; arthritis; benign prostatic hypertrophy; cancer; childbirth; childhood parasites; children's health; colic; conjunctivitis; diabetes; ear infections; emphysema; female health; fibrocystic breast disease; gout; hay fever; headaches; hemorrhoids; hypertension; insomnia; male health; menopause; menstrual cramps; obesity and weight management; osteoporosis; parasitic infections; pinworms; pneumonia; postpartum care; pregnancy; pregnancy and childbirth; premenstrual syndrome; prostatitis; respiratory conditions; sexually transmitted diseases; strep throat; uterine fibroids; and vaginal infection

Robert Charm, MD, a gastroenterologist, recommends colon hydrotherapy for the following reasons:

In the course of many years of performing hundreds of colonoscopies, one is impressed by the incomplete cleansing, especially in people over 50 who have diverticula.

Approximately 25% to 35% of all colonoscopies demonstrating diverticula will demonstrate retained fecaliths in the diverticula.

The age of these fecaliths and the bacterial and heavy metal content could be a significant factor in tendencies to cancer, migraine headaches, arthralgias, fatigue, dermatitis, and other chronic "essential diseases."

Ron Kennedy, MD, recommends colon hydrotherapy for prevention of colon problems. In a 1992 letter to the California Health and Human Services Committee, he states, " I have studied the practice of colon hydrotherapy over the last two years and I have come to the conclusion that it is a valuable procedure which, in trained hands, is as safe as any procedure performed on the human body can be. It is also, in my opinion, extremely useful as a method of preventing serious colon disease."

John Borduk, MD, states, " I have found colonic hydrotherapy to be very useful in some of my patients." He reports that on a 31-year-old patient with terrible constipation that was given the gastroenterologists' diagnosis of "colonic inertia" that "In spite of attempts with many different laxative regimens, she was unable to move her bowels any more than one or two times per month. A regular regimen of colonics (2 to 3 times per week at first) has now normalized her bowels." Dr. Borduk also reports that both ulcerative colitis and irritable bowel syndrome seem to respond very well to colon hydrotherapy.

Paul Flashner, MD, believes that "a significant percentage of patients who suffer with chronic illness have some degree of colonic dysbiosis–imbalanced and pathologic colonic flora which creates a toxic and immune stress on the body." This "colonic dysbiosis" may play a role in many disease conditions, such as fibromyalgia, chronic fatigue syndrome, rheumatoid arthritis, food and seasonal allergies, and migraine headaches, just to name a few examples.

Dr. Flashner concludes, "With a proper dietary regime, appropriate supplementation, and the use of colon hydrotherapy, normal balance in the colon can be restored and disease states will significantly improve if not completely resolve the body's natural immunity and healing abilities can once again flourish."

Research Base

Risk and Safety

There has been only one study on colon hydrotherapy that the author is aware of after 1940, and that study was designed to test the effects of colon hydrotherapy on serum electrolytes by John R. Colline, ND (Assistant Professor, National College of Naturopathic Medicine), Paul Mittman, ND (Director of Research, National College of Naturopathic Medicine), and Mara Katlaps, BA. The study results showed that no patients experienced any clinically significant complications during or after the course of treatments. The researchers also noted that "variances in both serum sodium and chloride levels were significant: chloride at the 0.5 level, and sodium at the .01 level. While statistically significant, neither the means nor the individual serum levels dropped to values which would be considered clinically significant."

Even with these findings, many physicians routinely recommend the oral intake of an electrolyte solution, such as Energize, following a colon hydrotherapy session.

Efficacy

Before this study, in 1927 R. G. Snyder, MD, and S. Fineman, MD, reported success in treating "certain cases of subacute and chronic arthritis" with colonic irrigations. They reported, "Following the addition of this form of treatment to the older well-known therapy of the disease, the clinical results have been definitely improved."[12]

An additional report in 1935 by Jacob Gutman, MD, validated this idea. Dr. Gutman concluded, "The desirability of the removal from the colon of all toxic products, whether of bacterial or metabolic origin, is indisputable; hence cleansing of the colon by the best means at our disposal should occupy a very important part in the treatment of arthritis."[13]

Although there have not been any recent peer-reviewed studies documenting the efficacy of colon hydrotherapy the large volume of empiric data documented for thousands of years for the use of enemas, clysters, and now colon hydrotherapy continues to grow. Patient after patient continue to report that simply feeling better.

Druglike Information

Safety

Colon hydrotherapy, when practiced appropriately with an I-ACT trained and certified therapist using equipment currently registered with the FDA, provides the greatest opportunity for safety and the absolute lowest chance of risk.

Presently, Florida is the only state in the nation that registers colon hydrotherapists. In response to a query to check complaints regarding colon therapy and colonic irrigation the State of Florida Department of Business and Professional Regulation reported on March 25, 1997 that in more than 5 years, "We have received no complaints during this time period involving injury or the spread of infection to a consumer following this type of procedure."[14]

Contraindications

The following is a list of known contraindications:

- Uncontrolled hypertension
- Congestive heart failure
- Aneurysm
- Severe anemia
- Gastrointestinal hemorrhage
- Gastrointestinal perforation
- Severe hemorrhoids
- Renal insufficiency
- Cirrhosis
- Carcinoma of the colon
- Fissures and fistulas

- Abdominal hernia
- Recent colon surgery (less than 3 months)
- Pregnancy (first and third trimester of pregnancies, because colonotherapy may induce labor)

Drug or Other Interactions

Colon hydrotherapy is not known to act or react with any drugs or medication.

Adverse Reactions

As with any cleansing process of the body the possibility exists that the patient may have a slight healing crisis manifesting in short-term flu-like symptoms. These symptoms usually pass within 3 to 4 hours and generally occur only after the first colon hydrotherapy session in a series. It is for this reason that the therapist generally recommends a series of 12 sessions: for example, two sessions in the first week (on subsequent days); two sessions in the second week (also on subsequent days); and then a single session per week for the remainder of the series.

Pregnancy and Lactation

Colon hydrotherapy is not recommended during the first or third trimester of pregnancy. The physician should exercise extreme caution during those trimesters. Use moderate caution by limiting the duration and water temperature of the colonotherapy session for women in the second trimester of pregnancy.

Trade Products

Modern colon hydrotherapy equipment should be manufactured through compliance with strict FDA guidelines that dictate rigorous accountability. The FDA-registered equipment features temperature and pressure regulation and controls. It provides water filtration systems and in most cases has ultraviolet filtration to eliminate any bacteria in the city water supply, and these units are designed with appropriate back-flow prevention valves. These units should be plumbed to meet all local ordinances.

To ensure patient safety, this equipment is designed for use with disposable (single-use only) speculae or rectal tubes. If the therapists use the stainless steel speculum (reusable), it is strongly recommended by I-ACT that the reusable speculum be cleaned in a disinfectant solution and rinsed thoroughly. The speculum then should be autoclaved for a minimum of 30 minutes. Finally, the autoclave unit should be inspected every 3 months by a certified inspector with the records on the inspection maintained and available for patient review upon request.

We only have listed the manufacturers that provide currently cleared FDA-registered colon hydrotherapy equipment. This equipment falls under two classifications: closed and open systems. Both types of equipment are completely odor-free. The type of equipment is solely a therapist preference.

The following manufacturers are listed alphabetically:

Clearwater Colon Hydrotherapy
PPC-101 of (HC-2000) (closed system)
Tel: (813) 726-7782

Colon Therapeutics Research
Jimmy John (open system)
Tel: (409) 963-0300

Dotolo Research
Toxygen Model BSC-UV (closed system)
Tel: (800) 237-8458

Specialty Health
Hydrosan Plus (closed system)
Tel: (602) 582-4950

Tiller
MIND BODY LIBBE (open system)
Tel: (800) 939-1110

Transcom S. L.
(Closed system)
Tel: 011 (344) 453-1033

Self-Help versus Professional

Enemas have been used by individuals for thousands of years, but when seeking a more complete cleansing using colon hydrotherapy the patient should seek the assistance of a trained and certified colon hydrotherapist.

Visiting a Professional

After selecting a certified colon hydrotherapist the patient should be given a short questionnaire and shown around the facility while being afforded the opportunity to have any and all questions answered. The therapist should make you feel comfortable, and the facility should be clean and neat. When you are ready for the session, you will be ushered into the session room and instructed in the proper method of draping and how to insert the rectal tube or speculum. You will be left as you prepare yourself for the session. When you are ready the therapist will reenter the room. You will be completely draped (with a sheet or gown), and your dignity will be maintained at all times. When you are ready the therapist will start the gentle flow of water, and when you need to release simply let the therapist know. You may then release the softened fecal material, which flows, odor-free, through a viewing tube into the sewer.

The therapist might work on energy points of your body during the session, talk to you about how to properly breathe, show you how to manipulate your abdominal muscles to achieve greater releases, work reflex points on your feet, or simply be there to assist you during the session.

After 30 to 40 minutes the session will end, and you will be instructed in how to remove yourself from the colon hydrotherapy equipment and where the restroom is located. Especially during the first few sessions, make sure you know where the restroom is because there usually will be a small amount of water left in the colon that may make a quick trip to the restroom advisable. After your session, you might consider taking an electrolyte-replacing drink. Your physician may recommend that you take acidophilus or bifidus to rejuvenate the friendly bacteria in your intestinal tract.

Credentialing and Training

The International Association for Colon Hydrotherapy (I-ACT), a member of the National Organization of Certifying Agencies, is the only agency currently providing national and international certification of colon hydrotherapists. It has three levels of certification: foundation, intermediate, and advanced (instructor) levels. This training is provided by I-ACT certified instructors or I-ACT certified schools. Contact I-ACT at (210) 366-2888 or check their internet referral service at www.i-act.org for recommendations of certified therapists in your area.

Presently, only one state in the U.S., Florida, requires registration. Numerous other states have been provided with draft legislation.

At a minimum the individual seeking a colon hydrotherapyy session should: 1) seek a certified colon hydrotherapist (trained and certified by I-ACT); 2) seek a colon hydrotherapist that uses equipment currently registered with the FDA; and 3) seek a colon hydrotherapist that uses disposable speculae or rectal nozzles, or ensure that the stainless steel (reusable) speculum is properly cleaned and sterilized.

Associations

The International Association for Colon Hydrotherapy (I-ACT)
PO Box 461285
San Antonio, TX 78246
Tel: (210) 366-2888
Fax: (210) 366-2999
E-mail: iact@healthy.net
www.i-act.org

Suggested Reading

1. Duggan S: *Edgar Cayce's guide to colon care*, Virginia Beach, Va, 1995, Inner Vision.
   Provides information and insight into colon hydrotherapy, the practice, procedures, and reason for the process as found in the readings of Edgar Cayce. Includes actual case histories from Edgar Cayce's files.

2. Haas EM: *Staying healthy with the seasons*, Berkeley, Calif, 1981, Celestial Arts.
   Describes the relationship between man and nature, as well as the Chinese system of medicine. Provides information on diet and exercise and how the needs vary with the time of year and seasons.

3. Jensen B: *Tissue cleansing through bowel management*, Escondido, Calif, 1998, self-published.
   A 7-day cleansing program is described along with relevant information about the process of cleansing the body from the inside out. Case histories also are included.

4. Walker N: *Colon health: the key to a vibrant life*, 1979, Norwalk Press.
   A review of the anatomy of the processes of the digestive system. A discussion about constipation and its effects on many other organs of the body with rationale why the colon (the body's sewer system) should be kept clean.

5. Weinberger S: *Healing within: the complete colon health guide*, Healing Within Products.
   A description of the anatomy of the colon and the reasons the colon may need attention. Information on colon hydrotherapy and various cleansing programs are provided.

6. Tiller WT: *Are you a toxic waste site?* San Antonio, MIND BODY Institute.
   A compilation of commonly asked questions and answers about the digestive system, diet, and the history, process, and procedure of colon hydrotherapy.

7. Medsker D, Medsker B: *A layperson's guide to colon hydrotherapy*, Quinby, SC, Medsker Publishing.
   A short booklet that tells the prospective patient anything they may want to know about colon hydrotherapy. Provides understanding about the procedure and good health care practices.

Refererences

1. Bettman OL: *A pictorial history of medicine*, Springfield, Ill, 1956, Charles C. Thomas.
2. Thompson CJS: *The mystery and art of the apothecary*, London, 1929.
3. Garrison FH: *Introduction to the history of medicine*, Philadelphia, 1924.
4. Hellmuth N: FLAAR Photo Archive at BCC, "Castillo Bowl." (Late classic shows a remarkable scene of crazed dancers; one grasps an enema clyster.)
5. Hippocrates (Adams F, translator): *On regimen in acute diseases*, appendix 19, extracted from The Internet Classics Archive.
6. Daremberg C, translator: *Oeuvers anatomique, physiologiques et medicales de Galen*, vol 2, chapter XI, Paris, 1854-56.
7. de Graaf R: *De vovorum organis generationi inservientibus, de clysteribus, et de usu siphonis in anatomia*, Leyden and Rotterdam, 1668.
8. Lieberman W: The enema, *Rev Gastroenterol*, 13(May-June).
9. Friedenwald J, Morrison S: History of the enema with some notes on related procedures, *Bull History Med* 3:254, 1940.

10. Kellogg JH: Should the colon be sacrificed or may it be reformed? *JAMA* 68(26):1957-1959, 1917.

11. Wiltsie JW: *Chronic intestinal toxemia and its treatment,* Baltimore, 1938, William & Wilkins.

12. Snyder RG, Fineman S: A clinical and roentgenologic study of high colonic irrigations as used in the therapy of subacute and chronic arthritis, *Am J Roentgenol* 27(1):27-43, 1927.

13. Gutman J: The arthritides and colon therapy, *Arch Phys Ther, X-Ray, Radium,* Mar 162-178, 1935.

14. Letter from the State of Florida Department of Business and Professional Regulation, Suzanne Lee, Senior Management Analyst II, March 25, 1997.

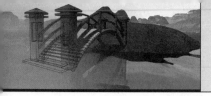

Color Therapy

THERESE M. DONNELLY

Origins and History

That color affects us all is an undoubted fact. Its significance has been investigated and the results used in merchandising, selling, home decorating, the workplace environment, industry, plant growth, nutrition, physics, physiology, psychology, ecclesiasticism, and art. In fact, color is so much a part of our lives that we tend to take it for granted.

Humanity's efforts to heal with light are as old as recorded history, but the foundations of modern color theory rest with scientists of the seventeenth century. Sir Isaac Newton (1642-1727), with his famous prism experiments, was the first to show that light is a mixture of all the colors of the visible spectrum. He reinforced this finding by proving that when the seven-color band was passed through a reversed prism, the colors recombined to form white light.

The celebrated German writer Johann Wolfgang von Goethe studied the phenomena of color for 20 years before publishing *Zur Farbenlehre (Theory of Colors)* in 1810. Goethe identified the three primary colors, red, blue, and yellow, and it was he who first described the psychologic effects of color.

A major influence of the nineteenth century was Edwin Babbitt. Born in New York in 1828, Babbitt produced his masterpiece "Principles of Light and Color" in 1878. Babbitt was a color enthusiast who explored color's effects in healing (chromotherapeutics), chromoculture of vegetable life, and color science.

Investigations continued into the twentieth century with Neils Finsen of Denmark being awarded the Nobel Prize for his discovery that sunlight healed *lupus vulgaris*. Ghadiali Dinshah (1873-1966), a naturalized American from India, worked for many years researching the effects of color, developing colored filters and lamps, and applying his scientific knowledge to the application of color in physical disease. His work probably is the most extensive and detailed of any this century. Regrettably, Dinshah was discredited as a result of an attack by the established medical order of the day. It is difficult to discern whether this attack was directed at him personally (perhaps deservedly in view of his claim to several fanciful titles) or whether it was solely aimed at his work. His science was in fact soundly based on the discoveries of Goethe and Newton, and Dinshah did receive some support from members of the medical profession, in particular, Dr. Kate Baldwin, a senior surgeon at the Women's Hospital in Philadelphia. In spite of this support, in 1947 the U.S. government saw fit to destroy most of Dinshah's equipment and written records. Although discredited for many years, the U.S. government's Office of Alternative Medicine (as of 1994) lists the Dinshah Health Society as an information source.

Contemporary with Dinshah was Dr. Harry Riley Spitler, who developed the clinical science termed *syntonics* in the 1920s. Spitler believed that bodily disorders were the result of imbalances in the nervous and endocrine systems and that by applying light through the eyes, balance could be restored. His work, updated and reorganized in the 1960s by Dr. Charles Butts, continues today.

It was not until the discovery of penicillin in 1938 and the subsequent development of antibiotics that light and color were largely eclipsed as methods of treatment. Phototherapy has, however, enjoyed a resurgence with the identification of Seasonal Affective Disorder (SAD) and the resultant wealth of research into the use of bright light to alleviate depression.

Mechanism of Action According to Its Own Theory

Color therapy can be described as the use of wavelengths of the energy of light to assist the body in self-healing. Therapy today falls broadly into three categories: psychologic, Eastern influenced, and physical.

Psychologic

Color is used to identify states of mind and negative stress. When a patient prefers or detests a certain shade or tone, it has to do with both the properties inherent in that color plus the patient's energy status at that moment. When a patient is drawn towards a color, its energy is needed for psychologic balance and healing.

Eastern Influenced

These days color therapy embraces Eastern influences plus intuitive and mystical thinking. Mystics view light as the one creative and unifying force of the universe and much current thinking among complementary therapists is that human beings are bodies of light, and their disorders therefore are amenable to treatment with light. Credence also is given to the use of intuition in discerning a patient's difficulties and selecting treatment.

The origin of much of today's therapy lies in Hindu, Tibetan, and Chinese teachings. Hinduism, for example, teaches that there are seven main *chakras* (Sanskrit for *wheel*), or energy centers, and each is associated with underlying organs and processes. In a state of health the energy of the chakras can be seen to spin with clear, translucent colors by those individuals said to be sensitive enough to see them. Treatment consists of directing the appropriate colors to the chakras to correct deficiencies in the underlying organs.

Physical

Physical healing is encouraged by directing colored light toward diseased areas of the body or the eyes. In conventional medical treatment, phototherapy and photochemotherapy are used in current dermatologic practice. For example, ultraviolet light has been used in the treatment of psoriasis and blue light has been shown to be effective in the treatment of hyperbilirubinemia in newborns.

Biologic Mechanism of Action

Color is a property of light. Light from the sun consists of many different electromagnetic waves of energy. The earth's atmosphere protects the earth's surface from receiving all but a small portion of these wavelengths, and only a very small portion of these can be seen by the human eye. Blue, yellow, and red are recognized as the primary colors. The secondary colors are formed by mixing equal parts of two primaries. When a secondary color is mixed with one of the primary colors next to it, a third or tertiary color is produced. Tertiary colors, when mixed with black and white, become the quaternary colors. Further combining produces thousands of hues. When an object appears to be a certain color, it is because it reflects one color and absorbs all others.

We record color as a sensation. Light falls upon the light receptor cells of the retina, which convert the light into electric pulses. The hypothalamus is stimulated by these pulses and transmits regulating instructions to both the pineal and pituitary glands. The pituitary gland responds to the impression of light by stimulating other endocrine glands into action as it deems appropriate. Research has shown that red stimulates the adrenal glands with the effects of raising blood pressure and pulse rate. Red therefore is considered to have an "exciting" effect on the nervous system, especially on the sympathetic branch of the autonomic nervous system.

Demographics

Color therapy in its different forms is found worldwide but especially in Europe, North America, Australia, and New Zealand.

Forms of Therapy

Although color therapy falls broadly into three categories, they do overlap. The following are some of the methods currently employed:

Psychologic

LUSCHER COLOR TEST

A Swiss professor of psychology, Dr. Max Luscher, developed a color test as a diagnostic aid. It was introduced to psychologists and physicians at the International Congress of Psychology, Lausanne, Switzerland in 1947 and has since become a widely accepted method of diagnosis. The principle of Luscher's system is that accurate psychological information can be gained from a person by observing the colors they choose or reject. For example, should a person choose darker colors, this suggests a need for peace and rest with release from psychological and physiological stress. The full test consists of 73 colors requiring 43 selections to be made, providing a wealth of information.

COLOR IMAGERY

If a patient is attracted to the uses of color healing a clinical hypnotherapist can use color imagery with a hypnotized patient. A patient can also use color in visualization and self-hypnosis.

MINDCOLOR

This Australian practice is designed to help people communicate with their subconscious minds to uncover hidden difficulties and strengths. Patients are asked to formulate a question and hold the question in their mind while selecting a single color or two-color combination from among 84 selections provided. Interpretations, including suggestions for future action, are supplied for each of the colors chosen.

Eastern Influenced

AURA-SOMA THERAPY

Of the Eastern-influenced therapies, Aura-soma is the most structured. It has been in existence for just over 10 years and is described as a "soul" therapy. Ninety-four dual-colored bottles of essential oils and herb extracts are the basis of the system. The patient is asked to choose four bottles and from this choice Aura-soma is said to shed light on the "true inner self." A trained practitioner guides the patient through the significance of the choices both in terms of the order of the selection and the color combination within each bottle.

COLORPUNCTURE

For more than 3000 years Chinese physicians have treated their patients with acupuncture. Fine needles are inserted into the skin at points along invisible energy paths or *meridians* with the intention of restoring an unimpeded flow of energy to internal organs and processes. Following experiments with Kirlian photography, which records the electromagnetic fields of living things, Peter Mandel developed a system of treating patients by focusing small *colorzone* lamps on acupuncture points and other areas of the body.

Physical

Although it is the ultraviolet portion of sunlight that has so far proven to be the most biologically active in the treatment of such conditions as tuberculosis, rickets, and the production of vitamin D in the skin, complementary therapy practitioners claim to have produced notable effects using color directed at diseased organs. The following methods can be employed.

BABBITT'S METHOD

Babbitt invented a chromodisc, a cone-shaped device made of tin with a diameter of about 5 inches at the small end, where a frame was installed to hold a colored glass lens. The chromodisc was hand-held for a few minutes as close to the skin as possible, allowing sunlight or artificial light to stream through the large end of the cone and pass through the colored lens onto the skin. In addition to describing treatment for specific disorders, such as blue light for burns, Babbitt ventured the following general recommendations:

> 1. For nervous excitability, hot or inflammatory conditions, fevers, acute pains, etc., *the BLUE is the proper glass to use, as this admits the violet, indigo and blue, and a portion of the fine trans-violet.*
> 2. For arousing the arterial blood, warming cold extremities, etc., *the RED glass is excellent, but should also have more or less of the YELLOW glass, which really transmits a greater variety of warm rays than the red, as we have seen.*
> 3. For arousing nervous action, warming up and thawing out, so to speak, hard negative inflammations, and vitalizing a cold, chronic condition, *the YELLOW glass is best.*

THE SPECTRO-CHROME SYSTEM

Ghadiali Dinshah was influenced by reading Babbitt's work. Dinshah introduced his system of healing with colored filters, Spectro-Chrome, in 1920. Spectro-Chrome is said to function not by penetrating the skin but by affecting the electromagnetic field surrounding the body which in turn, transmits the altered energy to the cells. The body is divided into 22 areas and colors or color combinations are recommended for each area. In the early 1900s Dinshah experimented on chemical elements with the newly invented spectroscope. He eventually felt able to assign a color to each element, such as calcium = orange. Thus the color orange was employed in the treatment of bone disorders. His therapy always has been considered complementary to conventional treatment.

SYNTONICS

The syntonic approach (optometric phototherapy) uses the prescription of frequencies of light to balance the autonomic nervous system through the eyes. This approach mainly is used by optometrists to heal visual dysfunctions, such as strabismus and convergence.

Indications and Reasons for Referral

Patients can be drawn to psychologic color treatment when they are emotionally distressed but cannot identify the reasons for it. They seek guidance and self-understanding. Treatment with color for physical disorders may be sought when patients have become disillusioned with other therapy and are attracted to the healing potential of color. It also can be applied where there is a good possibility that it will enhance the effect of current drug regimen, such as employing dark blue alongside drugs for hypertension. It also could be used experimentally when all other treatment has been shown to have a minimal curative effect. Its appeal rests in its intrinsic attractiveness, simplicity, cost-effectiveness, and absence of side effects.

Office Applications

Color therapy can be recommended as complementary to conventional treatment as follows:

Top level: *A therapy ideally suited for these conditions*
Seasonal Affective Disorder

Second level: *One of the better therapies for these conditions*
Depression

Third level: *A valuable adjunctive therapy for these conditions*
Stress

Practical Applications

Because of its gentle, stress-free action, it is worth using color with virtually any physical disorder, particularly if the patient is drawn to this form of treatment. It is unlikely to do any harm (except as mentioned in "Risk and Safety") and may prove highly beneficial. The treatment regimens documented by both Babbitt and Dinshah can provide guidance as to which colors to select until definitive research results are available.

The color can be applied above the skin or directly to the eyes. Commercially available or homemade light sources can be used. Alternatively, a collection of color cards can be used. Patients select a color and focuses on it for as long as they feel is necessary. Depending on the severity of the energy imbalance, it may take as long as 30 minutes before a sense of irritation begins to be felt as the saturation point for a color's vibration is reached.

Research Base

Evidence Based

There is a wealth of evidence to support the psychologic effects of color and Dr. Max Luscher's "Luscher Color Test" contains ample evidence of this.[1]

In conventional medical practice the use of blue light in the treatment of hyperbilirubinemia has been proven by many researchers, including Vreman et al with their study "Light-Emitting Diodes: A Novel Light Source for Phototherapy."[2] Creamer and McGregor of St. John's Institute of Dermatology in London published a paper in January 1998 entitled "Photo (Chemo) Therapy: Advances for Systemic or Cutaneous Disease," exploring the value of light as a treatment.[3] Griffiths of the University of Manchester (UK) published a paper in July 1998 on "Novel Therapeutic Approaches to Psoriasis"[4] and in October 1998 *The Archives of General Psychiatry* ran four articles on light therapy.[5-8]

Where treatment of a broader spectrum of disorders is concerned the evidence is largely anecdotal and this area needs the attention of researchers.

Risk and Safety

From the point of view of the complementary therapist, research is needed to define exactly what the dangers of exposure to some colors might be when used with physical disorders. Clearly, it would be wise to avoid prolonged exposure of patients with hypertension to large amounts of red. Similarly, dark blue or black would be best avoided for patients suffering from depression.

Efficacy

It has yet to be established what percentage of the population would benefit from this type of therapy. However, because light has a neurobiologic effect on all people, well-structured research could reveal widespread benefits.

Other

Research in the agricultural field lends support to the potential for color as a therapy in humans, as the following examples show:

1. In 1997 researchers at the School of Agriculture and Forest Science at the University of Wales (UK) used red and blue light to establish whether these would increase activity and reduce locomotion disorders in meat chickens. They showed that in 108 chicks walking, standing, aggression, and wing stretching all increased in intensity when reared from day 1 to 35 in red light. Where blue light was used, there was a high incidence of gait abnormalities.[9]

2. Michael Kasperbauer, a researcher at the U.S. Agricultural Research Service Center in Florence, South Carolina, showed that using red plastic sheeting under tomato and cotton plants produced a 15% to 20% higher yield than plants grown over traditional black or clear plastic. Also, turnips grown under blue plastic had an improved flavour when compared with those grown under green sheets. Analysis of those grown under the blue plastic revealed that they had higher concentrations of glucocinolates and vitamin C (glucosinolates being the compounds which give turnips and horseradish their traditional "bite"). Kasperbauer and his team also have investigated the link between color and pest control. Michael Orzolek of Pennsylvania State University proved that aphids and the plant viruses they transmit are generally attracted to yellow and repelled by red and blue. This finding echoes the work of Babbitt a century earlier when he wrote, "The electrical colors which are transmitted by blue glass often destroy the insects which feed upon plants."

Future Research Opportunities and Priorities

Research could focus on the clinical efficacy of color therapy and the neurobiologic mechanism of action. Extensive anecdotal evidence of the value of color therapy in the treatment of countless physical disorders over many decades deserves to be revisited. However, this evidence needs to be subjected to rigorous scientific research to establish (or otherwise) a sound basis for color therapy. Developing instruments for applying color could provide a commercial incentive for clinical trials.

A major resource for researchers is the Faber Birren Collection of Books on Color, which was presented to Yale University in 1971. Faber Birren was a leading authority on color and the collection's holdings are the most extensive to be found anywhere. A complete online bibliography can be found at the Yale University Library website.

Druglike Information

Warnings, Contraindications, and Precautions

If a patient is taking prescription drugs, warning labels should be read to ensure that no side effects are induced if the patient's skin is subjected to bright light.

Trade Products

The following two types of experimental equipment are currently available:

1. Color therapy eyewear: This is worn with the intention of affecting cellular and hormonal changes to bring the cells of the body into balance. Nonprescription colored sunglasses with acrylic lenses are supplied in seven colors. They are sold through the Mineral Connection Inc. online store at www.mineralconnection.com.
2. A "Circle of Color" projector lamp can be purchased from New Zealand at the approximate cost of $695 (NZ$) from www.altered.states.co.nz. The lamp is supplied along with five color slides and handbooks.

In addition, the nine Roscolene filters needed for Spectro-Chrome therapy can be purchased from the following retailer:

Samarco
PO Box 153008
Dallas, TX 75315
Tel: (214) 421-0757

Self-Help versus Professional

Where physical or psychologic disorders are concerned, it is preferable for a diagnosis to be made by a qualified medical practitioner, and it is essential should there be the least suggestion of a serious problem. A qualified therapist then can be sought to administer color treatment. However, most forms of color therapy lend themselves to self-application, enabling patients to assume an active role in restoring and maintaining their state of well-being.

Visiting a Professional

Visiting a color therapist should be an enjoyable and relaxing experience. The treatment room needs to be warm and the chair or couch should be comfortable. The therapist should write a case history, taking into consideration any diagnosis made by a qualified medical practitioner and any drugs the patient is taking. Unless psychologic therapy is being sought the patient probably will need to remove some clothing to expose the treatment area. While the color is being applied the patient can either relax quietly or take the opportunity to discuss anxieties and problems with the therapist. The diagnosis and method of treatment will determine the length of therapy sessions. Research should establish definitive treatment times.

Credentialing

The forms of color therapy used by complementary therapists today, such as colorpuncture, Aura-soma, and mindcolor, all have been established independently of any licensing body. The originators of each system lay down their own criteria for training, practice, and accreditation.

Training

There is no single, recognized training body or licensing authority for color therapy. The originators of each method have established their own training programs with wide variations in content, as listed here.

Colorpuncture training information, equipment, and international addresses are available from the following organizations:

Energetic Verlag GmbH
Hildestrasse 8, D-76646
Bruchsal, Germany
Tel: 49-7251-800135
Fax: 49-7251-800155

Mindcolor training details and information can be obtained by writing to the following organization:

What's Motivational Training
PO Box 283
Mt. Beauty, Victoria 3699, Australia
Tel: 03-5754-4965

For details of Aura-soma worldwide training courses and practitioners, contact www.aura-soma.co.uk/Programs/Courses.

There is a website for Syntonics at www.syntonicphototherapy.com.

What to Look for in a Provider

Given that most therapists are either self-taught or trained by organizations with independent training programs, it probably is wisest to choose a provider with a recognized qualification in another related field who is using color as an adjunct to other treatment. A qualified counselor, registered nurse, psychologist, or medical practitioner would be ideal choices.

Barriers and Key Issues

The promising work of the early part of the twentieth century was overtaken by the arrival of penicillin and other antibiotics. Color therapy with its (then) slow treatment times compared unfavorably with the speed and simplicity of antibiotics. Coupled with a lack of recognized research protocols, color therapy lost favor. As a cost-effective, simple, stress-free treatment it deserves to be revisited. It is a form of therapy that readily lends itself to being proven effective or otherwise. Lamps and color filters are available for trials. Clinical trials would establish the most suitable colors for a particular disorder, the optimum treatment times, and whether color should be applied directly to the skin or eyes. Unsubstantiated claims for color's effectiveness deter its acceptance by the medical profession. Only through rigorous testing is color therapy likely to be recognized in mainstream medicine.

Associations

The establishment of the new National Center for Complementary and Alternative Medicine in the U.S., supported by $50 million funding appropriated by Congress, holds out the possibility of competent research studies into the value of color as a treatment modality. Their address is as follows:

NCCAM Clearinghouse
PO Box 8218
Silver Spring, MD 20907-8218
Tel: (888) 644-6226
Toll-Free: (888) 644-6226
Fax: (301) 495-4957
E-mail: nccam-info@altmed.od.nih.gov
www.altmed.od.nih.gov/nccam

In the UK a point of contact for complementary therapists is as follows:

The British Holistic Medical Association
179 Gloucester Place
London NW1 6DX
Tel: 0171 262 5299
E-mail: bhma-sec@bhma.org.uk
www.users.dircon.co.uk/~bhma-sec

The Dinshah Health Society supplies educational material in the form of books, videos and case histories about Spectro-Chrome.

The Dinshah Health Society
PO Box 707
Malaga, NJ 08328
Tel: (609) 692-4686
www.wj.net/dinshah

Suggested Reading

1. von Goethe JW: *Theory of colors*, Cambridge, Mass, 1987, The M.I.T. Press.
   Here are more than 400 pages of detailed observations of color phenomena. Because it is broken down into nearly 1000 numbered paragraphs, it is a good book for dipping into. Many of Goethe's statements can be readily verified with brief experiments.
2. Babbitt ED: *The principles of light and color,* Secaucus, NJ, 1967, The Citadel Press.
   There were 560 pages in Babbitt's original text and this has been reduced to good effect by the editing of Faber Birren. It is a classic study of the science of color and its application as a healing power.
3. Dinshah D: *Let there be light,* Malaga, NJ, 1997, Dinshah Health Society.
   This is a practical manual compiled by Darius Dinshah from his father's work.. There is much in this book that medical practitioners will find unappealing; nevertheless, it contains detailed information on which colors to apply to 400 diagnosed disorders and would make a useful starting point for a researcher.

Bibliography

Allanach J: *Colour me healing*, Rockport, Mass, 1997, Element Books.

Avery DH: A turning point for seasonal affective disorder and light therapy research? *Arch Gen Psychiatry* 55:863-864, 1998.

Boyce N: Rainbow growing, *New Scientist*, 24 October 1998.

Evans YD: *Mindcolour*, Mt. Beauty, Australia, 1997, What's Motivational Training.

Gregory RL: *Eye and brain—the psychology of seeing*, 1990, Weidenfeld and Nicholson.

Hunter ME: *Healing imagery*. In Hammond CC, editor: *Handbook of hypnotic suggestion and metaphors*, New York, 1990, W.W. Norton, for the American Society of Clinical Hypnosis.

Reyner JH: *The universe of relationships*, 1960, Vincent Stuart.

Walker M: *The power of color*, Wayne, NJ, 1991. Avery.

Wirz-Justice A: Beginning to see the light, *Arch Gen Psychiatry* 55:861-862, 1998.

References

1. Luscher M: *The Luscher color test,* 1970, Jonathan Cape.

2. Vreman HJ et al: Light-emitting diodes: a novel light source for phototherapy, *Pediatr Res* 44(5):804-809, 1998.

3. Creamer D, McGregor J: Photo (chemo)therapy: advances for systemic or cutaneous disease, *Hosp Med* 59(1):23-27, 1998.

4. Griffiths CE: Novel therapeutic approaches to psoriasis, *Hosp Med* 59(7):539-542, 1998.

5. Lewy AJ et al: Morning vs. evening light treatment of patients with winter depression, *Arch Gen Psychiatry* 55(10):890-896, 1998.

6. Eastman CI et al: Bright light treatment of winter depression: a placebo-controlled trial, *Arch Gen Psychiatry* 55(10):875-882, 1998.

7. Terman M, Terman TS, Ross DC: A controlled trial of timed bright light and negative air ionization for treatment of winter depression, *Arch Gen Psychiatry* 55(10):875-882, 1998.

8. Avery DH: A turning point for seasonal affective disorder and light therapy research? *Arch Gen Psychiatry* 55(10):863-864, 1998.

9. Prayinto DS, Phillips CJ, Stokes DK: The effects of color and intensity of light on behavior and leg disorders in broiler chickens, *Poul Sci* 76(12):1675-1681, 1997.

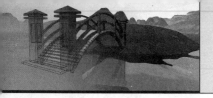

Detoxification Therapy

ELSON M. HAAS

DONALD W. NOVEY

Origins and History

Detoxification is a term well known to health professionals. In a mainstream medical context, "detox" often refers to a monitored and medicated withdrawal from substance dependence, including alcohol, narcotics, opioids, sedatives or hypnotics, and others. It implies cleansing from a harmful substance, safe passage through a withdrawal reaction, and a fresh start if a healthier lifestyle is maintained.

In a natural medicine setting, detoxification has a similar meaning, but the offending substances are generally byproducts of packaged, processed and "fast" foods, including refined sugars and flours, fried foods, sweets, caffeinated beverages, dairy products, meats, preservatives, and other food additives. In a broader context, it also includes cleansing from the subtle accumulation of chemicals inherent to an industrialized society, including pesticides, hydrocarbons, and heavy metals. These are often absorbed by inhalation, skin contact, or as contaminants in the foods we eat. The word *toxin*, in a natural medicine context, refers less to actual poisons and more to the presence of accumulated waste products on both a cellular and organ-system level.

Detoxification relies on the body's inherent ability to cleanse itself if given the opportunity. The process of detoxification therefore involves three aspects: initiating the cleansing process with a program that avoids toxin intake; facilitating elimination of waste products; and easing back into a healthier diet and lifestyle while rebuilding the body's nutrition.

Accumulating dirt is a part of life. Just as a house needs frequent cleaning, so do we. How badly we eat, or how poorly we maintain our lifestyle affects the speed with which we reaccumulate stress and metabolic strain. Consider the value of a vacation, and how fast we become "stressed out" again when we return. Similarly, in our fast-paced lives, the reaccumulation of toxins is almost inevitable. But, we can slow the process by maintaining a healthy lifestyle, and we can "clean the house" with detoxification. The degree of detoxification required depends upon the damage done. Therefore, detoxification can occur in many levels of intensity, from a 1-day event, to a carefully monitored setting weeks in length, depending on the desired effect and depth of cleansing.

Equally important to the physical process of detoxification is an educational component. The individual undergoing detoxification needs to be clearly informed on what the

---

THE NONTOXIC DIET[1]

Eat organic foods whenever possible.

Drink filtered water.

Rotate foods, especially common allergens such as milk products, eggs, wheat, and yeast foods.

Practice food combining. Minimize protein and starch combos to help optimum digestion (ch 9-10 under food combining. Seasons: use table from seasons book).

Eat a natural, seasonal cuisine.

Include fruits, vegetables, whole grains, legumes, nuts, and seeds. For omnivarians, add some lowfat or nonfat dairy products, fresh fish (not shellfish), and organic poultry.

Cook in iron, stainless steel, glass, or porcelain cookware.

Avoid or minimize the use of red meats, cured meats, organ meats, refined foods, canned foods, sugar, salt, saturated fats, coffee, alcohol, and nicotine.

---

process involves, what it will feel like, and what is needed to maintain its beneficial effects.

Mechanism of Action According to Its Own Theory

Detoxification relies on three primary tenets of naturopathy:

1. The primary cause of disease is the accumulation of unnecessary wastes that are not properly eliminated, resulting in toxin retention and subsequent disease.
2. The body is designed to support optimal function. Listen to its signals.
3. Given the proper environment, the body has the power to heal itself and return to its normal healthy state.

Cleansing or detoxification is only one part of a trilogy of nutritional action; the others being building, or toning, and balancing, or maintenance. A regular, balanced diet devoid of excess necessitates less intensive detoxification. Our body has a daily elimination cycle, mostly carried out at night and in the early morning up until breakfast. When we eat a congesting diet higher in fats, meats, dairy products, refined foods, and chemicals, detoxification becomes more important, particularly to those who eat excessively, and to those who eat excessively at night.

Our individual lifestyle provides clues for deciding how and when to detoxify. If we have any symptoms or diseases of toxicity and congestion, we will likely benefit from detoxification practices. It is like a vacation for our body and digestive tract. Common toxicity symptoms include headache, fatigue, congestion, backaches, aching or swollen joints, digestive problems, allergy symptoms, and sensitivity to environmental agents such as chemicals, perfumes, and synthetics.

SEASONAL VEGETABLE SUGGESTIONS[1]

Try steaming basic combinations that include some root vegetables, tubers, stems, leafy greens, and vegetables from vines such as zucchini, green beans, and peppers.

Spring:
Asparagus; baby carrots; spring garlic; red chard; beets; leeks; broccoli; wild greens such as mustard, sorrel, or collard, with a steamed artichoke.

Summer:
Zucchini; new potatoes; green beans; carrots; onion; beets and beet greens; yellow squash; bell pepper; and eggplant.

Autumn:
Broccoli; cabbage; potato; celery; spinach; cauliflower; onion; carrots; chard; and sugar peas.

Winter:
Broccoli; cabbage; potato; kale; spinach; chard; butternut squash; onion; cauliflower; collard greens; and Jerusalem artichoke

To season, add a bit of sea salt, vegetable salt, or a good garlic salt without additives, or cayenne for warmth. Better Butter (see "The Detox Diet Daily Menu Plan") is a must for the Alkaline-Detoxification Menu Plan, as it prevents deficiencies of essential fatty acids. The mixture of butter and cold-pressed canola oil provides all the fatty acids to nourish and support the tissues.

The naturopathic approach applies commonsense programs for health that first looks at lifestyle as a method to promote healing, then to natural therapies, and finally to pharmaceutic drugs and surgery. Pharmaceutic drugs or surgery are appropriate when a situation is acute or severe, or if natural therapies are not working.

Detoxification centers on gastrointestinal function, but it is supported by attention to facilitating all of the body's routes of excretion. This is explained in more detail in "Forms of Therapy."

Biologic Mechanism of Action

The presence of toxins as a cause of disease in the naturopathic sense is only a less obvious form than that recognized by mainstream medicine. Accumulation of wastes leads to many pathologic states. Chronic renal failure, for example, is rapidly lethal unless uremic waste products can be eliminated by renal or peritoneal dialysis. Advanced cirrhosis leads to hepatic coma and death as metabolic byproducts accumulate. Macular degeneration is thought to involve the accumulation of lipofuscins, waste products of rapid retinal cell membrane turnover.

Elsewhere in this text, marginal nutritional deficiencies are discussed. These are less extreme than classic deficiency syndromes and do not display the end-stage symptoms and signs known to most health care professions, yet they cause a myriad of disease manifestations. Logically speaking, marginal nutritional deficiencies are likely to be more common than outright deficiency states. Similarly, the marginal accumulation of waste products is likely to be more common as a contributing factor to dysphoria and dysfunction than overt organ system failure.

On a biochemical level, detoxification is a continuous metabolic process operating on a number of enzymatic pathways. Optimal function of these enzyme systems is dependent upon adequate intake of nutrients. Nutritional depletion therefore leads to inadequate metabolic function, and further buildup of waste chemicals, often referred to naturopathically as *toxicity and stagnation*. The body's natural detoxification process is overloaded when input of waste is increased, as in dietary indiscretion, or by exposure to environmental chemicals, which must also be detoxified. The processes may also be slowed by rerouting of the body's physiologic priorities to accommodate stress reactions.

Forms of Therapy

Detoxification programs are often used to assist a transition from an unhealthy lifestyle to a healthier one. Such programs are quite useful to catalyze change and inspire individuals to effectively alter their lifestyle for the better.

As a treatment approach, detoxification often applies to the elimination of some modern-day abuses: Sugar, Nicotine, Alcohol, Caffeine, and Chemicals, often referred to as "SNACCs." For alcohol and chemicals (substance abuse), naturopathic practices often serve as adjunctive therapy to mainstream detoxification protocols.

Detoxification can also be performed as a maintenance procedure to better prepare for changes of seasons, for improved stamina, and for resistance to illness.

Regardless of the reason, detoxification follows a rather standard set of steps. These consist of the following:

1. Initiating the cleansing process. This begins with either:
   a. Elimination of the offending substance(s). This may require supportive medical therapy to modify the withdrawal response, particularly for alcohol and drug dependence.
   b. Application of a formal cleansing technique. This is a signal to the body to begin its own elimination cycle in a more intensive fashion than in daily life. These triggers classically range in levels of intensity, listed from slowest to fastest acting.
      1. Reduce daily ingestion of offending foods, such as sugar, fried foods, meats and dairy products, and increase intake of more nourishing ones.
      2. Limit diet to (again, in order of increasing extremes):
         • Fruits, vegetables, whole grains, nuts, seeds and legumes (see boxes)
         • Raw foods
         • Fruits and vegetables alone
      3. Fasting techiques (again, in order of increasing extremes):
         • Fruit and vegetable juices
         • Specific juice diets
         • Water alone

THE DETOX DIET DAILY MENU PLAN[1]

Upon rising:
Two glasses of water (filtered or spring), one glass with half a lemon squeezed into it.

Breakfast:
One piece of fresh fruit (at room temperature), such as an apple, pear, banana, a citrus fruit, or some grapes. Chew well, mixing each bite with saliva.

Fifteen to 30 minutes later: one bowl of cooked whole grains, specifically millet, brown rice, amaranth, quinoa, or buckwheat.

For flavoring, use 2 tablespoons of fruit juice for sweetness, or use the Better Butter mentioned below with a little salt or tamari for a savory taste.

Lunch (Noon-1 PM):
One to two medium bowls of steamed vegetables; use a variety, including roots, stems, and greens. For example, potatoes or yams, green beans, broccoli or cauliflower, carrots or beets, asparagus, kale, chard, and cabbage. Be sure to chew well!

Dinner (5-6 PM):
Same as lunch.

Make Better Butter by mixing a quarter-cup of cold-pressed canola oil into a soft (room temperature) quarter-pound of butter; then place in dish and refrigerate. Use about 1 teaspoon per meal or a maximum of 3 teaspoons daily.

Special drinks (11 AM and 3 PM):
One to 2 cups veggie water, saved from the steamed vegetables. Add a little sea salt or kelp and drink slowly, mixing each mouthful with saliva.

Before retiring:
Consume no additional foods after dinner. Drink only water and herbal teas, such as peppermint, chamomile, pau d'arco, or blends.

---

    c. The key to proper detoxification is to individualize the program. The individual's general health, physiologic balance, energy level, and current lifestyle are important factors. If unsure where to begin, start with the basic diet and gradually intensify toward juice fasting. Take a few days for each step and, if the individual feels fine, move to the next level of cleansing, as described above.

2. Facilitating elimination through normal routes of excretion:

    a. Gastrointestinal: As the majority of waste is eliminated gastrointestinally, this process is accelerated during detoxification. Supplements to facilitate colon cleansing are useful to help elimination keep pace with excretion into the gut. Such supplements consist of psyllium seed husk (with extra water intake), herbal or pharmaceutic laxatives, and betonite clay in small amounts. Enemas are also used, particularly during juice or water fasting. The lower the caloric intake of the fast, the more frequent enemas will be needed, up to once daily. Failure to address increased gastrointestinal excretion often results in increased discomfort during the period of detoxification and sometimes even a flare of existing illness symptoms, such as headaches, irritability, and fatigue.

b. Renal: Increased fluid intake facilitates the excretion of water-soluble wastes. Mainstream medicine considers this inherently when a person with a common cold is told to "drink plenty of fluids." The physician knows that a viral infection creates waste products that result in the myalgias and malaise of a viral syndrome. Very comfortably, we think of these as toxins being washed out by the increased fluids. The process of detoxification will often increase the sense of thirst, signaling the body's need for increased fluids. Needless to say, increased fluids are contraindicted in individuals with organ system failure such as renal insufficiency or congestive heart failure.

c. Dermal: The skin is an important, yet often unrecognized organ of elimination. The skin is constantly shedding its squames, something most of us have experienced if rubbing our skin after a shower. Dry brushing the skin with an appropriate skin brush prior to shower or bathing can facilitate this desquamation. Some will also use a washcloth or loofah sponge during the bath or shower as well.

d. Respiratory: Breathing clean air, as simple as it sounds, is another part of detoxification. This is particularly facilitated by a relaxing walk near a body of water such as a lake, river or, if nearby, the ocean. If no water area is nearby, a walk in any nonurban area will do.

e. Lymphatics: As the lymphatics drain tissue spaces, they are an important route for elimination. Lymphatic drainage is facilitated by gentle exercise or stretching, and by massage therapy. A massage is a very pleasant addition to the detoxification process.

f. Mental and Emotional: Although not technically an organ of elimination, mental and emotional recovery is also important. During the detoxification process, the individual will often need more time for relaxation, reflection, and sleep. Some will add yoga or tai chi to their detoxification regimen. For more formal alcohol or drug detox programs, counseling and group therapy are time-tested components needed for successful abstinence.

3. Supplementation

a. Certain supplements are appropriate for detoxification programs. In specific programs for elimination of nicotine, caffeine and alcohol, certain nutrients can ease withdrawal symptoms. Specific programs of supplementation vary with the reason for detoxification. Some examples of supplement regimens are listed in the table "Examples of Nutrient Programs."

b. For straight juice cleansing or water fasts, supplements are not as important as selected nutrients or herbs to facilitate the detoxification process. From a natural medicine perspective, these consist of the following:

1. Supplemental potassium (low doses)
2. Extra fiber with olive oil to clear toxins from the colon
3. Sodium alginate from seaweed to bind heavy metals

Examples of Nutrient Programs[1]

	General	Sugar	Drugs	Caffeine	Nicotine
Water	2½ to 3 qt	2 to 3 qt	2 to 3½ qt	=	2 to 3 qt
Fiber	20 to 40 g	=	=	15 to 20 g	15 to 45 g
Vitamin A	5000 to 7500 IU		5000 to 10,000 IU	=	10,000 to 15,000 IU
Beta-carotene	15,000 to 30,000 IU		20,000 to 40,000 IU	15,000 to 25,000	20,000 to 40,000 IU
Vitamin D	200 to 400 IU		=	400 IU	200 to 400 IU
Vitamin E	400 to 1000 IU	200 to 800 IU	=	400 to 800 IU	=
Vitamin K	200 mcg		300 mcg	=	100 to 300 mcg
Thiamine (B1)	10 to 25 mg	25 to 100 mg	=	75 to 150 mg	100 to 200 mg
Riboflavin (B2)	10 to 25 mg	25 to 100 mg	=	50 to 100 mg	=
Niacinamide (B3)	50 mg	50 to 100 mg	50 to 1000[1]	150 to 100 mg	100 to 1000 mg[1]
Pantothenic acid (B5)	250 to 500 mg	250 to 1000 mg	=	500 to 1000 mg	250 to 1000 mg
Pyridoxine (B6)	10 to 25 mg	25 to 100 mg	=	50 to 100 mg	50 to 150 mg
Pyridoxal-5-phosphate			25 to 50 mg	=	25 to 75 mg
Cobalamine (B12)	50 to 100 mcg	100 to 250 mcg	=	100 to 200 mcg	200 to 1000 mcg
Folic acid	400 to 800 mcg	=	800 mcg	400 to 800 mcg	800 to 2000 mcg
Biotin	200 mcg		300 mcg	=	200 to 500 mcg
Choline			500 to 1000 mg		500 to 1000 mg
PABA					500 to 1500 mg
Inositol			500 to 1000 mg		
Vitamin C	1 to 4 g	2 to 10 g	=	2 to 6 g	3 to 12 g
Bioflavinoids	250 to 500 mg	=	=	=	=
Calcium	600 to 850 mg	650 to 1200 mg	=	800 to 1000 mg	850 to 1250 mg
Chromium	200 mcg	200 to 500 mcg	=	200 to 400 mcg	200 to 500 mcg
Copper	2 mg		2 to 3 mg	=	2 to 4 mg
Iodine	150 mcg		=	=	150 to 250 mcg
Iron			10 to 20 mg[2]	0 to 30 mg[2]	10 to 30 mg[2]

=, same as previous column.
1, increase dose slowly;
2, men: 0 to 15 mg, women: 15 to 30 mg, monitor blood count;

4. Apple cider vinegar in water (1 tbsp. vinegar to 8 oz. hot water) to reduce mucus. Lemon juice may also be used instead.
5. Blue-green algae, spirulina, or chlorella to improve energy and stamina during fasting

4. Returning to a healthier diet and lifestyle: Detoxification is a natural way to push the "reset" button in the body to return to a state of better health. Once there, it must be maintained. The box "Important Elements of Healthy Eating" lists some of the strategies used to maintain good gastrointestinal health, which leads to general well-being.

Examples of Nutrient Programs—cont'd

	General	Sugar	Drugs	Caffeine	Nicotine
Magnesium	300 to 500 mg	400 to 800 mg	=	500 to 800 mg	5000 to 1000 mg
Manganese	5 to 10 mg	=	=	=	5 to 10 mg
Molybdenum	300 mcg		150 to 300 mcg	300 to 500 mcg	300 to 600 mg
Potassium	300 to 500 mg		100 to 500 mg	300 to 600 mg	200 to 500 mg
Selenium	300 mcg	200 to 300 mcg	=	=	200 to 400 mg
Silicon	100 mg		50 to 150 mg	50 to 100 mg	50 to 150 mg
Vanadium	300 mcg	200 to 400 mcg	=		150 to 300 mcg
Zinc	30 mg	30 to 60 mg	=	=	30 to 75 mg
Coenzyme Q10					50 to 100 mg
Optional					
L-amino acids	0.5 to 1.0 g	1.0 to 1.5 g	=	0.5 to 1.5 g	1000 to 2000 mg
L-cysteine	250 to 500 mg		=		500 to 1500 mg
DL-methionine	250 to 500 mg				
L-glycine	250 to 500 mg				
L-glutamine	0.5 to 1.0 g	=	250 to 1000 mg		
Psyllium seed	2 to 4 tsp				
Flaxseed oil	2 to 4 caps	=	=		4 to 6 caps
Acidophilus culture	2 × 10⁹				
Detox formula herbs	4 to 6 caps				
Olive oil	3 to 6 tsp				
Liquid chlorophyll	2 to 4 tsp				
Apple cider vinegar	1 to 2 tbsp				
Adrenal glandular		100 to 200 mg		50 to 150 mg	
Goldenseal root			3 to 6 caps		
Potassium bicarbonate				600 to 1000 mg³	
Herb teas				3 cups daily	
Blue-green algae				400 to 2000 mg	

3, Can use alka-seltzer effervescent antacid, one tablet 2 to 3 times daily

Demographics

Detoxification is a practice commonly applied by practitioners trained in this method. Historically, this includes naturopaths, naprapaths, herbalists, some chiropractors, bodyworkers, and holistically trained medical doctors.

Detoxification is practiced by cultures the world over, as fasting and cleansing are humanity's oldest form of therapy.

IMPORTANT ELEMENTS OF HEALTHY EATING[1]

Eat natural, wholesome foods, particularly fresh fruits, vegetables, whole grains, and vegetable proteins (legumes, nuts, and seeds).

We are what we eat—put only quality foods into your body. Reduce refined foods, sugar, excess fatty and rich foods, and foods with additives or synthetic coloring.

Drink no more than 4 oz. of liquids with meals, as it can dilute the digestive juices.

Chew your food thoroughly, eat in a relaxed environment, and never eat while upset.

Get sufficient fiber in your diet by eating the majority of your foods from item #1 above, or by taking additional psyllium husk and flaxseed meal.

Drink 6 to 8 glasses of water daily, plus herbal teas.

Use nutritional supplements and herbs as appropriate. Supplement your digestive function as needed with hydrochloric acid, digestive enzymes, and pancreatic products.

Moderate your use of alcohol, caffeine, and nicotine. Use caution with excessive use of prescription, over-the-counter, and recreational drugs.

Exercise. If you don't yet have an exercise program, set one up. Do it regularly and with the right combination of activities that will provide strength, flexibility, endurance, and enjoyment.

Maintain regular elimination. Your diet, exercise, and stress levels should allow your bowels to move at least once or twice daily. After illness or antibiotic use, replace friendly gastrointestinal flora by taking probiotics (acidophilus and other positive digestive bacteria). If this is not sufficient to restore normal digestion and elimination, and your Gi function stays irregular for more than a few weeks, seek the advice of a health care practitioner.

Indications and Reasons for Referral

Detoxification is often performed for the following reasons:

Prevent disease	Rest the organs	Slow aging
Reduce symptoms	Purification	Improve flexibility
Treat disease	Rejuvenation	Improve fertility
Support lifestyle changes	Weight loss	Enhance the senses
Cleanse the body	Clear skin	

In general, detoxification programs often make people more aware of what they are doing when they eat. Patients who follow detoxification programs often claim to feel more creative, motivated, productive, relaxed, energetic, relationship-focused, and environmentally attuned.

Office Applications

The illnesses that may respond to detoxification therapy are those which are, at least in part, exacerbated by congestion, stagnation, and toxicity. Not all of the diagnoses listed here are related solely to toxicity, nor will they be completely cured by detoxification. Still, many conditions are created or accelerated by nutritional abuses and can be alleviated by eliminating the related toxins and following simple nutritional guidelines.

Abscesses	Heart disease
Acne	Hemorrhoids
Allergies	Hepatitis
Alzheimer's disease	Hypertension
Arthritis	Infections
Asthma	Kidney stones
Atherosclerosis	Menstrual disorders
Bronchitis	Mental illness*
Cancer*	Migraine headache
Cataracts	Multiple sclerosis
Cirrhosis	Obesity
Colds	Pancreatitis
Colitis	Parkinson's disease
Constipation	Peptic ulcer
Diabetes	Pneumonia
Diverticulitis	Prostate disease
Drug addiction	Sinusitis
Eczema	Stroke*
Emphysema	Tension headache
Fatigue**	Thrombophlebitis
Fibrocystic breast disease	Uterine fibroids
Gallstones	Vaginitis
Gout	Varicose veins

Practical Applications

Our bodies have natural cleansing cycles when they want a lighter diet, more liquids, and a greater elimination than intake. This occurs daily (usually from the night until midmorning, about an hour after we wake) and it may occur weekly and more commonly for a few days per month. Women, in particular, are aware of this natural cleansing time with their menstrual cycle. In fact, many women feel better both premenstrually and during their periods if they follow a simple cleansing program of more juices, greens, lighter foods, and herbs.

Seasonal changes are key times of stress when we need to reduce our outer demands and consumption and listen to the way our inner world mirrors the natural cycles. Spring is the key time for detoxification; autumn is also important. A 1 or 2-week program at these times is particularly beneficial. In spring, we may eat more citrus fruits, fresh greens, juices, or the Master Cleanser lemonade diet (see the box "Fasting Aids"). In autumn, we may dine on harvest fruits, such as apples or grapes, and seasonal vegetables. An abundance of fresh fruits and vegetables are appropriate for summer; and whole grains, legumes, vegetables, and soups best simplify our diet in winter.

---

*Fasting is not recommended with cancer, nutritional deficiencies, or motor disorders that could affect swallowing.
**Fatigue may be caused by either toxicity or deficiency.

FASTING AIDS[1]

Spring Master Cleanser

2 tbsp. fresh lemon or lime juice

1 tbsp. pure maple syrup (up to 2 tbsp if calories are not an issue)

1/10 tsp. cayenne pepper

8 oz. spring water

Mix and drink 8 to 12 glasses throughout the day. Eat or drink nothing else except water, laxative herb tea, and peppermint or chamomile tea. Keep the cleanser in a glass container (not plastic) or make it fresh each time. Rinse your mouth with water after each glass to prevent the lemon juice from hurting the enamel of your teeth.

*Autumn Rejuvenation Ration (a cleansing and nourishing soup)**

3 cups spring water

1 tbsp ginger root, chopped

1 or 2 tbsp miso paste (do not boil)

1 or 2 stalks green onion, chopped

Cilantro, to taste, chopped

1 or 2 pinches cayenne pepper

2 tsp. olive oil

Juice of ½ lemon

Boil water. Add ginger root. Simmer 10 minutes. Stir in miso paste to taste. Turn off burner. Then add green onion, some cilantro, cayenne, olive oil, and lemon juice. Remove and cover to steep for 10 minutes. May vary ingredient portions to satisfy flavors.

*From Bethany Argisle as printed in *The Detox Diet*[1]

Druglike Information

Safety

Detoxification of short duration is safe if performed by a well-informed individual or under the guidance of a skilled practitioner. Longer periods of detoxification, over 1 to 2 weeks, entail some risk of nutritional deficiencies and electrolyte imbalances and require careful monitoring by a trained health care practitioner.

Warnings, Contraindications, and Precautions

The detoxification diets listed in this discussion are not appropriate for individuals with heart disease, extreme fatigue, underweight conditions, or peripheral vascular disease. More complete, in-depth fasting programs may release even greater amounts of toxicity. Releasing too much toxicity can make people feel sicker. If this happens, they need to increase fluids and eat normally again until they feel better. Individuals with cancer need to be very careful about how they detoxify, and often they need regular, quality nourishment. Fasting should only be done under the care of an experienced physician. All people should avoid fasting just prior to surgery, and should wait 4 to 6 weeks before detoxifying after it.

Adverse Reactions

Most adverse effects of the detoxification process occur when the body's attempt to self-cleanse is not matched by an appropriate rate of elimination. When this imbalance occurs, it is referred to as a *healing crisis*. During this period, preexisting symptoms often flare and may be accompanied by fever, fatigue, nausea, headache, and skin rashes. Increasing elimination with the methods mentioned in "Forms of Therapy" often assist in reducing these responses.

Pregnancy and Lactation

Pregnant and lactating women should avoid heavy detoxification, although they can usually tolerate mild programs that should only be undertaken with the guidance of a qualified practitioner.

Self-Help versus Professional

Simple diet modification or a single-day fast can be performed by almost anyone. Detoxification of short duration is safe if performed by a well-informed individual or under the guidance of a skilled practitioner. Longer periods of detoxification, over 1 to 2 weeks, entail some risk of nutritional deficiencies and electrolyte imbalances and require careful monitoring by a trained health care practitioner.

Visiting a Professional

When setting up an initial detox or cleansing program, the practitioner could evaluate each individual with a health history, physical examination, biochemical tests, dietary analysis, and other tests, such as for salivary hormone measurements, stool ecology and function, whole blood mineral analysis, intestinal permeability, and detoxification profiles. By interpreting patients' current symptoms and disease as a result of their diet, lifestyle, and genetic patterns, and by then considering their current health goals, a plan can be created together. As is true with any healing process, the plan must be reevaluated and fine-tuned to the individual to make it work optimally over time.

Credentialing

No formal credentialing exists for detoxification therapy.

Training

Training also varies in quality and formality. Courses on the subject are often available in schools of naturopathy, chiropractic, bodyworkers, and others, as well as courses available for less formally licensed practitioners. Many of the common principles of detoxification are clearly described in lay publications.

What to Look for in a Provider

The practitioner should have extensive experience with methods of detoxification. A medical background is preferred, particularly if the individual wishes to pursue a prolonged period of detoxification or has significant concurrent illness.

Barriers and Key Issues

Perhaps the greatest barrier to the use of detoxification is that its primary philosophy is seemingly contrary to that of mainstream medicine. The process of detoxification, more than almost any other healing technique, illustrates the power of the human body to return to or move closer to a baseline state of health. The therapy seems more like "not doing" rather than doing. It implies that disease results when the body has an obstacle to natural good health and that, if the obstacle is removed, good health returns. Instead of treating illness, as mainstream medicine would with the assistance of medications and procedures, the body is "untreated" of its accumulated wastes, leaving what was there originally: good health.

Such a radical perspective often comes crashing into conventional thought in such a simple scenario as a common cold. According to mainstream medicine, the rhinovirus causes nasal vasodilatation and therefore rhinorrhea, the typical "runny nose." Whereas according to natural medicine theory, the body is releasing its excess mucus at the convenient opportunity of the viral infection. According to mainstream medicine, the rhinorrhea is treated by suppression, using an oral decongestant. According to more naturopathic thought, eliminating the mucus removes the need for the body to expel it through the nose. A short fast, or abstinence from dairy products and wheat for a few days may be all that is needed to decrease the nasal symptoms until the viral infection subsides spontaneously.

Associations

American Association of Naturopathic Physicians
601 Valley St. Suite 105
Seattle, WA 98109
Tel: (206) 298-0126
Fax: (206) 298-0129
E-mail: webmaster@naturopathic.org
www.naturopathic.org/Welcome

Suggested Reading

1. Haas EM: *The detox diet*, Berkeley, Calif, 1996, Celestial Arts.
   A how-to and when-to guide for cleansing the body.
2. Haas EM: *Staying healthy with nutrition*, Berkeley, Calif, 1992, Celestial Arts.
   A complete guide to diet and nutritional medicine.
3. Haas EM: *The staying healthy shopper's guide*, Berkeley, Calif, 1999, Celestial Arts.
   Addresses the chemical and toxicity concerns in our food system. Gives recommendations
   on how to feed your family safely by learning to avoid additives, preservatives, pesticides,
   pathogens, processed foods, and more.
4. Fuhrman J: *Fasting—and eating—for health: a medical doctor's program for conquering disease*,
   Glendale, Calif, 1998, Griffin Trade Paperback.
   A combination of classic fasting techniques with modern medical research to provide a
   complete diet and fasting program applicable to assist treatment of many medical disorders.

References

1. Haas EM: *The detox diet*, Berkeley, Calif, 1996, Celestial Arts.

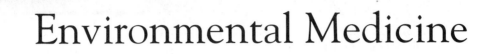

Environmental Medicine

GARY R. OBERG

Origins and History

The current medical care model has an impressive track record of performance for helping generally well patients who get acute and self-limiting illnesses, such as infectious diseases and trauma. This model has assumed for many years that good health is the natural homeostatic state of the human body. The environment is seen as an essentially benign place that generally has little effect on health, and the diet is simply a passive source of metabolic fuels for the body's inherently stable metabolic functions. Therefore when physicians are looking for the cause of a *chronic* disease, this same assumption is applied and the potential roles of the environment and diet are superficially acknowledged, but their true importance in chronic disease is neither appreciated nor effectively accommodated in actual practice.

Yet during the past several decades, there has been a burgeoning growth in the incidence of more complex and chronic diseases in our population. Unfortunately, application of the current medical model to these diseases seems to be resulting in a rapidly increasing cost for their care, accompanied by a rapidly decreasing satisfaction with the quality of life that results from this care. In an effort to find the explanation for this unacceptable and puzzling situation, a group of clinicians from various specialties banded together in the 1960s and formed a medical society that has evolved into the American Academy of Environmental Medicine (AAEM). These physicians noted, as many have, that increased chronicity of illness and multiple organ system involvement consistently and significantly decrease response rates to treatment. They determined that such treatment failures seemed to result when too much emphasis was placed on the nature of the disease and its symptomatic treatment and not enough attention on the causes and why the disease developed in the first place. To correct this situation, these physicians formed a new, more comprehensive, cause-oriented model for the diagnosis, treatment, and prevention of chronic disease, called the *Model of Environmental Medicine*.

The new model has its roots in the ancient traditions of both Western and Eastern medicine. In more recent times it has been influenced by research on the physiologic effects of prolonged exposure to cumulative stresses,[1,2] as well as systems analysis[3] and chaos theory.[4] The knowledge base used in this model is a standard composite of modern basic sciences and clinical disciplines.

Mechanisms of Action According to Its Own Theory

The time has come to give the study of the responses that the living organism makes to its [diet and] environment the same dignity and support which is being given at present to the study of the component parts of the organism . . . Overemphasis on a reductionist approach will otherwise lead biology and medicine into blind alleys.

   Rene Dubos

The model of environmental medicine is based on the growing appreciation that the human body is constantly coping with its dynamic environment by means of a number of inherited, built-in, complexly interacting, and usually reversible biologic mechanisms and systems. These systems are designed to maintain overall homeodynamic (not homeostatic) functioning among all biologic mechanisms. Their ongoing adjustments are unique to the individual and change continually over time.

According to this model, substances in the diet or environment are appreciated as being potential stressors, capable of contributing to destabilization of homeodynamic functions, therefore causing disease. The term *homeodynamic functioning* is preferred because it reflects the fact that maintenance of health and function is an active rather than passive process. Categories of potential external stressors would include organic inhalants such as dusts, molds, pollens, and danders; the myriad of manmade and naturally occurring chemicals; the diet and the many substances in it; infectious organisms; and physical phenomena such as radiation, heat, cold, humidity, vibrations, noise, electromagnetic fields, and so on. Categories of potential internal stressors would include psychologic stresses, genetic limitations, malnutrition, dysfunctioning biologic mechanisms, and others. Treatment strategies must be individualized and customized for each patient.

The Model of Environmental Medicine

OPTIMAL HEALTH is a sustained state of optimal physical, neuro/cognitive, psychologic, and social well-being. It is achieved and sustained by an active, ongoing expenditure of metabolic energy to insure a homeodynamic stability of interacting biologic functions despite the dynamically changing potential for disruption from all environmental and internal stressors.

ENVIRONMENTALLY-TRIGGERED ILLNESSES (ETI) are the adverse consequences that result when the homeodynamic interactions among biologic functions are compromised by external or internal stressors. These stressors may range from severe acute exposure to a single stressor, to cumulative relatively low-grade exposures to many stressors over time. The resultant dysfunction is dependent on the patient's genetic makeup, nutrition and health in general, stressors, degree of exposure to them, and effects of six fundamental biologic governing principles: total load, level of adaptation, bipolarity of responses, spreading phenomenon, switch phenomenon, and individual susceptibility (biochemical individuality).

ENVIRONMENTAL MEDICINE is the proactive, comprehensive, cause-oriented, and cost-effective strategic approach to medical care dedicated to the recognition, management, and prevention of the adverse consequences resulting from ETI.

Recognition of ETI is accomplished by use of a chronologic, sufficiently detailed, environmentally and diet-focused history designed to accurately detect the various clinical patterns generated by the involvement of specific stressors and the dynamic interactions resulting from the previous governing principles. A positive history then is supplemented as indicated by an appropriate physical examination, laboratory testing to assess the functional status of the patient's biologic mechanisms, medical imaging techniques, diagnostic surgical techniques, and endorsed diagnostic testing techniques.

Management of appropriately identified ETI is by use of the endorsed treatment techniques of comprehensive patient education about the nature of the illness, correction of abnormal nutritional, metabolic, and psychologic dysfunctions, immunotherapy, reasonable elimination of identified stressors, and symptomatic drugs and surgery where appropriate.

Prevention of ETI is achieved by the skillful proactive application of the concepts and principles of environmental medicine. This would include the adoption of appropriate lifestyles that specifically minimize exposures to identified stressors as much as practical, provide less contaminated air, food, and water, and insure ongoing optimal nutrition and metabolic functioning and optimal physical, neuro/cognitive, psychologic, and social well-being.

The ultimate long-term goal of appropriate diagnosis and treatment is the cost-effective attainment and sustaining of optimal physical, neuro/cognitive, psychologic, and social well-being. This includes the return to a preillness level of functioning and improved tolerance to stressors that previously caused adverse reactions. Through education, patients should develop and adopt appropriate lifestyles to prevent the recurrence and development of new illnesses.

Biologic Mechanism of Action

The proactive and preventive strategies of environmental medicine are applied through a conventional sequence. This begins with a comprehensive environment and diet-focused medical history, physical examination, and diagnostic testing. It proceeds to a hypothesis of the condition's origins and concludes with an effective match between suggested treatments and a beneficial response by the patient.

There are several major requirements that must be met for all patients to benefit most effectively and consistently from the concepts and modalities of environmental medicine, as follows:

1. The physician must know how and when to supplement the current model with the environmental medicine model, as dictated by the needs of each patient. This involves determining when symptomatic drugs alone may be appropriate, and when it is necessary to also actively seek the actual nature of the disease with the goal of identifying and correcting its actual causes.

2. When treating acute and self limited diseases, it is appropriate to look for fixed name disease diagnoses to guide the choosing of appropriate symptomatic drugs. The drugs may be used to buy time until the body's own homeodynamic functions recover from the acute illness and restore health again.

3. When treating more chronic and complex illnesses, it is more useful to think in terms of identifying dysfunctions in specific biologic mechanisms; for example, defects in insulin, glucose, and glycosalation control; activation of chronic proinflammatory pathways, and so on. The goal is to repair discovered dysfunctions to return the mechanisms to their homeodynamic state, restoring health.

4. The physician must be able to identify and test for the complex range of possible external and internal stressors that can contribute to ETI.

5. The physician must understand the functioning of the body's many biologic mechanisms and appreciate how they all interact inextricably in the "web of life." The physician must be able to assess the functional status of these mechanisms and their interactions with appropriate tests.

6. The physician must appreciate the true complexity of the relationships between biologic mechanisms and the environment and diet as they interact in health and disease. As one astute old physician put it, "Mother Nature ain't playing checkers! She's playing chess!"

7. To ascertain the causes of disease and to understand the dynamic ongoing clinical manifestations of an evolving illness, the physician must effectively apply the six fundamental biologic principles of environmental medicine while obtaining the patient's chronologic history.

8. A reasonable effective treatment plan must accommodate the patient's individual list of stressors, functional status of biologic mechanisms, level of understanding, as well as the patient's resources. Treatment modalities should be those that will be the most cost-effective, convenient, and efficacious for restoring the patient to good health and preventing further disease.

9. The physician must try to discover the dynamic nature of each patient's illnesses and then must be able to teach this to the patient in a clear and useful manner. After all, the word *doctor* comes from the Latin verb *docere*, which means "to teach." There is no more powerful way for the patient to control chronic disease than to understand its very nature and be able to manipulate its causes to reverse and prevent it. This will be best achieved by an ongoing and dynamic partnership between a well-motivated, effectively educated patient and a physician and staff who are well trained and experienced in the discipline of environmental medicine.

Forms of Therapy

The most effective and cost-efficient therapies will be *proactive* and stress early assessments and interventions to maintain optimal physical, emotional and cognitive, and psychologic health and spiritual well-being. The short and long-term forms of therapy must be customized for each and every patient and may consist of any combination of the following categories of treatment modalities:

1. *Patient education:* On the nature of the illness, its treatment, and future prevention.
2. *Therapeutic customized diets:* Whole food diets and nutriceuticals designed to reverse specific nutritional deficiencies, provide optimal nutrition, and accommodate specific diet-related problems such as food-born toxins, food allergies, and food intolerances.
3. *Nutritional supplements:* Vitamins, minerals, amino acids, fatty acids, and other specific nutrients provided to help correct or optimize specific biologic mechanism functions such as detoxification, antioxidation, and antiinflammatory pathways.
4. *Immunotherapies:* Customized vaccines made up of specific inhalants, foods, chemicals, and others. May be taken by subcutaneous injection or sublingually.
5. *Psychotherapies:* Specific modalities to attain and sustain optimal neuro/cognitive, psychologic, social, and spiritual well-being.
6. *Detoxification therapies:* Specific oral and parenteral nutritional protocols, heat depuration, massages, and exercises, and so on, designed to detoxify indicated patients contaminated with various types of xenobiotics such as pesticides, volatile organic hydrocarbons, heavy metals, and others.
7. *Environmental controls:* Protocols to achieve clean air, water, and food by the elimination or minimization as practical of specific environmental stressors, such as organic inhalants and chemicals and physical phenomena.
8. *Pharmaceutics:* All symptomatic drugs are routinely used as needed to provide symptomatic relief from symptoms while the underlying causes of an illness are being found and corrected. However, the potential for adverse reactions when using drugs must always be remembered.

Demographics

There are hundreds of physicians (MDs and DOs) who have been trained in environmental medicine to varying degrees by attending the continuing medical education courses of the American Academy of Environmental Medicine (AAEM). They may be found in almost any medical specialty, scattered throughout all parts of North America and Europe. AAEM has a directory of these physicians. See "Associations." There also are many clinicians in all specialties who have independently appreciated various aspects of environmental medicine and incorporated various insights or modalities into their practices.

Patients seeking an environmental medicine approach to their chronic and complex medical problems come from all walks of life, all ages, both sexes, and many different cultural groups.

Indications and Reasons for Referral

Referral to a physician well trained and experienced in environmental medicine should be considered anytime a patient or physician wishes to try to find the actual causes behind a chronic or complex illness rather than just continue to treat it with symptomatic drugs. All organ systems commonly are involved with illnesses that may respond well to the environmental medicine approach. See "Office Applications."

A referral might be particularly helpful if a patient's illness is chronic, consists of multiple symptoms in multiple organ systems, exhibits patterns that fluctuate over time (especially if the patterns are known to result from biologic mechanisms dysfunctioning as a result of exposures to environmental inhalants, chemicals, or diet), or has not responded satisfactorily to a symptomatic multiple drug approach.

Office Applications

This list illustrates only some of the potentially extensive range of adverse health effects that have been associated with Environmentally Triggered Illnesses (ETI) as defined in this discussion. By listing a disease name here, it is not implied that it is *always* the result of ETI. However, the physician should be alert to the possibility and consider evaluating the patient for an ETI connection if indicated by an appropriate history.

Where an illness does involve an ETI component, therapy to correct the contributing causes of the illness should always rank as the number one choice, ahead of any other therapy that is just symptomatic, although symptomatic therapies are appropriate adjuncts. All of the following diseases and symptoms listed are documented in the published peer-reviewed medical literature to be *potentially* results of the mechanisms of ETI[2,5]:

- Systemic illnesses: Alcoholism, obesity, and tobacco use
- Cardiovascular disorders: Migraine headaches, arrhythmias, vasculitis, thrombophlebitis, hypertension, angina, myocardial infarctions, edema, and fluid retention syndromes
- Eye, ear, nose, and throat disorders: Conjunctivitis, eczema of the eyelids, blurring of vision, photophobia, laryngeal edema, Meniere's disease, recurrent otitis media, rhinitis, frequent colds, sinusitis, vertigo, hearing loss, tinnitus, and pressure in the ear
- Pulmonary disorders: Asthma, certain pneumonias, and chronic bronchitis
- Endocrine dysfunction: Thyroid dysfunction, premenstrual syndrome, and fibrocystic breast disease
- Gastrointestinal disorders: Aphthous stomatitis, gastric and duodenal ulcers, chronic gastritis, irritable bowel syndrome, infantile enterocolitis, eosinophilic gastroenteritis, regional ileitis, ulcerative colitis, certain malabsorption syndromes, and gut flora dysbiosis
- Hematologic disorders: Certain anemias and thrombocytopenia
- Genitourinary disorders: Glomerulonephritis, nephrotic syndrome, chronic cystitis, recurrent vaginitis, enuresis, dysmenorrhea, infertility, and vulvodynia
- Neurologic disorders: Fatigue, certain seizure disorders, sleep disorders, Parkinson's disease, Alzheimer's disease, multiple sclerosis, and various cognitive and memory disorders

- Neurobehavioral and psychiatric disorders: Attention deficit disorder, manic-depressive illness, somatoform disorders, sexual dysfunction, eating disorders, schizophrenia, panic disorders, irritability, anxiety, and chronic fatigue
- Rheumatologic disorders: Lupus erythematosus, scleroderma, myalgia and arthralgia, fibromyalgia, rheumatoid arthritis, and other arthritides
- Musculoskeletal disorders: Muscle spasm headaches
- Skin disorders: Eczema, urticaria, angioedema, sclerodema, and dermatitis herpetiformis
- Cancer

Practical Applications

Appropriate indications and applications for both the current and the environmental medicine models are routinely and simultaneously found in every medical practice. A physician must know how to identify those patients who will benefit from each model and should be able to provide all indicated care or refer the patient elsewhere, as determined by the physician's expertise and experience. This involves determining when simply identifying and treating a disease after the fact with symptomatic drugs may be appropriate and when it is necessary to actively and deliberately seek the actual nature of the disease with the goal of identifying and correcting its actual causes.

A simple ranking of conditions responsive to this form of therapy is as follows. As with all alternative therapies, use of environmental medicine does not preclude the use of mainstream medical therapies in addition.

Top level: *A therapy ideally suited for these conditions*

Asthma; cancer (adjunctive therapy); gut flora dysbiosis; irritable bowel syndrome; Meniere's disease; rhinitis; and somatoform disorders

Second level: *One of the better therapies for these conditions*

Attention deficit disorder; chronic bronchitis; chronic fatigue; dermatitis herpetiformis; dysmenorrhea; eczema; enuresis; fatigue; fibrocystic breast disease; fibromyalgia; infantile enterocolitis; laryngeal edema; migraine headaches; muscle spasm headaches; myalgia and arthralgia; premenstrual syndrome; recurrent otitis media; regional ileitis; rheumatoid arthritis; sinusitis; ulcerative colitis; and urticaria

Third level: *A valuable adjunctive therapy for these conditions*

Alcoholism; Alzheimer's disease; angina; angioedema; anxiety; aphthous stomatitis; arrhythmias; certain anemias; certain malabsorption syndromes; certain pneumonias; chronic cystitis; chronic gastritis; conjunctivitis; eating disorders; eczema of the eyelids; edema and fluid retention syndromes; eosinophilic gastroenteritis; frequent colds; gastric and duodenal ulcers; glomerulonephritis; hearing loss; hypertension; infertility; irritability; lupus erythematosus; manic-depressive illness;

multiple sclerosis; myocardial infarctions; nephrotic syndrome; obesity; other arthritides; panic disorders; Parkinson's disease; pressure in the ear; recurrent vaginitis; schizophrenia; scleroderma; sexual dysfunction; thrombocytopenia; thrombophlebitis; thyroid dysfunction; tinnitus; various cognitive and memory disorders; vasculitis; vertigo; and vulvodynia

Research Base

Evidence Based

There are literally dozens of books and thousands of articles in the world peer-reviewed scientific literature that provide the database about the nature of the interactions between humans and their environment in health and disease or provide support for the concepts and modalities as promulgated by the discipline of environmental medicine. The reader is referred to "Suggested Reading" and "References" at the end of this discussion.

Basic Science

The information that delineates the molecular and physiologic basis behind the nature of the "web of life" as used in environmental medicine is discussed in depth by Rea[6] and Pischinger.[7] Capra discusses how these concepts actually apply at all levels of life.[4]

Risk and Safety

The practice of environmental medicine is a strategic comprehensive approach to medical care. It is not a limited modality of therapy for one or more specific purposes. The safety and risks of its application to ill patients is directly related to the medical skills of the practitioner to proceed wisely and effectively in the evaluation and treatment, as well as the severity and complexity of the patient's illness. This is true for all medical care models.

Efficacy

All illnesses whose causes include those involved with ETI will improve to some degree, within the patient's capacity to correct dysfunctioning mechanisms, if the specific causes can be properly identified and corrected as much as possible. As the physician's depth of medical knowledge and level of clinical skills in environmental medicine modalities increases, the treatment outcome for a wider scope of applicable illnesses will improve concomitantly.

Future Research Opportunities and Priorities

Much more research is needed in this area. Such topics relate to cost-effectiveness, nutritional needs in health and disease, responses to natural and synthetic environmental chemicals, epidemiology of ETIs, and systems interactions.

Druglike Information

The comprehensive treatment modalities of environmental medicine make use of all pharmaceutics, nutraceutics, dietary supplements, dietary manipulations, and so on, as indicated for each case. The appropriate way to use all of these substances is beyond the scope of this overview discussion.

Self-Help versus Professional

The therapies involved with environmental medicine range in complexity from entirely safe and simple to potentially very dangerous and quite complicated. Whether any particular therapy may be self-administered or used only under the care of a trained health professional will be best determined by an ongoing and dynamic partnership between a well-motivated, effectively educated, and responsible patient and a physician and staff who are well trained and experienced in the discipline of environmental medicine.

Visiting a Professional

It is very helpful to tell the patient that the environmental medicine physician will want to know everything the patient can remember about when, where, and under what circumstances the different symptoms have occurred, the order in which they have evolved, and the results of how they have been evaluated and treated up to that point, because a chronologic, sufficiently detailed, environmentally and diet-focused history is the most important and revealing part of an evaluation. This history may be taken by having the patient fill out a comprehensive history form before the visit or by an interview with the physician or staff member at the first visit. The final history then is supplemented as indicated by an appropriate physical examination. A typical first visit takes from half an hour to 1.5 hours. Appropriate laboratory testing to assess the functional status of the patient's biologic mechanisms (some combination of blood, saliva, urine, hair, or stool specimens), medical imaging techniques, and endorsed diagnostic testing techniques (skin tests and others) also may be performed at the first visit or scheduled for another time. After the physician has a complete picture about the full nature of the patient's problems, a comprehensive treatment plan then will be devised.

Subsequent management usually includes comprehensive patient education about the nature of the illness and correction of dysfunctions by a variety of medical, nutritional, and psychologic modalities. Once prescribed, the program generally is carried out by the physician's staff, with ongoing monitoring by the physician as needed. Communication with the patient's other physicians (if any) is required to coordinate all care being given.

Through education, patients should develop and adopt appropriate lifestyles to prevent the recurrence and development of new illnesses. This goal will be best achieved by an ongoing and dynamic partnership between a well-motivated, effectively educated patient and a physician and staff who are well trained and experienced in the discipline of environmental medicine.

Credentialing

The American Academy of Environmental Medicine (AAEM) feels that the most effective form of medical care based on this model can be provided by an MD or DO, because these practitioners have the medical licensure to carry out all aspects of a potentially comprehensive evaluation and treatment plan. Patients should be careful to determine the credentials and professional experience of anyone from whom they seek medical advice.

Training

The American Academy of Environmental Medicine (AAEM) provides a comprehensive, ACCME-accredited continuing medical education program dedicated to train physicians in all aspects of environmental medicine. Its continuing medical education activities are based upon the Core Curriculum of Environmental Medicine, which is determined by the ABEM/IBEM. AAEM has different levels of membership based on the member's level of training in the field. There also are several nonphysician categories of membership. All questions concerning AAEM and its physician education program or other functions should be addressed to the academy at its central office (see "Associations").

Other medical or health care provider organizations with varying levels of accreditation may provide educational activities about different aspects of the discipline, according to their educational goals and objectives. But only AAEM is currently providing a full and comprehensive program in this discipline, endorsed by this discipline's accrediting board, the ABEM and IBEM.

The American and International Boards of Environmental Medicine (ABEM and IBEM) are independent organizations with two missions: 1) to grant board certification in the field of environmental medicine; and 2) to establish educational and training criteria for those individuals wishing to prepare themselves as experts in the field of environmental medicine. Applications and other information may be obtained from the Executive Secretary of the Boards at the address provided in "Associations." The ABEM and IBEM are not members of the American Board of Medical Specialties.

What to Look for in a Provider

The reader may determine if any particular physician has credentials or training in environmental medicine from the AAEM and ABEM/IBEM by contacting these organizations. Also, AAEM has published *Practice Guidelines for the Field of Environmental Medicine*. Readers can call physicians and ask them about their practices and whether these guidelines are followed in their practices.

Barriers and Key Issues

We have not inherited the Earth from our Fathers; we are borrowing it from our Children.

Old Amish Saying

There already is sufficient scientific support to warrant all physicians to at least become familiar with the concepts of environmental medicine and how they enhance the cost efficiency and quality-of-life response in the treatment of chronic complex illnesses.

However, it is difficult for physicians to embrace a comprehensive medical model that is different from what they are used to. But all physicians have the same goal for their patients: they want them to get better. When they are aware of the credible scientific evidence to support the superior efficacy of a different way of treating the patient, physicians will take the time to learn it if there are also good educational opportunities to be exposed to the new ways.

Associations

The American Academy of Environmental Medicine
American Financial Center, Suite 625
7701 East Kellogg Ave.
Wichita, KS 67207
Tel: (316) 684-5500
Fax: (316) 684-5709
E-mail: aaem@swbell.net
www.aaem.com

The Executive Secretary, ABEM/IBEM
American and International Boards of Environmental Medicine
65 Wehrle Dr.
Buffalo, NY 14225
Tel: (716) 837-1380
Fax: (716) 833-2244

Suggested Reading

Each of the following selections and references listed here has been chosen because it provides a comprehensive review of its topic and a significant compilation of literature sources supporting different aspects of the discipline of environmental medicine.

1. Beasley JD, Swift J: *The Kellogg report: the impact of nutrition, environment, and lifestyle on the health of Americans,* Annandale-on-Hudson, N.Y., 1989, The Institute of Health Policy and Practice, The Bard College Center.
   A comprehensive and eloquent treatise on the value of preventive medicine concepts.
2. Brostoff J, Challacombe SJ: *Food allergy and intolerance,* Philadelphia, 1987, Bailliere Tindall.
   Excellent chapters on treatment strategies for food-related illnesses.

3. Dickey LD, editor: *Clinical ecology,* Springfield, Ill, 1976, Charles C. Thomas.

   The original physician textbook containing AAEM's initial concepts on environmental medicine. Still an invaluable source of clinical experience, although the name "Clinical Ecology" was dropped many years ago.

4. The British Society for Allergy and Environmental Medicine, The British Society for Nutritional Medicine Subcommittee: *Effective medicine in clinical practice.* Obtain from the BSAENM, PO Box 28, Totton, Southampton SO40 2ZA, England. Fax number from the U.S.: 011-44-1703-813912.

   This text of 20 superbly referenced chapters presents a current comprehensive overview of the practices of environmental medicine as endorsed by the AAEM and BSAENM.

References

1. Selye H: The general adaptation syndrome and the diseases of adaptation, *J Allergy* 17:231-398, 1946.

2. Randolph TG: *Human ecology and susceptibility to the chemical environment,* Springfield, Ill, 1962, Charles C. Thomas.

3. von Bertalanffy L: The theory of open systems in physics and biology, *Science* 111:23-29, 1950.

4. Capra F: *The web of life,* New York, 1996, Anchor Books.

5. Ashford NA, Miller CS: *Chemical exposures: low levels and high stakes,* ed 2, New York, 1998, Van Nostrand Reinhold.

6. Rea WJ: *Chemical sensitivity,* vols 1-4, Boca Raton, Fla, 1992-1996, CRC Press.

7. Pischinger A: *Matrix and matrix regulation: basis for a holistic theory in medicine,* English edition, Brussels, 1991, Haug International.

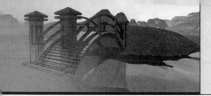

Fasting

ANDREAS BUCHINGER

Origins and History

In a modern world, where we wish to understand all things in concrete scientific terms, the term *fasting cure* sounds antiquated. To get closer to its meaning, consider the definition used by Dr. Otto Buchinger I, one of the leading proponents of fasting. The word stem *cure* has four Latin meanings: 1) *curare*, to heal; 2) *integer*, wholeness; 3) *salus*, to hail; and 4) *sanctus*, holy. The essence of fasting was defined as such, and so were the duties of a physician who practiced the fasting cure. Holistic medical practitioners should strive for these four principles, because the profession of a doctor originally comes from priesthood. In fact, from early times, doctor and priest were one and the same; the duty of a physician and the practice of religion were closely intertwined. Drs. Buchinger I and II (the author's grandfather and father) had and have worked toward this ideal.

From a historical perspective, the original reasons for fasting involved issues of faith, as medical reasons for fasting were not even considered in early times. People frequently talk about fasting motivated by Christian, Islamic, or Buddhist beliefs. Judaism, an even older religion than Christianity, includes many essential elements of fasting in its practice. In theologic terms, *fasting* means a way back to God (after violations of His commandments) and asking for forgiveness for offending God. Many religions, when examined, have a component of fasting involved. Therefore fasting and turning the self to God belonged together: fasting and having a dialogue with God, not out of self-interest, but also for the fellow human beings.

In Judaism, one particularly well known fast is that of Yom Kippur. It is interesting to note that in the beginning, Hebrew children, pregnant women, older adults, and the sick were excluded from fasting (a precursor of today's medical "contraindications"). In one chapter of the Talmud, there are 31 double-paged instructions for fasting. The "early Christians" modified the existing fasting practices into today's well-known fasting rituals in church. Muslims (following the Koran) practice the Ramadan during the ninth Islamic lunar year, with nothing to eat and to drink from sunrise to sunset, while drinking and eating (sometimes too much) from sunset to sunrise (combined with religious practices). Mekka pilgrims fast during the pilgrimage.

Medical fasting, however, was already part of the fasting rituals in early times. There is a saying in an old Egyptian papyrus (3600 years old) found by E. Smith, "The man eats too much! He lives on one-fourth of what he eats; the doctors live on the remaining three-fourths." How true! In ancient Egypt, fasting was used to prepare for the Isis Mysteries, a religion present during the early Roman Empire. In ancient Greece, people prepared for the Eleusinian rite by fasting. The Pythian in Delphi could ask the Oracle after 24 hours of fasting. The Inca and Aztec priests knew of and practiced fasting.

In 1724 Father Bernhard of Malta directed the first "fasting treatment" using light, air, water, and enema. He observed his patients closely and varied his fasting treatments individually. Dr. Linda Burfield-Hazzard already worked with methods very similar to today's practice at the end of the nineteenth century, using fasting (tea and water) supported by enemas, water application, and gymnastics, as did Dr. Tanner and Dr. Dewey. All three were American physicians.

In 1911, because of a severe case of gallbladder disease and poststreptococcal arthritis, Dr. Otto Buchinger I turned to Dr. Möller of Dresden and Dr. Riedlin of Freiburg. Dr. Buchinger was treated by both doctors, who used fasting to effect a cure, which was like a wonder at that time. Inspired by this transformation, Dr. Otto Buchinger I opened the first holistic medical clinic in Witzenhausen-Werra, south of Hannover, in 1920. The clinic was relocated in 1935 to Bad Pyrmont (with its spa tradition for nearly 2000 years), where the clinic has been ever since. In April 1996 the clinic celebrated its seventy-fifth anniversary. Great credits were due to Dr. Otto Buchinger II, born in 1913 (son of Dr. Buchinger I), who had established naturopathic treatment (especially with fasting as an integral part) after the end of the Second World War. It was he who developed the diet plans that still are used today. He published and lectured to many physicians across Germany and abroad. He gave his opinions in the media about holistic medicine (homeopathy, phytotherapy, Kneippism, nutrition and vegetarianism, nonsmoking, antialcoholism, fasting therapy, and so on). Even today at 85, he still practices his holistic approach with individual patients. The principles of fasting described in this chapter refer to the Buchinger approach.

Mechanism of Action According to Its Own Theory

Fasting

Sometimes doctors who use fasting in their treatment are accused of prescribing a so-called "nothing" diet. This accusation only comes from doctors who have never dealt with fasting. Fasting, for example, is nothing other than applied physiology. Fasting in no way means "hunger" and it does not mean "suffering." The word *hunger* can be applied in situations in many third-world countries, but we understand it by "appetite" at best. If people are starving against their will (due to crop failures, war, and so on), we can call that hunger, but this differs from a controlled medical fast.

Healing From Within

The human body is actually not created to be healthy but is well-equipped to survive; it always works toward the maintenance of homeostasis. Trauma (whether emotional, psychic, or physical, such as the way an individual eats) produces defense reactions steered by the subconscious, which tries to restore homeostasis to the traumatized body. Here only "on-or-off" reactions are possible. Our subconscious cannot decide or plan for the future; it only works here and now. It is obvious that sometimes these traumatic events can lead to undesirable results of the defense reactions; that is, disease or sickness.

Fasting, among other classic natural therapies, works on the root of the disease or incorrect behavior. According to Paracelsus (1493-1541), healing originates from the "doctor inside" (*Archaeus* or the "spirit of life"); we also recognize the "wisdom of nature." The *Qi* of the Chinese medicine and the "divine creative power" of the religions are sometime needed. In English we call that *innate intelligence* or just *innate*. One traces the concept of *innate* back to the embryonic stage of human development and it becomes immediately clear that we should be in awe of this higher wisdom or inborn intelligence that guides our life. The power that has created the body also can heal it in most cases.

It is important to point out that the human represents a unit of body, mind, and soul. The "doctor inside," divine power, or inborn intelligence is active in each of these three. If an individual only treats the symptoms of a disease or looks at a human by the sector (not as one single unit of body, mind, and soul), then that individual cannot bring about healing in the long run or at least does not do the human justice in the total being and approach the root of the disease.

Fasting is a valuable component in detoxification, the mechanisms of which are discussed in greater detail in that specific therapy.

Biologic Mechanism of Action

What Happens in the Body During Fasting?

The sugar supply of the body in liver, muscles, and other tissues lasts only 24 hours. Shortly after fasting begins, the body begins to metabolize fat storage, predominantly triglycerides. These fat depots are sometimes visible in the abdomen and neck. The triglycerides are broken down into glycerin and fatty acid molecules, from which the body can gain energy. Fatty acids are turned into ketone bodies that the body can tolerate, provided the individual drinks enough fluids to eliminate them through the kidneys. An alkalizing agent also can be given to speed up this process. Uric acid, which increases during fasting, also must be considered. If necessary, it can be treated by taking medications. The lay concept of *impurities removal* or *elimination of toxins* is rather unsatisfying to the scientific mind. It really means the elimination or metabolism of substances such as aging enzymes, environment pollutants, and others.

The body also reaches into its protein reserves, from which the glycogenic amino acids are used to generate energy. After 14 days the body automatically downregulates this process. We know that surplus enzymes and protein supplies (from excessive protein intake) are transformed to glucose (sugar). Practical experiences have demonstrated that muscle is strengthened and trained when fasting is combined with sports. If necessary, protein (in the form of buttermilk) is given to patients who do especially strenuous exercises during fasting. Minerals also are supplemented, particularly a combination of potassium and magnesium. With fasting, a sense of well-being follows and the individual feels increasingly relieved: physical and spiritual stress are "thrown overboard," so to speak. The individual often becomes more receptive to the inputs of the senses, such as music, arts, literature, and nature, and has a more active mind. The individual can show a normalization of previously elevated laboratory values (for example, cholesterol, gamma GT, and others), so that fasting also is ideal in reducing risk factors.

Forms of Therapy

Fasting consists of the following:

1. Plenty of fluids (a total of 3 liters per day). This can consist of mineral water, herbal and fruit teas, fasting broth, and fruit juices (for kidney care).
2. Regular exercise (gymnastics, condition training, swimming, hiking, and others)
3. Careful medical surveillance, such as extensive medical history taking, physical examination, laboratory investigations, and baseline EKG. In medical fasting, no fasting is allowed without baseline data. Empathy for the patient also is key in these interactions.
4. Cleansing of the bowels at the beginning of the fast (Glauber's salt and other alternatives)
5. Prescription of phytotherapy, homeopathy, massage, and Kneipp treatments (herbal or mineral baths)
6. Holistic lifestyle advice
7. Nutrition advice and cooking tips
8. Diet plans based on natural foods

Fasting always is a voluntary act and the duration of fast is limited. Fasting should never be used for weight reasons only, to get rid of the "fat," so to speak. Although weight loss is the nicest effect of minor importance, fasting primarily is an opportunity for the application of classic naturopathy.

Lifestyle Counseling

In addition, a healthy diet contributes to the maintenance of well-being; it also represents a self-awareness. The patterns and attitude of eating are discussed with the patient in details, who also receives them in writing. The holistic lifestyle advice which the patient receives during the treatment affects life and social surroundings, so that the patient is more open and responsive to dialogues. The doctor can therefore deal with the patient as an individual more effectively. The goal for the patient is to eat more vegetables and less animal fats (except butter) in the future. Furthermore, the patient is advised not to smoke; there are plenty of scientific arguments against smoking. Alcohol intake should be limited because alcohol prevents the breakdown of fats, increases blood pressure, and damages organs such as the brain and liver. Plans for exercises (regular and persistent) should be firmly implemented. Contrary to the unrestricted eating that often follows ritualistic fasting, medical fasting is a "reset" button to start a healthier lifestyle.

Demographics

Practitioners with knowledge of fasting are most prevalent in Europe, especially Germany, Austria, and Switzerland.

The types of patients who come to a formal fasting facility such as the Buchinger Clinic are between the ages of 40 and 70 years (there are a few regular patients in their 30s), with more women than men (60% to 40%).

Cultures and peoples using fasting as a therapy are diverse. The individuals who use fasting typically are better educated and in the occupations of academia, business, or the health professions.

Typical patients who apply for the remedial fasting are mostly self-employed, have risk factors, and are seriously interested in the maintenance of their health. The most important points are: interest, self-empowerment, and motivation of the patient. People who are not willing or cannot be motivated should not fast.

Indications and Reasons for Referral

Preventive Fasting Dealing with Risk Factors

Conditions include: hyperlipidemias; hypertension (see "Warnings"); obesity; smoking; alcohol use (see "Warnings"); binging behavior; sedentary lifestyle; and psychosocial stress and states of exhaustion.

Therapeutic Fasting in Existing Diseases

DISEASES OF THE MUSCULOSKELETAL SYSTEM Rheumatoid arthritis; psoriatic arthritis; osteoarthritis; degenerative diseases of the spinal column; and muscular and ligamental complaints (tendomyopathies).

METABOLIC DISORDERS Metabolic syndrome (overweight, impaired glucose tolerance, hypertension, lipid disorder); adult onset (type 2, noninsulin dependent) diabetes mellitus; hyperuricemia and gout; and fatty liver (from nutrition, diabetes, lipid disorders, or alcohol; see "Warnings").

DISEASES OF THE DIGESTIVE SYSTEM Disorders of the stomach and the intestines (for example, functional diseases such as nervous stomach syndrome and irritable bowel syndrome, but also simple gastritis); constipation; and diverticulosis.

OTHER FREQUENT DISEASES Skin diseases (psoriasis, acne, allergic skin diseases, and lichen simplex chronicus); respiratory system (hay fever and bronchial asthma); and menopausal disorders.

Practical Applications

A simple ranking of conditions responsive to this form of therapy is as follows. As with all alternative therapies, use of fasting does not preclude the use of mainstream medical therapies in addition (with the restriction of prescription medications during fasting).

Top level: *A therapy ideally suited for these conditions*

Constipation; fatty liver; hypertension; lipid disorders; obesity and weight management; osteoarthritis; rheumatoid arthritis and psoriatic arthritis; and sleep apnea

Second level: *One of the better therapies for these conditions*

Diabetes type 2 (noninsulin dependent diabetes mellitus); metabolic syndrome (Reaven's syndrome); gastrointestinal disorders; irritable bowel syndrome; binging; and tendomyopathies

Third level: *A valuable adjunctive therapy for these conditions*

Allergies; asthma; back pain; bronchitis; candidiasis; colds and flu; diverticulosis and diverticulitis; hay fever; and headaches

Research Base

Much of the medical literature on fasting is in untranslated German but is listed here for reference purposes.

Evidence Based

Otto Buchinger II[1] gave a comprehensive overview of the knowledge of the impact of fasting on the immune system, regarding his experiences from his own private hospital as well as the results of other researchers, including clinical and experimental research work. Kjeldsen-Kragh et al[2] described a controlled trial of fasting and 1-year vegetarian diet in rheumatoid arthritis, stating that fasting followed by a 1-year vegetarian diet is effective in the treatment of rheumatoid arthritis. Kuhn[3] demonstrated the holistic effect of remedial fasting on patients with seropositive rheumatoid arthritis.

Wilhelmi de Toledo[4] confirmed the efficacy of fasting in acute and chronic infections, allergies, and autoimmune diseases and its dependence upon early treatment, properly selected duration of fasting, and correct fasting method. Carlson et al[5] followed blood glucose levels and plasma concentration of free fatty acids glycerol, cholesterol, phospholipids, and triglycerides in a group of 12 men participating in a 10-day walk of 50 kilometers per day without food.

Fahrner[6] states that essential hypertension is secondary to civilizational changes of eating habits and conditions of life and work. Remedial fasting affects all facets of the etiopathogenesis of essential hypertension. The harmonic order of all regulative mechanisms of the blood circulation can be restored in most cases. Kuhn[7] discusses the holistic value of fasting therapy in the treatment of patients with diseases of the cardiovascular system. Luetzner[8] described a controlled 2-year study illustrating feasible methods that can be applied to combine science and dietitics into theoretic and practical treatment models. Schrag[9] describes the application of remedial fasting according to Buchinger in four cases of overweight patients with type 2 diabetes.

Basic Science

Takahashi[10] states that in aging mice, fasting helps to clear brain and liver tissue from aging (degraded) enzymes, suggesting the possibility of prolonged life expectancy.

Aly[11] performed blood and urine assays in patients undergoing long-term fasting from 10 to 36 days.

Risk and Safety

Kienzle[12] speaks about the possible (not dramatic) protein loss during a fast and the physiology of glucose buildup using triglycerides and the glucoplastic amino acids. He states that regular exercises (fitness training) during the fast can cause a decrease in the body fat mass and that sporadic use of buttermilk can be helpful, depending on the individual condition.

There always is the argument of irreversible loss of protein when it comes to fasting. With this statement the author shows that sufficient protein reserves for an appropriate fasting are available in the major part of people.[13] Wilhelmi de Toledo and Luetzner discuss the issue of whether fasting is dangerous. They explore the issue of protein loss and whether enough protein can be stored and recalled for this purpose. Some of the therapeutic effects of fasting cannot be explained without accepting the necessity of eliminating stored proteins in a selective catabolic way, showing the extreme capability of the body for self-regulation.[14]

Efficacy

There are no large-scale studies on fasting, but a significant level of experience has developed over the past 80 years. Some articles are available on different aspects of the impact of fasting. Luetzner describes a clinical and controlled 2-year study with 425 patients. Fasting causes the most drastic decrease of blood lipid levels. Fasting influences not only the patient's metabolism but also eating (nutritional) habits.[15]

As mentioned previously, hypertension often has a favorable response to fasting. Overweight and obesity can be treated with fasting but is not the primary method of treatment. In general, men will lose 5 to 7 kg and women will lose 3 to 5 kg in the first week of fasting. During a 3-week treatment a patient might loose about 10 kg, but this can vary significantly. However, after fasting the patient often is much more conscious of health, weight, and eating habits, which can contribute to maintaining a more ideal weight.

Other

Peper[16] assessed pre and postinterviews on corporal and emotional behavior and experienced changes in 52 patients who did at least 3-week inpatient remedial fasting treatment according to Buchinger, Mayr, or Schroth.

Future Research Opportunities and Priorities

More research is needed. However, the total number of beds in the few "classical fasting clinics" amounts to no more than 400 beds. As always, funding is the issue. This represents a problem with fasting, as no product sales result from its successes.

Druglike Information

Safety

Unsupervised fasts of 2 days in duration generally are safe. However, longer fasts, particularly if more than 5 days, require the supervision of a health professional experienced in this form of therapy.

True medical fasting is undertaken in a closely monitored and professional medical setting. Using the Buchinger method, it is best supervised by trained physicians who also have experienced a fast themselves. A complete medical evaluation is performed, followed by baseline testing of those patients who should be checked before undergoing fasting treatment. The medical history-taking is basic, followed by physical examination and studies including erythrocyte sedimentation rate, complete blood count with differential, urinalysis, fasting blood sugar, serum cholesterol (high or low-density lipoprotein) and triglycerides, liver functions (SGOT/SGPT/G-GT), electrolytes (sodium, potassium, and calcium), uric acid, blood urea nitrogen and creatinine, resting EKG with rhythm strip, and EKG stress testing, if indicated. Other investigations may include the following: abdominal ultrasonography, gastric or colonic endoscopy, and thyroid function testing. These investigations also can be helpful in order to see improvements resulting from fasting therapy. Most (positive) changes should be visible after a 3-week-long fasting treatment.

Warnings, Contraindications, and Precautions

Extended fasting (lasting for more than 48 hours) is contraindicated in the following conditions:

Alcoholism
Alzheimer's disease
Anorexia nervosa and bulimia
Emaciation
Epilepsy
Extensive carcinomas and metastatic cancers
HIV-positive patients or patients with AIDS
Insulin-dependent (type 1) diabetes mellitus
Kidney failure
Liver disease (except fatty liver)
Ongoing use of prescription medications (patient needs to be weaned off first)

Patients with serious chronic infection, such as tuberculosis

Pregnancy and lactation

Schizophrenia

Small children and very older adults

States of malnutrition

Adverse Reactions

Some discomfort may be felt during fasting. Some relates to the inherent ketosis that occurs. These are more common at the onset of a fast and include headache, nausea, insomnia, and dizziness, lightheadedness, and palpitations. Other reactions relate to the phenomenon of detoxification and include increased body odor, increased discharge from mucous membranes, skin rashes and dry skin, and arthralgias and myalgias. Yet others are a direct effect of decreased caloric intake, such as hunger (transient), cold intolerance, and constipation.

Pregnancy and Lactation

As mentioned previously, fasting is contraindicated for patients who are either pregnant or lactating.

Self-Help versus Professional

Short fasts are commonly practiced without supervision. However, a fast of any significant length or in cases of ongoing illness should be supervised by a medical professional familiar with fasting techniques.

Any individual wishing to attempt a prolonged fast should check first with a physician. It is highly advisable not to fast when the individual is under significant life stressors or time pressures.

Visiting a Professional

When a medically supervised fast is desired, the following scenario is typical of a specialized facility.

Course of Fasting

The fast often begins with a "relief" day, using a monodiet of fruit, natural brown rice, or potato or potato purée. The actual fasting begins the next day with a laxative (mostly mineral salts or a laxative tea). The bowels of a fasting person should be empty. During fasting an enema (or sauerkraut juice) is applied every 2 days alternating with a liver *wet pack*. Doctor's visits or consultations occur two times per week.

The *length of fasting* does not depend on the time available but on the following:

1. Whether the patient wants to fast as an ambulatory patient (without medical attendance); a recommended maximum fasting period in this case is 7 or 8 days;
2. Whether the patient wants to fast therapeutically because of diseases; and
3. Whether the patient wants to fast prophylactically (symptom prevention).

In the latter two situations the physician will recommend a period of fasting depending on the circumstances.

During the fast the patient must consume 3 liters of fluids each day (mineral water, juice, fruit teas, or buttermilk). Vegetable broth is taken at lunch.

The last day of fasting is also the day of breaking the fast (often called "breakfast day"). To prepare the gastrointestinal tract for the food to come, a gentle fruit is introduced. This often consists of an apple, chewed for half an hour at 11:00 AM and another at 2:00 PM, followed by a potato-vegetable soup at 6 PM.

In the postfasting days that follow (usually a minimum of 4 days) the patient begins with retraining in chewing to attempt to break the longstanding habit of gulping down food too quickly. This also is a process of self-awareness.

Achieving and Maintaining Health

After patients have gone through the fasting process, they are able recognize the pattern of behavior which makes them sick and to correct it in the future and put an end to the behavior that consumes health passively.

Credentialing

Credentialing is specific to country and state. It usually is tied to a preexisting medical licensure. In the U.S., no formal credentialing exists for medical fasting therapy.

Training

No formal training exists in the U.S. It does exist in Germany and is described as follows:

1. Training consists of 3 months in a private hospital, such as the "Klinik Dr. Otto Buchinger" (something like an internship) plus the courses (lectures and seminars). After training, applicants receive the additional designation "naturopathy," which can be used in the future in their formal designation of skills.
2. To receive the diploma in fasting, applicants who have undergone training also can just practice in the previously-mentioned "Klinik" (or other similar clinics) for not less than 1 month, together with participation in seminars (including self-experience in fasting under supervision), lectures, and so on. Parts of the seminars mentioned in (1) are needed and recognized for the training of fasting.

In Germany, the address (for both modalities) is as follows:

ZÄN
Alfredstrasse 21
D – 72250 Freudenstadt
Germany
Tel: +49 - (0) 7441-2151
Fax: +49- (0) 7441-8783

From there information will be given. This organization also offers lists of doctors practicing naturopathy and fasting. To participate in these courses, hospital experience (internship) for more than 1 year is required (basically knowledge in internal medicine).

What to Look for in a Provider

The type of provider depends on the degree of ongoing medical illness the individual already possesses. A greater amount of ongoing illness warrants formal medical expertise, in addition to training in fasting. In the U.S., these providers often are associated with holistic health centers.

In European countries the reader should look for the previously mentioned diplomas to choose a quality provider of this therapy. "ZÄN" in Freudenstadt, Germany gives addresses of providers of this therapy in other parts of the European countries (and sometimes Canada). If a reader receives addresses from ZÄN, these therapists are working according to professional standards.

Barriers and Key Issues

The concern over fasting-induced loss of protein reserves is ever present in the eyes of conventional medicine. The experience of the author is that such concerns are not justified. Monetary issues also are a barrier to the use of medical fasting, as conventional medicine often sees it as a "nontherapy" where nothing is administered, therefore requiring no reimbursement. As naturopathy becomes marketable in mainstream medical settings and hospitals, conventional hospitals again may provide fasting methods in a naturopathic ward. In Germany, this already is occurring.

Associations

Tree of Life Rejuvenation Center
Gabriel Cousens, MD
PO Box 1080
Patagonia, AZ 85624
Tel: (520) 394-2520 or (520) 394-2769
Fax: (520) 394-2099
www.treeofliferejuvenation.com

Naples Institute for Optimum Health and Healing
2335 Tamiami Trail N.
Naples, FL 34103
Tel: (941) 649-7551
Toll-Free: (800) 243-1148
Fax: (941) 262-4684
www.NaplesInstitute.com

Hippocrates Health Institute
1443 Palmdale Court
West Palm Beach, FL 33411
Tel: (561) 471-8876
Toll-Free: (800) 842-2125
Fax: (561) 471-9464
www.hippocratesinst.com

Suggested Reading

1. Boe E, Cott A, Jerome BA: *Fasting: the ultimate diet*, Mamaroneck, NY, 1997, Hastings House.

2. Fuhrman J: *Fasting—and eating—for health: a medical doctor's program for conquering disease*, Glendale, Calif, 1998, Griffin Trade Paperbacks.

3. Shelton H: *The hygenic system, fasting and sunbathing*, vol 3, San Antonio, 1934-1963, Dr. Shelton's Health School.

• In German only:

1. Buchinger O (I): *Das Heilfasten und seine Hilfsmethoden*, Stuttgart, Hippokrates.
   This book is the classical literature on fasting.

2. Buchinger O (II): *Das heilende Fasten*, Wiesbaden, A. Jopp.

3. Fahrner H: *Fasten als Therapie*, Stuttgart, Hippokrates.
   This book is nearly like a textbook of fasting, including experience with fasting throughout about 30 years of practice.

4. Kuhn C: Fasten—physiologie und methodische notwendigkeiten, *Aerztezeitschrift fuer Naturheilverfahren* 7:569-576.
   The metabolic changes (gluconeogenesis, ketoacidosis) and their compensation mechanisms are described to reduce any prejudice regarding fasting according to Buchinger. For any fasting free of crisis, it is absolutely necessary to pay attention to some important methodic necessities.

5. Wilhelmi-Buchinger M, editor: *Die Buchinger-Methode*, Munich, DTV Ratgeber.

References

1. Buchinger O (II): Heilfasten zur Steigerung der Abwehrkraefte, *Physikalische Medizin und Rehabilitation* 9:267-270, 1972.

2. Kjeldsen-Kragh J et al: Controlled trial of fasting and 1-year vegetarian diet in rheumatoid arthritis, *Lancet* 338(8772):899-902, 1991.

3. Kuhn C: Fasten bei rheumatoider Arthritis, *Aeztezeitschrift fuer Naturheilverfahren* (offprint) 9:702-714, 1988.

4. Wilhelmi de Toledo F: Therapeutisches Fasten nach Buchinger und Immunsystem: Erfahrung und Hypothesen, *Aerztezeitschrift fuer Naturheilverfahren* 5:331-341

5. Carlson LA et al: Blood lipid and glucose levels during a ten-day period of low-calorie intake and exercise in man, Karolinska Hospital, Stockholm, p.624-634, 1967.

6. Fahrner HA: Fasten als Grundlage einer ganzheitsmedizinischen Behandlung der essentiellen Hypertonie, *Aerztezeitschrift fuer Naturheilverfahren* 7:532-542, 1988.

7. Kuhn C: Zeitschrift fuer Allgemeinmedizin 63:437-440, 1987.

8. Luetzner H: Intensiv-und Langzeitdiaetetik bei metabolischem Syndrom, *Aerztezeitschrift fuer Naturheilverfahren* 12:872-879, 1994.

9. Schrag S: Diabetestherapie mit Heilfasten, *Aerztezeitschrift fuer Naturheilverfahren* 10:769-806, 1992.

10. Takahashi R, Goto S: Influence of dietary restriction on accumulation of heat-labile enzyme molecules in the liver and brain of mice, *Arch Biochem Biophys* 257(1):200-206, 1987.

11. Aly KO et al: Chemical studies on blood and urine in long-term fasting, *Biologisc Medicin* (Sweden) 2:23-29, 1981.

12. Kienzle P: Eiweissgabe beim Fasten ist von Fall zu Fall zu entscheiden, *Natura Med* 5:518-521, 1990.

13. Fahrner H: Der 'physiologische Eiweissspeicher' zur Ueberberbrueckung von Nahrungslosigkeit im Fasten – eine Utopie? *Aerztezeitschrift fuer Naturheilverfahren* 1:42-48, 1992.

14. Wilhelmi de Toledo F, Luetzner H: Kritisches zum Fasten, *Therapeutikon* 6:655-664, 1991.

15. Luetzner, Lipidstoffwechsel und Atherosklerose, *Therapeutikon* 3(4):204-214, 1989.

16. Peper E et al: Stationaeres Heilfasten, *Praevention-Rehabilitation* 3:129-136.

Juice Therapy

STEVE MEYEROWITZ

Origins and History

The vitamin supplement industry is booming. Consumers are buying more and more nutritional products as an alternative to drugs. But where do supplements come from? Plants have been the source of medicines for thousands of years. Our earliest drugs—aspirin, penicillin, quinine—all came from botanic sources. Juices are special because they behave like supplements but are naturally concentrated whole foods. Nutrients in foods coexist with numerous other factors that enhance and enable their function. Once isolated, they may not work as well. Albert Szent-Györgyi, Nobel prize winner and discoverer of vitamin C, found that the complex structure of "C" in peppers was more effective than the chemically isolated "vitamin C."[1] When we isolate nutrients from foods, we risk dissipating its effectiveness. But juices bring us a full spectrum of thousands of chemicals in perfect balance. Hippocrates, the "father of modern medicine," is famous for saying, "Let your food be your medicine and your medicine be your food." Where basic nutrition and health maintenance is concerned, whole, natural foods are best. Where health restoration and detoxification are needed, juices, as concentrated whole foods, make the best supplements.

Biologic Mechanism of Action

Juices are concentrated nutritional elixirs. Incorporating juices into the diet provides a vast array of tastes and flavors, enough to appeal to all tastes. Imagine eating a meal of spinach, parsley, sprouts, tomatoes, lemon, celery, radishes, green pepper, and cucumber. Ordinarily, considering the woeful state of Americans' digestion, we would be lucky to digest half of it. But once the cellulose is separated from the liquid portion of these vital foods, even those with weak digestion will be able to absorb and assimilate its maximum food value. The advantage of properly extracted and filtered juice is that it demands little to no digestive effort from the stomach. This condensing of pounds of valuable foods into a single glass while simultaneously maximizing assimilation is what makes drinking juices so advantageous. One pound of carrots, for example, makes 10 ounces of carrot juice. Even the most frail person could easily drink that in about 1 minute. But who can consume a pound of carrots? Yet the enzymes, water-soluble vitamins, minerals, and trace elements in those carrots are condensed into a glass of fresh-squeezed carrot juice.

Concentration is, admittedly, the concept behind vitamins. But vitamins are still not equivalent to raw fruit and vegetable juices. Vitamins involve several steps of processing along their journey from a botanic to a tablet. Many of those steps involve destructive forces like heat, chemical solvents, additives, excipients like sweeteners, stabilizers, coloring agents, fillers such as talc, binders, and more. This is a far cry from a fresh glass of vegetable juice. Yet, according to our precept from Hippocrates—that nourishing and healing are inextricable—then the purest, freshest, most concentrated natural foods are the finest healers.

Fiber—Yes or No?

Many wonder about the value of drinking juice. After all we have heard about its benefits, why eliminate it? Certainly, we approve of whole foods and fiber. But one does not exclude the other. Juices extract the vital nutrients in plants and make them more readily available for absorption. The fiber in whole foods is both therapeutic and necessary for a healthy digestive tract. But they are not mutually exclusive. Eat as many fresh, whole fruits and vegetables as desired and think of concentrated raw fruit and vegetable juices as supplements or medicines.

Forms of Therapy

This section describes practical information on the use of juices, including mechanisms of action according to its own theory.

Kinds of Juices

PASTEURIZED VERSUS FRESH

Bottled juices must be pasteurized to have a shelf life. This boiling process sanitizes the juice to protect against salmonella, E. coli, and other disease organisms. Unfortunately, enzymes and many vitamins are destroyed in the process and other nutrients are altered in ways that make them less bioavailable. Generally speaking, the vitality of the fresh product is gone, along with all the energetics that engender fresh foods with their healing power. Yes, they taste good, but they are mostly sugar, flavor, and water. They arguably could be better than nothing, but they are no match for the fresh-squeezed version.

FRUIT JUICES

The most widely consumed juices in the world are fruit juices, with orange and apple juice being the best sellers. Other top sellers are grapefruit, grape, prune, and cranberry. Tomato juice also is a best seller in the U.S., but it is considered a vegetable even though tomatoes are technically classified as fruits.

As a group, fruits are basically cleansing foods. Their high water content flushes the digestive tract and kidneys and thus are purifying for the blood.

Citrus fruits are strong solvents. Lemon is the strongest, followed by lime, pineapple, and grapefruit. All have a purging effect on the liver and gall bladder. Pineapple contains the enzyme bromelain, which encourages the secretion of hydrochloric acid that helps to digest protein.

Grape, although only a subacid fruit, also is a powerful cleanser. When making fresh grape juice, use the natural seeded variety. Concord style grapes are the most potent. Use organically grown varieties whenever possible to avoid the high antifungal and pesticide sprays on this fruit. It may be necessary to dilute this juice for sugar-sensitive patients (see "Contraindications").

Apples also are excellent intestinal brooms. They contain malic, elginic, and galacturonic acids, which help remove impurities. Pectins help prevent the putrefaction of protein by softening the stool and maintaining a quicker transit time. For this reason, apples are good bulking agents, gently pushing through the digestive tract. A monodiet of apples sometimes is recommended for this reason. In other words, only apples are eaten for the day. While this may sound radical to some, it is not difficult. Apples are filling and satisfying with digestive and cleansing benefits. Green apples have the lowest sugar content and thus may be desirable for sugar-sensitive patients.

Cranberry is an excellent diuretic as is the rind of watermelon. Your juicing machine can turn this ordinarily discarded portion into a therapeutic juice. The rind does not contain sugars that the rest of the watermelon provides.

Prune and apricot juice help to soften the stool and promote peristalsis. As stone fruits, however, these juices cannot be used with a juice extractor. Prune juice is made by soaking the fresh fruit in water. This is one fruit where purchasing the bottled juice is recommended.

When to Take Fruit Juices Fruit juices can be taken any time of day. They are good in the morning before breakfast, for lunch, or as an after-dinner snack. One way to think of juices is as meals. Have as much as you like, but do not gorge yourself with juice, just as you would not gorge yourself with food. A 10 to 16-ounce serving is average. Fruit juices can be alternated with other juices throughout the course of the day. One or two fruit juices per day should suffice.

Fruit Juice Recipes Mix the following either half-and-half or in any proportion that tastes right:

- Apple and watermelon
- Apple and prune
- Apple and pear
- Apple, pear, and pineapple
- Apple and cranberry
- Apple and grape
- Orange and grapefruit

CARROT COMBINATION JUICES

Prior to 1960, carrot juice was not well known. Today, there are nearly 1000 juice bar and smoothie chain stores that, like Starbucks, are franchised around the country. In addition to its image as a healthful drink, cancer research about the benefits of beta-carotene and antioxidants has even further broadened its popularity.

Benefits of Carrot Combinations   The qualities of these juices often are described using the terminology of natural medicine. Carrot juices are energy drinks. They provide caloric power for a sense of vigor. Because they are stimulating, they are good to have in the morning or daytime hours. Depending on the combinations, they can have many specific physiologic benefits. Beet juice, for example, is a wonderful stimulant for the liver. Parsley juice is considered a blood purifier and also a diuretic. Sweet potato is an alkalinizer of the bloodstream and a mineralizer that also contains an enzyme for diabetics. Cabbage is a wonderful juice for the stomach that is soothing for ulcers and gas. Cucumbers stimulate the kidneys. Watermelon's high alkaline fluid content neutralizes acids and flushes toxins out of the kidneys. Spinach stimulates peristalsis. Aloe vera, which is a plant more than a vegetable, is a wonderful detoxifier of the bloodstream and lymphatic system. Refer to the box "Recipes for Carrot Juices" for suggested carrot juice combinations.

RECIPES FOR CARROT JUICES*

Carrot	*Carrot*	*Carrot*	*Carrot*	*Carrot*	*Carrot*
Spinach	*Parsley*	*Spinach*	*Beet*	*Celery*	*Spinach*
Beet	*Cucumber*	*Carrot tops*	*Broccoli*	*Cilantro*	*Kale*
Cabbage	Radish	Aloe vera	Celery	*Garlic*	Red pepper
Carrot	*Carrot*	*Carrot*	*Carrot*	*Carrot*	*Carrot*
Beet	*Apple*	*Celery*	*Celery*	*Tomato*	*Parsley*
Green pepper	*Alfalfa sprouts*	*Beet*	*Beet*	*Celery*	*Spinach*
Cucumber	*Watermelon*	*Spinach*	Spinach	Spinach	Kale
Parsley	*Rind*	*Cabbage*			
	Ginger	Green Pepper			

*Italicized print indicates a larger quantity than the others listed.

How Much—How Often—What Proportions?

There are overeaters and perhaps overdrinkers as well. Generally, between 10 and 16 ounces of juice is an average portion. But gorging on juice is symptomatic of an imbalance just as gorging on food. The most common overdrinkers to look out for are the patients with undiagnosed hypoglycemia and candida. These people will most likely be taking carrot juice undiluted or with other sugary vegetables like beets.

For routine supplementation, one or two drinks per day is average. But if used therapeutically, there are programs that recommend as much as one drink per hour. Regarding proportions, carrot typically makes up at least 40% of these recipes. Mix the other vegetables to taste, similar to regular cooking. Strong herbals such as ginger or garlic need as little as one clove to be tasted. When used therapeutically the dosing of garlic or ginger may be increased to as many cloves as can be tolerated and still be palatable.

About Mixing Fruits and Vegetables

Ordinarily, fruits and vegetables are considered poor food combining. But the combining rules for solid foods do not always apply for liquids. Juices are mostly water and the versatility of mixing different liquids is much greater than that of solids. The main exception is the mixing of acid fruits such as lemon, grapefruit, and orange. Acid fruits can curdle other juices and, with some exceptions, usually are mixed among themselves.

GREEN JUICES

Although some of our carrot combinations had greens in them, green juices are all green. Green juices are healing, stabilizing, and calming. They have a relaxing and centering effect. For a quick "pick-me-up," drink a carrot juice. But for long-term energy, take a green juice. If you are restless or feeling mentally scattered, drink green juice. Green juice is a quieting drink that is usually taken in the evening. It is perfect when you are exhausted. With ingredients like lemon, ginger, garlic, and cayenne, these green drinks can make the user pucker or gasp. It is the closest thing to a natural cocktail. In fact, today's juice bars are not unlike their alcohol counterparts. After all, both have bartenders who mix drinks according to the customers' preferences. The only difference is that one *detoxifies* the liver while the other damages it.

These drinks are blood cleansers, body tonifiers, nerve tonics, alkalinizing agents, and mineralizers. And the recipes are adjustable (see the box "Green Juice Recpies"). The core ingredients are at the top of the list. The optional ingredients start from the third item on down. Feel free to add or subtract from this recipe. Don't forget to include other important greens such as radish, parsley, green pepper, or leafy sprouts such as alfalfa, buckwheat, lettuce, and sunflower greens.

GREEN JUICE RECIPES

Celery, cucumber, tomato, green pepper, and garlic
Celery, tomato, green pepper, cilantro, and garlic
Celery, spinach, tomato, cabbage, dill, and lemon
Celery, spinach, tomato, cabbage, dill, lemon, garlic, ginger, cayenne, and tamari

---

Although tamari (brewed soy sauce) is not a juice, it is a strained liquid that does not add any solids. It is added as a flavor enhancer much like a dressing on a salad. Green juices are the liquid equivalent of salads. The sodium in these vegetables helps counter sugar cravings. If too many carrot or fruit juices are taken, using green drinks will help balance blood sugar.

Green juices should be taken much more sparingly than carrot or fruit juices, probably no more than once per day. Eight or 10 ounces, sipped slowly, is entirely adequate.

CHLOROPHYLL: THE MOST THERAPEUTIC INGREDIENT

Chlorophyll is the chemical formed by the chloroplast cells of green plants. It is at the beginning of the food chain and forms the basis for most animal foods. Chlorophyll is the *plasma* of green plants. Amazingly, this "blood of plants" is structurally similar to hemin, part of hemoglobin (see the structural formulas in the illustration). The primary distinction is that chlorophyll is bound by an atom of magnesium and hemin is bound by iron. Chlorophyll has long been famous for its ability to heal infected and ulcerated wounds. Tissue cell activity and its normal regrowth are increased by using chlorophyll.[2] It is an important medicine for healing bleeding gums, canker sores, trench mouth, pyorrhea, gingivitis, and even sore throat. Chlorophyll has the unique ability to be absorbed directly through the mucous membranes, especially those of the nose, throat, and digestive tract. It makes a great mouthwash and an excellent dentifrice, especially when used in powder form. Chlorophyll's unique ability to kill anaerobic, odor-producing bacteria is one reason for its effectiveness in countering bad breath, body odor, and acting as a general antiseptic. Unlike many drugs, chlorophyll has never been found to be toxic at any dose.

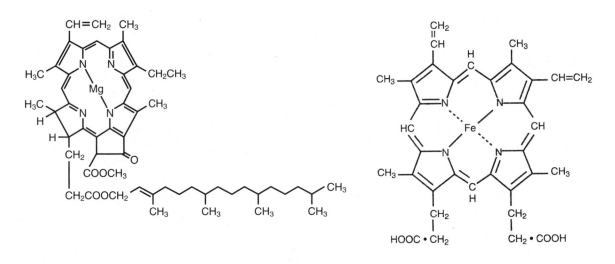

Chlorophyll [$C_{55}H_{72}MgN_4O_5$] and Hemin [$C_{34}H_{32}FeN_4O_4$].

Chlorophyll also may provide some resistance to low level radiograph radiation from hospital equipment, televisions, computer screens, transmitters, and microwaves. No area is totally radiation-free. Experiments on guinea pigs in the 1950s demonstrated that radiation poisoned guinea pigs recovered when chlorophyll-rich vegetables were added to their diet.[3] The U.S. Army repeated this experiment with broccoli and alfalfa and obtained similar results.[4]

WHEATGRASS JUICE

Wheatgrass is a popular juice available in juice bars and natural food stores nationwide. Unlike vegetable juices, it is taken in 1-ounce glassfuls. To give you some idea of its potency, it is similar to drinking an ounce of garlic juice. Although part of the 9000-member family that includes the variety grown on lawns, wheatgrass and its cousin barley grass are grown especially for nutritional purposes. These nutritional grasses are one of our finest sources of chlorophyll. In addition, grasses contain many other important pigments, including carotenoid: alpha-carotene and beta-carotene, xanthophylls, and zeaxanthin, to name a few. These milder pigments are overshadowed by the dark green color of chlorophyll, but they are present nonetheless. There are up to 18,000 units of beta-carotene per ounce of grass. This precursor of vitamin A has significant immune-enhancing properties including the promotion of T-cells.[5] High levels of this antioxidizing nutrient are associated with reduced cancer risk and cardiovascular disease.[6]

Another important vitamin and antioxidant abundant in grass is vitamin E. Grasses have a water-soluble form of E called *a-tocopherol succinate*, which has the ability to increase production of prolactin and growth hormone in the pituitary gland.[7] Grasses also are abundant sources of quality vitamin K, the blood-clotting vitamin. Grass juice can inactivate mutagenic substances found in agricultural chemicals, fertilizers, and food additives.[8]

Dr. T. Shibamoto of the University of California, discovered a powerful new antioxidant in barley grass called 2"-0-GIV. This new isoflavonoid is soluble in water and fats and is highly stable. This means it is capable of permeating both the fat and aqueous cell membranes to fully protect the cell from the damaging effects of oxidation. According to Shibamoto, 2"-0-GIV is more potent than vitamins E and C, but when taken together the effects are profound.[9] Barley grass has all three in good quantity. Tests have shown it is a preventative for arteriosclerosis and is just as effective as the prescription drug Probutol for this disease, without any side effects.[10]

Barley and wheat grass are both abundant, inexpensive sources of superoxide dismutase (SOD). This is a powerful antioxidant and antiaging enzyme. SOD is a proven antiinflammatory for arthritis, edema, gout, and bursitis.[8] Dr. K. Kubota of the Science University of Tokyo also found two glycoproteins, D1G1 and P4D1, which work alongside SOD but are more heat stable. All three have antiinflammatory action that is superior to aspirin.[11]

If fresh grass juice is not locally available, powdered wheat and barley grass products are on the shelves of natural food stores nationwide. Since all research was done with these powders, they stand a viable nutritive and therapeutic form of the juice. Powdered grass juice products are carefully processed to preserve as many enzymes as possible. Fresh-squeezed wheat grass juice is rich in enzymes, protein, phytochemicals, chlorophyll, carotenoids, fatty acids, and trace; it is a worthy supplement.

COLOR JUICES AND FOODS

Much can be said about the individual nutritional characteristics of these wonderful fruit and vegetables, but truly, it is hard to remember all the things that they each do. One way to simplify the healing properties of these foods and juices is by designing drinks and foods around color.

Red food speeds up circulation, creates fire, yang energy (Chinese medicine), and heats up the body, including hands and feet. Tomatoes, cherries, red cabbage, red peppers, hot peppers, cranberry, watermelon, radish, wheat, and rye are some examples.

Orange food is antispasmodic and is excellent for pains and cramps. It helps strengthen the lungs in polluted environments. Emotionally, it facilitates joy and expansiveness. It promotes vitality and mental clarity. Oranges, carrots, apricots, pumpkin, sesame, and pumpkin seeds are orange foods.

Yellow food is a motor stimulant, useful for a morning "pick-me-up." It strengthens nerves and digestion and helps constipation. Lemon, lime, pineapple, grapefruit, apple, peach, banana, papaya, mango, yellow squash, corn, and butter are some of these.

Green food is a blood cleanser, bactericide, nutrifier, and natural tranquilizer. All green leafy vegetables and sprouts, wheat grass, and avocado are in this class.

Blue food is for headaches and spiritual and mental work. It is yin and cool and includes blueberry, plum, grape, potato, celery, parsnip, asparagus, and nuts.

Indications and Reasons for Referral

A simple ranking of conditions responsive to this form of therapy is as follows, listed in order of effectiveness per category. As with all alternative therapies, use of juice therapy does not preclude the use of mainstream medical therapies in addition.

Allergic: Hay fever, hives, and asthma

Digestive disorders: Constipation, liver detox, ulcers, and gallstones

Arthritis (rheumatism)

Skin diseases: Eczema, acne, psoriasis, ulcers, and boils

Miscellaneous: High and low blood pressure, bronchitis, obesity, insomnia, inflammation, arteriosclerosis, and migraine headaches

Practical Applications

Traditionally, most juicing machines were sold by health food stores and juice bars. However, in the mid-1990s, infomercials by Jay Kordich, "the Juiceman," elevated sales into the mainstream. Juicers now can be purchased wherever appliances are sold. Most juice lovers can be found in the hundreds of juice and smoothie franchise stores sprinkled around the country. These consumers lean toward an alternative lifestyle or use juices as an alternative to a heavy lunch. The nutritional attributes of fresh-squeezed vegetable juice is part of its appeal.

Juice therapy is partly nutritional maintenance, prevention, detoxification, and treatment. It is the therapy of choice in managing a person's intestinal health—digestion, absorption, and nutrient intake are essential. This approach underlies the treatment of almost all chronic illnesses, degenerative diseases, and complex constellation syndromes such as fibromyalgia, chronic immune deficiency syndrome, and cancer.

Certain juice combinations are often recommended for particular conditions, in addition to conventional medical therapy (see the box "Home Juicing Remedies").

HOME JUICING REMEDIES

Cold fighter	Carrot, lemon, radish, ginger, garlic
Hay fever reliever	Carrot, celery, radish, ginger
Immune booster	Carrot, celery, parsley, garlic
Memory booster	Carrot, parsley, spinach, kale
Stress reliever	Carrot, celery, kale, parsley, broccoli, tomato
Headache helper	Carrot, celery, parsley, spinach
Detoxifier	Apple, beet, cucumber, ginger
Antioxidant cocktail	Carrot, orange, green pepper, ginger
Anticholesterol	Carrot, parsley, spinach, garlic, tobasco sauce
Liver cleanser	Carrot, apple, beet, parsley
Gallstones	Lemon juice (include "limonene" from white pit)
Laxative	Lemon in hot water, first thing in morning
Electrolyte balance	Celery
Liver detox	Wheat grass
Antiinflammatory	Barley grass juice powder
Digestive	Pineapple, papaya
Arthritis	Wheat grass, all greens

Druglike Information

Warnings, Contraindications, and Precautions

AVOID JUICING

The following make great smoothies but are not juices. They are blended fruits. Juicing machines commonly separate the pulp from the water content of the fruit. However, in the fruits listed here, this is cannot be done. They are not concentrated and a pound of bananas, even if run through a juicer, still weighs and digests like a pound of bananas, only in liquid form. These smoothies do not share the same therapeutic benefits as concentrated juice extracts. Avoid the following fruits for juice therapy. You can still enjoy them simply as fruits.

- Papaya
- Honeydew
- Coconut
- Peach
- Banana
- Plum and prune
- Strawberry
- Apricot
- Cantaloupe
- Avocado

SWEETS

Patients with problems with low blood sugar, hypoglycemia, diabetes, candida, or other sugar-sensitive conditions should avoid sweet juices just as they avoid sweet foods. Cravings for carrot, orange, watermelon, grape, and other sweet juices often is an indication of a sugar-sensitive condition.

ALLERGIES AND OTHER SYMPTOMS

Please be aware of the following:

1. Choose organic fruits whenever possible because pesticide sprays can be fairly heavy on certain fruits, such as grapes.
2. Do not gorge yourself with juice just as you would not gorge yourself with food.
3. Do not be alarmed if a patient reports urine or stool discoloration from red (such as beet) or green (such as wheat grass) juices.
4. After extended intake of carrot juice, the skin (but not the sclera) can turn yellow or orange from excessive carotene intake. If this occurs, switch to green juices or reduce dosage.
5. Watch out for berries and other allergic fruits. Many people have allergies to berries. Be cautious: allergic foods also are allergic juices. Have patients monitor themselves for allergic reactions like itchy eyes or skin. The only exception is wheat grass. The grass blades have none of the allergic glutinous properties of the grain. Therefore an allergy to wheat does not automatically imply an allergy to wheatgrass.

Be aware of the symptoms of detoxification Be careful not to confuse elimination symptoms with allergic symptoms. People tend to eliminate in a manner resembling a flare of their chronic illnesses. Thus, those with tendencies to recurring skin rashes will likely have an aggravation of such symptoms on an intensive juice therapy program. This phenomenon is called *detoxification*, a release of internal residues triggered by a stimulus to the body to begin cleansing. An intensive release associated with intense symptoms is called a *healing reaction*.

However, patients who drink too much too soon with any of these potent juices may report an excitation of symptoms from too much detoxification. Reduce the dosage and frequency to ameliorate the symptoms but do not discontinue the program. Doctors must balance the rate of detoxification with the rate of elimination. Not all elimination is through the digestive tract. But colonotherapy or even enemas can accelerate the cleansing and reduce symptoms. Promote the use of other eliminative avenues, such as the lungs with aerobic exercise, the kidneys with drinking plenty of water, the skin through stimulation by sunlight, fresh air, bathing, and massage. This is not a painless process. Typically a lifetime of bad diet and lifestyle habits such as stress or smoke has generated these conditions. A certain amount of discomfort is part of the restorative process and can be expected.

Keep Juices Fresh Freshly made juices are highly perishable. Any contact with light, heat, and air, even at room temperature, starts the process of oxidation. It only is a matter of time before the delicious-tasting juice turns sour. The general rule is juice it and drink it. How-ever, cold storage and use of thermoses will extend the life of fresh juice.

Don't Forget Water! Juices make kidneys work. To give them a rest, drink water. Water is a superb solvent, flushing agent, and cleanser and contains natural electrolytes—the acids, bases, and salts that conduct our bioelectric current through our nervous system. Choose pure water from a pure water appliance such as a distiller or carbon block purifier.

Blenders and Bottles Blenders make purees, not juices. Because of their high speed, blenders tend to oxidize the juice, thereby devitalizing it. Also, avoid the temptation of bottled juices. They are boiled, sweet, flavored waters and are not alive with the nutrition you want.

Trade Products, Administration, and Dosage

TYPES OF JUICERS

Price and ease of use are the two foremost factors to consider when buying a juicing ma-chine. Clean-up and ease of use make all the difference in a patient's ability to continue the therapy. Regular use is the secret to success with juice therapy. Juicing only once per week because it is too inconvenient will not provide much benefit, even if the juicer is state-of-the-art.

All machines have to be assembled and disassembled for use. The centrifugal machines usually have a cutter blade, a clutch, bowl, and cover to remove and clean. They often come with disposable paper filters, similar to a coffee-maker, that make cleaning quite easy. The triturators have a cutter blade, screen, screen housing, and juicer body. In either case, about three or four parts will have to be rinsed to clean and reassemble the machines. For juicing more than half a gallon at a time, the pulp-ejector machines are slightly more ad-vantageous. This process expels the pulp continuously during the juicer operation. The other juicers collect the pulp in the spinning basket, which has to be emptied every 1 or 2 quarts. This is often not an issue unless the user wishes to juice large quantities.

MAJOR JUICER MANUFACTURERS

Although manufacturers are listed here many of the following juicers can be ordered through local health food stores:

Omega Juicer
PO Box 4523
Harrisburg, PA 17111
Tel: (800) 633-3401
Fax: (717) 561-1298

Manufactures fruit, vegetable, and wheatgrass juicers with centrifugal, twin gear, and pulp ejectors, in stainless steel and plastic; heavy duty models; 5 and 10-year warranties; made in the U.S.; citrus attachments. Basic juicer in $200 price range. Excellent customer service.

Miracle Exclusives, Inc.
64 Seaview Blvd.
Port Washington, NY 11050
Tel: (516) 621-3333
Toll-Free: (800) 645-6360
Fax: (516) 621-1997
E-mail: Miracle-exc@juno.com
http://www.miracleexclusives.com

Imports fruit, vegetable, and wheatgrass juicers with both centrifugal and pulp ejectors, light duty and heavy duty. All are clean, modern kitchen appliances imported from Europe and very affordable. Excellent customer service.

L'Equip
555 Bolser Ave.
Harrisburg, PA 17043.
Tel: (717) 730-7100
Toll-Free: (800) 816-6811
Fax: (717) 730-7200
E-mail: Jpascotti@aol.com

U.S. manufacturer of fruit, vegetable, and wheatgrass, pulp-ejecting juicers.

Champion Juicer
Plasteket Manufacturing
6220 E. Highway 12
Lodi, CA 95240
Tel: (209) 369-2154
Fax: (209) 369-2455

A large U.S. manufacturer of a triturator type pulp ejector juicer that is versatile. It also grinds nuts and seeds into nut butter, makes frozen fruit sherbet, grates vegetables; there is even an attachment for grinding grains into flour. Heavy duty. 5 year warranty. List price $250.

WHOLESALE JUICER DISTRIBUTORS

If you wish to provide juicers to your patients, you can order any of the previous machines, wholesale, one at a time, from the following distributors. This is only a small selection of the many quality distributors available:

Albion Enterprises
3233 Coffee Lane #H
Santa Rosa, CA 95403
Tel: (707) 528-1473
Toll-Free: (800) 248-1475
Fax: (707) 528-0608
www.albionjuicer.com

ACME Equipment
1024 Concert Ave.
Springhill, FL 34609
Tel: (352) 688-0157
Toll-Free: (800) 882-0157
Fax: (352) 683-7740

TJ Plus
5631 East Morning Star Rd.
Cave Creek, AZ 85331
Tel: (602) 488-7808
Toll-Free: (888) 243-6450
Fax: (602) 488-7895
E-mail: sales@juicebars.com
http://www.juicebars.com

Barriers and Key Issues

Fruits, vegetables, and grasses are not drugs. Natural products are not easily patented and because the costs of bringing a new product up for FDA approval is in the hundreds of millions of dollars, juice therapy simply remains out of the realm of commercial drugs and thus is relegated to home use and folk medicine. Nevertheless, nature is the original source of modern medicine. Pharmacopoeias of ancient Egypt, Babylonia, Greece, and China were based on food. The twelfth-century Jewish physician and philosopher Maimonides recommended chicken soup as a remedy for asthma. Garlic, mustard seed, and other herbs and spices were used medicinally for centuries. And what child doesn't know that "an apple a day keeps the doctor away." Many modern pharmaceutics actually are synthetic replications of botanic products. Quinine from the cinchona tree was the only remedy for malaria for more than 300 years. Penicillin, our first antibiotic, comes from mold. Aspirin is synthetic salicylic acid derived from the bark of the willow tree.

In spite of our high technology, researchers today still look to nature for ideas and synthesize natural compounds. If nature is the source of all these miraculous medicines, why has it not earned our confidence?

Suggested Reading

1. Meyerowitz S: *Juice fasting and detoxification: use the healing power of fresh juice to clean up and feel great,* Summertown, Tenn, 1999 Book Publishing.
   Fasting is easier than you think. Here is a step by step guide to the use of raw fruit and vegetable juices and other potent drinks while fasting for the purposes of detoxification. Some fasts are as short as 1 day.
2. Meyerowitz S: *Power juices, super drinks,* Summertown, Tenn, 2000 Book Publishing.
   A review of common health conditions with dietary suggestions and effective juice,

smoothie, and tea recipes. Also the latest research on the health benefits of 40 different fruits and vegetables. For other books by the author, visit him at www.Sproutman.com

3. Kordich J: *The Juiceman's power of juicing*, New York, 1994, Warner.
No one speaks about the healing power of fresh juices with as much zest as the Juiceman himself, Jay Kordich.

4. Calbom C, Keane M: *Juicing for life: a guide to the health benefits of fresh fruit and vegetables*, Garden City Park, NY, 1992.

5. Heinerman J: *Heinerman's encyclopedia of healing juices*, 1994, Prentice Hall.

Other Resources and Associations

Tree of Life Rejuvenation Center
Gabriel Cousens, MD
PO Box 1080
Patagonia, AZ 85624
Tel: (520) 394-2520 or (520) 394-2769
Fax: (520) 394-2099
www.treeofliferejuvenation.com
A medical doctor's holistic health center that includes juice therapy, wheatgrass, and fasting retreats.

Naples Institute for Optimum Health and Healing.
2335 Tamiami Trail N.
Naples, FL 34103
Tel: (941) 649-7551
Toll-Free: (800) 243-1148
Fax: (941) 262-4684
www.NaplesInstitute.com
A health resort that uses juice therapy.

Hippocrates Health Institute
1443 Palmdale Court
West Palm Beach, FL 33411
Tel: (561) 471-8876
Toll-Free: (800) 842-2125
www.hippocratesinst.com
A health resort that uses juice therapy.

Green Foods Corporation
320 North Graves Ave.
Oxnard, CA 93030
Tel: (800) 777-4430
Fax: (805) 983-8843
E-mail: gfc@greenfoods.com
www.greenfoods.com
Makers of *Green Magma* barley grass juice.

The Sprout House*
Tel: (760) 788-4800
Toll-Free: (800) SPROUTS
Fax: (760) 788-7979
E-mail: info@SproutHouse.com
www.SproutHouse.com
A source of professionally grown wheat grass for making fresh squeezed juice at home. Ships nationwide overnight. Also sells juicers, grass juicers, and sprouters

References

1. Szent-Gyoergyi A: *Living state and cancer,* Workshop of the National Foundation for Cancer Research and Marine Biological Lab, Woods Hole, Mass.

2. Rudolph T: *Chlorophyll, nature's green magic,* San Gabriel, Calif, 1957, Nutritional Research Publishing.

3. Lourou M, Lartigue O: The influence of diet on the biological effects produced by whole body irradiation, *Experientai* 6:25, 1950.

4. Colloway DH, Calhoun WK, Munson AH: *Further studies on reduction of X-irradiation of guinea pigs by plant materials,* Quartermaster Food and Container Institute for the Armed Forces Report N.R. 12-61, 1961.

5. Murata T et al: Effect of long-term administration of beta-carotene on lymphocyte subsets in humans, *Am J Clin Nutr* 60(4):597-602, 1994.

6. Gaziano JM: Antioxidant vitamins and cardiovascular disease, *Proc Assoc Am Physicians* 111(1):2-9, 1999.

7. Badamchian M et al: Isolation of a Vitamin E analog from a green barley leaf extract that stimulates release of prolactin and growth hormone from rat anterior pituitary cells in vitro, *J Nutr Biochem* 5:145-150, 1994.

8. Hagiwara Y: Effect on the several food additives, agricultural chemicals, and carcinogens. Presented to the 98th Annual Assembly of Pharmaceutical Society of Japan, April 5, 1978.

9. Osawa T et al: A novel antioxidant isolated from young green barley leaves, *Agri Food Chem* 40:1135-1138, 1992.

10. Hagiwara Y et al: Studies on the constituents of green juice from young barley leaves effect on dietary induced hypercholesterolemia in rats, *J Pharm Soc Jpn* 105(11), 1985.

11. Kubota K, Matsuoka Y, Seki H: Isolation of potent antiinflammatory protein from barley leaves by faculty of Pharmaceutical Sciences, Science Univ. of Tokyo, Japan, *Jpn J Inflammat* 3(4), 1983.

*This company is owned by the author.

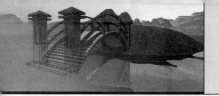

Iridology

HARRI WOLF*

Origins and History

Conventional medical diagnosis enables the doctor to analyze and determine the presence of certain diseases only when clinical signs and symptoms appear. *Iridology*, sometimes referred to as *iris diagnosis*, offers the practitioner a glimpse of certain problems or abnormalities occurring in the human body through indications shown in the iris of the eye long before the clinical symptoms of disease are manifest. To the iridologist, prevention of disease and the early detection of the risk for pathology are of paramount importance.

The iris, a multilayered membrane with a surface diameter of approximately 12 mm, is one of the most complex tissue structures of the human body. For the iridologist, this makes it an ideal microstructural analogue, or field, for preliminary analysis of a person's state of health, adaptive abilities, hereditary and congenital features. The results of a slit lamp examination of the iris can lead to the recommendation of a customized healthcare plan (diet regimen, nutrition, physical activity, therapeutics, and others) with the hope of preventing the physical expression of the disease process.

The first reference by a physician to iridology as a diagnostic procedure was made by Phillipus Meyens in his book, *Chiromatica Medica,* published in Dresden in 1670. He actually described a topography in which certain iris segments represented certain organs and tissue systems. The acknowledged founder of iridology in its present form was the Hungarian physician, Dr. Ignatz Von Peczely (1822-1911). In 1881 Von Peczely published *Discoveries in the Field of Natural Science and Medicine: Instruction in the Study of Diagnosis from the Eye.* In it he described a methodology he based on several decades of comparative study. Von Peczely was the first to teach that certain iridic phenomena were related to organic disease and that from the localization of such phenomena an observer can infer the localization of the disease. He mapped out the first iris topography in which every organ was represented in a corresponding iris *reaction field* (author's term).

Von Peczely's contemporary, the Swedish pastor Niels Liljequist, a talented naturopath, introduced a 284-page text and an atlas with 258 monochrome and 12 colored iris draw-

*The author would like to extend his heartfelt appreciation to the following: Justine Amadeo and Michael R.J. Roth for critique and editing; Jon Miles for his assistance with references, insights, and technical advice; Dr. Donald Novey for his editorial advice and encouragement; and Drs. Pierre Fragnay and Daniele Lo Rito for their insights and demographic contributions.

ings. Liljequist was recognized for his elaboration of iris topography in reference to the back, chest, and sexual organs.

The German Pastor Felke (d. 1926) had a major influence on iridology because of his development of compound homeopathy as a therapeutic methodology to address specific iris indications. This approach is very evident in iridology practice in Western Europe today. The Pastor Felke Institute, one of Germany's leading centers for iridologic research and education, stands as a monument to this pioneer.

Modern iridology bears the stamp of several Germans, notably Josef Angerer of Munich (d. 1994), who pioneered the analysis of the pupillary border, and Josef Deck of Ettlingen (d. 1989). Dr. Deck's two volumes, *Elements of Irisdiagnosis* and *Differentiation of the Iris Signs*, are recognized as the profession's standard texts throughout the world. Most modern European authors of iridology attended the courses in irisdiagnosis, which Dr. Deck conducted for decades in Ettlingen.

Bernard Jensen, a chiropractor from Escondido, California, is recognized as one of the leading proponents of iridology in the U.S. Up until the last decade, when European iridology gained prominence, he was basically the only source of training in this field in America. His teachings represent a mixture of turn-of-the-century notions about iris color (that their origin lies in exposure to chemicals such as arsenic, bismuth, lead, and others) and the toxemia-based interpretation and treatment of illness developed by Kellogg, Christopher, and numerous others in the "Natural Hygiene" schools of thought. By combining iris interpretation with natural food dietary regimens and detoxification procedures, Jensen made iridology practical as a clinical methodology. The main drawback to his approach was the suggestion that the iris can rapidly change in response to therapeutic treatment, a notion that has not yet been supported by any scientific evidence.

Meanwhile, the scientific observations of German, French, Russian, and Italian researchers in the past 50 years have led to detailed topographic mappings and a taxonomy of features that includes many correlations with disease processes.

Mechanism of Action According to Its Own Theory

Many health care practitioners believe that the body is always in touch with the environment through various "gates" or projection zones, such as the eyes, ears, nose, and mouth. In iridology, the projection zone (the iris) is used purely for a diagnosis that assumes a correspondence between different features of the iris and referred regions of the body. These features include the qualitative and quantitative properties of pigment distribution.

Most of the diagnostic field of the iris is ultra-fine human connective tissue. The numbers, shapes, composition, and location of lacunae, crypts, and trabeculae follow a unique pattern for each individual, much like the patterns of whorls in fingerprints. On the basis of the holistic principle, which states that each part of the body contains information about all other parts of the body, iridologists equate the microstructure (iris) with the unique constitutional dispositions and other properties of the macrostructure (body). Still at issue is the degree to which the iris is subdivided into reaction fields that correspond to particular organ and tissue systems, and the accuracy of the various maps developed over the past century (see the chart).

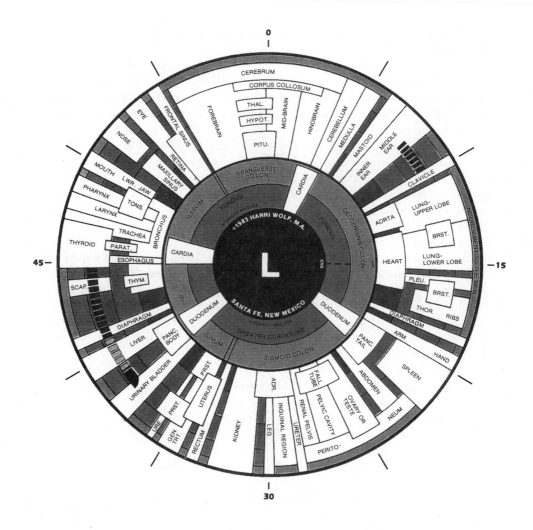

The structural correspondence between iris tissue and organ systems seems credible because of the fact that the iris is formed in the initial phase of embryonic development as part of the mid-brain. The question of how and why changes in the iris occur was first addressed by the neurologist Dr. Walter Lang of Heidelberg. Lang claimed that "iris topography corresponds to the anatomic subdivision of the sympathetic nervous system." His theory states that afferent autonomic nerve impulses from the various organs and tissues of the body reach the anterior thalamic nucleii of the mid-brain, which acts as a "filing cabinet" for information on all anatomic conditions. This information is then relayed to the muscles, stroma, and blood vessels of the irides.[1]

Typically, the iris starts out with a clear blue color. Throughout life, color is added to the iris through melanogenesis. It soon becomes some variation of brown in the more melanized individual or remains blue in the less melanized one. The color may be added in

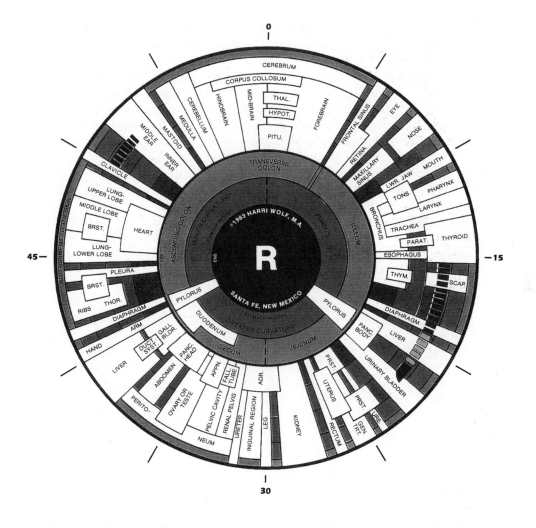

spots or in diffuse patterns and is cumulative. Iridologists assert that pigment deposits indicate that the body is in a defensive posture and that the color, density, and position of pigments may be clues to identifying pathogenesis and specific organ involvement. Ophthalmologists, on the other hand, consider colored spots to be no more significant than the freckles on an individual's face (ruling out the possibility of hemorrhagic pigment related to iris trauma or malignant melanoma).

E.S. Velchover of the Russian People's Friendship University studied more than 2000 people in clinics in Moscow and Alma Ata. He claims that pigment spots increased with age and with the development of different diseases. He observed no pigment patches in the irides of a majority of healthy children and asserts that every inflammatory, traumatic, toxic, or any other pathologic process accompanied by a pain syndrome influences the appearance and development of pigment spots in certain areas of the iris. He also concluded that, despite the fact that local pigmentation of the iris is connected topographically with certain pathology, the presence of pigmentation by itself does not reveal the inner character and mechanism of the disease.[2]

Russian researchers have more recently added a new vista in iris exploration by suggesting that the iris functions to protect the body from the energetic influence of light. The mechanism, though still conceptual and unproven, can be described as follows.

As a pathologic process develops, the pain impulses coming from the origin of dysfunction reach specific topographic chromatophores in the iris via the trigeminal-reticular centers. They then produce a spasm of local vessels, resulting in tissue hypoxia and nutritional disturbances. By analogy with cicatrization in myocardial infarction, the corresponding group of iris chromatophores turns into a distinctive, functionally inefficient, hyperpigmented patch. But such patches of pigmented melanoblasts, situated in the anterior border layer of the iris, act to protect the body from one of the most active energetic irritants of the environment (light), thus protecting the organs affected by the disease.

It also has been postulated that if an organ requires additional stimulation, a defect in the iris stroma is formed, allowing greater transmission of light.[3] This would support the belief that inherited organic weaknesses are represented by fibrous separation (rarefaction) and lacunae clusters in the iris stroma. These iris properties would allow light impulse to penetrate past the superficial iris stroma and follow the reverse pathway back to the organs needing it.

This rather revolutionary concept is exciting to proponents of iridology because it suggests that the iris is not simply a gauge but also an active exteroreceptor with a role to play in the healing process, bringing about the necessary condition of rest or stimulation of the weakened organs. Velchover,[2] Fragnay,[4] and Makarchuk[3] describe the use of lasers of varying color spectrum directed at certain iris projection zones to stimulate healing in the corresponding organ(s).

Biologic Mechanisms of Action

Genetics provides evidence of the holistic or holographic principle in many ways. Doctors routinely apply this principle when they examine the eyes to watch for systemic disease. Analysis of the microvasculature of the retina can yield important information about a person's circulatory system in much the same way as the iris stroma tells the iridologist about the body's mesenchyme.

Mainstream medicine unknowingly has been using one aspect of iridology for years by observing the cornea. A predominant feature of Wilson's disease, a disorder of copper metabolism, is the Kayser-Fleischer ring of the peripheral cornea. Rouhuainen et al[5] demonstrated that old age and high low-density lipoprotein (LDL) cholesterol concentration were associated with the presence of corneal arcus. Pe'er et al[6] showed that the corneal arcus is more frequent in men and the positive correlation between the size of corneal arcus and the levels of cholesterol and LDL in men. Iridologists have long recognized the significance of the corneal arcus in relation to hyperlipidemia and its accompanying cardiac risk. In fact, the corneal arcus, although not really an iris sign, is the leading indicator of the lipemic diathesis, an iris constitutional subtype classified by Deck.[7]

Forms of Therapy

There are several interpretive models under different names employed by iridologists around the world. Most often the word *iridology* is included as part of the name. These include *constitutional iridology* (emphasizing the German approach) and *medical iridology* (used by doctors in Italy and France to set them apart from nonmedical practitioners). The primary emphasis in these European approaches is to identify constitutional types and various pathologic dispositions based on iris structure, morphology, and overall pigment distribution.

Each model was developed to work in conjunction with a particular therapeutic principle. Naturopaths might use constitutional iridology because it is congruent with their therapeutic approaches, which include phytotherapy (herbalism) and nutrition. Homeopaths, who also are concerned with the psychologic characteristics of their patients, might use it along with one of several psychosomatic approaches. Applied Iridology is the name given to an approach that incorporates several interpretive models, physical and psychologic, for application in conjunction with a variety of therapies, both traditional and complementary.

Demographics

There may be as many as 10,000 iridologists in the U.S. and Canada, but only about 150 have completed training in the European approach and are either self-employed as clinicians or serve as consultants in chiropractic, naturopathic, acupuncture, and medical clinics with a holistic and preventive orientation. The rest attended home-study courses and seminars in the so-called Jensonian model (named after B. Jensen), are generally self-employed, and use iridology in conjunction with herbal, dietary, detoxification, and vitamin therapy.

Pierre Fragnay, MD, president of the French Iridology Association, puts the number of qualified iridologists in Western Europe at about 1500, with an average of 20% in conventional medical practice. The rest are naturopaths, herbalists, nutritionists, acupuncturists, homeopaths, and physical therapists. Daniele Lo Rito, MD, the scientific director of the Italian Iridology Association, estimates the number of medical iridologists in Europe at about 500. In Russia, where only medical doctors are certified as iridologists, the number of practitioners is estimated at 5000.[3] There are very few medical doctors practicing iridology in the U.S. Of these, most received their medical and iridologic education in Western Europe or Russia.

Most practitioners agree that the majority of iridology patients are between 35 and 65 years of age and are seeking ways to prevent the onset of disease, are interested in identifying underlying sources of physical discomfort, or are referred by a primary care practitioner. Patients who seek the help of an iridologist tend to want to have control and be responsible for their own health care.

The author is unaware of any studies describing the demographics of iridology patients.

Indications and Reasons for Referral

Iridology is preeminently suited for identifying genetic weaknesses and functional problems after the onset of symptoms but before the onset of defining physical, laboratory, or radiographic signs. For instance, a person complaining of fatigue, low back pain, and mental dullness may have negative laboratory and radiographic findings, whereas an iridology exam might reveal functional (preclinical) problems in the liver and intestines that are leading to autointoxication. A detoxification regimen followed by nutritional support then would be recommended to alleviate the patient's symptoms.

Sometimes the iridologist may discover indications of a potential problem and recommend further investigation through a different modality, such as applied kinesiology, Chinese pulse diagnosis, or a medical diagnostic procedure. For example, in this case the iridologist also may notice markings associated with a strong disposition to tissue change in the genital tract and recommend a visit to the gynecologist to rule out an insidious disorder.

Before selecting a pharmaceutic protocol, the doctor might want to consult an iridologist to identify inherent weaknesses so that adverse drug reactions can be avoided. For example, if known possible side effects to a particular drug are nausea and vomiting, it would be valuable to know if the stomach lining of the patient is vulnerable.

Iridology has shown itself to be most helpful in the area of gastrointestinal and associated dysfunction (liver, gallbladder, pancreas). It is an excellent source of information for the doctor who recognizes the importance of promoting a healthy gastrointestinal environment and proper digestive function to avoid the onset of disease.

Research Base

In addition to the studies cited previously,[1,2,7] there have been a number of papers published in peer-review journals that describe studies revolving around iris diagnosis, including those by Whitling,[8] Berdonces,[9] Steutzer,[10] Bjornsen,[11] and Allen and Wolf.[12] Medical recognition of the usefulness of iris examination has been published in the *Archives of Neurology* by Gladstone[13] and the *American Journal of Ophthalmology* by Holz et al.[14] Other references are found in "Suggested Reading."

Evidence Based

Several studies published in medical journals concluded that iridology is not a useful diagnostic aid.[15,16] Iridologists criticized these studies on the following grounds:

1. Iris exams are best performed in vivo using specialized microscopes. The participating iridologists should have rejected interpretations by photographic images, most of poor quality.
2. Iridology does not claim to see either the presence of gallstones (Knipshild) or the elevation of creatinine in the urine because of kidney malfunction (Simonet al). It is concerned with the unique components of a person's constitution that, when combined with other intrinsic and extrinsic factors, may lead to gallstones or kidney

disease. Therefore it appears that the iridologists, in their zeal, and the medical screeners, in their bias, were testing iridology on the wrong merits and suppositions.

Iridologists scored better in a study by H.D. Whitling.[8] Although accepting the restrictions of a limited study sample, the researchers concluded that the data suggested a possible ability for iridology to assess specific organ involvement in chronically ill individuals.

The burden of proof to support the effectiveness, usefulness, and importance of iridology is, of course, on the iridologists. Studies are needed in the natural history of iris color change throughout life. Also, a base line must be established through population studies in all areas of the world to develop demographic and epidemiologic profiles of color and texture distribution. Finally, there must be unbiased examination of clinical correlates from the empiric data.

Druglike Information

Trade Products

Iridology has benefited greatly from developments in photographic and digital technology. Most medical iridologists in Europe use a specialized microscope called an *iridoscope* or a slit lamp with a camera attachment. Most slit lamp manufacturers provide the necessary accessories for iris photography (Zeiss, Kodac, Kowa, and others). Expanded Enterprises of Tustin, California pioneered iris photography and, through its affiliation with Dr. Bernard Jensen, became the leading manufacturer of specialized iris cameras. Lena Medical Photo, formerly of Laguna Beach, California, produced the forerunner in hand-held iris cameras. Recently, Polaroid introduced an instant camera, the Polaroid Macro 5 SLR, which even comes with instructions specifically written for iris photo application.

Miles Research of Poway, California has been developing instruments for digital photography and analytical software for years. It also is setting up groupware systems for collaborative work in both clinic and laboratory. Various companies that sell iridology instruments, books, charts, and related materials are listed as follows.

TRADE PRODUCT SELLERS AND MANUFACTURERS

Expanded Enterprises (cameras, digital cameras, and software)
235 South A St.
Tustin, CA 92780
Tel: (714) 921-1548
Fax: (714) 544-9614
E-mail: eyecam7@aol.com
http://eyecamera.com

Iridology Educational Services (books and charts)
PO Box 31013
Seattle, WA 98103
Tel: (206) 282-6604

MD Jones Enterprises (books, charts, and Polaroid iris photo systems)
27672 E. Tomball Pkwy
Tomball, TX 77375
Tel: (281) 351-4372
E-mail: MDJones@iridology.com

Miles Research (digital cameras, computerized analysis systems, and software)
15045 Eastvale Rd.
Poway, CA 92064
Tel: (619) 679-8505
Fax: (619) 679-4955
E-mail: jon@memoryplace.com
www.milesresearch.com

Natural Books and Products (books and charts)
1718 E. Valley Pkwy
Escondido, CA 92027
Tel: (888) 743-1790

Wolf & Associates* (books, charts, and instructional videos)
1278 Glenneyre #153
Laguna Beach, CA 92652
Tel: (888) 886-8985
Fax: (949) 362-4959
E-mail: Bobbarobba@aol.com

Visiting a Professional

Upon entering an iridologist's office, a patient might notice an array of wall charts depicting various mappings of iris topography. There also will be credentials and professional licenses on display. The patient is directed to a chair and asked to fill out a form that inventories past personal and family medical history, current symptoms, dietary and exercise habits, and social, psychologic, familial, and occupational stresses. Following a review of the form, the practitioner directs the patient to the examination area.

The iridologist normally examines the iris by direct view with an illuminated magnifier or, in the case of a European-style practitioner, a slit lamp. Often photographic images are acquired using a specially designed iris camera. These then are stored in a patient's file for reference. The iris textural and chromatic features are inspected and analyzed using one or several interpretive models. Predispositions and somatic and psychologic constitutional factors that are evident from the iris patterns are noted and considered to design a customized therapeutic protocol. If the iridologist is employed as a consultant, the interpretation is forwarded to the primary care physician for subsequent health planning.

---

*This company is owned by the author.

What to Look for in a Professional

The referring physician should be certain that the iridologist is certified by the International Iridology Research Association or the Institute for Applied Iridology.

In choosing an iridologist, it is important to seek out the qualities expected of any health care professional, including professional attire and manner, professional office environment and hygienic examination area, and a detailed explanation of the procedure and the findings.

Credentialing

There is no city, state, or federal licensing for iridologists in the U.S. Some lay iridologists have been prosecuted under state laws for unlicensed medical practice because the act of diagnosis, in many states, requires physician licensure. The definition of physician also varies from state to state and, in some states, includes naturopathic physician.

Training

In Europe, iridology is included in the curriculum at naturopathic medical colleges as a diagnostic modality. These same schools offer iridology training as part of continuing education (CE) for physicians and usually award a diploma in medical iridology to graduates upon completion of an oral and written examination. Practitioners generally practice under licenses to diagnose granted by city or national governments.

In the U.S., courses leading to certification in Applied Iridology are offered by the Institute for Applied Iridology (IAI), directed by the author, which also has a European chapter based in Urbino, Italy. Classes, taught by a variety of instructors, are held at regional centers throughout the U.S. and usually take place over the course of several weekends (72 hours). Because Applied Iridology is an open system into which many therapeutic modalities can be incorporated, the IAI attracts many licensed or certified health care providers who have fulfilled the prerequisite requirements, including courses in anatomy, physiology, and pathology. Certificates are awarded upon completion of a written examination and an oral presentation before a faculty panel, several of whom are both physicians and iridologists.

The International Iridology Research Association (IIRA) has been promoting European iridology in the U.S. since its inception in 1981. Most of its members are certified in one of the alternative health care modalities, which include herbology, nutrition, massage therapy, chiropractic, and naturopathic medicine. The John Bastyr College of Naturopathic Medicine in Seattle, Washington offers an elective course in iridology for students enrolled in its 4-year naturopathy program. Various other organizations offer training in iridology, principally in the form of home-study courses, but generally do not meet the standards set by the European schools, IAI, or NIRA. Some of the leading manufacturers of herbal combination formulas, especially multi-level marketing companies, offer weekend seminars in iridology and urge its use to identify problems that might be addressed by particular formulas. This practice, so prevalent in the U.S., is frowned upon by many professionals who see a conflict of interest that could lead such practitioners to overdiagnose to sell more products.

Institute for Applied Iridology* (IAI)
PO Box 301
Laguna Beach, CA 92652
Tel: (888) 886-8985
E-mail: wolf1angel@aol.com
www.AppliedIridology.com

College of Herbs and Natural Healing
16 England's Lane
Primrose Hill
London NW34TG
E-mail: Collherb@hotmail.com

Advanced Iridology Research
The Natural Healing Centre
55 Beverly Rd.
Hull, East Yorkshire
England HU37XL
E-mail: Johnherbal@hotmail.com

Barriers and Key Issues

In the U.S., iridology generally has been used by amateurs lacking any serious background in health care or health education and little, if any, background in anatomy, physiology, and the basics of pathology. Many received their "certifications" following attendance at a single weekend seminar. As a result the field became cluttered with anecdotal information, erroneous and outdated beliefs, and oversimplification. A lack of scientific and professional conduct, sometimes bordering on fanaticism and arrogance, has contributed to the perception of iridology as little more than gazing into a crystal ball or interpreting the bumps on the head (phrenology).

Because orthodox medicine does not value phenomena that are too subtle to detect with instrumentation, it has trouble accepting the concept of information referral through the autonomic nervous system, acupuncture meridians, and other hypothesized energy pathways throughout the body. It also has difficulty with the idea that health status can be indicated in patterns appearing in the iris, or for that matter, any other part of the body (such as the ear, tongue, or feet) that has a corresponding mapping relationship to the whole body.

The status of iridology will rise if more scientific workers turn their attention to it and insist on carrying out rigorous research. Protocols and standards in methodology and technology must be established and fostered by the recruitment of biomedical experts who can provide the necessary technical resources.

---

*The author is director of this school.

Associations

Only those associations that correspond in the English language are listed.

Canadian Neuroptic Institute
2078 Wascana
Regina, SK
S4T-4J7 Canada
E-mail: techsupp@cnri.edu
http://www.neuroptic.com

Iridologists International
24360 Old Wagon Rd.
Escondido, CA 92027

International Iridology Research Association (IIRA)
William Fullerton, PhD
PO Box 1442
Solana Beach, CA 92075
Tel: (888) 682-2208

The European Society of Iridologists Ltd (UK)
Bournemouth, UK
E-mail: iridology@iridology.co.uk
http://www.iridology.co.uk/

Suggested Reading

1. Deck J: *Elements of irisdiagnosis* (translated from German), Ettlingen/Karlsruhe, Germany, 1965, Institute for Fundamental Research in Iris Diagnosis.
   This standard text in European schools describes the principle constitutional types and subtypes as well as the meanings of common iris markings and pigmentations.
2. Deck J: *Differentiation of iris markings* (translated from German), Ettlingen/Karlsruhe, Germany, 1980, Institute for Fundamental Research in Iris Diagnosis.
   This also is a standard text in European schools. The emphasis of this text is on the interpretation and differentiation of iris signs within the context of correct identification of constitutional predispositions. It contains excellent photos and illustrations.
3. Kriege T: *Fundamental basis of irisdiagnosis* (translated from German), Romford, Essex, 1969, L.N. Fowler.
   This is an excellent introduction to the German style of iridology. Consideration is given to specific organ and tissue system problems and their common iris indications. Black and white iris photos are used to illustrate case studies.
4. Wolf H: *The iris and the constitution*, Laguna Beach, Calif, 1997, Wolf & Associates.
   Although recognizing the importance of Deck's constitutional typing system as the center point for European iridology, this workbook also offers a glimpse at common variations in constitutional typing as derived from the author's clinical experience. Color photos demonstrate common iris patterns associated with various constitutional traits.

5. Wolf H: *Iris instructional analysis, V 1-4*, Laguna Beach, Calif, 1996, Wolf & Associates.
This set of four workbooks, with 80 accompanying iris slides, was designed to show the correlation between iris indications and the medical histories of patients. Volume 1 is fairly general; Volume 2 emphasizes digestive disorders; Volume 3 focuses on cardiac and circulatory problems; and Volume 4 highlights the criteria used for selecting the iris signs most relevant to the case at hand.

Bibliography

Angerer J: *Handbook of irisdiagnosis*, Saulgan, Germany, 1953, Haug.

Deck J: *Fundamentals of irisdiagnosis*, Ettlingen/Karlsruhe, Germany, 1965, Institute for Fundamental Research in Iris Diagnosis.

Jensen B: *The science and practice of iridology*, Escondido, Calif, 1952, Jensen's Nutritional and Health Products.

Liljequist P: *Om Irisdiagnostik* (in German only), Leipzig, Germany, 1897, Kruger.

Makarchuk IY: Modern aspects of iridoreflexology, *Bexel Medical News*, Seoul, South Korea, Dec. 1996.

Newsome D, Lowenfeld I: Iris mechanics II, influence of pupil size on details of iris structure, *Am J Ophthalmol* 71(2):553-573, 1971.

Peczely I: *Discoveries in the field of natural science and medicine: instruction in the study of diagnosis from the eye*, Budapest, 1880, KgL.

Velchover ES, Romashov FN: *Opportunities and errors in iridology*, Laguna Beach, Calif, 1992, IAI.

Velchover ES: The basis of computer irisdiagnostics, *Bexel Medical News*, Seoul, South Korea, 1996.

Velchover ES, Damurrina IN: Iridosomatic relationship, *Bexel Medical News*, Seoul, South Korea, June, 1997.

References

1. Lang W: *The anatomical and physiological basis for eyediagnosis* (in Germany only), Ulm, Germany, 1954, Haug Verlag.

2. Velchover ES: *Iridiagnostika* (in Russian only), Moscow, 1988, Meditchina.

3. Makarchuk IY: Examination of the influence and application of a spectral beam on patients' irides, *Bexel Medical News*, Seoul, South Korea, 1997.

4. Fragnay P: *Curing with color* (in Italian and French only), Lyon, 1998, International School of Chromo-Reflexology.

5. Rouhiainen P et al: Association of corneal arcus with ultrasonographically assessed arterial wall thickness and serum lipids, *Cornea* 12(2):142-145, 1993.

6. Pe'er J et al: Association between corneal arcus and some of the risk factors for coronary artery disease, *Br J Ophthalmol* 67(12):795-798, 1983.

7. Deck J, Vida F: *Clinical evidence of organ and disease signs in the iris* (in Germany only), Ulm, Germany, 1954, Haug.

8. Whitling HD: *An evaluation of iridology as an assessment tool for nurse clinicians*, Rochester, New York, 1981, School of Nursing, University of Rochester.

9. Berdonces JL: An iridologic study of hospitalized respiratory patients (a proposal for the use of the statistical method in iridology), *Iridol Rev* 2(1), 1988.

10. Stuetzer PH: Iris constitutions: iridology and the detection of precancerous conditions, *Iridol Rev* 1(1), 1987.

11. Bjornsen NL: Correlation between human iris patterns and certain physiological conditions (abstract), *Iridol Rev* 2(1), 1988.

12. Allen MD, Wolf H: Correlating applied iridology and applied kinesiological findings, *International College of Applied Kinesiology (ICAK) Collected Papers*, Jan:1, 1979.

13. Gladstone R: Development and significance of heterochromia of the iris, *Arch Neurol* 21 (Aug):184-191, 1969.

14. Holz FG et al: Pigmentation as a risk factor for age-related macular degeneration, *Am J Ophthalmol* 117:19-23, 1994.

15. Simon A, Worthen DM, Mitas JA: An evaluation of iridology, *JAMA* 242(13):1385-1389, 1979.

16. Knipschild P: Looking for gall bladder disease in the patient's iris, *BMJ* 297(6663):1578-1581, 1988.

Quartz Crystal Therapy

EILEEN NAUMAN

Origins and History

Quartz is one of the two most common chemical elements in the earth's crust. Quartz has the chemical formula SiO_2 and is the second most abundant mineral after feldspar. Quartz comes in many varieties. Sometimes minor impurities, such as lithium, sodium, potassium, and titanium may be present.

On a more personal, metaphysical, and spiritual level, the use of crystals, according to Native American heritage, is one of the oldest healing forms on earth. The medicine woman Oh Shinnah Fast Wolf, of Apache and Mohawk lineage, is considered one of the best teachers regarding crystals and gem healing therapy. How a quartz crystal is used on an energetic and catalytic spiritual level is based on the training the person has received. Some people are taught how to use them based on a (Native American) lineage handed down from generation to generation. Others follow their own intuition to begin working with them. Still others work in a more pseudoscientific manner to use them as a catalyst for a healing. The individual may be self-taught or attend a school, workshop, or seminar to garner information on how to use quartz crystal.

Mechanism of Action According to Its Own Theory

From a Native American perspective it is believed that all things, animate and inanimate, contain energy. Each one has the capacity to heal us, providing the organism wants to share it with us. All humans have an energy system. When a gem works *with* a person, there is a definite energy exchange. The quartz crystal then becomes a catalyst, energetically speaking, of triggering this cascade of changes throughout the person on every level simultaneously or in a hierarchy of cure: spirit, mind, emotional, and physical. Quartz crystal works on this premise, stimulating the body to heal itself from an energetic level.

Biologic Mechanism of Action

The biologic mechanism of action is unknown at this time.

Demographics

Crystal facilitators diverge in their belief systems. There is no governing body or board that an individual can access for such information. Nor is there a single comprehensive directory from which to obtain that information. Various ways to find a crystal facilitator are to contact an author who has written a book on quartz crystal healing, go to a New Age bookstore, or search the Internet.

Individuals who are metaphysically or more spiritually inclined and understand the connection between their aura and all things surrounding them are more inclined to think of using crystal therapy. Those individuals who do not want to use conventional drugs or those who try to reduce their drugs are open to this therapy. Those who love stones (rocks) in general are very drawn to considering the use of quartz crystal as a treatment. Where there is a passion for stones or gems, there is almost always a passion for using quartz crystal therapy.

Forms of Therapy

Crystal therapy is as varied as the training of the crystal facilitator. Generally, a six-sided crystal is used. But some people prefer the Marcel Vogel four-sided crystal for a healing session. There are many different rituals (a *ritual* is something created in the moment) and ceremonies (a *ceremony* is something that has been handed down through the generations, such as a Native American word-of-mouth practice or oral tradition). The ritual or ceremony that is being used is predicated on the crystal therapist who is using it. No one method is superior for crystal therapy.

Some crystal facilitators use colored rough or tumbled stones along with crystal healing. Many times, colored gemstones or colored crystals are placed on the front of the person who is lying in a prone position, and each gemstone or crystal is placed over a major *chakra* (an energy station equivalent to an electric substation) such as the brow, throat, heart, stomach, or abdomen region. For the head, the stone is usually placed a few inches from the skull. For the root chakra, which is at the base of the spine, a gemstone is placed on the lower abdominal area. At other times, colored stones or crystals may be placed in a specific pattern around the individual while the work is being done. Again, it does not matter which way is used. In the author's opinion, all ways and methods of quartz crystal therapy are equally effective.

Depending on training and heritage, different techniques are used. In a Native American approach, *smudging* may be employed before or after a session. Singing (tone) or a drum or rattle may be used. The drum promotes mental relaxation. A rattle is used to break up energy blocks in the aura. The crystal is used to attract the debris left in the wake of the rattle, which acts like a hammer smashing into a glass. One or more songs may be sung. Certain music may be played during the session. Again, all methods are equally effective. A crystal session may last from 5 minutes to several hours, depending on the practitioner, the style of healing used, the problems the patient has, and how long it takes to clear the energy (auric) field of these blocks and debris. Each crystal therapist has a personal style and training.

Indications and Reasons for Referral

Quartz crystal therapy has a value in almost all clinical situations. It can be very effective in acute conditions such as colds, flu, and soft tissue trauma. Crystal should be considered in all patients who have a chronic condition in which expensive treatments and long-term management of medications and therapy is required. Many patients with cases of arthritis, stress-related diseases, immunosuppression, fatigue, and gastrointestinal disorders should be considered for quartz crystal therapy. Although many patients can reduce or eliminate many of their medications after crystal treatment, it is not realistic to expect a cure in all cases. Crystal therapy should be viewed as an adjunct in the management of these conditions.

Quartz crystals can address spiritual, mental, emotional, and physical problems. They are destressors and strongly support the immune system. Patients who are highly sensitive to conventional medications and experience side effects are frequently often attracted to the use of crystals. Users of crystals tend to be individuals with a belief that "things from nature" can heal them. The warmth, attention, and genuine care of the crystal facilitator helps to open the healing process for the patient.

Office Applications

A simple ranking of conditions responsive to this form of therapy is as follows. As with all alternative therapies, the use of quartz crystal therapy does not preclude the use of mainstream medical therapies in addition.

Top level: *A therapy ideally suited for these conditions*
Stress

Second level: *One of the better therapies for these conditions*
Radiographic radiation exposure

Third level: *A valuable adjunctive therapy for these conditions*
Arthritis; back pain; colds; colitis; headache; lung problems; migraine headaches; nerves; nervousness; neurologic corrections; pain; rheumatism; sciatica; tendonitis; and wound healing

Practical Applications

Many individuals appreciate being taught how to use the crystal so that they can continue to perform daily therapy on themselves on an as-needed basis. This puts an element of healing and control back into the individual person's hands, which always aids the healing process.

Research Base

Evidence Based

No formal research exists on crystal healing. The following are examples of unstructured and uncontrolled experiments involving the use of crystals. The results have been assessed subjectively in many cases. The terminology of these experiments shows the energy realm in which crystals are purported to operate. However, they suggest that the presence of crystals affects their environment.

1. In 1985 the West Coast Conference of the American Society of Dowsers at the University of California in Santa Cruz drank regular and crystal-charged water. Crystal-charged water is made by placing a quartz crystal in water overnight, then removing the crystal and either drinking or using the charged water in some way. A test of each subject's energy fields using dowsing rods was taken beforehand. The fields on the test subjects were detected 12 inches from the body. A drink from regular water show little change after 1 minute. Drinking the crystal-charged water showed a dramatic change in the energy field. The detectable field expanded to 15 feet or more only 45 seconds after drinking the charged water.

2. Two saucers with seeds to sprout were used. One saucer contained plain water. The second saucer's water was charged with a 2-inch clear quartz crystal inside a 1-gallon jug for 24 hours. The charged water's seeds sprouted 1 day earlier with a deeper green color and grew to twice the height as the seeds in the regular saucer.

3. Two roses were cut and placed in separate vases, one with plain water and one with crystal-charged water. The rose in plain water wilted in 5 days. The one in charged water lasted 21 days.

4. Crystal slices placed under milk cartons showed an average spoilage time of 27 days instead of the normal 7 to 10 days.

5. Crystals placed in a swimming pool or spa seem to inhibit algae growth and decrease the need for chemicals.

6. At a booth at the New York State Fair in 1980, Dael Walker tested peoples' ability to heal themselves. A total of 234 people attempted the test of holding a quartz crystal over an area of claimed physical pain or stiffness. Of these, 227 said they had significant reduction in pain or stiffness.

Efficacy

The person must be willing to work on root causes of the problem. If not, then crystal treatment will only be a temporary and not permanent solution to their symptoms. If the person is willing to work on the deeper issues, the core issue, then crystal healing will be 50% efficient. If not, there will be minor improvement or temporary improvement, and then symptoms will reappear.

Future Research Opportunities and Priorities

Some valuable studies for this type of therapy would include the following areas: 1) research to show the effectiveness of crystal in alleviating pain in an individual person; and 2) a test to show the ways in which quartz crystal therapy acts to alleviate or reduce stress in an individual person.

Druglike Information

Safety

Crystals can only work to put something back into harmony or balance; they will not imbalance.

Drug or Other Interactions

No illnesses or medical conditions are able to render quartz crystal therapy ineffective to the individual user.

Adverse Reactions

General response to a quartz crystal healing is that the person feels better and more in balance. Sometimes during the therapy the person will have a release of emotions, usually crying, although there can be contact with a great sense of euphoria and joy. There can be physical reactions after crystal therapy, such as nausea or vomiting. Headache and skin rashes also can occur. After such a reaction, which may last 1 or 2 days, there often is a feeling or sensation of more calm or peacefulness. Some report an increase in energy and productivity after a crystal healing session. Food habits and cravings also may change to healthier ones.

Trade Products, Administration, and Dosage

There is no labeling involved with crystal healing. A major healing usually is performed once per week. For acute conditions and symptoms, the crystal may be used every 15 minutes until relief is obtained.

Self-Help versus Professional

All people, with a little training, can use crystals on themselves. Crystals often are used on people, animals, and plants. Crystals can be used safely for acute ailments and conditions. However, other types of medical therapy also may be needed, depending on the severity of the problem. In cases of chronic disease, the services of a crystal facilitator are advisable.

Visiting a Professional

For both acute and chronic cases, a past and present medical history form is filled out. The time taken with a patient is between 1 and 1.5 hours. Case-taking usually consists of a patient sitting in the office with the facilitator. In brief, an "aura assessment" is performed and the hot and cold or textured spots in the energy field are noted on the form. If the practitioner is unable to see the aura, an assessment may be made on the basis of symptoms. The crystal healing is continued until the patient no longer has any symptoms of the chief complaint remaining.

This information shared here is only *one* way to conduct a crystal healing; there are many other ways and methods. All of them work. The tradition in which the crystal facilitator is trained will dictate that framework. The following method comes through training with Oh Shinnah Fast Wolf, an Apache medicine woman. It is *not* the only crystal method of healing; there are many that cannot be mentioned here because of lack of space. Routinely, smudging or incense is involved and a feather (or hand) is used, as well as New Age or drum music being played.

1. A candle is lit before a crystal healing session. This symbolizes light and protection for the facilitator and patient. The patient sits on a stool in the center of a room, if possible. If patients are too sick to sit up, then they are treated from their bed.

2. *Smudging* involves the smoke from sage (or possibly incense) being wafted across the patient to "cleanse" the aura in preparation for the crystal healing.

3. The patient is asked to take as deep a breath as possible into the abdomen and to release that breath through the mouth. This is done three times.

4. An aura assessment is then taken. With the palms, the practitioner begins about 1 foot above the head and feels the energy emanating from the aura. Normal field energy is not hot or cold; nor is it textured. When slowly bringing the palms down over the center of the head, the practitioner will run into resistance, which will feel like touching an invisible top of a balloon. This often is felt physically. This is where the crystal healing will take place.

5. The crystal being used is then *programmed*.

6. The facilitator will sometimes choose a second colored gemstone (usually faceted or tumbled, but sometimes rough) and place it in the patient's left hand for the duration of the healing.

7. Facilitators "ground" themselves before the healing.

8. The facilitator then visualizes a white or gold "bubble" of protection over them.

9. The tip of the crystal is held about 6 inches from the patient's physical body. The facilitator then refers to the diagram and begins to execute a crystal healing. No area worked on in the energy field is left open or disturbed after a crystal has been used in it. Instead, each area is smoothed back down. This is called *unruffling the fields*. The smudge stick is lit once more, and the person is smudged again.

10. The facilitator then takes the stone from the patient's left hand. The facilitator then runs the hands, palms open and toward the patient, to feel and assess the areas

cleansed by the quartz crystal. There should be no sensation of hot or cold and no texture. The treated area should feel the same temperature as the person's aura in general and feel very smooth. If this occurs, then the crystal healing was a success.

Credentialing

There is no single, governing body for crystal healing in the United States. A crystal facilitator's qualifications may best be judged by a list of references, many years of practice, and the addition of formal medical training to assist in differentiating emergency from non-emergency medical conditions.

Training

There is no organized quartz crystal schooling in the U.S. There certainly are many workshops or seminars offered but not from one main source. Authors of books on the subject also serve as excellent contacts. At this point in time, a search of the Internet may be the best way to locate individuals familiar with crystal therapy. There is one school among them:

Crystal Awareness Institute
c/o The Energy Medicine Association
PO Box 5287
Kingwood, TX 77325
Tel: (281) 510-3972
http://www.energymedicineassn.com/dael/

The following is additional international information derived from the Internet that does offer some kind of schooling in crystal healing:

The Isle of Avalon Foundation (school)
2-4 High St., Glastonbury
BA6 9DU, Somerset, Great Britain.
Tel: 44 (0)1458 833933/831518
Fax: 44 (0)1458 831324
E-mail: ioaf@glastonbury.co.uk
http://www.glastonbury.co.uk/whatson/crystal-healing.htm

In Harmony Traders (workshop)
20 Palm St.
Cooya Beach, North Queensland, 4871, Australia
Tel: 61 18 18 7679
Fax: 61 70 98 2031
E-mail: newage1@ozemail.com.au
http://www.ozemail.com.au/~harmony8/crystal.html

Aesclepius (correspondence course)
PO Box 5944
Asheville, NC 28813
E-mail: asclepus@netcomuk.co.uk
http://www.netcomuk.co.uk/~asclepus/crystal_healing_correspondence.htm

What to Look for in a Provider

The best way to determine if a crystal facilitator is good is through a list of patient referrals. Has the facilitator published any articles or books? Does the facilitator conduct workshops or seminars? From a human point of view, does the facilitator's manner promote trust between the patient and facilitator? Does the facilitator demonstrate care and interest? (Please see "Credentialing.")

Barriers and Key Issues

An awareness of this modality is a position that few health professionals have a chance to acquire. One recommended approach is to invite crystal facilitators to speak and give case histories to acquaint health practitioners with the methodology.

Associations

The International Association of Crystal Healing Therapists (IACHT) was established 1986. The IACHT is a member of the Association of Crystal Healing Organizations (ACHO) and the British Complementary Medicine Association (BCMA). It was formed to promote the use of crystals for healing and self-realization.

IACHT
PO Box 344
Manchester M602EZ UK
Tel: (44) (0)161 702 8191
Fax: (44) (0)161 799 6420
E-mail: info@iacht.co.uk
http://www.iacht.co.uk/index.htm

Crystal Facilitators Directory:
http://www.netcomuk.co.uk/~asclepus/chusa.htm

Suggested Reading

1. Milewski JV, Harford VL: *The crystal sourcebook: from science to metaphysics,* Santa Fe, 1987, Mystic Crystal Publications.

2. Nauman E, Gent R: *Crystals and colored stones*, Cottonwood, Ariz, 1988, Blue Turtle.
3. Raphaell K: *Crystal enlightenment: the transforming properties of crystals and healing stones*, vol 1, New York, 1985, Aurora Press.
4. Walker D: *The crystal healing book*, Pacheco, Calif, 1988, The Crystal Company.

Internet Resources

1. http://www.crystalinks.com/crys.html
2. http://www.crystalinks.com/chakra_balancing.html

Reflexology

DONALD A. BISSON

Origins and History

Reflexology is a focused pressure technique, usually directed at the feet or hands. It is based on the premise that zones or reflex areas exist in the hands or feet that correspond to all organs, glands, and systems of the body. Stimulation of these reflex areas assists the body to biologically correct, strengthen, and reinforce itself.

The oldest documentation of the use of reflexology is found in Egypt. Early Egyptian artists observed and recorded scenes of daily life, which included the medical practices of the times. Ed and Ellen Case of Los Angeles toured Egypt in 1979. During their travels, they discovered and brought back an ancient Egyptian papyrus scene depicting medical practitioners treating the hands and feet of their patients in 2500 BCE. The tomb of Ankhmahor (a physician of high esteem) at Saqqara is where the scene depicting the practice of reflexology is to be found.

Chinese civilization developed reflexology a little later. Zone therapy was practiced later in Europe and spread from country to country.

Dr. William Fitzgerald (1872-1942) is credited with being the founder of modern reflexology. He discovered zone therapy as practiced by the "Red Indians." Several tribes of Native Americans used pressure to the feet as a source of healing. Jenny Wallace, a full-blooded Cherokee Indian from North Carolina says the clan of her father (Bear Clan) believe feet are important: "Your feet walk on the earth and through this your spirit is connected to the universe. Our feet are our contact with the Earth and the energies that flow through it."

Dr. Fitzgerald's studies brought about the development and practice of reflexology in the U.S. His medical degree came from the University of Vermont in 1895. He practiced in Boston, then in London at a nose and throat hospital, then in Vienna where he discovered the art of pressure therapy. He returned to the U.S. to Hartford (St. Francis Hospital, Nose and Throat division) and found that pressure in the nose, mouth, throat, tongue, hands, feet, joints, and others deadened definite areas of sensation and relieved pain. This led to the discovery of zone therapy. Dr. Joe Shelby Riley of Washington, D.C. studied many therapies, including surgery, physiotherapy, chiropractic, zone therapy, osteopathy, naturopathy, electrotherapy, and color and light therapy. Dr. Riley used this method in his practice for years.

Eunice Ingham (1879-1974) worked with Dr. Riley as his therapist in the early 1930s in Florida. Because doctors were not interested in reflexology, she contributed greatly in helping people help themselves with this method. She shared her techniques and knowledge with many. In 1938 her book *Stories the Feet Can Tell* was published and in 1951 she wrote *Stories the Feet Have Told*. In the 1960s, she wrote *Stories the Feet Are Telling*. She died in 1974 and her nephew Dwight Byers is still carrying on her work.

Mildred Carter was another renowned woman in the world of reflexology. Her book *Helping Yourself with Foot Reflexology* sold 500,000 copies, bringing greater recognition to reflexology.

Mechanism of Action According to Its Own Theory

Reflexology is based on the premise that there are zones and reflexes on different parts of the body, which correspond to and are relative to all parts, glands and organs of the entire body. The manipulation of specific reflexes removes stress, placing the body in a parasympathetic healing state and enabling the disharmonies to be released by a physiologic change in the body. With stress removed and circulation improved, the body is allowed to return to a state of homeostasis.

Reflexology demonstrates the following four main benefits:

1. Relaxes with the removal of stress
2. Enhances circulation
3. Assists the body to normalize metabolisms naturally
4. Complements all other healing modalities

When the reflexes are stimulated, the body's natural electric energy works along the nervous system and meridian lines to clear any blockages on those lines and in the corresponding zones.

A treatment seems to break up deposits (felt as a sandy or gritty area under the skin) that may interfere with this natural flow of the body's energy.

Reflexologists do not diagnose medical conditions. The only diagnosis made is a tender reflex. Nor are any disharmonies in any area of the body diagnosed other than in the reflexes. Just as organs overlap in the body, so do reflexes overlap on the feet. Tender reflexes indicate some disharmony in related parts, glands, or organs, but reflexology does not tell this specifically.

Similarly, reflexologists do not prescribe medications. The therapeutic intervention is limited to "working the reflexes."

In a forward for author Dwight C. Byers in *Better Health with Foot Reflexology*, Ray C. Wunderlich Jr., MD, stated the following:

Foot reflexology stands the test of patient acceptance as a valid means of making one feel good, relaxing, and functioning better than he otherwise would. As such foot reflexology qualifies as an important adjunct for health care . . . . There are 7200 nerve endings in each foot. Perhaps this fact, more than any other, explains why we feel so much better when our feet are treated. Nerve endings in the feet have ex-

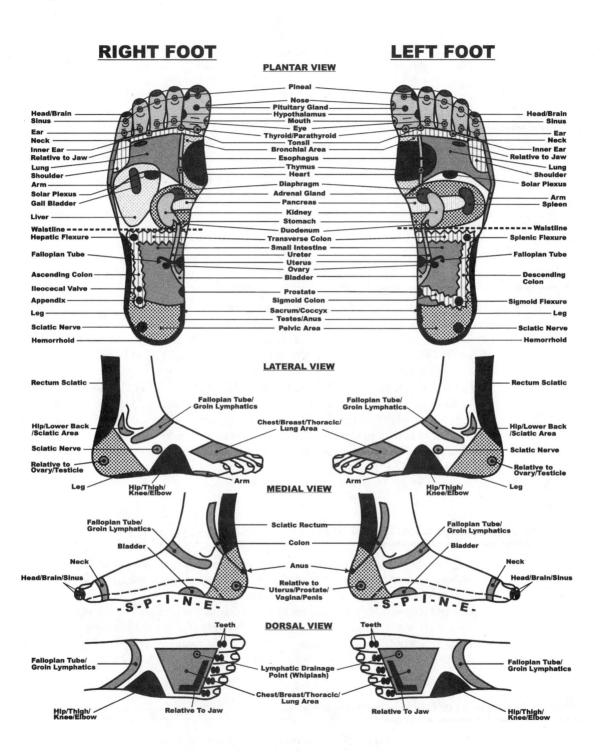

RIGHT FOOT   **LEFT FOOT**

PLANTAR VIEW

Pineal
Nose
Pituitary Gland
Hypothalamus
Mouth
Eye
Thyroid/Parathyroid
Tonsil
Bronchial Area
Esophagus
Thymus
Heart
Diaphragm
Adrenal Gland
Pancreas
Kidney
Stomach
Duodenum
Transverse Colon
Small Intestine
Ureter
Uterus
Ovary
Bladder
Prostate
Sigmoid Colon
Sacrum/Coccyx
Testes/Anus
Pelvic Area

Head/Brain
Sinus
Ear
Neck
Inner Ear
Relative to Jaw
Lung
Shoulder
Arm
Solar Plexus
Gall Bladder
Liver
Waistline
Hepatic Flexure
Fallopian Tube
Ascending Colon
Ileocecal Valve
Appendix
Leg
Sciatic Nerve
Hemorrhoid

Head/Brain
Sinus
Ear
Neck
Inner Ear
Relative to Jaw
Lung
Shoulder
Solar Plexus
Arm
Spleen
Waistline
Splenic Flexure
Fallopian Tube
Descending Colon
Sigmoid Flexure
Leg
Sciatic Nerve
Hemorrhoid

LATERAL VIEW

Rectum Sciatic
Hip/Lower Back/Sciatic Area
Sciatic Nerve
Relative to Ovary/Testicle
Leg
Hip/Thigh/Knee/Elbow
Arm

Fallopian Tube/Groin Lymphatics
Chest/Breast/Thoracic/Lung Area

Fallopian Tube/Groin Lymphatics

Rectum Sciatic
Hip/Lower Back/Sciatic Area
Sciatic Nerve
Relative to Ovary/Testicle
Leg
Arm
Hip/Thigh/Knee/Elbow

MEDIAL VIEW

Fallopian Tube/Groin Lymphatics
Bladder
Neck
Head/Brain/Sinus
-S-P-I-N-E-

Sciatic Rectum
Colon
Anus
Relative to Uterus/Prostate/Vagina/Penis

Fallopian Tube/Groin Lymphatics
Bladder
Neck
Head/Brain/Sinus
-S-P-I-N-E-

DORSAL VIEW

Teeth
Fallopian Tube/Groin Lymphatics
Hip/Thigh/Knee/Elbow
Relative To Jaw
Lymphatic Drainage Point (Whiplash)
Chest/Breast/Thoracic/Lung Area

Teeth
Fallopian Tube/Groin Lymphatics
Relative To Jaw
Hip/Thigh/Knee/Elbow

tensive interconnections through the spinal cord and brain with all areas of the body. Surely the feet are a gold mine of opportunity to release tension and enhance health.

Forms of Therapy

Reflexology is performed on the feet, although some practitioners do work on the hands, ears, and the body in general. Some practitioners use other forms of modalities in conjunction with reflexology, such as chakral reflexology (energy work), color reflexology (color visualization), and gems. Some practitioners are known to work with instruments (electrical or mechanical), particularly in the Asian countries, although instrument usage generally is discouraged or banned in North America.

Demographics

The number of trained reflexologists in any given area is usually proportional to the area population: the higher the density, the more reflexologists can be found.

Certified reflexologists usually can be found in the Yellow Pages listing under "Reflexology" or "Holistic Health." Practitioners sometimes can be found under "Massage" although a distinction is made between massage and reflexology.

Referrals of certified reflexologists usually can be obtained from a reflexology organization. Referrals can also be found at those Internet sites that are mentioned later in this discussion.

Types of people seeking reflexology treatments are of all ages, but approximately 70% are women. These people are usually health conscious and wish to explore alternatives. The vast majority of patients usually realize the benefits of reducing stress from a reflexology treatment, which in turn minimizes physical symptoms. Usually after a treatment, a patient is more apt to talk about mental health issues.

Indications and Reasons for Referral

Usually referrals are made in conjunction with other existing forms of therapy to supplement ongoing medical treatments. Reflexology has been known to help patients deal with events such as side effects of cancer chemotherapy.

Reflexology may be performed on everyone, from the newborn to the aged. It can be used for a general "tune-up" or in a very sick body. It can be used throughout pregnancy care and presurgically and postsurgically. In all cases, common sense should be used in selecting this therapy.

Office Applications

A simple ranking of conditions responsive to this form of therapy is as follows. As with all alternative therapies, use of reflexology does not preclude the use of mainstream medical therapies in addition.

Top level: *A therapy ideally suited for these conditions*

Allergies; restless leg syndrome; back pain; bladder infection; bronchitis; childbirth; children's health; chronic fatigue syndrome; chronic pain; colic; constipation; diarrhea; ear infections; female health; fever; gastritis; hay fever; headaches; insomnia; irritable bowel syndrome; male health; menopause; menstrual cramps; mental health; periodic leg movement syndrome; postpartum care; pregnancy and childbirth; premenstrual syndrome; sleep disorders; stomachache; and stress

Second level: *One of the better therapies for these conditions*

Addictions; Alzheimer's disease; arthritis; asthma; candidiasis; cataracts; chicken pox; childhood parasites; chlamydia; colds and flu; colitis and Crohn's disease; conjunctivitis; diabetes; diverticulosis and diverticulitis; endometriosis; gastrointestinal disorders; general ear pain; glaucoma; gout; hearing disorders; heart disease; hemorrhoids; hyperactivity; hypertension; impotence; lazy eye; measles; menorrhagia; obesity and weight management; osteoarthritis; osteoporosis; otitis media; pneumonia; preconception; prostatitis; respiratory conditions; rheumatoid arthritis; sinusitis; sleep apnea; strep throat; trichomonas; ulcers; vaginal, viral, and bacterial infections; vision disorders; and yeast infections

Third level: *A valuable adjunctive therapy for these conditions*

AIDS; amenorrhea; benign prostatic hypertrophy; cancer; cervical cancer; emphysema; fibrocystic breast disease; genital warts; gonorrhea; hearing loss; herpes; lung cancer; macular degeneration; Meniere's disease; multiple sclerosis; mumps; night blindness; ovarian cancer and cysts; parasitic infections; pinworms; poor eyesight; prostate cancer; retinal detachment; retinopathy; sexually transmitted diseases; syphilis; tinnitus; and uterine fibroids

Practical Applications

Frequency of Visits

When a patient ask when the next visit will be, the therapist explains the treatment will go on working for 5 or more days. Beyond this, the practitioner cannot guess the patient's needs. Have patients attune themselves to their own body needs and decide when and if they should return for another treatment. They may wish to return in 1 week, 1 month, or 6 months. We have no way to measure the amount of stress they have gathered or the state of their bodies since the last visit. Therapists who say "I want to see you three times a week for 6 months" are considering their own pockets instead of the true needs of the patient.

Length of Treatment

A complete treatment is always performed. Depending on the practitioner's level of experience and the patient's needs, sessions will last between 30 and 50 minutes.

Pressure

Reflexes are worked according to body disharmonies. Stress removal is first priority, followed by improved circulation, and then attention paid to reflexes relative to body needs. Common sense dictates when less pressure is required.

Communication with the patient is essential. Ask if the pressure is too light or too great. It is important to remember that the reflexes need to be located and deeply worked. Massaging or pampering the foot may feel good but does nothing to stimulate the reflexes and begin the body's natural process of healing. Well-worked reflexes prove to the patient the necessity of pressure by the renewed harmony brought to the body. The practitioner always works *within* the pain tolerance threshold of the individual.

Therapy Setting

The optimum location is a quiet, relaxing environment with the patient comfortably seated on a recliner chair, which is best because the practitioner and patient can see eye-to-eye. In reality, reflexology can be administered anywhere, sitting up as well as lying down. Receiving the therapy when necessary is more important than waiting for optimum treatment conditions.

Research Base

Evidence Based

Organized research material is not yet available.

Efficacy

Organized research material is not yet available, but rate of success is usually 75%.

Druglike Information

Actions and Pharmacokinetics

Reflexology is known to help the body eliminate wastes efficiently.

Tenderness is an expected sensation during reflexology. It can be caused by the following:1) tension (can affect all reflexes); 2) injury or illness; 3) surgery (both presurgery and postsurgery); 4) general or specific stress; 5) drugs (prescription or nonprescription; they numb reflexes); 6) corns, calluses, heel spurs, and others; and 7) Piriformis syndrome.

The following benefits may be noticed after a reflexology session or sessions:

1. Improved urination: In addition, the patient may experience a temporary increase in urine flow.

2. Improved digestion: Relaxation puts the body into the parasympathetic state, thereby improving digestion. It also may bring improved appetite and a more settled feeling after eating.
3. Heightened sense of energy: The "system runs cleaner" and organ function is "reset" to optimum function.
4. Pain release: From relaxation of nerves and muscles.

Warnings, Contraindications, and Precautions

Pressure on the corresponding reflex areas should be decreased for heart problems, blood problems, high blood pressure, epilepsy, and diabetes. In diabetic patients, overstimulation of the corresponding reflexes may cause the pancreas to start producing insulin again and thus cause a high level of insulin when the patient uses artificial insulin. Watch for the sweet breath odor during treatment, which would indicate ketosis. If this occurs, stop the treatment session immediately.

After surgery, a patient can expect to find tender reflexes in areas corresponding to surgical work done. Even with surgically removed organs, the reflex points for the organs still can be tender. Similarly, after an accident, serious illness, or recent fracture, reflexology treatments could show tender reflexes relating to accidents or illnesses. Do not work too hard on areas representing recent fractures.

Be aware of the patient's medications and side effects. If unsure about the adverse reactions, look them up. Side effects may show up in the treatment. For example, a side effect of a particular medication may affect the kidneys, thus the kidney reflexes may be tender. Analgesics may affect the tenderness of all reflexes so it may appear that the patient is in good health. Always be aware of possible medication side effects.

As many local disorders or systemic diseases have manifestations on the feet, the practitioner should be well acquainted with common foot disorders. These include Achilles' tendonitis; pes planus (flat feet); tinea pedis (athletes foot); bunions; calluses; clubfoot; diabetic foot changes; peripheral vascular disease; corns; edema and its causes; muscle cramps; gangrene; gout; hammer toes; ingrown toenails; osteoarthritis and rheumatoid arthritis; deep vein thrombophlebitis; plantar warts; shin splints; plantar fasciitis; skin ulcerations and their causes; and varicose veins.

Drug or Other Interactions

No research is available.

Adverse Reactions

Possible reactions include the following:

1. *Cold sensation:* The patient may feel cold because of relaxation.
2. *Taste in mouth:* The patient may have a bad taste due to cleansing of toxins.

3. *Perspiration:* Detoxification may cause perspiration from a release of excess fluids.

4. *Mucus formation:* Detoxification may occur from clogged sinuses, ileocecal valve, or small intestines. The gall bladder may increase secretion of bile, causing an overlubrication of the small intestine manifesting as loose bowel movements.

5. *Diarrhea or frequent bowel movements:* Stimulation of the liver, gall bladder, or digestive tract may normalize bowel functions or cause cleansing activity.

6. *Fatigue:* It is suggested that the patient rest after the treatment. The body has switched into a parasympathetic nervous state for rest and repair, so the body often feels sleepy.

7. *Headache and nausea:* This is caused by cleansing of toxins, especially in the liver.

8. *Eyes watering:* This is from cleansing of the lacrimal glands in the eyes.

9. *Rash:* This can occur from release of toxins through the body's largest elimination organ, the skin.

10. *Gas release (burping):* This is from toxin elimination and improved stomach and bowel functions.

Pregnancy and Lactation

The therapist should avoid overstimulating the reflexes to the reproductive organs in the first trimester. This increases the risk of abortion or miscarriages.

Reflexology may improve lactation.

Trade Products, Administration, and Dosage

Not applicable.

Self-Help versus Professional

Ten percent of reflexologists are usually self-taught and apply the therapy to family members only. Professional reflexologists are preferable because they are trained to apply the techniques properly and be aware of common medical conditions.

Visiting a Professional

The encounter usually occurs in a relaxed but professional environment. The session begins with a health history. The patient often is asked to sign a consent form accepting responsibility for the treatment. The practitioner then performs a thorough foot examination. The practitioner then works on the patient's bare feet, if possible. Classical music often is played during the session, and conversation is encouraged. Oil is used only on the feet at the *end* of the treatment to offer a reward to reflexes. The practitioner works within a time frame whereby the patient does not feel rushed and has time for questions.

Credentialing

No formal credentialing exists for reflexology. Certification is provided by certain educational institutions specializing in this training.

Training

There are many schools of reflexology who can provide adequate training that ranges from 100 to 1000 hours of instruction. Look for a school that is established and, if possible, recognized by the local governing body.

The following listing is operated by the author and is one example of specialized training locations for reflexology:

Ontario College of Reflexology
PO Box 220
New Liskeard, Ontario P0J 1P0, Canada
Tel: (705) 647-5354
Toll-Free: (888) OCR-FEET
Fax: (705) 647-0719
E-mail: ocr@ocr.edu
www.ocr.edu

What to Look for in a Provider

Look for a therapist who is certified or registered as a qualified reflexologist by a reputable organization. Also, select a reflexologist who presents a professional attitude. There is a difference between a therapist who works out of a basement in a home and one who maintains a business clinic with staff.

Barriers and Key Issues

The main barriers of this therapy seem to be that the profession is not yet organized on a large scale, although attempts have been made in smaller communities. There is a need for the reflexology profession to become self-regulated. When mainstream medical personnel accept that reflexology will help reduce or minimize stress, which in turn will reduce or minimize physical symptoms, it will become more widely accepted.

Associations

International Institute of Reflexology
PO Box 12642
St. Petersburg, FL 33733

Reflexology Association of California
PO Box 641156
Los Angeles, CA 90064
E-mail (Bobbi Warren): california_girl@my-dejanews.com

Reflexology Research by Kevin Kunz
PO Box 35820
Albuquerque, NM 87176
Tel: (888) 777-9911
Fax: (505) 344-0246
E-mail: footC@aol.com
www.reflexology-research.com

International Institute of Reflexology—Canada
c/o Philip Pittman
190 Athabasca St., Oshawa
ON, L1H 7J1, Canada
Fax: (905) 576-0447
E-mail: iirpit@idirect.com

Association of Reflexologists
27 Old Gloucester St.
London WC1N 3XX, England
Tel: 44 990 673320
www.reflexology.org/aor/

Reflexology Association of Australia
PO Box 366
Cammeray, NSW 2062, Australia
Tel: 61 02 4721 4752
Fax: 61 02 9631 3287

(Danish Reflexologists Association)
Forenede Danske Zoneterapeuter
Chr. Winthervej 13
DK-6000 Kolding, Denmark
Tel: 45 7550 1250
Fax: 45 7550 7447
E-mail: info@fdz.dk

Rwo-Shr Health Institute International
Room 1902, Java Commercial Centre
128 Java Rd.
North Point, Hong Kong

Reflexology Association of Japan
Akasaka TS Building, 5-1-36
Akasaka, Minato-ku, Tokyoto, 107, Japan
Tel: 81 3 3585 9100
Fax: 81 3 3585 2250

Chinese Society of Reflexologists
Xuanwu Hospital, Capital Institute of Medicine
Chang Chun Street, Beijing, China
Tel: 86 1 338687

Internet Resources

1. Ontario College of Reflexology
   http://www.ocr.edu/linkorgn.htm*
2. Reflexology journal based in Australia:
   www.reflexologyworld.com

Suggested Reading

1. Carter M, Weber T: *Healing yourself with foot reflexology*, New York, 1997, Prentice Hall Trade.
   Mildred Carter was one of the original authors who invented the term *reflexology* and has popularized this healing art in America and all over the world for the past 40 years.
2. Byers DC: *Better health with foot reflexology*, St Petersburg, Fla, 1987, Ingham Publishers.
   After Eunice Ingham's many books published on reflexology, her nephew has carried on her work with this book.
3. *The complete guide to foot reflexology, revised*, New Mexico, 1993, Reflexology Research Project.
   Very well known authors based in New Mexico, who have published many books (translated into many languages) that are very well illustrated and informative.
4. Kunz K, Kunz B: *Hand and foot reflexology—a self-help guide*, New York, 1992, Prentice Hall Trade.
   An excellent book for Reflexology self-help.
5. Issel C: *Reflexology: art, science, and history*, Sacramento, Calif, 1996, New Frontier.
   An excellent book of research on the history of reflexology and a compilation of different reflexology methodologies used around the world.

---

*This site is operated by the author.

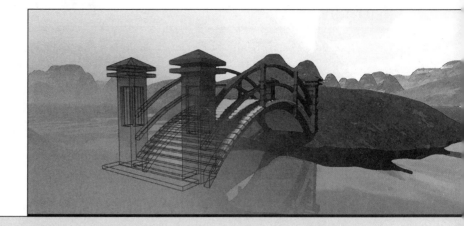

Health Conditions and Suggested Therapies

Introduction

Many health professionals desire a guide to determine which nontraditional therapies are applicable to selected diagnoses. This section provides an extensive array of diagnoses and a prioritized listing of therapies applicable to each diagnosis. To explain how this section may be used, it is necessary to describe its design and construction.

Each contributor was given an identical list of diagnoses and asked to rank them as the diagnoses applied to that particular form of therapy. The contributor could add additional diagnoses or delete ones irrelevant to that form of therapy. The top three levels of each rank listing are present in each respective chapter. In this section, all diagnosis rank lists are combined into a single listing, which provides rank-ordered therapy suggestions for a composite list of diagnoses.

The ranking of suggested therapies fall into five levels, as follows:

Level 1: A therapy ideally suited for this condition

Level 2: One of the better therapies for this condition

Level 3: A valuable adjunctive therapy for this condition

Level 4: One of a number of useful adjunctive therapies for this condition

Level 5: Equal among many adjunctive therapies for this condition

This list may be appropriately used as long as the following caveats are applied:

1. These therapies are often adjuncts to mainstream medical therapy. Some are listed for acute and life-threatening diagnoses. In these instances, their use would logically follow whatever standard medical care is required to create a safe and stable environment, after which other therapies can then be applied. This "team approach" to medical care is important in applying the best of many forms of therapy for the benefit of the patient.

2. A number of contributors did not provide rank listings for their respective therapies. These therapies are in many cases useful for the diagnoses represented in this section. The unranked therapies are:

Art Therapy	Imagery
Biofeedback	Latin American Community-Based Practices
Antineoplastons	Micronutrients
Aromatherapy	Bonnie Prudden Myotherapy
Aston-Patterning	Native American Medicine
Biological Dentistry	Naturopathic Medicine
Detoxification Therapy	Nutritional Oncology
Environmental Medicine	Polarity Therapy
Enzyme Therapy	Reflexology
Fasting	Rolfing
Flower Essences	Spiritual Healing and Prayer
Herbal Medicine	Yoga

Please refer to each individual discussion for recommendations for these forms of therapy.

3. Some diagnoses have only one or two associated therapies. In these cases, either few contributors listed them, or one or two contributors added this diagnosis to their listing. This does not mean other therapies are not applicable to a particular diagnosis. In some cases, such as in homeopathy, the listing of diagnoses was curtailed only because of space limitations.

4. Within each level for a particular diagnosis, therapies are listed alphabetically.

5. The precise level of the suggested therapy is less important than whether it is listed in the top three levels. Some individual contributors may rank their therapy higher than others. Use this listing as a general indicator, not as a precise instrument.

With these cautions in mind, the reader will find an extensive listing of diagnoses and suggestions as to the choice of applicable therapies for each diagnosis. This listing is notable in that each selection has been chosen and ranked by representatives of each profession according to their profession's consensus experience with each diagnosis.

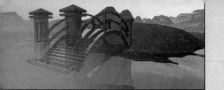

Conditions and Suggested Therapies

Abdominal injury: *Level 3*—Homeopathy

Abscess: *Level 1*—Homeopathy

Accidents of any kind: *Level 2*—Flower essences, homeopathy

Acne: *Level 1*—Homeopathy

Acute diseases: *Level 1*—Homeopathy

    Level 3—Flower essences

Acute grief reactions: *Level 1*—Poetry Therapy

Addictions: *Level 1*—Reiki, Tai Chi

    Level 2—Colon hydrotherapy, flower essences, hypnotherapy (to prevent relapse), light therapy, neuro linguistic programming, poetry therapy, reflexology, traditional Chinese herbal medicine, therapeutic touch

    Level 3—Acupressure, acupuncture, Ayurveda, Bowen technique, CranioSacral therapy, dance/movement therapy, environmental medicine, homeopathy, music therapy, yoga

    Level 4—Feldenkrais method, massage therapy

    Level 5—Chiropractic, fasting, magnetic field therapy, Qi Gong

Adhesive capsulitis: *Level 2*—Osteopathic medicine

Adjustment disorder with depressed mood: *Level 2*—Poetry therapy

Adolescent identity issues: *Level 2*—Poetry therapy

Agoraphobia: *Level 1*—Homeopathy

AIDS: *Level 2*—Bowen technique, hypnotherapy, Qi Gong, reiki, shamanism

    Level 3—Acupuncture, Ayurveda, colon hydrotherapy, dance/movement therapy, environmental medicine, massage therapy, music therapy, reflexology, Tai Chi, traditional Chinese herbal medicine

    Level 4—Acupressure, chiropractic, yoga

    Level 5—Feldenkrais method, magnetic field therapy

Alcoholism: *Level 3*—Environmental medicine

Allergic reaction: *Level 3*—Homeopathy

Allergies: *Level 1*—Acupuncture, applied kinesiology, Ayurveda, environmental medicine, homeopathy, neuro linguistic programming, reflexology, traditional Chinese herbal medicine

    Level 2—Bowen technique, colon hydrotherapy, flower essences, hypnotherapy, light therapy, magnetic field therapy, Qi Gong, Tai Chi, therapeutic touch

    Level 3—Acupressure, fasting, Rosen method, yoga

    Level 4—Chiropractic, Feldenkrais method, reiki

    Level 5—Dance/movement therapy, massage therapy

Allergies or hay fever with proven heavy metal intoxication: *Level 1*—Chelation therapy

Alzheimer's disease: *Level 1*—Chelation therapy (with proven heavy metal intoxication)

    Level 2—Ayurveda, magnetic field therapy, music therapy, reflexology, reiki

    Level 3—Colon hydrotherapy, dance/movement therapy, environmental medicine, homeopathy

Level 4—Acupressure, acupuncture, quartz crystal therapy, massage therapy

Level 5—Chiropractic, Qi Gong

Amenorrhea: *Level 1*—Applied kinesiology, Ayurveda, homeopathy, hypnotherapy (emotional causation), reiki

Level 2—Acupressure, environmental medicine, traditional Chinese herbal medicine

Level 3—Acupuncture, dance/movement therapy, reflexology, yoga

Level 4—Chiropractic, colon hydrotherapy, Feldenkrais method fasting, massage therapy, Qi Gong

Amyotrophic lateral sclerosis: *Level 3*—Chelation therapy

Anaphylactic reaction: *Level 2*—Homeopathy

Anemias (selected): *Level 3*—Environmental medicine

Anesthesia reaction: *Level 2*—Homeopathy

Anger, uncontrolled: *Level 1*—Homeopathy

Level 2—Flower essences

Angina pectoris: *Level 2*—Homeopathy

Level 3—Bowen technique, environmental medicine

Level 5—Color therapy

Angioedema: *Level 3*—Environmental medicine

Ankle sprain: *Level 1*—Bowen technique

Level 2—Acupressure

Anterior knee pain: *Level 2*—Osteopathic medicine

Anxiety: *Level 1*—Acupressure, dance/movement therapy, Feldenkrais method (for chronic), homeopathy, relaxation therapy

Level 2—Flower essences, light therapy, massage therapy, meditation (for generalized)

Level 3—Environmental medicine, osteopathic medicine, quartz crystal therapy

Aphthous stomatitis: *Level 3*—Environmental medicine

Appendicitis: *Level 3*—Homeopathy

Arrhythmia: *Level 2*—Homeopathy

Level 4—Flower essences

Arrhythmias: *Level 3*—Environmental medicine

Arteriosclerosis: *Level 4*—Quartz crystal therapy

Arteriosclerotic occlusive disease: *Level 1*—Chelation therapy

Arthritis: *Level 1*—Alexander technique, Ayurveda, fasting, flower essences (rheumatoid or osteoarthritis), homeopathy (rheumatoid or osteoarthritis), macronutrients, orthomolecular medicine, Rosen method, therapeutic touch

Level 2—Acupressure, Bowen technique (for severe), chiropractic, environmental medicine, magnetic field therapy, reflexology, reiki, Tai Chi, traditional Chinese herbal medicine, yoga

Level 3—Acupuncture, applied kinesiology, Bonnie Prudden myotherapy, colon hydrotherapy, quartz crystal therapy, Feldenkrais method, Hellerwork, massage therapy, meditation (including fibromyalgia), Qi Gong

Level 4—Dance/movement therapy

Asperger's disorder: *Level 1*—Dance/movement therapy

Asthma: *Level 1*—Alexander technique, Ayurveda, environmental medicine, homeopathy, orthomolecular medicine, reiki

Level 2—Bonnie Prudden myotherapy, Bowen technique, colon hydrotherapy, Hellerwork, hypnotherapy, light therapy, magnetic field therapy, neuro linguistic programming, osteopathic medicine, Qi Gong, reflexology, reiki, Rosen method, Tai Chi, traditional Chinese herbal medicine, yoga

Level 3—Acupressure, acupuncture, applied kinesiology, dance/movement therapy, fasting, flower essences, macronutrients, massage therapy

Level 4—Feldenkrais method, meditation

Level 5—Chiropractic, color therapy, Trager approach

Atherosclerosis (prevention): *Level 3*—Meditation

Atherosclerosis or arteriosclerosis: *Level 1*—Ayurveda

Attention deficit disorder: *Level 1*—Ayurveda, CranioSacral therapy, homeopathy, light therapy

Level 2—Dance/movement therapy, environmental medicine, flower essences

Level 3—Dance/movement therapy

Autism: *Level 1*—Dance/movement therapy, Feldenkrais method, music therapy, Tai Chi

Level 2—CranioSacral therapy, environmental medicine, light therapy, magnetic field therapy

Level 3—Ayurveda, homeopathy

Level 4—Acupuncture, flower essences, massage therapy, orthomolecular medicine, reflexology

Level 5—Acupressure, chiropractic, colon hydrotherapy

Back pain: *Level 1*—Applied kinesiology, Alexander technique, Ayurveda, Bonnie Prudden myotherapy, chiropractic, Feldenkrais method, flower essences, Hellerwork, hypnotherapy, magnetic field therapy, reflexology, Rosen method, Tai Chi, therapeutic touch, yoga

Level 2—Acupressure, acupuncture, colon hydrotherapy, homeopathy, massage therapy, reiki, traditional Chinese herbal medicine

Level 3—CranioSacral therapy, quartz crystal therapy, environmental medicine, fasting, light therapy, Trager approach

Level 4—Dance/movement therapy, Qi Gong

Level 5—Neuro linguistic programming

Balance problems: *Level 1*—Feldenkrais method

Bed wetting: *Level 1*—Bowen technique

Belching: *Level 1*—Homeopathy

Bell's palsy: *Level 2*—Bowen technique

Level 3—Osteopathic medicine

Benign prostatic hypertrophy: *Level 1*—Ayurveda, homeopathy

Level 2—Environmental medicine, magnetic field therapy, Tai Chi, traditional Chinese herbal medicine

Level 3—Acupressure, colon hydrotherapy, reflexology

Level 4—Acupuncture, orthomolecular medicine, Qi Gong, reiki

Level 5—Chiropractic, fasting

Benign vocal cord nodules: *Level 2*—Hypnotherapy

Bingeing: *Level 2*—Fasting

Bipolar and unipolar mood disorders: *Level 1*—Dance/movement therapy

Bites and stings (animal, insect, reptiles): *Level 1*—Homeopathy

Bleeding: *Level 3*—Homeopathy

Level 4—Flower essences

Blephartis: *Level 1*—Homeopathy

Level 4—Flower essences

Blindness: *Level 5*—Homeopathy

Blood clots: *Level 2*—Homeopathy

Level 4—Flower essences

Blurring of vision: *Level 4*—Environmental medicine

Boils: *Level 1*—Homeopathy

Bone, ailments of: *Level 1*—Homeopathy
    Level 3—Flower essences
Botulism: *Level 1*—Homeopathy
Breast pain (PMS, mastitis, lactation, engorgement): *Level 1*—Bowen technique
Breathing disorders: *Level 2*—Flower essences, homeopathy
Bronchitis: *Level 1*—Ayurveda, homeopathy, reflexology, Tai Chi
    Level 2—Bowen technique, colon hydrotherapy, environmental medicine (for chronic), light
        therapy, magnetic field therapy, Qi Gong, traditional Chinese herbal medicine,
        therapeutic touch
    Level 3—Acupressure, applied kinesiology, environmental medicine, fasting, flower essences,
        massage therapy, reiki, yoga
    Level 4—Acupuncture, Alexander technique
    Level 5—Chiropractic
Bruises: *Level 1*—Homeopathy
    Level 3—Flower essences
Bruxism: *Level 1*—Homeopathy
    Level 4—Flower essences
Burns: *Level 4*—Quartz crystal therapy
    Level 5—Color therapy
Bursitis: *Level 1*—Homeopathy
    Level 2—Flower essences
Cancer: *Level 1*—Dance/movement therapy (for emotional sequelae), environmental medicine,
        macronutrients, shamanism
    Level 2—Ayurveda (for early stages), Qi Gong, reiki, therapeutic touch
    Level 3—Ayurveda (for late stages), colon hydrotherapy, Feldenkrais method, meditation, music
        therapy, reflexology, Tai Chi, traditional Chinese herbal medicine, yoga
    Level 4—Acupressure, acupuncture, Alexander technique, magnetic field therapy, massage
        therapy (if not contraindicated)
    Level 5—Chiropractic, CranioSacral therapy, neuro linguistic programming, orthomolecular therapy
Candidiasis: *Level 1*—Ayurveda
    Level 2—Colon hydrotherapy, environmental medicine, homeopathy, reflexology, traditional
        Chinese herbal medicine
    Level 3—Fasting, hypnotherapy, light therapy
    Level 4—Acupuncture, reiki
    Level 5—Acupressure, chiropractic, massage therapy, Qi Gong
Carbon monoxide poisoning: *Level 3*—Homeopathy
Cardiac arrest: *Level 3*—Homeopathy, meditation (for prevention)
Cardiac arrhythmias: *Level 1*—Hypnotherapy
Cardiovascular disease: *Level 2*—Homeopathy
    Level 4—Flower essences
Carotid artery disease: *Level 1*—Chelation therapy
Carpal tunnel syndrome: *Level 1*—Acupressure, Bowen technique, homeopathy
    Level 2—Osteopathic medicine
    Level 3—Flower essences, Trager approach
Cataracts: *Level 1*—Flower essences, light therapy
    Level 2—Reflexology, Tai Chi
    Level 3—Ayurveda, homeopathy, traditional Chinese herbal medicine
    Level 4—Acupuncture, environmental medicine
    Level 5—Acupressure, chiropractic, colon hydrotherapy, Qi Gong, Tai Chi, reiki

Catarrh, chronic: *Level 5*—Color therapy

Central nervous system diseases: *Level 2*—Homeopathy
Level 3—Flower essences

Cerebral concussion: *Level 1*—Homeopathy

Cerebral hematoma: *Level 2*—Homeopathy

Cerebral palsy: *Level 1*—Feldenkrais method
Level 2—Bowen technique, hypnotherapy (for athetoid movements)

Cerebral vascular disease: *Level 1*—Chelation therapy

Cervical cancer: *Level 2*—Ayurveda, environmental medicine, Qi Gong, reiki, Tai Chi
Level 3—Colon hydrotherapy, reflexology, traditional Chinese herbal medicine
Level 4—Acupressure, acupuncture, massage therapy (if not contraindicated)
Level 5—Chiropractic, homeopathy

Cervical disease: *Level 3*—Hypnotherapy

Cervical strain or sprain: *Level 1*—Osteopathic medicine

Chancre sores: *Level 1*—Homeopathy

Chemical poisoning: *Level 3*—Homeopathy

Chickenpox: *Level 1*—Ayurveda, homeopathy
Level 2—Reflexology
Level 3—Magnetic field therapy, Tai Chi
Level 4—Acupuncture, colon hydrotherapy, environmental medicine
Level 5—Acupressure, chiropractic, reiki

Child behavior disorders: *Level 1*—Macronutrients

Childbirth: *Level 1*—Homeopathy, hypnotherapy (including postpartum care), reflexology, reiki
Level 2—Acupressure, Bonnie Prudden myotherapy, chiropractic, light therapy, music therapy, yoga
Level 3—Colon hydrotherapy, Hellerwork
Level 4—Acupuncture, Tai Chi
Level 5—Environmental medicine, neuro linguistic programming, Rosen method

Childbirth preparation: *Level 1*—Ayurveda

Childhood parasites: *Level 1*—Ayurveda, homeopathy
Level 2—Magnetic field therapy, reflexology, Tai Chi
Level 3—Colon hydrotherapy
Level 4—Environmental medicine
Level 5—Acupressure, acupuncture, chiropractic

Children's health: *Level 1*—Ayurveda, environmental medicine, homeopathy, reflexology, yoga
Level 2—Reiki, Acupressure, dance/movement therapy
Level 3—Applied kinesiology, Hellerwork, acupuncture, Bonnie Prudden myotherapy, colon hydrotherapy, flower essences, massage therapy
Level 4—Chiropractic, Qi Gong
Level 5—Magnetic field therapy

Chlamydia: *Level 2*—Reflexology
Level 3—Ayurveda
Level 4—Acupuncture, environmental medicine, reiki
Level 5—Acupressure, chiropractic, colon hydrotherapy

Cholecystitis: *Level 1*—Homeopathy

Chronic fatigue syndrome: *Level 1*—Acupressure, applied kinesiology, Ayurveda, Feldenkrais method, homeopathy, hypnotherapy, magnetic field therapy, Qi Gong, reflexology, reiki, Rosen method, shamanism, Tai Chi, therapeutic touch

Level 2—Alexander technique, Bowen technique, colon hydrotherapy, environmental medicine, macronutrients, yoga

Level 3—Acupuncture, Bonnie Prudden myotherapy, chiropractic, CranioSacral therapy, light therapy, massage therapy, neuro linguistic programming, Trager approach

Level 4—Fasting

Chronic obstructive pulmonary disease: *Level 1*—Homeopathy

Level 3—Osteopathic medicine

Level 4—Flower essences

Chronic pain: *Level 1*—Alexander technique, Bonnie Prudden myotherapy, Bowen technique, Feldenkrais method, flower essences, Hellerwork (musculoskeletal pain), homeopathy, hypnotherapy, magnetic field therapy, reflexology, reiki, Tai Chi, therapeutic touch

Level 2—Acupressure, chiropractic, macronutrients, meditation, Trager approach, yoga

Level 3—Acupuncture, applied kinesiology, colon hydrotherapy, environmental medicine, massage therapy, music therapy, Qi Gong

Level 4—Dance/movement therapy, neuro linguistic programming, osteopathic medicine

Chronic pain and fibromyalgia: *Level 1*—Ayurveda

Ciliary spasm: *Level 1*—Hypnotherapy

Circulation disorders: *Level 1*—Homeopathy

Level 2—Flower essences

Circulation, poor: *Level 3*—Acupressure

Closed head injuries: *Level 1*—Feldenkrais method

Coccyx pain: *Level 1*—Bowen technique

Cognitive and memory disorders (selected): *Level 3*—Environmental medicine

Cold and flu: *Level 1*—Applied kinesiology, Ayurveda, Bowen technique, homeopathy, macronutrients, orthomolecular medicine, Qi Gong

Level 2—Colon hydrotherapy, magnetic field therapy, reflexology

Level 3—Acupressure, acupuncture, quartz crystal therapy, environmental medicine, fasting, flower essences, Tai Chi

Level 4—Quartz crystal therapy, reiki

Level 5—Chiropractic, color therapy, massage therapy

Cold sores: *Level 1*—Homeopathy

Colic: *Level 1*—Ayurveda, Bowen technique, environmental medicine, homeopathy, magnetic therapy medicine, reflexology

Level 2—Acupressure, massage therapy, reiki, Rosen method, Tai Chi

Level 3—Acupuncture, applied kinesiology, Bonnie Prudden myotherapy, chiropractic, colon hydrotherapy

Collagen vascular disease: *Level 3*—Chelation therapy, macronutrients

Coma: *Level 2*—Homeopathy

Level 4—Quartz crystal therapy

Compulsive disorders: *Level 1*—Homeopathy

Concussion: *Level 1*—Bowen technique

Conduct disorder: *Level 1*—Dance/movement therapy

Confusion: *Level 1*—Homeopathy

Congenital torticollis: *Level 4*—Osteopathic medicine

Congestive heart failure: *Level 2*—Homeopathy

Level 3—Flower essences

Conjunctivitis: *Level 1*—Ayurveda, homeopathy, light therapy

Level 2—Reflexology, Tai Chi, yoga

Level 3—Acupressure, colon hydrotherapy, environmental medicine, flower essences, reiki
Level 4—Acupuncture
Level 5—Chiropractic
Connective tissue disorders: *Level 1*—Homeopathy
Level 2—Flower essences
Constipation: *Level 1*—Applied kinesiology, Ayurveda, colon hydrotherapy, fasting, homeopathy, macronutrients, reflexology, reiki, Tai Chi, yoga
Level 2—Bowen technique, Hellerwork, Rosen method
Level 3—Acupressure, acupuncture, Bonnie Prudden myotherapy, environmental medicine, Feldenkrais method, magnetic field therapy, massage therapy, neuro linguistic programming Qi Gong
Level 4—Chiropractic
Level 5—Color therapy
Cornea disorders: *Level 3*—Flower essences, homeopathy
Coronary artery disease: *Level 1*—Chelation therapy
Cough: *Level 1*—Homeopathy
Cramps: *Level 1*—Homeopathy
Crohn's disease: *Level 2*—Environmental medicine
Croup: *Level 1*—Homeopathy
Cuts: *Level 1*—Homeopathy
Cystitis: *Level 1*—Ayurveda (for chronic), homeopathy, reflexology
Level 2—Ayurveda, colon hydrotherapy, traditional Chinese herbal medicine
Level 3—Dance/movement therapy, environmental medicine (for chronic), magnetic field therapy
Level 4—Acupressure, acupuncture, environmental medicine, fasting, reiki, Tai Chi
Level 5—Chiropractic
Cysts: *Level 1*—Homeopathy
Dacryocystitis: *Level 1*—Homeopathy
Degenerative disc disease: *Level 3*—Osteopathic medicine
Dehydration: *Level 2*—Homeopathy
Delirium: *Level 1*—Homeopathy
Delusions: *Level 1*—Homeopathy
Dental phobia: *Level 1*—Hypnotherapy
Depression: *Level 1*—Homeopathy
Level 2—Color therapy, flower essences, macronutrients, relaxation therapy
Level 3—Light therapy, osteopathic medicine
Level 4—Quartz crystal therapy
Dermatitis: *Level 1*—Homeopathy
Dermatitis herpetiformis: *Level 2*—Environmental medicine
Detached retina: *Level 3*—Flower essences, homeopathy
Developmental disabilities: *Level 2*—Music therapy
Diabetes mellitus: *Level 1*—Macronutrients, Ayurveda (for type 2-niddm)
Level 2—Chelation therapy, fasting (for type 2-niddm), magnetic field therapy, reflexology, yoga
Level 3—Acupressure, acupuncture, applied kinesiology, Ayurveda (for type 1), Bonnie Prudden myotherapy, colon hydrotherapy, homeopathy, hypnotherapy, massage therapy (if not contraindicated), Qi Gong, Tai Chi
Level 5—Chiropractic, CranioSacral therapy, orthomolecular medicine, reiki
Diarrhea: *Level 1*—Applied kinesiology, Ayurveda, colon hydrotherapy, homeopathy, macronutrients, reflexology

Level 2—Bowen technique, magnetic field therapy

Level 3—Acupressure, acupuncture, environmental medicine, massage therapy, Qi Gong, Tai Chi

Level 4—Chiropractic

Level 5—Color therapy

Digestive problem: *Level 2*—Bowen technique

Digestive problems: *Level 1*—Homeopathy

Dislocation: *Level 2*—Homeopathy

Diverticulosis and diverticulitis: *Level 1*—Ayurveda, homeopathy

Level 2—Colon hydrotherapy, magnetic field therapy, reflexology, therapeutic touch

Level 3—Acupressure, acupuncture, applied kinesiology, fasting, massage therapy, reiki, yoga

Level 4—Chiropractic, environmental medicine

Level 5—Qi Gong

Double vision: *Level 3*—Homeopathy

Drug overdose: *Level 2*—Homeopathy

Level 4—Flower essences

Dry eyes: *Level 1*—Homeopathy

Dysmenorrhea: *Level 1*—Hypnotherapy

Level 2—Environmental medicine

Level 3—Osteopathic medicine

Level 4—Meditation

Dyspareunia: *Level 1*—Hypnotherapy

Dysphasia: *Level 1*—Homeopathy

Dysthymic disorder: *Level 2*—Meditation

Dystonia: *Level 1*—Feldenkrais method

Level 3—Trager approach

Ear infection, otitis media, recurrent: *Level 2*—Environmental medicine

Ear infections: *Level 1*—Ayurveda, homeopathy, reflexology

Level 3—Acupressure, acupuncture, applied kinesiology, colon hydrotherapy, environmental medicine, Qi Gong

Level 4—Chiropractic

Level 5—Reiki

Ear infections, otitis media: *Level 1*—Ayurveda, CranioSacral therapy, homeopathy

Level 2—Reflexology, Tai Chi

Level 3—Acupuncture, chiropractic, environmental medicine, light therapy, magnetic field therapy, osteopathic medicine, Qi Gong

Level 4—Acupressure

Level 5—Colon hydrotherapy

Ear injuries: *Level 1*—Homeopathy

Ear pain, nonspecific: *Level 1*—Ayurveda, homeopathic, magnetic field therapy, Tai Chi

Level 2—Reflexology, reiki

Level 3—Acupressure, acupuncture, applied kinesiology, environmental medicine, Qi Gong

Level 4—Colon hydrotherapy

Level 5—Chiropractic, massage therapy

Ear pressure: *Level 3*—Environmental medicine

Ear problems: *Level 4*—Quartz crystal therapy

Earaches: *Level 1*—Homeopathy

Eating disorders: *Level 1*—Dance/movement therapies

Level 3—Environmental medicine

Eclampsia: *Level 3*—Homeopathy

Eczema: *Level 1*—Homeopathy

   Level 2—Environmental medicine, light therapy

Eczema of the eyelids: *Level 3*—Environmental medicine

Edema: *Level 1*—Homeopathy

   Level 3—Acupressure, environmental medicine

   Level 4—Flower essences

Embolism: *Level 3*—Homeopathy

Emotional disorders: *Level 1*—Flower essences, homeopathy

Emphysema: *Level 1*—Magnetic field therapy, Tai Chi

   Level 2—Alexander technique, Bowen technique, homeopathy, Qi Gong, yoga

   Level 3—Acupressure, acupuncture, applied kinesiology, Ayurveda, colon hydrotherapy, environmental medicine, Feldenkrais method, flower essences, reflexology, Rosen method

   Level 4—Chiropractic, quartz crystal therapy, massage therapy

Encopresis: *Level 1*—Homeopathy

Endocarditis: *Level 3*—Ayurveda

Endometriosis: *Level 1*—Ayurveda, homeopathy, magnetic field therapy

   Level 2—Environmental medicine, reflexology, reiki, therapeutic touch, yoga

   Level 3—Acupressure, acupuncture, applied kinesiology, light therapy

   Level 4—Chiropractic, colon hydrotherapy, massage therapy

   Level 5—CranioSacral therapy, dance/movement therapy

Enuresis: *Level 1*—Homeopathy, hypnotherapy

   Level 2—Environmental medicine

Eosinophilic gastroenteritis: *Level 3*—Environmental medicine

Epicondylitis: *Level 1*—Bowen technique

   Level 2—Osteopathic medicine

Epidural hematoma: *Level 2*—Homeopathy

Epilepsy: *Level 1*—Homeopathy

   Level 2—Hypnotherapy

   Level 3—Light therapy

   Level 4—Quartz crystal therapy, environmental medicine

   Level 5—Trager approach

Esophageal spasm: *Level 1*—Homeopathy

Esophagitis: *Level 1*—Homeopathy

Exhibitionism: *Level 1*—Homeopathy

Exposure to environmental poisons: *Level 2*—Homeopathy

Eye diseases: *Level 3*—Flower essences, homeopathy

   Level 4—Quartz crystal therapy

Eyesight, poor: *Level 1*—Light therapy

   Level 2—Magnetic field therapy, Tai Chi

   Level 3—Acupressure, acupuncture, neuro linguistic programming, reflexology

   Level 4—Chiropractic, environmental medicine, traditional Chinese herbal medicine

   Level 5—Ayurveda, colon hydrotherapy, massage therapy

Eye strain: *Level 1*—Homeopathy

Facet syndrome: *Level 1*—Osteopathic medicine

Family and marital dysfunction: *Level 2*—Poetry therapy

Fatigue: *Level 2*—Environmental medicine

Fatigue syndromes with proven heavy metal intoxications: *Level 2*—Chelation therapy

Fatty liver: *Level 1*—Fasting

Fears: *Level 1*—Homeopathy

    Level 2—Flower essences

Febrile convulsion: *Level 1*—Homeopathy

Female health: *Level 1*—Ayurveda, environmental medicine, homeopathy, Qi Gong, reflexology, reiki, shamanism, Tai Chi, therapeutic touch, yoga

    Level 2—Acupressure, light therapy, neuro linguistic programming

    Level 3—Acupuncture, applied kinesiology, Bonnie Prudden myotherapy, chiropractic, colon hydrotherapy, dance/movement therapy, flower essences, massage therapy

    Level 4—Quartz crystal therapy, fasting

    Level 5—Magnetic field therapy

Fever: *Level 1*—Homeopathy, reflexology, Tai Chi

    Level 2—Ayurveda, colon hydrotherapy, hypnotherapy, light therapy, magnetic field therapy, orthomolecular medicine

    Level 3—Acupressure, applied kinesiology

    Level 4—Acupuncture, quartz crystal therapy, environmental medicine, reiki

    Level 5—Chiropractic, massage therapy (if not contraindicated)

Fibrocystic breast disease: *Level 1*—Ayurveda, homeopathy, macronutrients, magnetic field therapy, Tai Chi, therapeutic touch

    Level 2—Environmental medicine, hypnotherapy

    Level 3—Acupressure, acupuncture, colon hydrotherapy, reflexology, reiki

    Level 4—Massage therapy

    Level 5—Chiropractic

Fibromyalgia: *Level 1*—Bowen technique, Feldenkrais method, homeopathy, hypnotherapy

    Level 2—Alexander technique, CranioSacral therapy, environmental medicine, massage therapy

    Level 3—Flower essences, osteopathic medicine, Trager approach

Fibrosis: *Level 1*—Homeopathy

Flatulence: *Level 1*—Ayurveda, homeopathy

Floaters: *Level 1*—Homeopathy

    Level 3—Flower essences

Food allergies: *Level 1*—Macronurtients

Food poisoning: *Level 1*—Homeopathy

Foot injuries: *Level 1*—Homeopathy

    Level 2—Flower essences

Foot pain: *Level 1*—Bowen technique

Fractures: *Level 1*—Homeopathy

    Level 3—Flower essences

    Level 5—Color therapy

Frost bite: *Level 1*—Homeopathy

Frozen shoulder (capsulitis, rotator cuff, arthritis): *Level 1*—Bowen technique

Gallbladder disease: *Level 1*—Homeopathy

Gallstones: *Level 1*—Homeopathy

    Level 4—Quartz crystal therapy

Gangrene: *Level 2*—Homeopathy

Gastric and duodenal ulcers: *Level 3*—Environmental medicine

Gastric ulcers: *Level 1*—Reiki

    Level 2—Hypnotherapy

Gastritis: *Level 1*—Ayurveda, homeopathy, reflexology

    Level 2—Colon hydrotherapy, environmental medicine, hypnotherapy, magnetic field therapy, Qi Gong, relaxation therapy, Tai Chi, yoga

Level 3—Acupressure, acupuncture, environmental medicine (for chronic), massage therapy, neuro linguistic programming, orthomolecular medicine

Level 4—Fasting

Level 5—Chiropractic

Gastroenteritis: *Level 1*—Homeopathy, reiki

Level 2—CranioSacral therapy

Gastrointestinal disorders: *Level 1*—Ayurveda, colon hydrotherapy, homeopathy, macronutrients, Tai Chi

Level 2—Environmental medicine, fasting, magnetic field therapy, Qi Gong, reflexology, yoga

Level 3—Acupressure, acupuncture, applied kinesiology, light therapy, massage therapy, neuro linguistic programming, osteopathic medicine

Level 4—Chiropractic

Level 5—Rosen method

Genital warts: *Level 1*—Homeopathy

Level 2—Magnetic field therapy

Level 3—Ayurveda, orthomolecular medicine, reflexology

Level 4—Acupuncture, environmental medicine

Level 5—Chiropractic, colon hydrotherapy

Gastroesophageal reflux: *Level 1*—Homeopathy

Level 2—Hypnotherapy

German measles (rubella): *Level 1*—Homeopathy

Glandular fever: *Level 5*—Color therapy

Glaucoma: *Level 2*—Homeopathy, light therapy, magnetic field therapy, reflexology, Tai Chi

Level 3—Acupressure, acupuncture, Ayurveda, environmental medicine

Level 4—Colon hydrotherapy, flower essences

Level 5—Chiropractic

Glomerulonephritis: *Level 1*—Ayurveda (for chronic)

Level 3—Ayurveda (for acute)

Level 4—Environmental medicine

Gonorrhea: *Level 2*—Homeopathy

Level 3—Ayurveda, reflexology

Level 4—Environmental medicine

Level 5—Acupuncture, chiropractic, colon hydrotherapy

Gout: *Level 1*—Ayurveda, homeopathy, Tai Chi

Level 2—Hypnotherapy, magnetic field therapy, reflexology

Level 3—Acupressure, applied kinesiology, colon hydrotherapy, environmental medicine, Qi Gong, yoga

Level 4—Acupuncture, reiki

Level 5—Chiropractic, massage therapy (locally contraindicated)

Graves' disease: *Level 2*—Hypnotherapy

Growing pains, children: *Level 1*—Homeopathy

Gut flora dysbiosis: *Level 1*—Environmental medicine

Habit management (smoking, obesity): *Level 1*—Hypnotherapy

Halitosis: *Level 2*—Homeopathy

Hallucinations: *Level 2*—Homeopathy

Hamstring and adductor strain: *Level 1*—Bowen technique

Hamstring strain: *Level 1*—Bowen technique, osteopathic medicine

Hay fever: *Level 1*—Applied kinesiology, Ayurveda, environmental medicine, homeopathy, neuro linguistic programming, reflexology

Level 2—Acupuncture, Bowen technique, magnetic field therapy, Qi Gong, Tai Chi

Level 3—Acupressure, colon hydrotherapy, fasting, flower essences, hypnotherapy, light therapy, orthomolecular medicine, yoga

Level 4—Quartz crystal therapy, massage therapy

Level 5—Chiropractic, color therapy, reiki, Rosen method

Head injury: *Level 1*—Homeopathy

Head lice: *Level 1*—Ayurveda

Level 2—Tai Chi

Level 3—Environmental medicine, homeopathy

Level 5—Acupuncture, chiropractic, colon hydrotherapy, reflexology

Head trauma: *Level 1*—Light therapy

Head or neck pain: *Level 1*—Feldenkrais method

Headache: *Level 1*—Applied kinesiology, Alexander technique, Bonnie Prudden myotherapy, chiropractic, CranioSacral therapy, environmental medicine, homeopathy, hypnotherapy, light therapy, magnetic field therapy, reflexology, reiki, relaxation therapy, Rosen method, therapeutic touch

Level 2—Flower essences, neuro linguistic programming, Tai Chi, Trager approach, yoga

Level 3—Acupressure, acupuncture, colon hydrotherapy, quartz crystal therapy, fasting

Level 5—Dance/movement therapy

Headaches, cluster: *Level 1*—Ayurveda

Headaches, cluster: *Level 1*—Ayurveda, Bowen technique, homeopathy, light therapy, osteopathic medicine

Level 2—Environmental medicine, flower essences, Qi Gong

Level 3—Quartz crystal therapy, flower essences, macronutrients, meditation

Level 5—Color therapy, Hellerwork

Headaches, tension: *Level 1*—Ayurveda, Hellerwork, homeopathy, osteopathic medicine, Qi Gong

Level 2—Environmental medicine, massage therapy

Level 3—Flower essences

Hearing disorders: *Level 1*—Dance/movement therapy

Level 2—Reflexology, shamanism, Tai Chi

Level 3—Acupressure, environmental medicine, homeopathy, Qi Gong, yoga

Level 4—Acupuncture, flower essences

Level 5—Chiropractic, colon hydrotherapy, reiki

Hearing disorders or tinnitis: *Level 3*—Ayurveda

Hearing loss: *Level 1*—Tai Chi

Level 2—Homeopathy

Level 3—Ayurveda, environmental medicine, music therapy, Qi Gong, reflexology

Level 4—Acupressure, acupuncture

Level 5—Chiropractic, colon hydrotherapy

Heart disease: *Level 1*—Macronutrients, Tai Chi

Level 2—Ayurveda, CranioSacral therapy, environmental medicine, homeopathy, magnetic field therapy, reflexology, reiki, therapeutic touch, yoga

Level 3—Acupuncture, applied kinesiology, colon hydrotherapy, dance/movement therapy, music therapy, Qi Gong

Level 4—Alexander technique, chiropractic, massage therapy (if not contraindicated)

Level 5—Acupressure, fasting, orthomolecular medicine, Rosen method

Heartburn: *Level 1*—Homeopathy

Heat cramps: *Level 2*—Homeopathy

Heat stroke: *Level 2*—Homeopathy

Hemochromatosis: *Level 1*—Chelation therapy

Hemolytic anemia: *Level 2*—Hypnotherapy

Hemophilia: *Level 5*—Homeopathy

Hemoptysis: *Level 3*—Homeopathy

Hemorrhage: *Level 3*—Homeopathy

Hemorrhoids: *Level 1*—Ayurveda, homeopathy, magnetic field therapy

    Level 2—Bonnie Prudden myotherapy, colon hydrotherapy, Hellerwork, Qi Gong, reflexology, reiki, yoga

    Level 3—Acupressure, acupuncture, applied kinesiology, hypnotherapy

    Level 4—Environmental medicine, massage therapy

    Level 5—Chiropractic, fasting

Hepatitis, acute: *Level 1*—Ayurveda

Hepatitis, chronic: *Level 1*—Ayurveda

Hepatitis and hepatitis c: *Level 1*—Ayurveda

Herniated disc: *Level 1*—Bowen technique

    Level 3—Osteopathic medicine

Herpes: *Level 2*—Hypnotherapy, magnetic field therapy, Tai Chi

    Level 3—Ayurveda, colon hydrotherapy, environmental medicine, reflexology, reiki

    Level 4—Acupressure, acupuncture

    Level 5—Chiropractic

Herpes simplex and zoster: *Level 1*—Homeopathy

Herpes zoster: *Level 1*—Homeopathy

    Level 4—Quartz crystal therapy

    Level 5—Color therapy

Hiccups: *Level 2*—Acupressure

High altitude sickness: *Level 1*—Homeopathy

Hip disease: *Level 2*—Homeopathy

Hip dislocation: *Level 3*—Homeopathy

Hoarseness: *Level 1*—Homeopathy

Hyperactivity: *Level 1*—Environmental medicine, light therapy, magnetic field therapy, yoga

    Level 2—Ayurveda, Bowen technique, reflexology, reiki

    Level 3—Acupressure, acupuncture, applied kinesiology, dance/movement therapy, Hellerwork, neuro linguistic programming, Tai Chi, Trager approach

    Level 4—Chiropractic, colon hydrotherapy, massage therapy, Qi Gong

Hyperplasias benign or malignant: *Level 3*—Hypnotherapy

Hyperreflexic bladder: *Level 2*—Hypnotherapy

Hypertension: *Level 1*—Ayurveda, fasting, Hellerwork, homeopathy, hypnotherapy, magnetic field therapy, reiki, Tai Chi, therapeutic touch, yoga

    Level 2—Chelation therapy, dance/movement therapy, Feldenkrais method, Qi Gong, reflexology, reiki, relaxation therapy, Rosen method

    Level 3—Acupressure, acupuncture, applied kinesiology, Alexander technique, Bonnie Prudden myotherapy, chelation therapy, chiropractic, colon hydrotherapy, environmental medicine, light therapy, meditation, osteopathic medicine, massage therapy (if not contraindicated)

    Level 4—CranioSacral therapy, orthomolecular medicine

    Level 5—Trager approach

Hyphema: *Level 3*—Homeopathy

Hypoglycemia: *Level 2*—Homeopathy

    Level 3—Flower essences

Hypothermia: *Level 2*—Homeopathy

Hypoxia: *Level 2*—Homeopathy

Idiopathic scoliosis: *Level 4*—Osteopathic medicine

Immune system boosting: *Level 3*—Acupressure

Impingement syndrome: *Level 2*—Osteopathic medicine

Impotence: *Level 1*—Reiki
    Level 2—Magnetic field therapy, Qi Gong, reflexology, Tai Chi, yoga
    Level 3—Acupressure, acupuncture, Ayurveda, Bonnie Prudden myotherapy environmental
        medicine, neuro linguistic programming
    Level 4—Colon hydrotherapy
    Level 5—Chiropractic, fasting, massage therapy, Rosen method

Incontinence (adult): *Level 2*—Homeopathy
    Level 3—Bowen technique

Indigestion: *Level 1*—Homeopathy
    Level 4—Quartz crystal therapy
    Level 5—Color therapy

Infant feeding difficulties: *Level 3*—Osteopathic medicine

Infantile enterocolitis: *Level 2*—Environmental medicine

Infection: *Level 2*—Homeopathy

Infertility: *Level 2*—Bowen technique, Qi Gong
    Level 3—Environmental medicine
    Level 4—Meditation

Influenza: *Level 1*—Homeopathy
    Level 3—Flower essences
    Level 5—Color therapy

Insect stings, all kinds: *Level 1*—Homeopathy

Insomnia: *Level 1*—Applied kinesiology, Ayurveda, homeopathy, hypnotherapy, magnetic field
        therapy, reflexology, yoga
    Level 2—Acupressure, acupuncture, Feldenkrais method, light therapy, massage therapy, reiki,
        Rosen method
    Level 3—Colon hydrotherapy, CranioSacral therapy, dance/movement therapy, environmental
        medicine, flower essences, meditation, Tai Chi, Trager approach
    Level 4—Quartz crystal therapy, Qi Gong
    Level 5—Chiropractic

Internal injuries: *Level 2*—Homeopathy

Intestinal disorders: *Level 1*—Homeopathy

Iritis: *Level 3*—Flower essences, homeopathy

Irritability: *Level 3*—Environmental medicine

Irritable bowel syndrome: *Level 1*—Applied kinesiology, Ayurveda, colon hydrotherapy,
        environmental medicine, Feldenkrais method, homeopathy,
        macronutrients, magnetic field therapy, reflexology
    Level 2—Acupuncture, fasting, hypnotherapy, massage therapy, osteopathic medicine, Qi
        Gong, relaxation therapy, Tai Chi, therapeutic touch, yoga
    Level 3—Acupressure, CranioSacral therapy, neuro linguistic programming, reiki
    Level 4—Bonnie Prudden myotherapy
    Level 5—Chiropractic

Jaw problems: *Level 2*—Acupressure

Joint pain: *Level 1*—Applied kinesiology

Kidney stone: *Level 2*—Bowen technique, homeopathy

Knee disorders: *Level 1*—Homeopathy
 Level 3—Flower essences
Knee pain: *Level 1*—Bowen technique
Knee trouble: *Level 4*—Quartz crystal therapy
Lactation (breast feeding): *Level 1*—Homeopathy
Lactation, diminished milk supply: *Level 1*—Ayurveda
Laryngeal edema: *Level 2*—Environmental medicine
Laryngitis: *Level 1*—Homeopathy
Laryngospasm: *Level 1*—Homeopathy
Lazy eye: *Level 1*—Light therapy, Tai Chi
 Level 2—Feldenkrais method, reflexology
 Level 3—Acupressure, acupuncture, Ayurveda, hypnotherapy
 Level 4—Chiropractic, environmental medicine
 Level 5—Colon hydrotherapy, magnetic field therapy
Lead, arsenic, or cadmium poisoning: *Level 1*—Chelation therapy
Life review in the elderly: *Level 1*—Poetry therapy
Lightning strike injury: *Level 2*—Homeopathy
Lipid disorders: *Level 1*—Fasting
Liver and gall bladder congestion and pain: *Level 2*—Bowen technique
Liver disease: *Level 2*—Homeopathy
Locomotor ataxia: *Level 2*—Homeopathy
Lower back disorders: *Level 2*—Flower essences, homeopathy
Lower back injury: *Level 2*—Flower essences, homeopathy
Lumbar strain or sprain: *Level 1*—Osteopathic medicine
Lung cancer: *Level 1*—Environmental medicine
 Level 2—Qi Gong, reiki, Tai Chi, yoga
 Level 3—Ayurveda, colon hydrotherapy, reflexology
 Level 4—Acupuncture, magnetic field therapy, massage therapy (if not contraindicated)
 Level 5—Acupressure, chiropractic
Lung disorders: *Level 1*—Homeopathy
 Level 3—Quartz crystal therapy, flower essences
Lupus erythematosus: *Level 3*—Alexander technique, environmental medicine
Lyme disease: *Level 1*—Homeopathy
 Level 2—Alexander technique
 Level 4—Flower essences
Lymph gland swelling: *Level 1*—Homeopathy
 Level 2—Flower essences
Lymphedema (lymphatic massage): *Level 1*—Massage therapy
Macular degeneration: *Level 1*—Flower essences, light therapy
 Level 2—Ayurveda, environmental medicine, magnetic field therapy, Tai Chi
 Level 3—Colon hydrotherapy, homeopathy, reflexology, yoga
 Level 4—Acupressure, reiki
 Level 5—Acupuncture, chiropractic
Malabsorption syndromes (selected): *Level 3*—Environmental medicine
Male health: *Level 1*—Ayurveda, environmental medicine, homeopathy, reflexology, shamanism, Tai Chi, therapeutic touch, yoga, Qi Gong (for prevention or wellness)
 Level 2—Acupressure, neuro linguistic programming, reiki
 Level 3—Applied kinesiology, chiropractic, colon hydrotherapy, light therapy, massage therapy
 Level 4—Acupuncture, fasting
 Level 5—Magnetic field therapy

Manic behavior: *Level 2*—Homeopathy
    Level 4—Flower essences
Manic depressive illness: *Level 2*—Homeopathy
    Level 3—Environmental medicine, flower essences
Masatoiditis: *Level 4*—Quartz crystal therapy
Measles: *Level 1*—Homeopathy
    Level 2—Reflexology
    Level 3—Ayurveda
    Level 4—Acupressure, acupuncture, colon hydrotherapy, environmental medicine
    Level 5—Chiropractic, reiki
Memory disorders: *Level 1*—Homeopathy
Meniere's disease: *Level 1*—Environmental medicine, homeopathy, hypnotherapy, magnetic field
                      therapy
    Level 2—Qi Gong, Tai Chi
    Level 3—Reflexology
    Level 4—Acupressure, acupuncture, chiropractic
    Level 5—Colon hydrotherapy, massage therapy, reiki
Menopause: *Level 1*—Ayurveda, homeopathy, reflexology, reiki
    Level 2—Dance/movement therapy, environmental medicine, hypnotherapy, magnetic field
        therapy, Tai Chi, therapeutic touch, yoga
    Level 3—Acupressure, acupuncture, chiropractic, colon hydrotherapy, CranioSacral therapy,
        flower essences, light therapy
    Level 4—Alexander technique, fasting, massage therapy, Qi Gong
Menorrhagia: *Level 1*—Ayurveda
    Level 2—Environmental medicine, hypnotherapy, reflexology, Tai Chi
    Level 3—Acupuncture, massage therapy
    Level 4—Acupressure, chiropractic, colon hydrotherapy, fasting, Qi Gong
    Level 5—Magnetic field therapy
Menstrual cramps: *Level 1*—Acupressure, Ayurveda, Bonnie Prudden myotherapy, Bowen
                  technique, homeopathy, hypnotherapy, magnetic field therapy,
                  reflexology, reiki, therapeutic touch, yoga
    Level 2—Chiropractic, environmental medicine, Hellerwork, massage therapy, Rosen method,
        Tai Chi
    Level 3—Acupuncture, applied kinesiology, colon hydrotherapy, Feldenkrais method, light therapy
    Level 4—Fasting, Qi Gong
Menstrual irregularity: *Level 3*—CranioSacral therapy
Mental health: *Level 1*—Homeopathy, reflexology, Tai Chi
    Level 2—Flower essences, music therapy, Qi Gong (for depression, anxiety; not recommended
        for bipolar disorder), reiki, yoga
    Level 3—Acupressure, acupuncture, Alexander technique, environmental medicine, magnetic
        field therapy, massage therapy, neuro linguistic programming
    Level 4—Colon hydrotherapy, Rosen method
    Level 5—Chiropractic, fasting, orthomolecular medicine
Mental retardation: *Level 3*—Dance/movement therapy
Mercury amalgams, problems with: *Level 2*—Homeopathy
Mononucleosis: *Level 1*—Homeopathy
Motion sickness: *Level 1*—Homeopathy
    Level 2—Acupressure
Motor limitations: *Level 1*—Feldenkrais method
Mouth disorders: *Level 1*—Homeopathy

Multiple chemical sensitivity syndrome: *Level 1*—Ayurveda

Multiple sclerosis: *Level 1*—Ayurveda, Feldenkrais method, homeopathy
   Level 2—Alexander technique, Bowen technique, magnetic field therapy, Qi Gong, yoga
   Level 3—Acupressure, Bonnie Prudden myotherapy, chelation therapy, colon hydrotherapy, environmental medicine, light therapy, macronutrients, reflexology, Trager approach
   Level 4—Dance/movement therapy, massage therapy, reiki
   Level 5—Acupuncture, chiropractic

Mumps: *Level 1*—Homeopathy
   Level 2—Magnetic field therapy, Tai Chi
   Level 3—Ayurveda, reflexology
   Level 4—Environmental medicine
   Level 5—Acupressure, acupuncture, chiropractic, colon hydrotherapy, reiki

Muscle injuries: *Level 1*—Homeopathy
   Level 3—Flower essences

Muscle spasm: *Level 1*—Osteopathic medicine
   Level 2—Light therapy

Muscular aches and pains: *Level 1*—Reiki

Muscular dystrophy: *Level 1*—Feldenkrais method
   Level 2—Bowen technique

Musculosketal pain: *Level 1*—Bowen technique
   Level 2—Relaxation therapy

Myalgia and arthralgia: *Level 2*—Environmental medicine

Myasthernia gravis: *Level 2*—Hypnotherapy
   Level 3—Homeopathy

Myocardial infarction: *Level 2*—Homeopathy
   Level 3—Environmental medicine

Myoclonus: *Level 2*—Hypnotherapy

Myofascial strain: *Level 1*—Osteopathic medicine

Myofascial syndromes: *Level 1*—Trager approach

Myopia: *Level 2*—Hypnotherapy

Myositis: *Level 1*—Osteopathic medicine

Nacolepsy: *Level 1*—Homeopathy, hypnotherapy

Narcotic overdose: *Level 2*—Homeopathy
   Level 4—Flower essences

Nausea: *Level 1*—Homeopathy
   Level 2—Acupressure
   Level 4—Quartz crystal therapy

Neck injuries: *Level 3*—Flower essences, homeopathy

Neck pain: *Level 1*—Acupressure
   Level 2—Trager approach
   Level 3—Light therapy

Nephrotic syndrome: *Level 3*—Environmental medicine

Nerve disorders: *Level 1*—Homeopathy
   Level 2—Flower essences

Neuralgia: *Level 1*—Homeopathy
   Level 3—Flower essences

Neurodermatitis: *Level 1*—Hypnotherapy

Neurologic conditions (These conditions will respond to varying degree over repeated series of sessions. Main goal is to improve quality of life): *Level 2*—Bowen technique

Neurologic corrections: *Level 3*—Quartz crystal therapy

Neurologic diagnoses (Parkinson's, dystonia, stroke, brain damage): *Level 3*—Alexander technique

Neurologic disorders: *Level 1*—Feldenkrais method
    Level 3—Music therapy

Neurologic insults: traumatic brain injury, stroke, Parkinson's disease: *Level 2*—Dance/movement therapy

Neuroses and psychoses: *Level 1*—Hypnotherapy

Night blindness: *Level 1*—Flower essences, homeopathy, light therapy
    Level 2—Environmental medicine, Tai Chi
    Level 3—Reflexology
    Level 4—Acupressure, Ayurveda
    Level 5—Acupuncture, chiropractic, colon hydrotherapy, reiki

Nose disorders: *Level 1*—Homeopathy

Nose injuries: *Level 1*—Homeopathy

Obesity: *Level 1*—Macronutrients
    Level 5—CranioSacral therapy

Obesity and weight management: *Level 1*—Applied kinesiology, Ayurveda, fasting, Tai Chi
    Level 2—Dance/movement therapy, neuro linguistic programming, reflexology, yoga
    Level 3—Acupressure, colon hydrotherapy, environmental medicine, light therapy, magnetic field therapy
    Level 4—Acupuncture, chiropractic, massage therapy, Qi Gong, reiki
    Level 5—Rosen method

Obsessive-compulsive disorder: *Level 2*—Homeopathy
    Level 4—Flower essences

Open head injuries: *Level 1*—Feldenkrais method

Orthopedic injuries: *Level 1*—Feldenkrais method

Osteoarthritis: *Level 1*—Alexander technique, colon hydrotherapy, fasting, magnetic field therapy
    Level 2—Acupuncture, Ayurveda, Bonnie Prudden myotherapy, chiropractic, CranioSacral therapy, Feldenkrais method, flower essences, homeopathy, hypnotherapy, massage therapy, reflexology, reiki, Rosen method, yoga
    Level 3—Acupressure, applied kinesiology, environmental medicine, light therapy, osteopathic medicine, Qi Gong
    Level 5—Color therapy

Osteoporosis: *Level 1*—Applied kinesiology
    Level 2—Alexander technique, Ayurveda, environmental medicine, Feldenkrais method, flower essences, homeopathy, reflexology, reiki, Tai Chi, yoga
    Level 3—Acupressure, chelation therapy, colon hydrotherapy, light therapy
    Level 4—Acupuncture, chiropractic, magnetic field therapy, Qi Gong, massage therapy (if not contraindicated)

Osteoporosis (prevention, role of stress in bone mineral loss): *Level 4*—Meditation

Other arthritides: *Level 3*—Environmental medicine

Ovarian cancer: *Level 1*—Environmental medicine
    Level 2—Qi Gong, reiki, therapeutic touch
    Level 3—Acupuncture, Ayurveda, colon hydrotherapy, reflexology
    Level 4—Acupressure, magnetic field therapy, massage therapy (if not contraindicated)
    Level 5—Chiropractic, homeopathy

Ovarian cysts: *Level 1*—Ayurveda, magnetic field therapy, therapeutic touch
    Level 2—Environmental medicine, homeopathy, hypnotherapy, Qi Gong, reiki
    Level 3—Acupuncture, colon hydrotherapy, reflexology
    Level 4—Acupressure, massage therapy
    Level 5—Chiropractic
Pain: *Level 1*—CranioSacral therapy
    Level 3—Quartz crystal therapy
    Level 5—Color therapy
Pain and discomfort, generalized: *Level 1*—Reiki
Pain and limitation postsurgery: *Level 1*—Bowen technique
Pain management: *Level 1*—Reiki
Pain of any kind: *Level 1*—Homeopathy
    Level 4—Flower essences
Palliative Care: *Level 2*—Music therapy
Panic disorder: *Level 1*—Homeopathy
    Level 2—Meditation, relaxation therapy
    Level 3—Environmental medicine, flower essences
Paralysis: *Level 3*—Homeopathy
    Level 4—Quartz crystal therapy
Paranoia: *Level 1*—Homeopathy
Parasitic infections: *Level 1*—Ayurveda
    Level 2—Colon hydrotherapy
    Level 3—Environmental medicine, homeopathy, reflexology, Tai Chi, orthomolecular medicine
    Level 4—Acupuncture, reiki
    Level 5—Acupressure, chiropractic
Parkinson's disease: *Level 1*—Reiki
    Level 2—Ayurveda, Bowen technique, homeopathy
    Level 3—Trager approach
Paruresis: *Level 1*—Hypnotherapy
Pedal edema: *Level 2*—Homeopathy
    Level 4—Flower essences
Pelvic disorders: *Level 1*—Homeopathy
Pelvic imbalances: tilt, leg length, hip pain and imbalance, inguinal and groin pain:
    Level 1—Bowen technique
Peptic ulcer disease: *Level 1*—Ayurveda, homeopathy, magnetic field therapy
    Level 2—Acupuncture, Qi Gong, reflexology, relaxation therapy, Tai Chi, traditional Chinese herbal medicine
    Level 3—Colon hydrotherapy, environmental medicine, light therapy
    Level 4—Massage therapy
    Level 5—Chiropractic, reiki, Rosen method
Periodic leg movement syndrome: *Level 1*—Homeopathy, hypnotherapy, magnetic field therapy, reflexology, Tai Chi, yoga
    Level 2—Acupressure, environmental medicine, Feldenkrais method, therapeutic touch
    Level 3—Acupuncture, Ayurveda, chiropractic, reiki, traditional Chinese herbal medicine
    Level 4—Bonnie Prudden myotherapy, colon hydrotherapy, massage therapy
Peripheral vascular disorders (selected): *Level 1*—Chelation therapy
Personality disorders (selected): *Level 1*—Hypnotherapy
Pertussis: *Level 2*—Homeopathy
Phantom limb pain: *Level 1*—Homeopathy

Pharyngitis: *Level 1*—Homeopathy
Pharyngitis, streptococcal: *Level 1*—Homeopathy
    Level 2—Ayurveda, light therapy, reflexology, Tai Chi, traditional Chinese herbal medicine
    Level 3—Colon hydrotherapy
    Level 4—Environmental medicine, reiki
    Level 5—Acupuncture, chiropractic
Phlebitis: *Level 2*—Homeopathy
Phobias: *Level 1*—Homeopathy
Photophobia: *Level 4*—Environmental medicine
Photosensitivity: *Level 1*—Homeopathy
Physical disabilities: *Level 3*—Music therapy
Pinworms: *Level 1*—Ayurveda
    Level 2—Colon hydrotherapy, magnetic field therapy, Tai Chi
    Level 3—Reflexology, traditional Chinese herbal medicine
    Level 4—Acupuncture, environmental medicine
    Level 5—Chiropractic, reiki
Piriformis syndrome: *Level 1*—Osteopathic medicine
Plantar fascitis: *Level 2*—Osteopathic medicine
Pleurisy: *Level 1*—Homeopathy
Pneumonia: *Level 1*—Ayurveda (for subacute or chronic), homeopathy
    Level 2—CranioSacral therapy, magnetic field therapy, reflexology, Tai Chi, traditional Chinese
        herbal medicine
    Level 3—Acupuncture, Ayurveda (for acute), colon hydrotherapy, environmental medicine (for
        selected), light therapy, osteopathic medicine, Qi Gong
    Level 4—Acupressure, flower essences, massage therapy
    Level 5—Chiropractic, reiki
Poison ivy or oak: *Level 1*—Homeopathy
Poisoning, any type: *Level 2*—Homeopathy
Polio: *Level 2*—Bowen technique
Porphyria: *Level 3*—Chelation therapy
Postmyocardial infarct care: *Level 1*—Ayurveda
Postpartum depression: *Level 1*—Ayurveda
Posttraumatic stress disorder: *Level 1*—Homeopathy
    Level 3—Flower essences
Postpartum bleeding: *Level 1*—Ayurveda
Postpartum care: *Level 1*—Feldenkrais method, homeopathy, magnetic field therapy, reflexology,
                Tai Chi, traditional Chinese herbal medicine
    Level 2—Acupressure, reiki
    Level 3—Acupuncture, chiropractic, colon hydrotherapy, environmental medicine, massage
        therapy, Rosen method, yoga
Postpartum recovery: *Level 1*—Hellerwork
Postpartum syndrome: *Level 2*—Alexander technique
Postsurgical tissue trauma: *Level 1*—Feldenkrais method
Posture problems: *Level 1*—Hellerwork
Preconception care: *Level 1*—Ayurveda, environmental medicine, therapeutic touch
    Level 2—Acupuncture, Qi Gong, reflexology, Rosen method, yoga
    Level 3—Acupressure, colon hydrotherapy, reiki
    Level 4—Traditional Chinese herbal medicine
    Level 5—Chiropractic, massage therapy

Pregnancy: *Level 1*—Reflexology, reiki, Tai Chi
   Level 2—Acupressure, chiropractic, music therapy, traditional Chinese herbal medicine, yoga
   Level 3—Bonnie Prudden myotherapy, colon hydrotherapy, Hellerwork, acupuncture (if patient seen prior and by a senior acupuncturist—usually contraindicated in pregnancy), massage therapy (if not contraindicated)
Pregnancy and childbirth: *Level 1*—Environmental medicine, homeopathy, reflexology, Tai Chi
   Level 2—Acupressure, dance/movement therapy, music therapy, traditional Chinese herbal therapy
   Level 3—Acupuncture, Alexander technique, Ayurveda, Bonnie Prudden myotherapy, colon hydrotherapy, osteopathic medicine, Rosen method, massage therapy (if not contraindicated)
   Level 4—Chiropractic, flower essences
Pregnancy-induced low back pain: *Level 1*—Bowen technique
Pregnancy-related discomfort: *Level 1*—Reiki
Pregnancy, difficult: *Level 1*—Therapeutic touch
Premenstrual syndrome: *Level 1*—Applied kinesiology, Ayurveda, Bowen technique, homeopathy, magnetic field therapy, reflexology, traditional Chinese herbal medicine, yoga, hypnotherapy
   Level 2—Acupressure, environmental medicine, light therapy, orthomolecular medicine, Tai Chi, therapeutic touch
   Level 3—Acupuncture, Bonnie Prudden myotherapy, chiropractic, colon hydrotherapy, flower essences, massage therapy, osteopathic medicine, Rosen method
   Level 4—Qi Gong
Prevention: *Level 1*—Qi Gong
Prostate: *Level 3*—Bowen technique
Prostatic cancer: *Level 1*—Environmental medicine
   Level 2—Ayurveda, Qi Gong, reiki, traditional Chinese herbal medicine
   Level 3—Acupuncture, colon hydrotherapy, reflexology
   Level 4—Acupressure, magnetic field therapy, massage therapy (if not contraindicated)
   Level 5—Chiropractic, homeopathy
Prostatitis: *Level 1*—Ayurveda, homeopathy
   Level 2—Magnetic field therapy, reflexology, Tai Chi, traditional Chinese herbal medicine
   Level 3—Acupuncture, colon hydrotherapy, environmental medicine, hypnotherapy, reiki
   Level 4—Acupressure, Qi Gong
   Level 5—Chiropractic, massage therapy
Psoriasis: *Level 1*—Homeopathy, reiki
   Level 2—Hypnotherapy, light therapy, meditation
   Level 5—Color therapy
Psoriatic arthritis: *Level 1*—Fasting
Psychiatric disorders (selected): *Level 1*—Reiki
Psychologic problems: *Level 2*—Flower essences, homeopathy
Psychoses: *Level 2*—Hypnotherapy
Psychosomatic disorders: *Level 1*—Feldenkrais method
Psychotic behavior: *Level 2*—Flower essences, homeopathy
Ptyalism: *Level 2*—Hypnotherapy
Pulmonary disease: *Level 1*—Homeopathy
Pulmonary edema: *Level 2*—Homeopathy
Puncture wounds: *Level 1*—Homeopathy
Pylonephritis: *Level 2*—Ayurveda

Raynaud's syndrome: *Level 1*—Homeopathy, hypnotherapy
    Level 3—Flower essences
Reactions to diagnoses of severe medical illnesses: *Level 1*—Poetry therapy
Reaven's syndrome (syndrome X): *Level 2*—Fasting
Rectum disorders: *Level 1*—Homeopathy
Reflex sympathetic dystrophy: *Level 3*—Osteopathic medicine
Rehabilitation, postsurgical: *Level 3*—Trager approach
Renal colic: *Level 2*—Homeopathy
Renal disorders: *Level 1*—Homeopathy
Repetitive strain injury: *Level 1*—Alexander technique
Repetitive stress injuries: *Level 1*—Feldenkrais method
    Level 2—Massage therapy
Respiratory conditions: *Level 1*—Alexander technique, Ayurveda, homeopathy, yoga
    Level 2—Acupuncture, Bowen technique, environmental medicine, magnetic field therapy, Qi
        Gong, reflexology, traditional Chinese herbal medicine
    Level 3—Acupressure, Bonnie Prudden myotherapy, colon hydrotherapy, flower essences,
        massage therapy, reiki
    Level 4—Chiropractic
Restless leg syndrome: *Level 1*—Applied kinesiology, homeopathy, magnetic field therapy,
        reflexology, Tai Chi
    Level 2—Acupressure, environmental medicine, Rosen method, traditional Chinese herbal
        medicine, therapeutic touch, yoga
    Level 3—Bonnie Prudden myotherapy, chelation therapy, massage therapy
    Level 4—Acupuncture, chiropractic, colon hydrotherapy, Feldenkrais method, Qi Gong
Retinal degeneration: *Level 2*—Homeopathy
    Level 3—Flower essences
Retinal detachment: *Level 2*—Light therapy
    Level 3—Acupuncture, reflexology
    Level 4—Traditional Chinese herbal medicine, Ayurveda
    Level 5—Acupressure, chiropractic, colon hydrotherapy, environmental medicine
Retinitis: *Level 2*—Homeopathy
    Level 3—Flower essences
Retinopathy: *Level 2*—Light therapy
    Level 3—Acupuncture, reflexology, traditional Chinese herbal medicine
    Level 4—Environmental medicine
    Level 5—Chiropractic, colon hydrotherapy, magnetic field therapy, Qi Gong
Retts' syndrome: *Level 1*—Music therapy
Rheumatic fever: *Level 2*—Homeopathy
Rheumatoid arthritis: *Level 1*—Ayurveda, colon hydrotherapy, fasting, homeopathy, Tai Chi, yoga
    Level 2—Alexander technique, CranioSacral therapy, environmental medicine, flower essences,
        hypnotherapy, magnetic field therapy, reflexology, reiki, traditional Chinese herbal
        medicine, therapeutic touch
    Level 3—Chelation therapy, acupuncture, Bonnie Prudden myotherapy, chiropractic, quartz
        crystal therapy, neuro linguistic programming, Qi Gong, massage therapy (if not
        contraindicated)
    Level 5—Color therapy, Rosen method
Rhinitis: *Level 1*—Environmental medicine
Rib sprain or strain: *Level 1*—Osteopathic medicine
Rocky Mountain spotted fever: *Level 1*—Homeopathy

Rotator cuff tendonitis: *Level 2*—Osteopathic medicine

Runner's knees: *Level 1*—Bowen technique

Sacral sprain: *Level 1*—Osteopathic medicine

Sacroiliac pain and imbalances: posttraumatic or related to pregnancy: *Level 1*—Bowen
technique

Salmonella: *Level 1*—Homeopathy

Schizophrenia: *Level 1*—Dance/movement therapy

   Level 2—Homeopathy

   Level 3—Environmental medicine

Sciatica: *Level 1*—Bowen technique

   Level 2—Homeopathy

   Level 3—Quartz crystal therapy, flower essences

Scleroderma: *Level 3*—Environmental medicine

Scoliosis: *Level 2*—Alexander technique, Bowen technique, Homeopathy

   Level 3—Flower essences

Seasickness: *Level 1*—Homeopathy

Seasonally activated depression: *Level 1*—Color therapy

Separation anxiety disorder: *Level 1*—Dance/movement therapy

Sepsis: *Level 2*—Homeopathy

Sexual dysfunction (male and female): *Level 2*—Homeopathy

   Level 3—Environmental medicine

Sexual impotence (gender nonspecific): *Level 2*—Hypnotherapy

Sexually transmitted diseases: *Level 2*—Homeopathy

   Level 3—Ayurveda, colon hydrotherapy, environmental medicine, reflexology, traditional
Chinese herbal medicine

   Level 4—Acupuncture

   Level 5—Chiropractic

Shin splints: *Level 1*—Bowen techniques

Shock, treatment of: *Level 3*—Flower essences, homeopathy

Shortness of breath (dyspnea): *Level 1*—Homeopathy

   Level 2—Flower essences

Shoulder dislocation: *Level 3*—Flower essences, homeopathy

Sinus congestion: *Level 2*—Bowen technique

Sinus disorders, acute and chronic: *Level 1*—Homeopathy

   Level 2—Flower essences

   Level 4—Quartz crystal therapy

Sinusitis: *Level 1*—Applied kinesiology, Ayurveda, Tai Chi

   Level 2—Acupuncture, CranioSacral therapy, environmental medicine, magnetic field therapy,
Qi Gong, reflexology, reiki, traditional Chinese herbal medicine, yoga

   Level 3—Hypnotherapy, light therapy, massage therapy

   Level 4—Chiropractic, colon hydrotherapy

Sinusitis, acute and chronic: *Level 1*—Homeopathy

   Level 2—Flower essences

Skin diseases: *Level 1*—Homeopathy

Skin diseases (acne and others): *Level 4*—Fasting

Sleep apnea: *Level 1*—Ayurveda, fasting, homeopathy, Tai Chi

   Level 2—Magnetic field therapy, reflexology, therapeutic touch, yoga

   Level 3—Acupuncture, applied kinesiology, hypnotherapy, traditional Chinese herbal medicine

   Level 4—Colon hydrotherapy, environmental medicine, massage therapy

   Level 5—Chiropractic

Sleep disorders: *Level 1*—Homeopathy, hypnotherapy, magnetic field therapy, reflexology, yoga
    Level 2—Ayurveda, Feldenkrais method, neuro linguistic programming, orthomolecular medicine, Tai Chi, traditional Chinese herbal medicine
    Level 3—Acupuncture, applied kinesiology, Alexander technique, flower essences, light therapy, reiki
    Level 4—Colon hydrotherapy, environmental medicine
    Level 5—Chiropractic, fasting
Sleep paralysis: *Level 1*—Hypnotherapy
Snakebite: *Level 2*—Homeopathy
Soft tissue injuries: *Level 1*—Homeopathy
Soft tissue fungal infections: *Level 2*—Light therapy
Somatoform disorders: *Level 1*—Environmental medicine
Spasms or strains: *Level 2*—Light therapy
Speech disorders: *Level 2*—Homeopathy
Spider bites: *Level 1*—Homeopathy
Spinal injury: *Level 2*—Flower essences, homeopathy
Spleen disorders: *Level 2*—Homeopathy
Spleen injury: *Level 1*—Homeopathy
Spondylolisthesis: *Level 3*—Osteopathic medicine
Sports injuries: *Level 1*—Applied kinesiology, Bowen technique, homeopathy
    Level 3—Flower essences
Sprains: *Level 1*—Homeopathy
Sprains (first and second degree): *Level 2*—Massage therapy
Sprains and strains: *Level 2*—CranioSacral therapy
Stammering: *Level 2*—Homeopathy
Sternocostal pain: *Level 1*—Bowen technique
Stiffness: *Level 4*—Quartz crystal therapy
Stomachache: *Level 1*—Applied kinesiology, Ayurveda, hypnotherapy, magnetic field therapy, reflexology
    Level 2—Acupuncture, colon hydrotherapy, Qi Gong, reiki, Tai Chi, traditional Chinese herbal medicine
    Level 3—Environmental medicine, massage therapy, neuro linguistic programming
    Level 4—Chiropractic
    Level 5—Fasting
Stomach disorders: *Level 1*—Homeopathy
    Level 4—Quartz crystal therapy
Strabismus: *Level 3*—Homeopathy
Strains: *Level 1*—Homeopathy
Strains (first and second degree): *Level 2*—Massage therapy
Stress: *Level 1*—Applied kinesiology, Ayurveda, quartz crystal therapy, dance/movement therapy, environmental medicine, Feldenkrais method, Hellerwork, homeopathy, hypnotherapy, magnetic field therapy, massage therapy, neuro linguistic programming, osteopathic medicine, Qi Gong, reflexology, reiki, Rosen method, Tai Chi, traditional Chinese herbal medicine, therapeutic touch, yoga
    Level 2—Colon hydrotherapy, light therapy
    Level 3—Acupuncture, Bonnie Prudden myotherapy, color therapy
    Level 4—Chiropractic
Stress disorders: *Level 1*—Relaxation therapy
Stress-induced dysfunction of the nervous system: *Level 1*—Reiki
Stress-related allergies: *Level 1*—Reiki

Stress syndromes: *Level 1*—Alexander technique

Stress, tension, sleep disorders: *Level 1*—Bowen technique

Stress-related illnesses: *Level 2*—Trager approach

Stroke: *Level 1*—Feldenkrais method, light therapy

    Level 2—Bowen technique, homeopathy

    Level 4—Quartz crystal therapy

Stroke (prevention): *Level 3*—Meditation

Styes: *Level 1*—Homeopathy

Substance dependence or abuse: *Level 2*—Meditation

Surgical (pre and postsurgical): *Level 1*—Homeopathy

Survivors of violence, abuse, or incest: *Level 1*—Poetry therapy

Syphilis: *Level 2*—Homeopathy

    Level 3—Ayurveda, reflexology, traditional Chinese herbal medicine

    Level 4—Environmental medicine

    Level 5—Acupuncture, chiropractic, colon hydrotherapy

Systemic lupus erythematosus: *Level 2*—Hypnotherapy

Teething: *Level 1*—Homeopathy

Temporomandibular joint syndrome: *Level 1*—Bowen technique, Feldenkrais method

    Level 2—Homeopathy, osteopathic medicine

    Level 3—Massage therapy

Tendomyopathies: *Level 2*—Fasting

Tendonitis: *Level 2*—Osteopathic medicine

    Level 3—Quartz crystal therapy

Thoracic outlet syndrome: *Level 2*—Osteopathic medicine

Thoracic sprain or strain: *Level 1*—Osteopathic medicine

Throat problems: *Level 4*—Quartz crystal therapy

Thrombocytopenia: *Level 3*—Environmental medicine

Thrombophlebitis: *Level 3*—Environmental medicine

Thyroid dysfunction: *Level 3*—Environmental medicine

Tick bite: *Level 2*—Homeopathy

Tinnitus: *Level 1*—Homeopathy, hypnotherapy, Qi Gong, Tai Chi

    Level 2—Ayurveda, Feldenkrais method, magnetic field therapy, traditional Chinese herbal medicine

    Level 3—Acupuncture, chiropractic, environmental medicine, flower essences, reflexology

    Level 4—Bonnie Prudden myotherapy

    Level 5—Colon hydrotherapy, reiki

Tobacco use: *Level 4*—Environmental medicine

Tonsillitis: *Level 1*—Homeopathy

Toothache: *Level 1*—Homeopathy

Torticollis: *Level 1*—Hypnotherapy

    Level 2—Bowen technique

Transitions from life to death: *Level 1*—Shamanism

Trauma (scar tissue from injury or surgery): *Level 1*—Hellerwork

Traumatic brain injury: *Level 3*—Music therapy

Traumatic injury: *Level 3*—Alexander technique

Trichomonas: *Level 2*—Ayurveda, reflexology

    Level 3—Environmental medicine, traditional Chinese herbal medicine

    Level 5—Acupuncture, chiropractic, colon hydrotherapy, reiki

Tuberculosis: *Level 4*—Quartz crystal therapy

Tumors: *Level 4*—Quartz crystal therapy

Turner's syndrome: *Level 1*—Dance/movement therapy

Ulcer: *Level 2*—Meditation

Ulcerative colitis: *Level 1*—Ayurveda, homeopathy
    Level 2—Bowen technique, environmental medicine, meditation
    Level 3—Quartz crystal therapy, Hellerwork

Ulcerative colitis and Crohn's disease: *Level 1*—Ayurveda, homeopathy
    Level 2—Colon hydrotherapy, environmental medicine, magnetic field therapy, massage
        therapy, reflexology, reiki, relaxation therapy, Tai Chi, yoga
    Level 3—Acupressure, applied kinesiology, Bonnie Prudden myotherapy, hypnotherapy, Rosen
        method
    Level 4—Acupuncture, chiropractic, fasting, Qi Gong
    Level 5—Feldenkrais method

Ulcerative colitis, acute: *Level 3*—Ayurveda

Ulcerative colitis, chronic or subacute: *Level 1*—Ayurveda

Upper respiratory infections: *Level 3*—Light therapy

Urethritis: *Level 1*—Homeopathy

URI or sinusitis: *Level 3*—Osteopathic medicine

Urinary tract infection, acute: *Level 2*—Ayurveda

Uticaria: *Level 1*—Homeopathy
    Level 2—Environmental medicine

Uterine and ovarian cancer: *Level 3*—Hypnotherapy

Uterine fibroids: *Level 1*—Ayurveda, homeopathy
    Level 2—Hypnotherapy, magnetic field therapy, traditional Chinese herbal medicine
    Level 3—Acupuncture, colon hydrotherapy, Qi Gong, reflexology, reiki
    Level 4—Massage therapy
    Level 5—Chiropractic

Vaccination alternative: *Level 1*—Homeopathy

Vaccination reactions: *Level 1*—Homeopathy

Vaginal infection: *Level 5*—Homeopathy

Vaginal infections: *Level 1*—Homeopathy
    Level 2—Ayurveda, environmental medicine, reflexology, Tai Chi, traditional Chinese herbal
        medicine
    Level 3—Acupuncture, colon hydrotherapy, environmental medicine, magnetic field therapy,
        reiki

Vaginismus: *Level 1*—Hypnotherapy

Valvular heart disease, acute or severe: *Level 3*—Ayurveda

Valvular heart disease, chronic or subacute: *Level 1*—Ayurveda

Varicose veins: *Level 5*—Color therapy

Vasculitis: *Level 3*—Environmental medicine

Vertigo: *Level 1*—Homeopathy
    Level 2—Osteopathic medicine
    Level 3—Environmental medicine

Violent behavior: *Level 2*—Flower essences, homeopathy

Viral and bacterial infections: *Level 1*—Ayurveda, homeopathy
    Level 2—Colon hydrotherapy, environmental medicine, magnetic field therapy, reflexology, Tai
        Chi, traditional Chinese herbal medicine
    Level 3—Acupuncture, flower essences, Qi Gong, reiki
    Level 5—Chiropractic

Vision disorders: *Level 1*—Flower essences, homeopathy, light therapy, Tai Chi
  Level 2—Ayurveda, magnetic field therapy, orthomolecular medicine, reflexology
  Level 3—Acupuncture, environmental medicine, Feldenkrais method, neuro linguistic programming, traditional Chinese herbal medicine
  Level 4—Quartz crystal therapy
  Level 5—Chiropractic, colon hydrotherapy, massage therapy
Vomiting: *Level 1*—Homeopathy
Vulvadynia: *Level 1*—Ayurveda
Vulvodynia: *Level 3*—Environmental medicine
Warts: *Level 1*—Homeopathy
  Level 3—Hypnotherapy
Wellness or health maintenance: *Level 1*—CranioSacral therapy
Whiplash: *Level 1*—Feldenkrais method, flower essences, homeopathy, Bowen technique
Wound healing: *Level 3*—Quartz crystal therapy
X-ray radiation: *Level 2*—Quartz crystal therapy
Yeast infections: *Level 1*—Homeopathy
  Level 2—Ayurveda, colon hydrotherapy, reflexology, traditional Chinese herbal medicine
  Level 3—Acupuncture, environmental medicine
  Level 4—Orthomolecular medicine
  Level 5—Chiropractic, massage therapy, reiki

Index

A

AAEM; *see* American Academy of Environmental Medicine (AAEM)

AATA; *see* American Art Therapy Association (AATA)

AATOM; *see* American Association for Teachers of Oriental Medicine (AATOM)

Academy for Guided Imagery, 65, 66

ACAOM; *see* Accreditation Commission for Acupuncture and Oriental Medicine (ACAOM)

Accreditation Commission for Acupuncture and Oriental Medicine (ACAOM), 215

Aconite, sources and uses of, 555*t*

Acquired immunodeficiency syndrome (AIDS), Qi Gong for, 235

Actions/pharmacokinetics
  of acupuncture, 198
  of antineoplastons, 502
  of aromatherapy, 659
  of chelation therapy, 512
  of enzyme therapy, 525-526
  of macronutrients, 571
  of micronutrients, 587
  of orthomolecular medicine, 611
  of reflexology, 784-785
  of Tai Chi, 225
  of therapeutic touch, 467
  of traditional Chinese medicine, 212

Acupoints, 179
  proving existence of, 183-184

Acupressure, 340
  applications of, 182
  associations on, 188
  credentialing in, 187
  demographics of, 181
  druglike information on, 185-186
  efficacy of, 184
  electric stimulation in, 183
  forms of, 181
  history of, 178-179
  in lactation, 186
  mechanisms of action of, 179-181

Acupressure—Cont.
  origins of, 178-179
  in pain control, 180-181
  in pregnancy, 186
  provider selection in, 187-188
  referral for, 181
  research on, 183-185
  risks in, 184
  safety of, 185
    research on, 184
  self-help versus professional approach to, 187
  trade products for, 186
  training in, 187
  warnings on, 185-186

Acupressure Institute, 187

Acupuncture, 191-202
  actions of, 198
  adverse reactions to, 198
  American style of, 195
  associations for, 200-201
  auricular, 194
  biologic dentistry and, 668
  classical, 195
  color, 157
    development of, 155
    referral for, 158
  credentialing in, 199-200
  demographics of, 196
  drug interactions with, 198
  druglike information on, 198
  EAV and, 194
  five-element, 194
  forms of, 194-196
  French energetics, 194
  history of, 191-192
  in Japanese herbal medicine, 194
  Korean hand, 195
  in lactation, 198
  mechanisms of action of, 192-194
  method of stimulation in, 195-196
  neuroanatomic, 194

Page numbers in italics indicate illustrations or boxes; *t* indicates tables.

Acupuncture—Cont.
  origins of, 191-192
  pharmacokinetics of, 198
  in pregnancy, 198
  provider selection in, 200
  referral for, 196-197
  research on, 197
  safety of, 198
  self-help versus professional approach to, 199
  trade products for, 198
  in traditional Chinese medicine, 194
  training in, 200
  in Vietnamese traditions, 195
  visiting professional in, 199
  warnings on, 198
Acupuncture points in Bowen technique, 373
Acupuncture system, magnets and, 165
Additives in foods, 571-572
Adverse reactions
  to acupuncture, 198
  to antineoplastons, 503
  to aromatherapy, 661-662
  to art therapy, 26
  to Aston-Patterning, 367
  to biologic dentistry, 673
  to chelation therapy, 512
  to colon hydrotherapy, 685
  to CranioSacral therapy, 388
  to detoxification therapy, 713
  to enzyme therapy, 527
  to fasting, 736
  to flower essences, 541
  to Hellerwork Structural Integration, 412
  to herbal medicines, 556-563t
  to homeopathy, 266
  to macronutrients, 572
  to magnetic field therapy, 171
  to micronutrients, 588-589
  to Native American Medicine, 297
  to neuro linguistic programming, 101
  to orthomolecular medicine, 612
  to poetry therapy, 109
  to quartz crystal therapy, 774
  to reflexology, 785-786
  to relaxation therapies, 124
  to Tai Chi, 226
  to therapeutic touch, 468
  to traditional Chinese medicine, 213
Aging
  diseases of, oxidants and, 601-602
  micronutrient deficiencies in, 580
AIDS (acquired immunodeficiency syndrome), Qi Gong for, 235
Alexander, FM, in Alexander Technique history, 350

Alexander Technique, 350-358
  applications of, 353
  associations for, 356
  barriers to, 356
  credentialing in, 355
  demographics of, 352
  efficacy of, 354
  history of, 350
  issues in, key, 356
  mechanisms of action of, 350-352
  origins of, 350
  provider selection in, 356
  referral for, 352-353
  research on, 353-354
  risks in, 354
  safety of, 354
  self-help versus professional approach to, 354-355
  training in, 356
  visiting professional in, 355
Alexander Technique International, 355
Allergies, Qi Gong for, 235
Aloe, sources and uses of, 555t
Aloe vera, use, interactions, adverse effects, and
    contraindications of, 556t
Alpha brain wave frequency, 33
Alternative medicine
  background on, 2-4
  basic principles of, 5-7
  conditions and treatments in, 794
  evidence on, dilemma of, 7-9
  integration of, into practice, 13-16
  in integrative cancer care, 627-628
  learning, 11-12
  unlearning and, 11-12
  working with medical community and, 14-15
Altschuler, Ira, in music therapy history, 86
Alzheimer's disease
  aromatherapy for, 656
  vitamin E and, 610
Amalgam, 667; see also Mercury amalgam in dentistry
AMBP; see Associated Bodywork and Massage Professionals
    (ABMP)
American Academy of Environmental Medicine (AAEM), 716
American Academy of Medical Acupuncture (AAMA), 196
American Academy of Medicine Acupuncture (AAMA), 200-
    201
American Art Therapy Association (AATA), 20
American Association For Teachers in Oriental Medicine
    (AATOM), 215
American Board of Chelation Therapy, 513
American Dance Therapy Association (ADTA), 42, 47, 48
American Music Therapy Association (AMTA), 89, 93
American Polarity Therapy Association (APTA), 431, 433

American Society for the Alexander Technique (ASAT), 355
American style of acupuncture, 195
AMTA; *see* American Music Therapy Association (AMTA)
Amygdala in aromatherapy, 652-653
Anasura, 144
Angerer, Josef, in iridology history, 757
Angiology, efficacy of enzymes in, research on, 523
Antagonism, balanced, in acupressure, 179-180
Antiangiogenic agents in cancer biotherapy, 625-626
Antidepressants, hypotension caused by, aromatherapy for, 656
Antidrugs in orthomolecular medicine, 607
Antiinflammatory effects of enzymes, research on, 522
Antineoplastons, 496-507
    actions of, 502
    administration of, 504
    adverse reactions to, 503
    applications of, 500-501
    barriers to, 506
    credentialing in, 505
    demographics of, 497
    dosage of, 504
    druglike information on, 501-504
    efficacy of, 499
    forms of, 497
    history of, 496
    issues on, key, 506
    in lactation, 504
    mechanisms of action of, 496-497
    origins of, 496
    pharmacokinetics of, 502
    in pregnancy, 504
    provider of, 505
    referral for, 497-498
    research on, 498-500
    risks of, 499
    safety of, 501-502
        research on, 499
    self-help versus professional approach to, 504
    trade products in, 504
    visiting professional in, 504-505
    warnings on, 502-503
Antioxidants, 596
    aging diseases and, 601-602
    cellular physiology and, 598-599
    dietary, actions of, 597t
    need for, 600
Anxiety
    aromatherapy for, 655
    meditation for, 77
    relaxation-induced, 123
    symptoms of, generalized, relaxation therapies for, research on, 122
Anxiety disorders, relaxation therapies for, research on, 121
APTA; *see* American Polarity Therapy Association (APTA)

Arndt-Schultz Law in homeopathy, 261
Arnica, use, interactions, adverse effects, and contraindications of, 556t
Aromatherapy, 651-666
    actions of, 659
    administration of, 662-663
    adverse reactions to, 661-662
    applications of, 654-658
    associations for, 664
    in Ayurveda, 250
    barriers to, 664
    credentialing in, 663-664
    demographics of, 653
    druglike information on, 659-661
    efficacy of, 659
    essential oils in, 651-666; *see also* Essential oils
    forms of, 653
    history of, 651
    interactions with, 661-662
    issues in, 664
    mechanisms of action of, 651-653
    origins of, 651
    pharmacokinetics of, 659
    in pregnancy, 662
    provider selection in, 664
    referral for, 653
    research on, 658-659
    risks of, 658-659
    safety of, 658-659
    self-help versus professional approach to, 663
    trade products in, 662
    visiting professional in, 663
    warnings on, 660-661
Art therapy, 20-31
    adverse reactions to, 26
    applications of, 23
    associations for, 28
    barriers to, 28
    credentialing in, 27
    definition of, 20
    demographics of, 23
    drug interactions with, 25
    druglike information on, 25-26
    efficacy of, 24
    forms of, 21-22
    history of, 20
    issues involving, 28
    mechanism of action of, 20-21
    origins of, 20
    outcome-based assessment of, 24
    populations served by, 23
    provider selection for, 27
    referral for, indications and reasons for, 22
    research base for, 24-25

Art therapy—Cont.
  risks of, 24
  safety of, 24
  self-help versus professional approach to, 26
  training in, 27
  visiting professional in, 26-27
Art Therapy Credentialing Board (ATCB), 27
Arteries, hardened, chelation therapy and, 509-510
Arteriosclerosis, chelation therapy and, 509-510
Arthritis, Qi Gong for, 236
Arthrokinetics, Aston, 364
Asanas in Yoga, 142, 143
ASAT; see American Society for the Alexander Technique
      (ASAT)
Ascorbic acid; see also Vitamin C
  actions of, 597t
Ashtang Hrdyam, 246
Assertiveness, neuro linguistic programming for, 98
Associated Bodywork and Massage Professionals (ABMP), 415
Associations
  for acupressure, 188
  for acupuncture, 200-201
  for Alexander Technique, 356
  for antineoplastons, 506
  for applied kinesiology, 648
  for aromatherapy, 664
  for art therapy, 28
  for Ayurveda, 256
  for biofeedback, 39
  for biologic dentistry, 676-677
  for Bonnie Prudden Myotherapy, 421
  for Bowen Technique, 378-379
  for chelation therapy, 513-514
  for chiropractic, 321-322
  for colon hydrotherapy, 687
  for color therapy, 699-700
  for CranioSacral therapy, 390-391
  for dance/movement therapy, 48
  for detoxification therapy, 714
  for environmental medicine, 726
  for enzyme therapy, 529
  for fasting, 738-739
  for Feldenkrais Method, 403
  for flower essences, 543-544
  for Hellerwork Structural Integration, 415
  for homeopathy, 270-272
  for hypnotherapy, 61-62
  for interactive guided imagery, 70
  for iridology, 767
  for juice therapy, 754-755
  for light therapy, 161
  for macronutrients, 574
  for magnetic field therapy, 173
  for massage therapy, 347

Associations—Cont.
  for meditation, 81-82
  for micronutrients, 592
  for music therapy, 94
  for Native American medicine, 299
  for naturopathic medicine, 282
  for neuro linguistic programming, 103
  for orthomolecular medicine, 614
  for osteopathic medicine, 335-336
  for poetry therapy, 111
  for Polarity Therapy, 433
  for Qi Gong, 242
  for quartz crystal therapy, 777
  for reflexology, 787-789
  for Reiki, 442
  for relaxation therapies, 125-126
  for Rolfing Structural Integration, 451
  for Rosen Method, 460-461
  for spiritual healing and prayer, 138
  for Tai Chi, 228
  for traditional Chinese medicine, 216
  for Trager approach, 481
  for Yoga, 150
Astanga, 144
Asthma
  Alexander Technique for, 352
  Qi Gong for, 235
Aston, Judith, in Aston-Patterning history, 359
Aston Paradigm, 359
Aston-Patterning, 359-370
  adverse reactions to, 367
  applications of, 366-367
  barriers to, 370
  credentialing in, 369
  demographics of, 365
  drug interactions with, 367
  druglike information on, 367-368
  forms of, 364-365
  history of, 359
  issues in, key, 370
  in lactation, 368
  mechanisms of action of, 360-364
  origins of, 359
  in pregnancy, 368
  provider selection in, 370
  referral for, 365
  research on, 367
  safety of, 367
  self-help versus professional approach to, 368
  trade products for, 368
  training in, 369
  visiting professional in, 368-369
  warnings on, 367

Astragalus, use, interactions, adverse effects, and contraindications of, 556*t*

Atherosclerosis
 antioxidants and, 598
 chelation therapy and, 510
 oxidants and, 598

Attitudes in integrative cancer care, 621

Attunement, 41

Aura in flower essences, 536

Auricular acupuncture, 194

Auroma-soma therapy, 693

Authentic movement, 42

Autogenic discharges from relaxation, 123

Autoimmune diseases, enzyme therapy for, 518-519

Autonomic nervous system rebalancing in Bowen technique, 373

Awareness in Alexander Technique, 351

Awareness Through Movement lessons in Feldendrais Method, 395-396

Ayurveda, 246-257
 applications of, 252
 associations for, 256
 barriers to, 256
 constitution in, 248-249
 credentialing in, 256
 demographics of, 251
 doshas in, 247-248
 druglike information on, 254-255
 efficacy of, 253
 forms of, 249-251
 history of, 246
 imbalance in, 248-249
 issues in, key, 256
 mechanisms of action of, 246-249
 origins of, 246
 principles of, 247-249
 provider selection in, 256
 referral for, 251-252
 research on, 252-253
 risks in, 253
 safety of, 253
 self-help versus professional approach to, 255
 trade products for, 255
 training in, 255
 visiting professional in, 255
 yoga and, 251

B

Babbitt, Edwin
 in color therapy history, 690
 in light therapy history, 154

Babbitt's method of color therapy, 694

Bach, Edward, in flower essence history, 535

Back pain, Alexander Technique for, 352

Balanced antagonism in acupressure, 179-180

Baldwin, Kate, in color therapy history, 690

Bandler, Richard, in neuro linguistic programming history, 96

Bar magnets, uses of, 167

Basmajian, John, in biofeedback history, 33

Bateson, Gregory, in neuro linguistic programming history, 96

Baths, aromatherapy by, 657

BCIA; *see* Biofeedback Certification Institute of America (BCIA)

BEAM; *see* Brain Electrical Activity Maps (BEAM)

Bearberry, use, interactions, adverse effects, and contraindications of, 556*t*

Behavioral music therapy, 88

Behavioral problems, aromatherapy for, 656

Belief Art Therapy Assessment (BATA), 26

Beliefs
 in integrative cancer care, 621
 limiting, neuro linguistic programming for, 98

Bereavement, aromatherapy for, 656

Bernhard, Father, in fasting history, 729

Bernheim, Hippolyte, in hypnotherapy history, 54

Bhakti Yoga, 142

Bibliotherapy, 105-113; *see also* Poetry therapy

Bikram, 144

Bilberry, use, interactions, adverse effects, and contraindications of, 556*t*

Bioavailability of enzyme therapy, 525

Biochemical individuality, 607

Biocompatible dentistry, 667; *see also* Biologic dentistry

Bioelectromagnetics applications in medicine, 153-175
 light therapy as, 154-163; *see also* Light therapy
 magnetic field therapy as, 164-175; *see also* Magnetic field therapy

Bioenergy, effects mediated by, radiation hormesis compared with, 490

Bioenergy therapies, 483-493
 history of, 483-490
 origins of, 483-490
 radiation for, 486-489

Biofeedback, 32-40
 associations on, 39
 barriers to, 38
 credentialing in, 37-38
 demographics of, 34
 druglike information on, 36
 forms of, 34
 history of, 32
 key issues in, 38
 mechanisms of action of, 33-34
 origins of, 32-33
 practical applications of, 34-35
 provider selection in, 38
 referral for, indications and reasons for, 34, 35*t*

Biofeedback—Cont.
  research on, 35-36
  risks of, 36
  safety of, 36
  self-help versus professional approach to, 36-37
  training in, 37-38
  visiting professional in, 37
Biofeedback Certification Institute of America (BCIA), 37
Biologic dentistry, 667-678
  associtions for, 676-677
  barriers to, 676
  credentialing in, 675
  demographics of, 669-670
  druglike information on, 671-673
  efficacy of, 671
  forms of, 669
  history of, 667
  issues in, key, 676
  in lactation, 673
  mechanisms of action of, 667-669
  origins of, 667
  in pregnancy, 673
  provider selection in, 675-676
  referral for, 670
  research on, 670
  risks in, 670-671
  safety of, 670-671
  self-help versus professional approach to, 673
  training in, 675
  visiting professional in, 673-674
  warnings on, 672-673
Biomagnetic fields, frequency-pulsing, trained healers and, 484
Biotherapy, cancer, 625-626
Black cohosh, use, interactions, adverse effects, and
    contraindications of, 556t
Bladder in traditional Chinese medicine, 205t
Blessed thistle, use, interactions, adverse effects, and
    contraindications of, 556t
Blood in traditional Chinese medicine, 204
Blood viscosity, influence of enzymes on, 522
Blue cohosh, use, interactions, adverse effects, and
    contraindications of, 557t
Body awareness in relaxation therapy, 119-120
  mechanism of action of, 116
Body fluids in traditional Chinese medicine, 204
Bodywork, 349-494
  Alexander Technique as, 350-358; see also Alexander
      Technique
  Aston-Patterning as, 359-370; see also Aston-Patterning
  Bonnie Prudden myotherapy as, 417-422; see also Bonnie
      Prudden myotherapy
  Bowen technique as, 371-380; see also Bowen technique
  categories of, 341t

Bodywork—Cont.
  CranioSacral therapy as, 381-392; see also CranioSacral
      therapy
  Feldenkrais method as, 393-406; see also Feldenkrais method
  Hellerwork Structural Integration as, 407-416; see also
      Hellerwork Structural Integration
  polarity therapy as, 423-434; see also Polarity Therapy
  Reiki as, 435-443; see also Reiki
  Rolfing Structural Integration as, 444-452; see also Rolfing
      Structural Integration
  Rosen Method as, 453-461; see also Rosen Method bodywork
  Therapeutic Touch as, 462-471; see also Therapeutic Touch
  Trager Approach as, 472-482; see also Trager Approach
Bonnie Prudden myotherapy, 417-422
  associations for, 421
  credentialing in, 420
  demographics of, 418
  druglike information on, 419
  forms of, 418
  mechanism of action of, 418
  provider selection in, 421
  referral for, 419
  training in, 421
  visiting professional in, 420
  warnings on, 419
Borage, sources and uses of, 555t
Botanic medicine in naturopathic medicine, 277
Bowen, Tom, in Bowen technique history, 371
Bowen technique, 371-380
  applications of, 374-375
  associations for, 378-379
  barriers to, 378
  credentialing in, 377
  demographics of, 374
  efficacy of, 376
  history of, 371
  issues in, key, 378
  mechanisms of action of, 371-373
  origins of, 371
  provider selection in, 378
  referral for, 374
  research on, 375-376
  risks in, 376
  safety of, 376
  self-help versus professional approach to, 377
  training in, 377-378
  visiting professional in, 377
Braid, James, in hypnotherapy history, 54
Brain Electrical Activity Maps (BEAM), 653
Breast cancer, nutritional deficiencies in, 625
Breast-feeding; see Lactation
Breath ethane in oxidant stress assessment, 600
Breath pentane in oxidant stress assessment, 600

Breathing
conscious, in relaxation therapy, 119
mechanism of action of, 115
pranayama, 143-144
problems with, Alexander Technique for, 352
in Rosen Method bodywork, 455, 457
British Medical Society in hypnotherapy history, 54
Bromelain in enzyme therapy, 520
Buchinger, Otto I, in fasting history, 728, 729
Buchinger, Otto II, in fasting history, 729
Burfield-Hazzard, Linda, in fasting history, 729
Button magnets, uses of, 167
Butts, Charles, in color therapy history, 691

C

Calamus, sources and uses of, 555t
Calendula, use, interactions, adverse effects, and
contraindications of, 557t
Cancer
efficacy of enzyme therapy for, research on, 524
environment and, 620
integrative care for, 618-636; see also Integrative cancer care
nutritional oncology for, 618-636; see also Oncology,
nutritional
oxidants and, 598-599
Qi Gong for, 235
Capsicum, use, interactions, adverse effects, and
contraindications of, 557t
Caraka Samhita, 246
Carbohydrates, simple versus complex, 567
Cardiovascular disorders
essential oils and, indications and applications methods for,
654t
meditation for, 77
from mercury vapor exposure, 668
β-carotene, actions of, 597t
Carotenoids, actions of, 597t
Carpal tunnel syndrome, Alexander Technique for, 352
Carrot combination juices, 744-745
Cascade theory of reward, nutrition and, 570
Cascara sagrada, use, interactions, adverse effects, and
contraindications of, 557t
Cat's claw, use, interactions, adverse effects, and
contraindications of, 557t
Cayenne, use, interactions, adverse effects, and
contraindications of, 557t
CCE; see Council on Chiropractic Education (CCE)
Cell adhesion molecules, modulation of, enzymes in, 522
Cellular effects of magnets, 165
Cellular physiology, oxidants and, 598-599
Center for Mindfulness in Medicine, Health Care, and Society,
80
Ceroid, oxidative stress and, 597

Certification Board for Music Therapists, 93
Certification in homeopathy, 268
Chakras
in aura, 536
in color therapy, 691
Chamomile, use, interactions, adverse effects, and
contraindications of, 557t
Chance, Marian, in dance/movement therapy history, 41
Chaparral
sources and uses of, 555t
warnings on, 540
Charcot, Jean, in hypnotherapy history, 54
Chaste tree berry, use, interactions, adverse effects, and
contraindications of, 562t
CHC; see Council for Homeopathic Certification (CHC)
Chelation, definition of, 508
Chelation therapy, 508-516
actions of, 512
adverse reactions to, 512
applications of, 511
associations for, 513-514
barriers to, 514
credentialing in, 513
demographics of, 510
druglike information on, 512-513
forms of, 510
history of, 508-509
issues in, key, 514
mechanisms of action of, 509-510
origins of, 508-509
pharmacokinetics of, 512
provider selection in, 514
referral for, 510-511
research on, 511-512
safety of, 513
self-help versus professional approach to, 513
training in, 513
visiting professional in, 513
warnings on, 513
Chemical additives in foods, 571-572
Chemotherapy side effects, essential oils and, indications and
applications methods for, 655
Chen Tai Chi, 221
Childbirth, natural, in naturopathic medicine, 278
Children, relaxation therapies with, 122
Chiropractic, 310-324
applications of, 315-316
associations for, 321-322
barriers to, 321
credentialing in, 319-320
demographics of, 312-313
forms of, 312
history of, 310
issues in, key, 321

Chiropractic—Cont.
  mechanism of action of, 311-312
  origins of, 310
  provider selection in, 321
  referral for, 313-315
  research on, 316-318
  risks in, 317-318
  safety of, 317-318
  self-help versus professional approach to, 318
  training in, 320-321
  visiting professional in, 318-319
Chitosan, 567
Chlorophyll in juices, 746
Cholesterol, 568
Chromodisc in color therapy, 694
Chymotrypsin in enzyme therapy, 520
Circulation, lymphatic, in Bowen technique, 373
Clarke, Norman, in chelation therapy history, 508
Classical acupuncture, 195
Clinical nutrition in naturopathic medicine, 277
Clysters, 679-689; see also Colon hydrotherapy
CNME; see Council on Naturopathic Medical Education
        (CNME)
Cognitive Art Therapy Assessment (CATA), 26
Cohosh
  black, use, interactions, adverse effects, and contraindications
        of, 556t
  blue, use, interactions, adverse effects, and contraindications
        of, 557t
Cold laser technologies, 157, 158
  development of, 155
Collaterals in Qi Gong, 232
College of Syntonic Optometry, 160-161
Colon hydrotherapy, 679-689
  adverse reactions to, 685
  associations for, 687
  contraindications to, 684-685
  credentialing in, 687
  demographics of, 681-682
  druglike information on, 684-685
  efficacy of, 683-684
  forms of, 681
  history of, 679-680
  interactions with, 685-686
  mechanisms of action of, 680-681
  origins of, 679-680
  in pregnancy, 685
  referral for, 682-683
  research on, 683-684
  risks in, 683
  safety of, 684
    research on, 683
  self-help versus professional approach to, 686
  trade products for, 685-686

Colon hydrotherapy—Cont.
  training in, 687
  visiting professional in, 686-687
Color acupuncture, 157
  development of, 155
  referral for, 158
Color imagery, 693
Color therapy, 154, 690-701
  applications of, 695
  associations for, 699-700
  in Ayurveda, 250
  barriers to, 699
  credentialing in, 698
  demographics of, 692
  druglike information on, 697
  Eastern-influenced, 691
    forms of, 693
  efficacy of, 696
  forms of, 692-694
  history of, 690-691
  issues in, key, 699
  mechanisms of action of, 691-692
  origins of, 690-691
  physical, 691-692
    forms of, 693-694
  practical applications of, 159
  provider selection in, 699
  psychologic, 691
    forms of, 692-693
  referral for, 158, 694
  research on, 695-696
  risks in, 696
  safety of, 696
  self-help versus professional approach to, 697
  trade products in, 697
  training in, 698
  visiting professional in, 698
  warnings on, 697
Colorpuncture, 693
  training in, 698
Colors, doshas and, 251t
Colorzone lamps focused on acupuncture points, 693
Coltsfoot, sources and uses of, 555t
Comfrey, sources and uses of, 555t
Community-based health care practices, 283-308
  Latin American traditional medicine as, 284-292; see also
        Latin American traditional medicine
  Native American medicine as, 293-300; see also Native
        American medicine
  shamanism as, 301-308; see also Shamanism
Complementary medicine, 4
  basic principles of, 5-7
  incorporating medical model in, 15-16
Complementation activation, decreased, enzymes in, 522

Compresses, aromatherapy by, 657
Concentration methods of meditation, 73
Conscious breathing in relaxation therapy, 119
    mechanism of action of, 115
Constitution in Ayurveda, 248-249
Contraindications; *see also*
        Warnings/contraindications/precautions
    to colon hydrotherapy, 684-685
Control, primary, in Alexander Technique, 351
Conversational prayer, 131
Coping, religious, 132
Coreopsis, warnings on, 540
Coronary artery disease, meditation for, 77
Council for Homeopathic Certification (CHC), 268
Council on Chiropractic Education (CCE), 320
Council on Naturopathic Medical Education (CNME), 280
Counseling, lifestyle, fasting and, 731-732
Cranberry, use, interactions, adverse effects, and
        contraindications of, 557t
CranioSacral, 340
CranioSacral therapy, 381-392
    adverse reactions to, 388
    applications of, 384-385
    associations for, 390-391
    barriers to, 390
    credentialing in, 389
    demographics of, 383-384
    drug interactions with, 388
    druglike information on, 387-389
    efficacy of, 387
    forms of, 383
    history of, 381
    issues in, key, 390
    in lactation, 388
    mechanisms of action of, 381-382
    origins of, 381
    in pregnancy, 388
    provider selection in, 390
    referral for, 384
    research on, 386-387
    risks in, 387
    safety of, 387-388
    self-help versus professional approach to, 389
    trade products for, 388-389
    training in, 389-390
    visiting professional in, 389
    warnings on, 388
Creative music therapy, 89
Credentialing
    in acupressure, 187
    in acupuncture, 199-200
    in Alexander technique, 355
    in antineoplastons, 505
    in applied kinesiology, 646

Credentialing—Cont.
    in aromatherapy, 663-664
    in art therapy, 27
    in Aston-Patterning, 369
    in biofeedback, 37-38
    in biologic dentistry, 675
    in Bonnie Prudden myotherapy, 420
    in Bowen technique, 377
    in chelation therapy, 513
    in chiropractic, 319-320
    in colon hydrotherapy, 687
    in color therapy, 698
    in CranioSacral therapy, 389
    in dance/movement therapy, 47
    in detoxification therapy, 713
    in environmental medicine, 725
    in enzyme therapy, 528
    in fasting, 737
    in Feldenkrais Method, 402
    in flower essence therapy, 542
    in Hellerwork Structural Integration, 414
    in homeopathy, 268
    in hypnotherapy, 60
    in interactive guided imagery, 69
    in iridology, 765
    in light therapy, 160-161
    in macronutrients, 573
    in magnetic field therapy, 172
    in massage therapy, 346
    in meditation, 80
    in micronutrients, 591
    in music therapy, 93
    in Native American medicine, 298
    in naturopathic medicine, 280
    in neuro linguistic programming, 101
    in orthomolecular medicine, 613
    in osteopathic medicine, 334
    in poetry therapy, 110
    in Polarity Therapy, 431
    in prayer/spiritual healing, 138
    in Qi Gong, 240-241
    in quartz crystal therapy, 776
    in reflexology, 787
    in Reiki, 441
    in relaxation therapies, 125
    in Rolfing Structural Integration, 450
    in Rosen Method bodywork, 459-460
    in shamanism, 306
    in Tai Chi, 227
    in Therapeutic Touch, 469
    in traditional Chinese medicine, 215
    in Trager Approach, 479
    in Yoga, 149

Curanderismo, 284; *see also* Latin American traditional medicine

Cytokine network regulation, enzymes in, 522

D

Dance/movement therapy
  administration of, 46
  associations for, 48
  barriers to, 48
  credentialing in, 47
  demographics of, 43
  dosage of, 46
  druglike information on, 46
  history of, 41-42
  issues in, key, 48
  lactation and, 46
  mechanisms of action of, 42-43
  origins of, 41-42
  practical applications of, 44
  in pregnancy, 46
  provider selection in, 48
  referral for, 43-44
  research on, 45-46
  safety of, 46
  self-help versus professional approach to, 47
  training in, 48
  visiting professional in, 47
  warnings on, 46
Dandelion, use, interactions, adverse effects, and
    contraindications of, 557t
de Graaf, Regnier, in colon hydrotherapy history, 679
Deck, Josef, in iridology history, 757
Decubitus ulcers, aromatherapy for, 656
Deep tissue bodywork in Hellerwork Structural Integration, 407
Deep tissue massage, 340
Deficiency(ies)
  in breast cancer, 625
  chromium, 607
  subclinical, 607
  taurine, 610
Dementia, aromatherapy for, 656
Demographics of users
  of acupressure, 181
  of acupuncture, 196
  of Alexander technique, 352
  of antineoplastons, 497
  of applied kinesiology, 641
  of aromatherapy, 653
  of art therapy, 22
  of Aston-Patterning, 365
  of Ayurveda, 251
  of biofeedback, 34
  of biologic dentistry, 669-670
  of Bonnie Prudden myotherapy, 418-419

Demographics of users—Cont.
  of Bowen technique, 374
  of chelation therapy, 510
  of chiropractic, 312-313
  of colon hydrotherapy, 681-682
  of color therapy, 692
  of CranioSacral therapy, 383-384
  of dance/movement therapy, 43
  of detoxification therapy, 709
  of environmental medicine, 720
  of enzyme therapy, 520
  of fasting, 732
  of Feldendrais Method, 396
  of flower essence therapy, 537
  of Hellerwork Structural Integration, 410
  of herbal medicine, 548
  of homeopathy, 261
  of hypnotherapy, 56
  of interactive guided imagery, 66
  of iridology, 761
  of Latin American traditional medicine, 286
  of light therapy, 157
  of macronutrients, 569
  of magnetic field therapy, 166
  of massage therapy, 341-342
  of meditation, 75
  of micronutrients, 582
  of music therapy, 89
  of Native American medicine, 294
  of naturopathic medicine, 278
  of neuro linguistic programming, 97-98
  of orthomolecular medicine, 608
  of osteopathic medicine, 329
  of poetry therapy, 108
  of Polarity Therapy, 426
  of prayer/spiritual healing, 132
  of Qi Gong, 234
  of quartz crystal therapy, 771
  of reflexology, 782
  of Reiki, 437
  of relaxation therapies, 120
  of Rolfing Structural Integration, 446
  of Rosen Method bodywork, 458
  of shamanism, 304
  of Tai Chi, 221
  of Therapeutic Touch, 464
  of traditional Chinese medicine, 209
  of Trager Approach, 474-475
  of Yoga, 145
Dental materials, health and, 667-668
Depression
  aromatherapy for, 656
  manic, from mercury vapor exposure, 669
Depressive symptoms, meditation for, 78

Dermatologic disorders, meditation for, 78

Dermatology, essential oils in, indications and applications methods for, 655*t*

Detox diet daily menu plan, 706

Detoxification therapy, 702-715
  adverse reactions to, 713
  applications of, 710-712
  associations for, 714
  barriers to, 714
  credentialing in, 713
  druglike information on, 712-713
  forms of, 705-708
  history of, 702-703
  issues in, key, 714
  in lactation, 713
  mechanisms of action of, 703-705
  origins of, 702-703
  in pregnancy, 713
  provider selection for, 714
  referral for, 710
  safety of, 712
  self-help versus professional approach to, 713
  training in, 714
  visiting professional in, 713
  warnings on, 712-713

Devil's claw, use, interactions, adverse effects, and contraindications of, 558*t*

Dewey, Dr., in fasting history, 729

Dhatus in Ayurveda, 248

Diabetes mellitus, Qi Gong for, 235

Dialogue in Hellerwork Structural Integration, 407

Diet, nontoxic, 703

Digestive enzymes, mechanisms of action of, 568-569

Dilts, Robert, in neuro linguistic programming history, 96

Dimercaptopropane sulfonate (DMPS) in chelation therapy, 509

Dinshah, Ghadiali
  in color therapy history, 690-691
  Spectro-Chrome of, 694

Dioscorides, Pedanios, in herbal medicine history, 545

Direction of energy in CranioSacral therapy, 383

Directions in Alexander Technique, 351

Disease prevention, Trager Approach for, 475

Disharmony, causes of, in traditional Chinese medicine, 205-206

DMPS in chelation therapy, 509

DMSA in chelation therapy, 509

DNA damage, free radical-induced, 600

Dong-quai, use, interactions, adverse effects, and contraindications of, 558*t*

Doshas in Ayurveda, 247-248
  colors and, 251*t*
  foods and herbs for, 250*t*

Drainage, lymph, manual, 340
  research on, 343

Drug or other interactions
  with acupuncture, 198
  with antineoplastons, 503
  with aromatherapy, 661-662
  with art therapy, 25
  with Aston-Patterning, 367
  with Ayurveda, 254
  with chelation therapy, 512
  with CranioSacral therapy, 388
  with enzyme therapy, 527
  with flower essences, 540-541
  with homeopathy, 266
  with hypnotherapy, 59
  with micronutrients, 589-590
  with Native American medicine, 297
  with neuro linguistic programming, 101
  with orthomolecular medicine, 612
  with quartz crystal therapy, 774
  with relaxation therapies, 124
  with Tai Chi, 226
  with therapeutic touch, 468
  with traditional Chinese herbal medicine, 212-213

Dying, care of, essential oils and, indications and applications methods for, 655*t*

Dynamical energy systems theory, 484
  radiogenic metabolism and, 489-490

Dysphoria, gender, neuro linguistic programming for, 98-99

E

Eastern-influenced color therapy, 691
  forms of, 693

Eating, healthy, elements of, 710

Echinacea, use, interactions, adverse effects, and contraindications of, 558*t*

Eclectic model of music therapy, 89

EDTA therapy, 508-516; *see also* Chelation therapy

Eicosapentaenoic acid (EPA), supplemental, 624-625

Elderly, micronutrient deficiencies in, 580

Electric stimulation in acupressure, 183

Electric stimuli in acupuncture, 195

Eleuthero, use, interactions, adverse effects, and contraindications of, 558*t*

Empacho in Latin American traditional medicine, 288

Endocrine disorders from mercury vapor exposure, 669

Endorphins in pain control, acupressure and, 180-181

Enemas, 679-689; *see also* Colon hydrotherapy

Energy
  direction of, in CranioSacral therapy, 383
  low, Qi Gong for, 236
  in touch-based healing, exploring concept of, 483-493; *see also* Bioenergy therapies

Energy cyst release, 383

Environment, cancer and, 620
Environmental dentistry, 667; *see also* Biologic dentistry
Environmental medicine, 716-727
    applications of, 721-723
    associations for, 726
    barriers to, 726
    credentialing in, 725
    demographics of, 720
    druglike information on, 724
    efficacy of, 723
    forms of, 719-720
    history of, 716
    issues in, key, 726
    mechanisms of action of, 717-719
    model of, 717-718
    origins of, 716
    provider selection in, 725
    referral for, 720-721
    research on, 723
    risks in, 723
    safety of, 723
    self-help versus professional approach to, 724
    training in, 725
    visiting professional in, 724-725
Environmentally-triggered illnesses, 717
Enzyme(s), digestive, mechanisms of action of, 568-569
Enzyme therapy, 517-534
    absorption of, 525-526
    actions of, 525
    adverse reactions to, 527
    applications of, 521
    associations for, 529
    bioavailability of, 525
    credentialing in, 528
    demographics of, 520
    distribution of, 526
    dose-response relationships in, 525
    drug interactions of, 527
    druglike information on, 525-528
    efficacy of, 523-524
    elimination of, 526
    forms of, 520
    history of, 517-518
    in lactation, 527
    mechanisms of action of, 518-520
    metabolism of, 526
    origins of, 517-518
    overdose of, 527
    pharmacokinetics of, 525-526
    in pregnancy, 527
    provider selection in, 529
    referral for, 521
    research on, 521-524
    risks of, 523

Enzyme therapy—Cont.
    safety of, 523
    self-help versus professional approach to, 528
    trade products in, 527-528
    training in, 528-529
    warnings on, 526-527
Ephedra, sources and uses of, 555t
Erethysm from mercury vapor exposure, 668
Ergonomics, Aston, 365
Erickson, Milton H.
    in hypnotherapy history, 54
    in neuro linguistic programming history, 96
Esdaile, James, in hypnotherapy history, 53
Espenak, L., in dance/movement therapy history, 42
Essential fatty acids (EFAs)
    mechanisms of action of, 567-568
    shortage of, 572
Essential oils, 651-666; *see also* Aromatherapy
    to avoid, 660t
    distributors of, 662
    indications for, 654-655t
    methods of application of, 654-655t
Ethane, breath, in oxidant stress assessment, 600
Ethnomedical illnesses, 287-289
Ethylene diamine tetraacetate (EDTA) therapy, 508-516; *see also* Chelation therapy
Evan in dance/movement therapy history, 42
Evening primrose, use, interactions, adverse effects, and contraindications of, 558t
Experimental design of alternative medicines, difficulties in, 8
Experimental therapies in integrative cancer care, 627-628
Extracellular fluid, magnets and, 165-166
Eyebright, use, interactions, adverse effects, and contraindications of, 559t

F

Facial fitness, Aston, 364
Facilitation, segmental, 332
Fascia in Bowen technique, 373
Fast Wolf, Oh Shinnah, in quartz crystal therapy history, 770
Fasting, 728-740
    adverse reactions to, 736
    applications of, 733
    associations for, 738-739
    barriers to, 738
    body reactions to, 730-731
    credentialing in, 737
    demographics of, 732
    druglike information on, 735-736
    efficacy of, 734
    forms of, 731-732
    healing from within and, 729-730
    history of, 728-729

Fasting—Cont.
  issues in, key, 738
  in lactation, 736
  lifestyle counseling in, 731-732
  mechanisms of action of, 729-731
  origins of, 728-729
  in pregnancy, 736
  provider selection in, 738
  referral for, 732
  research on, 733-735
  risks in, 734
  safety of, 735
    research on, 734
  self-help versus professional approach to, 736
  training in, 737-738
  visiting professional in, 736-737
  warnings on, 735-736
Fasting aids, 712
Fatigue, chronic, Qi Gong for, 235
Fats, mechanisms of action of, 567-568
Fatty acids
  essential
    mechanisms of action of, 567-568
    shortage of, 572
  saturated, mechanism of action of, 568
Fehmi, Les, in biofeedback history, 33
Feldendrais Method, 393-406
  applications of, 397
  associations for, 403
  barriers to, 402
  credentialing in, 402
  demographics of, 396
  efficacy of, 400-401
  forms of, 395-396
  history of, 393
  issues in, key, 402
  mechanisms of action of, 393-395
  origins of, 393
  provider selection in, 402
  referral for, 397
  research on, 397-401
  risks in, 400
  safety of, 400
  training in, 402
  visiting professional in, 401-402
Feldenkrais, Moshe, in Feldendrais Method history, 393
Felke, Pastor, in iridology history, 757
Fennel in Polarity Therapy, 430
Fenugreek
  in Polarity Therapy, 430
  use, interactions, adverse effects, and contraindications of,
    559t
Ferromagnets, 164
Feverfew, use, interactions, adverse effects, and
    contraindications of, 559t

Fiber(s)
  insoluble versus soluble, 567
  juice therapy and, 742
Fibromyalgia, Qi Gong for, 235
Fight-or-flight response, 114
Finsen, Neils, in color therapy history, 690
Fitness training, Aston, 364
Flat pad magnets, uses of, 167
Flavonoids, actions of, 597t
Flax in Polarity Therapy, 430
Flower essence therapy, 535-544
  adverse reactions to, 541
  applications of, 537-538
  associations for, 543-544
  barriers to, 543
  credentialing in, 542
  demographics of, 537
  dosage of, 541
  drug interactions with, 540-541
  druglike information on, 539-541
  efficacy of, 539
  forms of, 537
  history of, 535-536
  issues in, key, 543
  mechanisms of action of, 536-537
  origins of, 535-536
  preparing flower essence for, 539-540
  provider selection in, 543
  referral for, 527
  research on, 538-539
  risks in, 539
  safety of, 539
  self-help versus professional approach to, 542
  trade products for, 541
  training in, 542-543
  visiting professional in, 542
  warnings on, 540
Fluid(s)
  body, in traditional Chinese medicine, 204
  extracellular, magnets and, 165-166
Foster, Robert, in naturopathic medicine history, 276
Fo-ti, use, interactions, adverse effects, and contraindications of,
    559t
Free radical(s)
  definition of, 595
  DNA damage induced by, 600
French energetics acupuncture, 194
Frequency-pulsing biomagnetic fields, trained healers and, 484
Freud, Sigmund, in hypnotherapy history, 54
Fridovich, Irwin, in oxidative stress history, 595
Fruit juices, 742-743
  mixing vegetable juices with, 745
Functional Integration in Feldendrais Method, 396
Functional performance, Feldendrais Method in, 398-399
Futurehealth, biofeedback and, 37-38

G

Galen in colon hydrotherapy history, 679
Gallbladder in traditional Chinese medicine, 205t
Galvanism of mercury amalgam, 668
Garlic, use, interactions, adverse effects, and contraindications of, 559t
Gastrointestinal disorders
    essential oils and, indications and applications methods for, 654t
    fasting for, 732
    from mercury vapor exposure, 668
    Qi Gong for, 235
Gattefosse, Maurice, in aromatherapy history, 651
Gender dysphoria, neuro linguistic programming for, 98-99
Genogram in art therapy assessment, 26
Geriatrics, essential oils in, indications and applications methods for, 655t
Germander, sources and uses of, 555t
Ghadiali, D, in light therapy history, 154
Ginger, use, interactions, adverse effects, and contraindications of, 559t
Ginkgo, use, interactions, adverse effects, and contraindications of, 560t
Ginseng, use, interactions, adverse effects, and contraindications of, 560t
Glomerulonephritis, 518
Glutathione in protection against oxidative stress, 602
Goldenseal, use, interactions, adverse effects, and contraindications of, 560t
Goodheart, George, in applied kinesiology history, 638-639
Gorgias in poetry therapy history, 105
Gotu kola, use, interactions, adverse effects, and contraindications of, 560t
Grape seed, use, interactions, adverse effects, and contraindications of, 560t
Gravity, body balance and, 408
Green, Alyce, in biofeedback history, 32, 33
Green, Elmer, in biofeedback history, 32, 33
Green juices, 745-746
Greifer, Eli, in poetry therapy history, 105-106
Grinder, John, in neuro linguistic programming history, 96
Guided imagery
    interacive, 64-72
    interactive; see also Imagery, interactive guided
    music and, 88
Guild of Certified Feldenkrais Practitioners, 402
Gynocologic disorders, essential oils and, indications and applications methods for, 654t

H

Hahnemann, Samuel, in homeopathy history, 258-259
Hallucinations from mercury vapor exposure, 669
Hara diagnosis, 214

Harman, Denham, in oxidative stress discovery, 595
Hatha Yoga, 142
Hayashi, Chujiro, in Reiki history, 435
Headaches, relaxation therapies for, research on, 122
Healing
    from within, 729-730
    spiritual, 130-140; see also Prayer/spiritual healing
    touch-based, energy in, exploring concept of, 483-493; see also Bioenergy therapies
Health
    maintenance of, Trager Approach for, 475
    optimal, in environmental medicine, 717
    promotion of, Trager Approach for, 475
Hearing in traditional Chinese medicine, 206
Heart
    disease of
        oxidants and, 598
        relaxation therapies for, research on, 122
    in traditional Chinese medicine, 205t
Heavy metals, 577
Heller, Joseph, in Hellerwork Structural Integration history, 407-408
Hellerwork International, 415
Hellerwork Structural Integration
    adverse reactions to, 412
    applications of, 410-411
    associations for, 415
    barriers to, 415
    credentialing in, 414
    demographics of, 410
    druglike information on, 412
    efficacy of, 411
    forms of, 410
    history of, 407-408
    issues in, key, 415
    mechanism of action of, 408-409
    origins of, 407-408
    provider selection in, 414
    referral for, 410
    research on, 411
    safety of, 412
    self-help versus professional approach to, 412
    training in, 414
    visiting professional in, 413
Hematologic system, magnets and, 165
Hepatitis, Qi Gong for, 236
Herb(s)
    ayurvedic principles and, 254t
    in Polarity Therapy, 430
Herbal medicine, 545-564
    barriers to, 551
    demographics of, 548
    efficacy of, 551
    forms of, 547, 548t

Herbal medicine—Cont.
  history of, 545-546
  issues in, key, 551
  mechanisms of action of, 546-547
  origins of, 545-546
  referral for, 549
  research on, 549-551
  risks in, 550-551
  safety of, 550-551
  traditional Chinese, 203-218; see also traditional Chinese
      medicine (TCM), herbal
Herpes zoster, efficacy of enzyme therapy for, research on, 524
Heyer, Gustav, in Rosen Method history, 454
Heyer, Lucy, in Rosen Method history, 454
High velocity—low amplitude techniques in osteopathy, 328
Hippocampus in aromatherapy, 653
Hippocrates
  in juice therapy history, 741
  in massage therapy history, 338
  in naturopathic medicine history, 274
History/origins
  of acupressure, 178-179
  of acupuncture, 191-192
  of Alexander technique, 350
  of antineoplastons, 496
  of applied kinesiology, 638-639
  of aromatherapy, 651
  of art therapy, 20
  of Aston-Patterning, 359
  of Ayurveda, 246
  of bioenergy therapies, 483-490
  of biofeedback, 32-33
  of biologic dentistry, 667
  of Bonnie Prudden myotherapy, 417-418
  of Bowen technique, 371
  of chelation therapy, 508-509
  of chiropractic, 310
  of colon hydrotherapy, 679-680
  of color therapy, 690-691
  of CranioSacral therapy, 381
  of dance/movement therapy, 41-42
  of detoxification therapy, 702-703
  of environmental medicine, 716
  of enzyme therapy, 517-518
  of fasting, 728-729
  of Feldendrais Method, 393
  of flower essence therapy, 535-536
  of Hellerwork Structural Integration, 407-408
  of herbal medicine, 545-546
  of homeopathy, 258-260
  of hypnotherapy, 53-54
  of interactive guided imagery, 64-65
  of iridology, 756-757
  of juice therapy, 741

History/origins—Cont.
  of Latin American traditional medicine, 284
  of light therapy, 154-155
  of macronutrients, 566
  of magnetic field therapy, 164-165
  of massage therapy, 338
  of meditation, 73-74
  of micronutrients, 576-577
  of music therapy, 86
  of Native American medicine, 293
  of naturopathic medicine, 274-276
  of neuro linguistic programming, 96
  of orthomolecular medicine, 606
  of osteopathic medicine, 325
  of poetry therapy, 105-107
  of Polarity Therapy, 423
  of prayer/spiritual healing, 130
  of Qi Gong, 231
  of quartz crystal therapy, 770
  of reflexology, 779-780
  of Reiki, 435-436
  of relaxation therapies, 114-115
  of Rolfing Structural Integration, 444-445
  of Rosen Method bodywork, 453-455
  of shamanism, 301-302
  of Tai Chi, 219
  of Therapeutic Touch, 462
  of traditional Chinese medicine, 203
  of Trager Approach, 472
  of Yoga, 141-142
Hoffer, Abram, in orthomolecular medicine history, 606
Holistic dentistry, 667; see also Biologic dentistry
Homeodynamic functioning, 717
Homeopathic medicine in naturopathic medicine, 277
Homeopathy
  adverse reactions to, 266
  applications of, 262-264
  associations for, 270-272
  barriers to, 270
  certification in, 268
  credentialing in, 268
  demographics of, 261
  drug interactions of, 266
  efficacy of, 265
  forms of, 261
  history of, 258-260
  issues in, key, 270
  laws of, 259-260
  mechanisms of action of, 260-261
  origins of, 258-260
  provider selection in, 269-270
  referral for, 261-262
  research on, 264-265
  risks in, 265

Homeopathy—Cont.
  safety of, 265
  self-help versus professional approach to, 267
  trade products in, 266-267
  training in, 268-269
  visiting professional in, 267-268
  warnings on, 266
Hormesis
  in homeopathy, 260
  radiation, 485-486
    bioenergy mediated effects compared with, 490
Horney, Karen, in Rosen Method history, 453
Horse chestnut, use, interactions, adverse effects, and
    contraindications of, 561t
Hull, Clark, in hypnotherapy history, 54
Hydrotherapy in naturopathic medicine, 277
Hynes, Arleen, in poetry therapy history, 106
Hypertension
  borderline, aromatherapy for, 656
  meditation for, 77
  Qi Gong for, 235
    research on, 237
  relaxation therapies for, research on, 122
Hypnosis, 53; see also Hypnotherapy
Hypnotherapy, 53-63
  applications of, 57
  associations for, 61-62
  barriers to, 60-61
  credentialing in, 60
  demographics of, 56
  drug interactions of, 59
  druglike information on, 59
  efficacy of, 58
  forms of, 55-56
  history of, 53-54
  issues in, key, 60-61
  mechanisms of action of, 54-55
  neuro linguistic programming and, 97, 101
  origins of, 53-54
  precautions with, 59
  provider selection in, 60
  referral for, 56
  research on, 58
  risk of, 58
  safety of, 59
    research on, 58
  self-help versus professional approach to, 59
  tranining in, 60
  visiting professional in, 59-60
Hypnotic language, 57
Hypoglycemia, coreopsis for, 540
Hypotension, transient, aromatherapy for, 656
Hyssop, use, interactions, adverse effects, and contraindications
    of, 561t

I

I-ACT; see International Association for Colon Hydrotherapy
    (I-ACT)
IIRA; see International Iridology Research Association (IIRA)
Illnesses, environmentally-triggered, 717
IMA; see International Myotherapy Association (IMA)
Imagery
  directed, interactive guided imagery in, 67
  guided
    music and, 88
  insight-oriented, interactive guided imagery in, 67
  interactive guided
    applications of, 67-68
    associations on, 70
    barriers to, 70
    credentialing in, 69
    demographics of, 66
    efficacy of, 684
    forms of, 66
    history of, 64-65
    issues in, key, 70
    mechanisms of action of, 65-66
    origins of, 64-65
    provider selection in, 70
    referrals for, 67
    research on, 68-69
    risks in, 68
    safety of, 68
    self-help versus professional approach to, 69
    training in, 69
    visiting professional in, 69
  receptive, interactive guided imagery in, 67
Imagery, color, 693
Imbalance in Ayurveda, 248-249
Immune complexes, fragmentation of, enzymes in, 522
Immune modulation, nutritional pharmacology and, 624
Immune regulatory effects of enzymes, research on, 522
Immune system
  disorders of, from mercury vapor exposure, 669
  mercury amalgam and, 668
Immunoglobulins, 517
Immunologic changes, prayer and, 136
Infection(s)
  essential oils and, indications and application methods for,
    654t
  resistant, aromatherapy for, 656
  upper respiratory tract, aromatherapy for, 656
  vaginal, aromatherapy for, 655-656
Infertility, aromatherapy for, 656
Inflammation, efficacy of enzyme therapy for, research on, 523
Inhalation, aromatherapy by, 657
Inhibition in Alexander Technique, 351
Injuries, sports, aromatherapy for, 656

Insomnia
   aromatherapy for, 656
   relaxation therapies for, research on, 122
Institute for Applied Iridology, 765
Insulin, CranioSacral therapy and, 388
Integral, 144
Integrative cancer care, 618-636
   alternative/experimental therapies in, 627-628
   attitudes in, 621
   beliefs in, 621
   conclusion on, 628-629
   medical care in, 622-623
   modulating malignant terrain in, 619-620
   physical care in, 627
   stress care in, 627
   supplementation in, 624-626
   therapeutic nutrition in, 623-624
Integrative model of relaxation therapy, 123
Interactive guided imagery, 64-72; *see also* Imagery, interactive guided
Intercessory prayer, 132
   studies on effects of, 134-136
International Academy of Oral Medicine and Toxicology, 675, 676
International Association for Colon Hydrotherapy (I-ACT), 680, 681-682, 687
International Iridology Research Association (IIRA), 765
International Myotherapy Association (IMA), 421
Intestine in traditional Chinese medicine, 205t
Ion pumping cords, 195
Iridology, 756-769
   associations for, 767
   barriers to, 766
   credentialing in, 765
   demographics of, 761
   druglike information on, 763-764
   forms of, 761
   history of, 756-757
   issues in, key, 766
   mechanisms of action of, 757-760
   origins of, 756-757
   professional selection in, 765
   referral for, 762
   research on, 762-763
   training in, 765-766
   visiting professional in, 764
Irlen lens therapy, 157
Iron, marginal deficiency of, 580
Iron overload, 508
Irritable bowel syndrome, relaxation therapies for, research on, 122
Isometric muscle energy, direct, in osteopathy, 328, 329
Iyengar, BKS, in Yoga history, 142, 144

J

Japanese herbal medicine, acupuncture in, 194
Jensen, Bernrd, in iridology history, 757
Jin Shin style of acupressure, 181
Jing in traditional Chinese medicine, 204
Jin-Yuan Dynasty, acupuncture in, 191
Jnana Yoga, 142
Joint proprioreceptors in Bowen technique, 373
Juice therapy, 741-755
   applications of, 748, 749
   associations for, 754-755
   barriers to, 753
   carrot combination juices in, 744-745
   chlorophyll in, 746
   color of juices in, 747-748
   druglike information on, 749-753
   forms of, 742-748
   fruit juices in, 742-743
   green juices in, 745-746
   history of, 741
   issues in, key, 753
   juice kinds in, 742-745
   mechanisms of action of, 741-742
   mixing fruit and vegetable juices in, 745
   origins of, 741
   referral for, 748
   trade products for, 751-753
   warnings on, 749-751
   wheat grass juice in, 747

K

Kamiya, Joe, in biofeedback history, 33
Kampo, 210
Kapha dosha in Ayurveda, 248
   food and herbs for, 250t
Karma Yoga, 142
Kava-kava, use, interactions, adverse effects, and contraindications of, 561t
Kellogg, JH, in colon hydrotherapy history, 680
Kidneys in traditional Chinese medicine, 205t
Kinesiology, applied, 638-650
   applications of, 642-643
   associations for, 648
   barriers to, 647-648
   credentialing in, 646
   demographics of, 641
   druglike information on, 644
   efficacy of, 644
   forms of, 641
   history of, 638-639
   issues in, key, 647-648
   mechanisms of action of, 639-641
   origins of, 638-639

Kinesiology, applied—Cont.
  referral for, 641, 644
  self-help versus professional approach to, 645
  training in, 646-647
  visiting professional in, 645-646
Kinesthetic identification, 41
Kinetic family drawing test (KFD) in art therapy assessment, 26
Korean hand acupuncture, 195
Kramer, E., in art therapy history, 20
Kraus, Hans, in myotherapy history, 417
Kripalu, 144-145
Krishan in Yoga history, 142
Kundalini, 145

L

Lactation
  acupressure in, 186
  acupuncture in, 198
  antineoplastons in, 504
  Aston-Patterning in, 368
  biologic dentistry in, 673
  CranioSacral therapy in, 388
  dance/movement therapy in, 46
  enzyme therapy in, 527
  micronutrients in, 590
  neuro linguistic programming in, 101
  orthomolecular medicine in, 612
  reflexology in, 786
  Tai Chi in, 226
  traditional Chinese medicine in, 213
  Yoga in, 148
Lange, Hans, in myotherapy history, 417
Laser in acupuncture, 195-196
Laser therapy development, 155
Latin American traditional medicine, 284-292
  applications of, 289
  barriers to, 290-291
  demographics of, 286
  druglike information on, 290
  forms of, 286-287
  history of, 284
  issues in, key, 290-291
  mechanism of action of, 284-285
  origins of, 284
  referral for, 287-289
  safety of, 290
  self-help versus professional approach to, 290
  visiting professional in, 290
Lavandula angustifolia in aromatherapy, 652-653
Lavender, true, in aromatherapy, 652-653
Law of dilution and succession in homeopathy, 259-260
Law of similare in homeopathy, 259

Laws of cure in homeopathy, 260
Lead toxicity, 508
Leedy, Jack, in poetry therapy history, 106
Lerner, Arthur, in poetry therapy history, 106
Licorice
  in Polarity Therapy, 430
  sources and uses of, 555t
  use, interactions, adverse effects, and contraindications of, 561t
Life root, sources and uses of, 555t
Lifestyle counseling, fasting and, 731-732
Light therapy, 154-163
  applications of, 158-159
  associations on, 161
  barriers to, 161
  credentialing in, 160-161
  demographics of, 157
  efficacy of, 159
  forms of, 157
  history of, 154-155
  issues in, key, 161
  mechanisms of action of, 155-156
  origins of, 154-155
  referral for, 157-158
  research on, 159-160
  risks in, 159
  safety of, 159
  self-help versus professional approach to, 160
  training in, 160-161
  visiting professional in, 160
Liljequist, Pastor, in iridology history, 756-757
Limiting beliefs, neuro linguistic programming for, 98
Ling, Per Henrik, in massage therapy history, 338
Lipofuscin, oxidative stress and, 597
Liver
  oxidative damage to, 596
  in traditional Chinese medicine, 205t
Liver flush in Polarity Therapy, 430
Local-naturalistic mechanism of prayer effects, 130
Loeb, Carl, in light therapy history, 154
Looking in traditional Chinese medicine, 206
Lung(s)
  disorders of
    nitric oxide and, 599
    oxidative stress and, 599
    reactive oxygen species and, 599
  in traditional Chinese medicine, 205t
Luscher, Max, 692-693
Luscher color test, 692-693
Lust, Benedict, in naturopathic medicine history, 276
Lymph drainage, manual, 340
  research on, 343
Lymphatic circulation in Bowen technique, 373

M

M technique in aromatherapy, 663
α2-macroglobulin, interaction of proteolytic serum activity with, 521
Macrominerals, 577
Macronutrients, 566-575
  actions of, 571
  adverse reactions to, 572
  applications of, 570
  associations for, 574
  barriers to, 573-574
  credentialing in, 573
  demographics of, 569
  druglike information on, 570-572
  forms of therapy with, 569
  history of, 566
  issues in, key, 573-574
  mechanisms of action of, 566-569
  origins of, 566
  pharmacokinetics of, 571
  in pregnancy, 572
  referral for therapy with, 569-570
  safety of, 571
  self-help versus professional approach to, 572
  training in, 573
  visiting professional in, 573
  warnings on, 571-572
Macrophages in enzyme therapy, 518
Magnetic energy, therapeutic effects of, 484
Magnetic field therapy, 164-175
  adverse reactions to, 171
  applications of, 166-168
  associations for, 173
  credentialing in, 172
  demographics of, 166
  dose considerations in, 170
  druglike considerations on, 171-172
  efficacy of, 170
  history of, 164-165
  mechanisms of action of, 165-166
  origins of, 164-165
  pregnancy and, 172
  product availability for, 172
  provider selection in, 173
  referral for, 166
  research on, 168-171
  risks in, 170
  safety of, 170
  self-help versus professional approach to, 172
  training in, 173
  trials of, in humans by condition, 169t
  warnings for, 171
Magnetic fields, types of, 164
Mal de ojo in Latin American traditional medicine, 288

Malillumination, 155
Management in environmental medicine, 718
Manic depression from mercury vapor exposure, 669
Mantras in Ayurveda, 250
Manual healing methods, 309-348
  chiropractic as, 310-324; see also Chiropractic
  massage therapy as, 338-348; see also Massage therapy
  osteopathic medicine as, 325-337; see also Osteopathic medicine
Manual lymph drainage, 340
Marshmallow, use, interactions, adverse effects, and contraindications of, 561t
Massage, Aston, 364
Massage therapy, 338-348
  applications of, 342
  associations for, 347
  barriers to, 347
  categories of, 341t
  credentialing in, 346
  demographics of, 341-342
  druglike information on, 344
  forms of, 339-341
  history of, 338
  issues in, key, 347
  mechanisms of action of, 339
  origins of, 338
  provider selection in, 346
  referral for, 342
  research on, 343-344
  training in, 346
  visiting professional in, 345
  warnings on, 344
Maury, Marguerite, in aromatherapy history, 651
Mechanisms of action
  of acupressure, 179-181
  of acupuncture, 192-194
  of Alexander technique, 350-351
  of antineoplastons, 496-497
  of applied kinesiology, 639-641
  of aromatherapy, 651-653
  of art therapy, 20-21
  of Aston-Patterning, 360-364
  of Ayurveda, 246-249
  of biofeedback, 33-34
  of biologic dentistry, 667-669
  of Bonnie Prudden myotherapy, 418
  of Bowen technique, 371-373
  of chelation therapy, 509-510
  of chiropractic, 311-312
  of colon hydrotherapy, 680-681
  of color therapy, 691-692
  of CranioSacral therapy, 381-382
  of dance/movement therapy, 42-43
  of detoxification therapy, 703-705

Mechanisms of action—Cont.
    of environmental medicine, 717-719
    of enzyme therapy, 518-520
    of fasting, 729-731
    of Feldendrais Method, 393-395
    of flower essence therapy, 536-537
    of Hellerwork Structural Integration, 408-409
    of herbal medicine, 546-547
    of homeopathy, 260-261
    of hypnotherapy, 54-55
    of interactive guided imagery, 65-66
    of iridology, 757-760
    of juice therapy, 741-742
    of Latin American traditional medicine, 284-285
    of light therapy, 155-156
    of macronutrients, 566-569
    of magnetic field therapy, 165-166
    of massage therapy, 339
    of meditation, 74-75
    of micronutrients, 577-582
    of music therapy, 87-88
    of Native American medicine, 294
    of naturopathic medicine, 276
    of neuro linguistic programming, 97
    of orthomolecular medicine, 606-607
    of osteopathic medicine, 326-327
    of poetry therapy, 107
    of Polarity Therapy, 423-426
    of prayer/spiritual healing, 130-131
    of Qi Gong, 231-233
    of quartz crystal therapy, 770
    of reflexology, 780-782
    of Reiki, 436
    of relaxation therapies, 115-117
    of Rolfing Structural Integration, 445-446
    of Rosen Method bodywork, 455-457
    of shamanism, 302-303
    of Tai Chi, 219-221
    of Therapeutic Touch, 462-464
    of traditional Chinese medicine, 203-207, 208t
    of Trager Approach, 472-474
    of Yoga, 143-144
Medical care in integrative cancer care, 622-623
Medical community, working with, 14-15
Medical model
    incorporating, in complementary medicine practice, 15-16
    leaving, 10-12
Medicine
    nutritional, 576
    orthomolecular, 606-617; see also Orthomolecular medicine
Meditation, 73-85
    as adjunct to psychotherapy, 78
    for anxiety, 77

Meditation—Cont.
    applications of, 76
    associations on, 81-82
    barriers to, 81
    for cardiovascular disease, 77
    for chronic pain, 77
    concentration methods of, 73
    credentialing in, 80
    demographics of, 75
    for depressive symptoms, 78
    for dermatologic disorders, 78
    effects on neuroendocrine function, 74
    enhancing self-efficacy, 74-75
    forms of, 75
    history of, 73-74
    issues in, key, 81
    mechanisms of action of, 74-75
    mindfulness practices of, 73
    origins of, 73-74
    provider selection in, 81
    Qi Gong, 232
    referral for, 75
    in relapse prevention, 75
    relaxation therapies and, 115
    research on, 77-79
    risks in, 79
    safety of, 79
    self-help versus professional approach to, 80
    in stress reactivity attenuation, 74
    for substance abuse, 77
    training in, 80-81
    transcendental, 73
    visiting professional in, 80
    in yoga, 143
Meditative prayer, 131
Memory loss, aromatherapy for, 656
Menninger, Karl, in music therapy history, 86
Menopausal symptoms, aromatherapy for, 656
Menstrual problems, aromatherapy for, 656
Mentastics, 473, 474
Mercury amalgam in dentistry, 667
    acupuncture meridians and, 668
    adverse reactions to, 673
    galvanism of, 668
    immune system and, 668
    in lactation, 673
    in pregnancy, 673
    replacement of, health improvements from, 672t
    toxicity of, 667-668
Mercury exposure, organic, 669
Mercury toxicity, 508
Mercury vapor exposure toxicity, 668-669
Mercury-free dentistry, 667

Meridians
  in acupressure, 179
  acupuncture, 193
    biologic dentistry and, 668
    in Bowen technique, 373
    in colorpuncture, 693
    in Qi Gong, 232
Mesmer, Anton, in hypnotherapy history, 53
Metabolic disorders, fasting for, 732
Metabolism
  of enzymes, 526
  radiogenic, 488
    dynamical energy systems theory and, 489-490
Meyens, Phillipus, in iridology history, 756
Microcosmic orbit, 233
Micronutrients, 576-594
  actions of, 587
  adverse reactions to, 588-589
  applications of, 583-585
  associations for, 592
  barriers to, 591-592
  credentialing in, 591
  deficiencies of
    marginal, 578-582
      adverse effects of, 579
      clinical findings in, 581
      laboratory testing for, 581
      nail abnormalities in, 582t
      nutrient repletion for, 580
      stages of, 579t
  druglike information of, 587-590
  efficacy of, 586
  history of, 576-577
  intractions with, 589-590
  issues in, key, 591-592
  in lactation, 590
  mechanisms of action of, 577-582
  origins of, 576-577
  pharmokinetics of, 587
  practitioners using, demographics of, 582
  in pregnancy, 590
  provider selection in, 591
  research on, 585-587
  risks of, 586
  safety of, 587
    research on, 586
  self-help versus professional approach to, 590
  therapy with, forms of, 582
  trade products for, 590
  training in, 591
  visiting professional in, 590
  warnings on, 587-588
Midwifery in naturopathic medicine, 278

Milkthistle, use, interactions, adverse effects, and
    contraindications of, 561t
Mind-body interventions, 19-151
  art therapy as, 20-31; see also Art therapy
  biofeedback as, 32-40; see also Biofeedback
  dance/movement therapy as, 41-52; see also Dance/movement
      therapy
  hypnotherapy as, 53-63; see also Hypnotherapy
  interactive guided imagery as, 64-72; see also Imagery,
      interactive guided
  meditation as, 73-85; see also Meditation
  music therapy as, 86-95; see also Music therapy
  neuro linguistic programming as, 96-104; see also Neuro
      linguistic programming (NLP)
  poetry therapy as, 105-113; see also Poetry therapy
  prayer/spiritual healing as, 130-140; see also Prayer/spiritual
      healing
  relaxation therapies as, 114-129; see also Relaxation therapies
  yoga as, 141-151; see also Yoga
Mindcolor, 693
Mindfulness practice of meditation, 73
Minerals, 576-594; see also Micronutrients
Minimum dose in homeopathy, 259
Minor surgery in naturopathic medicine, 278
Möller, Dr., in fasting history, 729
Morrison, Morris, in poetry therapy history, 106
Motor control, Feldendrais Method in, 398-399
Mountain sun, 154
Movement, authentic, 42
Movement disorder, Trager Approach for, 475
Movement education, Aston, 364
Movement reeducation in Hellerwork Structural Integration,
    407
Movement therapy, 41-52; see also Dance/movement therapy
Movement-in-depth, 42
Moxabustion in acupuncture, 195
Muscle tension in Rosen Method bodywork, 455-456
Muscular disorders, essential oils and, indications and
    applications methods for, 655t
Musculoskeletal system
  disorders of, fasting for, 732
  pains in, Qi Gong for, 236
Music therapy, 86-95
  applications of, 90
  associations for, 94
  barriers to, 93-94
  behavioral, 88
  creative, 89
  credentialing in, 93
  definition of, 86
  demographics of, 89
  druglike information on, 92
  eclectic model of, 89
  efficacy of, 92

Music therapy—Cont.
  forms of, 88-89
  history of, 86
  issues in, key, 93-94
  mechanisms of action of, 87-88
  Nordoff-Robbins improvisational, 89
  origins of, 86
  provider selection in, 93
  referral for, 89-90
  research on, 90-92
  risks in, 92
  safety of, 92
  self-help versus professional approach to, 92
  training in, 93
  visiting professional in, 92-93
  warnings for, 92
Myofascial release
  in CranioSacral therapy, 383
  direct, in osteopathy, 328, 329
Myokinetics, Aston, 364
Myotherapy
  Bonnie Prudden, 417-422; see also Bonnie Prudden
      myotherapy
  definition of, 417

                        N
NACSCAOM; see National Accreditation Commission for
      Schools and Colleges of Acupuncture and Oriental
      Medicine (NACSCAOM)
Nadi in Ayurveda, 248
Nail abnormalities, nutritional deficiency and, 582t
NAMT; see National Association for Music Therapy (NAMT)
NAPT; see National Association for Poetry Therapy (NAPT)
National Accreditation Commission for Schools and Colleges of
      Acupuncture and Oriental Medicine (NACSCAOM),
      215
National Association for Music Therapy (NAMT), 86
National Association for Poetry Therapy (NAPT), 106, 110
National Association of Holistic Aromatherapy (NAHA), 664
National Board of Chiropractic Examiners, 315
  in credentialing, 319-320
National Center for Complementary and Alternative Medicine,
      699
National Certification Commission for Acupuncture and
      Oriental Certification Medicine (NCCAOM), 196,
      199-200
National Committee for Acupuncture and Traditional Oriental
      Medicine, 187
Native American medicine, 293-300
  adverse reactions to, 297
  applications of, 296
  associations 1for, 299
  barriers to, 299-300

Native American medicine—Cont.
  credentialing in, 298
  demographics of, 294
  druglike information on, 297
  forms of, 294-295
  history of, 293
  issues in, key, 299-300
  mechanism of action of, 294
  origins of, 293
  in pregnancy, 297
  provider selection in, 299
  referral for, 295-296
  research on, 296
  safety of, 297
  self-help versus professional approach to, 298
  training in, 298-299
  visiting professional in, 298
  warnings on, 297
Naturopathic medicine, 274-282
  applications of, 279
  associations for, 282
  barriers to, 281-282
  credentialing in, 280
  demographics of, 278
  forms of, 276-278
  healing principles of, 274-275
  history of, 275-276
  issues in, key, 281-282
  mechanism of action of, 276
  origins of, 274-276
  provider selection in, 281
  referral for, 278-279
  research on, 279
  self-help versus professional approach to, 279-280
  training in, 280-281
  visiting professional in, 280
Naumberg, M., in art therapy history, 20
NCCAOM; see National Certification Commission for
      Acupuncture and Oriental Certification Medicine
      (NCCAOM)
Needles, acupuncture, 195
Neigong, 233
Nervous system, magnets and, 165
Nettle, stinging, use, interactions, adverse effects, and
      contraindications of, 562t
Neuro linguistic programming
  adverse reactions to, 101
  applications of, 98-99
  associations for, 103
  barriers to, 102
  credentialing in, 101
  demographics of, 97-98
  druglike information on, 100-101
  efficacy of, 100

Neuro linguistic programming—Cont.
  forms of, 97
  history of, 96
  interactions with, 101
  issues in, key, 102
  mechanisms of action of, 97
  origins of, 96
  in pregnancy and lactation, 101
  provider selection in, 102
  referral for, 9
  research on, 99-100
  risks in, 100
  safety of, 100
  self-help versus professional approach to, 101
  training in, 102
  visiting professional in, 101
Neuroendocrine changes, prayer and, 136
Neuroendocrine function, effects of meditation on, 74
Neurologic disorders
  Alexander Technique for, 353
  from mercury vapor exposure, 669
  Trager Approach for, 475
Neurolymphatic points in Bowen technique, 373
Neuromuscular massage, 340
Neurosis, neuro linguistic programming for, 98
Newton, Sir Isaac, in color therapy history, 690
Nissen, Hartwig, in massage therapy history, 338
Nitric oxide, pulmonary disorders and, 599
NLP; see Neuro linguistic programming (NLP)
Nonlocal-naturalistic mechanisms of prayer effects, 130
Nontoxic diet, 703
Nordoff-Robins improvisational music therapy, 89
North American Academy of Magnetic Therapy, 173
Northern California Advisory Group on Mindfulness and
      Medicine, 80
Nutrient pharmacotherapy, 581
Nutrient programs, 708-709t
Nutrient repletion, 580
Nutrition
  clinical, in naturopathic medicine, 277
  therapeutic, in integrative cancer care, 623-624
Nutrition screening panel, sample tests of, 629
Nutritional medicine, 576
Nutritional oncology, 618-636; see also Integrative cancer care
Nutritional therapy, 606-617; see also Orthomolecular medicine

                              O

Olfaction in aromatherapy, 652-653
Oncology, nutritional, 618-636; see also Integrative cancer care
Optimal health in environmental medicine, 717
Optometric phototherapy, 694
Oral cavity disorders from mercury vapor exposure, 668
Orange Randolph in Polarity Therapy, 430

Organ systems in traditional Chinese medicine, 205
Oriental medicine practices, 177-244
  acupressure as, 178-190; see also Acupressure
  acupuncture as, 191-202; see also Acupuncture
  Qi Gong as, 231-244; see also Qi Gong
  Tai Chi as, 219-230; see also Tai Chi
  traditional Chinese herbal medicine as, 203-218; see also
      Traditional Chinese medicine (TCM)
Origins; see History/origins
Orthomolecular medicine, 606-617
  actions of, 611
  adverse reactions to, 612
  applications of, 608-610
  associations for, 614
  barriers to, 614
  credentialing in, 613
  demographics of, 608
  druglike information on, 611-612
  efficacy of, 610-611
  forms of, 607-608
  history of, 606
  interactions with, 612
  issues in, key, 614
  in lactation, 612
  mechanisms of action of, 606-607
  pharmacokinetics of, 611
  in pregnancy, 612
  provider selection in, 613
  referral for, 608
  research on, 610-611
  risks of, 610
  safety of, 611
      research on, 610
  self-help versus professional approach to, 612
  trade products for, 612
  training in, 613
  visiting professional in, 613
  warnings on, 611
Osmond, Humphrey, in orthomolecular medicine history, 606
Osteoarthritis, Alexander Technique for, 352
Osteopathic medicine
  applications of, 330-331
  associations for, 335-336
  barriers to, 335
  credentialing in, 334
  demographics of, 329
  efficacy of, 333
  history of, 325
  issues in, key, 335
  manipulative techniques in, 328-329
  mechanisms of action of, 326-328
  origins of, 325
  provider selection in, 335
  referral for, 329-330

Osteopathic medicine—Cont.
  research on, 331-334
  risks in, 333
  safety of, 333
  self-help versus professional approach to, 334
  training in, 334-335
  visiting professional in, 334
Ott, John, in light therapy history, 155
Oxidant challenge procedure in oxidant stress assessment, 600-601
Oxidative stress, 595-605
  aging diseases and, 601-602
  assessment of, 600-601
  atherosclerosis and, 598
  cellular physiology and, 598-599
  clinical conclusions on, 602-603
  lung conditions and, 599
  protection against, glutathione in, 602
  resistance to, 600
Oxygen, pathology induced by, 596-597

P

Pain
  back, Alexander Technique for, 352
  chronic
    Alexander Technique for, 352
    aromatherapy for, 654
    meditation for, 77
  control of, acupressure in, 180-181
  enzymes in reduction of, research on, 522
  management of, Feldendrais Method in, 398
  musculoskeletal, Qi Gong for, 236
  relief of, essential oils and, indications and applications methods for, 654t
  Trager Approach for, 475
Pain-gateway theory, 180
Palliative care, essential oils in, indications and applications methods for, 655t
Palmer, Daniel David, in chiropractic history, 310
Palpation in traditional Chinese medicine, 206-207
Panic disorders, relaxation therapies for, research on, 121
Panic symptoms, relaxation therapies for, research on, 122
Papain in enzyme therapy, 520
Paracelsus in hypnotherapy history, 53
Passion flower, use, interactions, adverse effects, and contraindications of, 562t
Passive volition, 33
Patanjali in Yoga history, 142
Pau d'arco, use, interactions, adverse effects, and contraindications of, 562t
Pauling, Linus
  in orthomolecular medicine history, 606
  in oxidative stress history, 595

Pediatrics, essential oils in, indications and applications methods for, 655t
Pentane, breath, in oxidant stress assessment, 600
Peppermint, use, interactions, adverse effects, and contraindications of, 562t
Performance enhancement, neuro linguistic programming for, 98
Pericardium in traditional Chinese medicine, 205t
Perls, Fritz, in neuro linguistic programming history, 96
Personal development, Trager Approach for, 475
Petitionary prayer, 131
Pharmacokinetics; see Actions/pharmacokinetics
Pharmacotherapy, nutrient, 581
Phobias
  neuro linguistic programming for, 98
  social, relaxation therapies for, research on, 122
Photodynamic therapy, 156
Phototherapy
  optometric, 694
  syntonic optometric, 157
    practical applications of, 159
    referral for, 157
Physical color therapy, 691-692
  forms of, 693-694
Physical medicine in naturopathic medicine, 277
Phytomedicines, 546; see also Herbal medicine
Pitta dosha in Ayurveda, 247
  foods and herbs for, 250t
Plantain, use, interactions, adverse effects, and contraindications of, 562t
Poetry therapy, 105-113
  adverse reactions to, 109
  applications of, 108
  associations for, 111
  barriers to, 111
  credentialing in, 110
  demographics of, 108
  druglike information on, 109
  forms of, 107
  history of, 105-107
  issues in, key, 111
  mechanism of action of, 107
  origins of, 105-107
  principles of, 106-107
  provider selection in, 111
  referral for, 108
  research on, 108-109
  safety of, 109
  training in, 111
  visiting professional in, 109-110
Points
  acupressure, 179
    proving existence of, 183-184
  acupuncture, in Bowen technique, 373
  neurolymphatic, in Bowen technique, 373

Pokeroot, sources and uses of, 555*t*

Polarity tea, 430

Polarity Therapy
applications of, 428-429
barriers to, 432
credentialing in, 431
demographics of, 426
druglike information on, 430
efficacy of, 429-430
forms of, 426
history of, 423
issues in, key, 432
mechanisms of action of, 423-426
origins of, 423
provider selection in, 431-432
referral for, 427-428
research on, 429-430
risks in, 429
safety of, 429
self-help versus professional approach to, 430
training in, 431
visiting professional in, 431

Position of release in CranioSacral therapy, 383

Posse, Nils, in massage therapy history, 338

Postisometric relaxation in osteopathy, 328-329

Postoperative treatment, efficacy of enzymes in, research on, 523

Postural problems, Alexander Technique for, 352

Pranayama breathing, 143-144

Prayer/spiritual healing, 130-140
applications of, 133
associations for, 138
credentialing in, 138
demographics of, 132
efficacy of, 137
forms of, 131-132
history of, 130
mechanisms of action of, 130-131
neuroendocrine and immunologic changes in, 136
origins of, 130
provider selection in, 138
referral for, 133
research on, 133-137
basic science-based, 136-137
evidence-based, 133-136
risks in, 137
safety of, 137
self-help versus professional approach to, 137
training in, 138
visiting professional in, 138

Precautions; *see* Warnings/contraindications/precautions

Pregnancy
acupressure in, 186
acupuncture in, 198
antineoplastons in, 504
aromatherapy in, 662

Pregnancy—Cont.
Aston-Patterning in, 368
biologic dentistry in, 673
colon hydrotherapy in, 685
CranioSacral therapy in, 388
dance/movement therapy in, 46
enzyme therapy in, 527
magnetic field therapy in, 172
micronutrients in, 590
Native American medicine in, 297
neuro linguistic programming in, 101
orthomolecular medicine in, 612
reflexology in, 786
Tai Chi in, 226
traditional Chinese medicine in, 213
Yoga in, 148

Premenstrual syndrome, aromatherapy for, 656

Prevention in environmental medicine, 718

Primrose, evening, use, interactions, adverse effects, and contraindications of, 558*t*

Probiotics, 577

Professional, visiting; *see* Visiting professional

Professionalized health care systems, 245-282
Ayurveda as, 246-257; *see also* Ayurveda
homeopathy as, 258-273; *see also* Homeopathy
naturopathic medicine as, 274-282; *see also* Naturopathic medicine

Proprioreceptos, joint, in Bowen technique, 373

Proteins, mechanism of action of, 567

Proteolytic enzyme metabolism, 526

Proteolytic serum activity, research on, 521

Prudden, Bonnie
in myotherapy history, 418
myotherapy of, 417-422; *see also* Bonnie Prudden myotherapy

Pryor, William, in oxidative stress history, 595

Psychologic color therapy, 691
forms of, 692-693

Psychologic disorders, essential oils and, indications and application methods for, 654*t*

Psychologic disturbances from mercury vapor exposure, 668

Psychologic effects, Feldendrais Method in, 399

Psychophysiology; *see also* Biofeedback
definition of, 32

Psychotherapy, meditation as adjunct to, 78

Psychotropics, art therapy and, 25

Push hands
mechanism of action of, 220
risk/safety of, 224

Pygeum, use, interactions, adverse effects, and contraindications of, 562*t*

Q

Qi
in acupuncture, 193
in traditional Chinese herbal medicine, 203, 204

Qi Gong
  applications of, 235-236
  associations for, 242
  barriers to, 241-242
  credentialing in, 240-241
  demographics of, 234
  druglike information on, 239
  efficacy of, 238-239
  forms of, 233-234
  history of, 231
  issues in, key, 241-242
  mechanisms of action of, 231-233
  origins of, 231
  provider selection in, 241
  referral for, 234-235
  research on, 485
  risks in, 238
  safety of, 238
  self-help versus professional approach to, 239
  training in, 240-241
  visiting professional in, 239-240
Qi Gong deviation syndrome, 238
Quality of life, Feldendrais Method and, 399
Quartz crystal therapy, 770-778
  adverse reactions to, 774
  applications of, 772
  associations for, 777
  barriers to, 777
  credentialing in, 776
  demographics of, 771
  druglike information on, 774
  efficacy of, 773
  forms of, 771
  history of, 770
  interactions with, 774
  issues in, key, 777
  mechanisms of action of, 770
  origins of, 770
  provider selection in, 777
  referral for, 772
  research on, 773-774
  safety of, 774
  self-help versus professional approach to, 774
  training in, 776-777
  visiting professional in, 775-776
Que, Bian, in acupuncture history, 191
Questioning in traditional Chinese medicine, 206

R
Radiation for bioenergy, 486-489
Radiation hormesis, 485-486
  bioenergy mediated effects compared with, 490
Radical oxidative damage; see also Oxidative stress
  discovery of, 595

Radiogenic metabolism, 488
  dynamical energy systems theory and, 489-490
Rama in biofeedback history, 32-33
Rare earth magnets, 164
Reactive oxygen species (ROS)
  atherosclerosis and, 598
  in oxidative stress, 595-596
  pulmonary disorders and, 599
Recognition in environmental medicine, 718
Referral
  for acupressure, 181
  for acupuncture, 196-197
  for Alexander technique, 352-353
  for antineoplastons, 497-498
  for applied kinesiology, 641
  for aromatherapy, 653
  for art therapy, 22-23
  for Aston-Patterning, 365
  for Ayurveda, 251-252
  for biofeedback, 34, 35t
  for biologic dentistry, 670
  for Bonnie Prudden myotherapy, 419
  for Bowen technique, 374
  for chelation therapy, 510-511
  for chiropractic, 313-315
  for colon hydrotherapy, 682-683
  for color therapy, 694
  for CranioSacral therapy, 384
  for dance/movement therapy, 43-44
  for detoxification therapy, 710
  for environmental medicine, 720
  for enzyme therapy, 521
  for fasting, 732
  for Feldendrais Method, 397
  for flower essence therapy, 537
  for Hellerwork Structural Integration, 410
  for herbal medicine, 549
  for homeopathy, 261-262
  for hypnotherapy, 56
  for interactive guided imagery, 67
  for iridology, 762
  for juice therapy, 748
  for Latin American traditional medicine, 287-289
  for light therapy, 157-158
  for macronutrients, 569
  for magnetic field therapy, 166
  for massage therapy, 342
  for meditation, 75
  for music therapy, 89-90
  for Native American medicine, 295-296
  for naturopathic medicine, 278-279
  for neuro linguistic programming, 99
  for osteopathic medicine, 329-330
  for poetry therapy, 108
  for Polarity Therapy, 427-428

Referral—Cont.
 for prayer/spiritual healing, 133
 for Qi Gong, 234-235
 for quartz crystal therapy, 772
 for reflexology, 782
 for Reiki, 437-438
 for relaxation therapies, 120-121
 for Rolfing Structural Integration, 447
 for Rosen Method bodywork, 458
 for shamanism, 304
 for Tai Chi, 222
 for Therapeutic Touch, 464-465
 for traditional Chinese medicine, 209-210
 for Trager Approach, 475-476
Reflex(es)
 spinal, segmental viscerosomatic, in Bowen technique, 373
 stretch, in Bowen technique, 372-373
Reflexology
 actions of, 784-785
 adverse reactions to, 785-786
 applications of, 782-784
 associations for, 787-789
 barriers to, 787
 credentialing in, 787
 demographics of, 782
 druglike information on, 784-785
 forms of, 782
 history of, 779-780
 interactions with, 785-786
 issues in, key, 787
 in lactation, 786
 mechanisms of action of, 780-782
 origins of, 779-780
 pharmacokinetics of, 784-785
 in pregnancy, 786
 provider selection in, 787
 referral for, 782
 research on, 784
 self-help versus professional approach to, 786
 training in, 787
 visiting professional in, 786
 warnings on, 785
Refocusing techniques in relaxation therapy, 117-118
 mechanism of action of, 115
Reich, Wilhelm, in Rosen Method history, 453
Reiki, 435-443
 associations for, 442
 credentialing in, 441
 demographics of, 437
 druglike information on, 438
 efficacy of, 439
 forms of, 436-437
 history of, 435-436
 mechanisms of action of, 436

Reiki—Cont.
 origins of, 435-436
 provider selection in, 441
 referral for, 437-438
 research on, 438-329
 safety of, 438
  research on, 439
 self-help versus professional approach to, 439
 teaching establishments in, 442
 training in, 441
 visiting professional in, 440-441
Reiter, R, in light therapy history, 155
Reiter, Sherry, in poetry therapy history, 106
Relapse prevention, meditation in, 75
Relaxation
 interactive guided imagery in, 67
 postisometric, in osteopathy, 328-329
Relaxation response, 114
Relaxation response model, research on, 123
Relaxation therapies, 114-129
 adverse reactions to, 124
  research on, 123
 applications of, 121
 associations for, 125-126
 barriers to, 125
 body awareness in, mechanism of action of, 116
 with children, 122
 conscious breathing in, mechanism of action of, 115
 credentialing in, 125
 demographics of, 120
 drug interactions with, 124
 drug therapy versus, 121
 druglike information on, 124
 efficacy of, 123-124
 forms of, 117-120
 history of, 114-115
 issues in, key, 125
 mechanisms of action of, 115-117
 meditation in, 115
 origins of, 114-115
 provider selection in, 125
 referral for, 120-121
 refocusing techniques in, 117-118
  mechanism of action of, 115
 research on, 121-124
 risks in, 123
 safety of, 124
  research on, 123
 self-help versus professional approach to, 1224
 training in, 125
 visiting professional in, 125
 warnings on, 124
Relaxation training, Trager Approach for, 475
Religious coping, 132

Religious coping strategies, 130-140; *see also* Prayer/spiritual
   healing
Rentsch, Oswald, in Bowen technique history, 371
Representational systems, 97
Research
   on acupressure, 183-185
   on acupuncture, 197
   on Alexander technique, 353-354
   on alternative medicines, finances of, 7-8
   on antineoplastons, 498-500
   on applied kinesiology, 644
   on aromatherapy, 658-659
   on art therapy, 24-25
   on Aston-Patterning, 367
   on Ayurveda, 252-253
   on biofeedback, 35-36
   on biologic dentistry, 670-671
   on Bowen technique, 375-376
   on chelation therapy, 511-512
   on chiropractic, 316-318
   on colon hydrotherapy, 683-684
   on color therapy, 695-696
   on CranioSacral therapy, 386-387
   on dance/movement therapy, 45-46
   on environmental medicine, 723
   on enzyme therapy, 521-524
   on fasting, 733-735
   on Feldendrais Method, 397-401
   on flower essence therapy, 538-539
   on Hellerwork Structural Integration, 411
   on herbal medicine, 549-551
   on homeopathy, 264-265
   on hypnotherapy, 58
   on interactive guided imagery, 68-69
   on iridology, 762-763
   on light therapy, 159-160
   on magnetic field therapy, 168-171
   on massage therapy, 343-344
   on meditation, 77-79
   on micronutrients, 583-585
   on music therapy, 90-92
   on Native American medicine, 296-297
   on naturopathic medicine, 279
   on neuro linguistic programming, 99-100
   on orthomolecular medicine, 610-611
   on osteopathic medicine, 331
   on poetry therapy, 108-109
   on Polarity Therapy, 429-430
   on prayer/spiritual healing, 133-137
      basic science-based, 136-137
      evidence-based, 133-136
   on Qi Gong, 237-239
   on quartz crystal therapy, 773
   on reflexology, 784
Research—Cont.
   on relaxation therapies, 121-124
   on Rolfing Structural Integration, 448
   on Rosen Method bodywork, 458
   on shamanism, 305
   on Tai Chi, 224-225
   on Therapeutic Touch, 466-467
   on Trager Approach, 477
   on Yoga, 145, 146-148
Respiratory tract
   disorders of
      essential oils and, indications and applications methods for,
         655t
      from mercury vapor exposure, 669
      reactive oxygen species and, 599
   upper, infections of, aromatherapy for, 656
Retinal hypothalamic pathway, 155-156
Retrolental fibroplasia, oxygen and, 597
Rheumatic diseases, efficacy of enzyme therapy for, research on,
   523-524
Rhyne's Gestalt art therapy, 22
Riedlin, Dr., in fasting history, 729
Risks
   in acupressure, 184
   in Alexander technique, 354
   in antineoplastons, 499
   in aromatherapy, 658-659
   in art therapy, 24
   in Ayurveda, 253
   in biofeedback, 36
   in biologic dentistry, 670-671
   in Bowen technique, 376
   in chiropractic, 317-318
   in colon hydrotherapy, 683
   in color therapy, 696
   in CranioSacral therapy, 387
   in environmental medicine, 723
   in fasting, 734
   in Feldendrais Method, 400
   in flower essence therapy, 539
   in herbal medicine, 550-551
   in homeopathy, 265
   in hypnotherapy, 58
   in interactive guided imagery, 68
   in light therapy, 159
   in magnetic field therapy, 170
   in meditation, 79
   in micronutrients, 584
   in neuro linguistic programming, 100
   in orthomolecular medicine, 610
   in osteopathic medicine, 333
   in Polarity Therapy, 429
   in prayer/spiritual healing, 137
   in Qi Gong, 238

Risks—Cont.
    in relaxation therapies, 123
    in Tai Chi, 224
    in Therapeutic Touch, 466-467
    in traditional Chinese medicine, 211
    in Yoga, 148
Ritualistic prayer, 131
Rolf, Ida P., in Rolfing Structural Integration history, 444
Rolfing Structural Integration, 444-452
    applications of, 447-448
    associations for, 451
    barriers to, 450
    credentialing in, 450
    demographics of, 446
    forms of, 446
    history of, 444-445
    issues in, key, 450
    mechanisms of action of, 445-446
    origins of, 444-445
    referral for, 447
    research on, 448
    self-help versus professional approach to, 449
    training in, 450
    visiting professional in, 449
ROS; *see* Reactive oxygen species (ROS)
Rosen, Marion, in Rosen Method history, 453
Rosen Method bodywork
    applications of, 458
    associations for, 460-461
    barriers to, 460
    credentialing in, 459-460
    demographics of, 458
    druglike information on, 459
    forms of, 457-458
    history of, 453-455
    issues in, key, 460
    mechanisms of action of, 455-457
    origins of, 453-455
    provider selection in, 460
    referral for, 458
    research on, 458
    self-help versus professional approach to, 459
    training in, 459-460
    visiting professional in, 459
    warnings on, 459
Rosen method bodywork, 453-461
Rosenthal, N, in light therapy history, 155
Rotating unipolar magnets, uses of, 167
Rush, Benjamin
    in music therapy history, 86
    in poetry therapy history, 105
Rutosid
    in enzyme therapy, 520
    metabolism of, 526

S

Safety
    of acupressure, 185
        research on, 184
    of acupuncture, 198
    of Alexander technique, 354
    of antineoplastons, 501-502
        research on, 499
    of aromatherapy, 658-659
    of art therapy, 25
        research on, 24
    of Aston-Patterning, 367
    of Ayurveda, 253
    of biofeedback, 36
    of biologic dentistry, 670-671
    of Bowen technique, 376
    of chelation therapy, 513
    of chiropractic, 317-318
    of colon hydrotherapy, 684
        research on, 683
    of color therapy, 696
    of CranioSacral therapy, 387-388
    of dance/movement therapy, 46
    of detoxification therapy, 712
    of environmental medicine, 723
    of fasting, 735
        research on, 734
    of Feldendrais Method, 400
    of flower essence therapy, 539
    of Hellerwork Structural Integration, 412
    of herbal medicine, 550-551
    of homeopathy, 265
    of hypnotherapy, 59
        research on, 58
    of interactive guided imagery, 68
    of Latin American traditional medicine, 290
    of light therapy, 159
    of macronutrients, 571
    of magnetic field therapy, 170
    of meditation, 79
    of micronutrients, 587
        research on, 584
    of music therapy, 92
    of Native American medicine, 297
    of neuro linguistic programming, 100
    of orthomolecular medicine, 611
        research on, 610
    of osteopathic medicine, 333
    of Polarity Therapy, 429
    of prayer/spiritual healing, 137
    of Qi Gong, 238
    of Reiki, 438
    of relaxation therapies, 124
        research on, 123

Safety—Cont.
    of Tai Chi, 225
        research on, 224
    of Therapeutic Touch, 466-467
    of traditional Chinese medicine, 211
    of Yoga, 148
Sahumerio in Latin American traditional medicine, 287
St. John's wort, use, interactions, adverse effects, and
        contraindications of, 562t
Salicylate challenge test in oxidant stress assessment, 601
Sassafras, sources and uses of, 555t
Satir, Virginia, in neuro linguistic programming history, 96
Saturated fatty acids, mechanism of action of, 568
Saw palmetto, use, interactions, adverse effects, and
        contraindications of, 562t
Schizophrenia, neuro linguistic programming for, 99
Schloss, Gil, in poetry therapy history, 106
Schoop, Trudi, in dance/movement therapy history, 41-42
Seasonal affective disorder, 155
    white light therapy for, 157, 158
Segmental facilitation, 332
Segmental viscerosomatic spinal reflexes in Bowen technique,
        373
Seifert in enzyme therapy history, 517
Self-efficacy, meditation enhancing, 74-75
Selye, Hans, on stress, 114
Shamanism, 301-308
    applications of, 304-305
    barriers to, 307
    credentialing in, 306
    demographics of, 304
    forms of, 303-304
    history of, 301-302
    issues in, key, 307
    mechanism of action of, 302-303
    origins of, 301-302
    provider selection in, 307
    referral for, 304
    research on, 305
    self-help versus professional approach to, 305-306
    training in, 306-307
    visiting professional in, 306
Shen in traditional Chinese medicine, 204-205
Shiatsu, 340
Shiatsu style of acupressure, 181
Shoe inserts with magnets, 167
Sies, Helmut, in oxidative stress history, 595-596
Silk-reeling pattern in Tai Chi, 221
Silver Drawing Test of Cognitive and Creative Abilities (STD)
        in art therapy assessment, 26
Single dose in homeopathy, 259
Sivananda, 145
Skin, dry flaky, aromatherapy for, 656
Smelling in traditional Chinese medicine, 206
Smoking cessation, neuro linguistic programming for, 98

Smudging in quartz crystal therapy, 771
Social phobia, relaxation therapies for, research on, 122
Society for Sensory and Neuronal Regulation (SSNR)
        biofeedback and, 37-38
SomatoEmotional release in CranioSacral therapy, 383
Soranus in poetry therapy history, 105
Spector, Sam, in poetry therapy history, 106
Spectro-Chrome system in color therapy, 694
Spinal reflexes, segmental viscerosomatic, in Bowen technique,
        373
Spinning magnets, uses of, 167
Spiritual healing, 130-140; see also Prayer/spiritual healing
Spitler, Harry Riley, in color therapy history, 691
Spitler, HR, in light therapy history, 155
Spleen in traditional Chinese medicine, 205t
Sports injuries
    aromatherapy for, 656
    Qi Gong for, 236
Sports massage, 340
Srotas in Ayurveda, 248
State-bound information, 55
Still, Andrew Taylor, in osteopathic history, 325
Stinging nettle, use, interactions, adverse effects, and
        contraindications of, 562t
Stomach in traditional Chinese medicine, 205t
Stone, Randolph, in Polarity Therapy history, 423
Strain injury, repetitive, Alexander Technique for, 352
Stress
    aromatherapy for, 655
    management of, neuro linguistic programming for, 98
    oxidative, 595-605; see also Oxidative stress
    Qi Gong for, 235
Stress care in integrative cancer care, 627
Stress reactivity, attenuation of, meditation in, 74
Stress reduction, interactive guided imagery in, 67
Stress response, Alexander Technique for, 352
Stretch reflex in Bowen technique, 372-373
Study design on alternatives medicines, inexperience in, 8-9
Substance abuse
    meditation for, 77
    relaxation therapies for, research on, 123
Sun Tai Chi, 221
Supernatural mechanisms of prayer effects, 130
Superoxide, 595
Supplementation in integrative cancer care, 624-626
Surgery
    efficacy of enzyme therapy in, research on, 523
    minor, in naturopathic medicine, 278
Sushrut Samhita, 246
Susto in Latin American traditional medicine, 287-288
Sutherland, William G., in CranioSacral therapy history, 381
Swedish massage, 338, 340
Syntonic optometric phototherapy, 157
    practical applications of, 159
    referral for, 157

Syntonics, 155, 694
Szent-Györgyi, Albert, in juice therapy history, 741

T

Tablework in Trager Approach, 473, 474
Tai Chi, 219-230
  actions of, 225
  adverse reactions to, 226
  applications of, 222-223
  associations for, 228
  barriers to, 228
  credentialing in, 227
  demographics of, 221
  drug interactions with, 226
  druglike information on, 225-227
  efficacy of, 225
  forms of, 221
  history of, 219
  issues in, key, 228
  in lactation, 226
  mechanisms of action of, 219-221
  origins of, 219
  pharmacokinetics of, 225
  in pregnancy, 226
  provider selection in, 228
  referral for, 222
  research on, 224-225
  risks in, 224
  safety of, 225
    research on, 224
  self-help versus professional approach to, 227
  trade products for, 226-227
  training in, 227-228
  visiting professional in, 227
  warnings on, 226
Taiji, 219-230; see also Tai Chi
Taijiquan, 219-230; see also Tai Chi
Takarta, Hawaya, in Reiki history, 435
Talking in Rosen Method bodywork, 454, 455, 457
Tang Dynasty, acupuncture in, 191
Tanner, Dr., in fasting history, 729
Taurine deficiency, 610
Taylor, Charles, in massage therapy history, 338
Taylor, George, in massage therapy history, 338
Tea, polarity, 430
Tea tree, use, interactions, adverse effects, and contraindications
     of, 562t
Terrain, malignant, modulating, 619-620
Therapeutic Touch, 462-471
  actions of, 467
  adverse reactions of, 468
  applicatiosn of, 465
  barriers to, 470
  credentialing in, 469

Therapeutic Touch—Cont.
  demographics of, 464
  druglike information on, 467-468
  efficacy of, 467
  forms of, 464
  history of, 462
  interactiosn of, 468
  issues in, key, 470
  mechanisms of action of, 462-464
  origins of, 462
  in pregnancy, 468
  provider selection in, 469-470
  referral for, 464-465
  research on, 466-467
  risks of, 466-467
  safety of, 466-467
  self-help versus professional approach to, 468
  training in, 469
  visiting professional in, 468
  warnings on, 467
Therapy, forms of
  of acupressure, 181
  of acupuncture, 194-196
  of antineoplastons, 497
  of applied kinesiology, 641
  of aromatherapy, 653
  of art therapy, 21-22
  of Aston-Patterning, 364-365
  of Ayurveda, 249-251
  of biofeedback, 34
  of biologic dentistry, 669
  of Bonnie Prudden Myotherapy, 418
  of chelation therapy, 510
  of chiropractic, 312
  of colon hydrotherapy, 681
  of color therapy, 692-694
  of CranioSacral therapy, 383
  of detoxification therapy, 705-708
  of environmental medicine, 719-720
  of enzyme therapy, 520
  of fasting, 731-732
  of Feldenkrais Method, 395-396
  of flower essences, 537
  of Hellerwork Structural Integration, 410
  of herbal medicine, 547
  of homeopathy, 261
  of hypnotherapy, 55-56
  of interactive guided imagery, 66
  of iridology, 761
  of juice therapy, 742-748
  of Latin American traditional medicine, 286-287
  of light therapy, 157
  of macronutrient therapy, 569
  of massage therapy, 339-341
  of meditation, 75

Therapy, forms of—Cont.
  of micronutrient therapy, 582
  of music therapy, 88-89
  of Native American medicine, 294-295
  of naturopathic medicine, 276-278
  of neuro linguistic programming, 97
  of orthomolecular medicine, 607-608
  of osteopathic medicine, 328-329
  of poetry therapy, 107
  of Polarity Therapy, 426
  of Qi Gong, 233-234
  of quartz crystal therapy, 771
  of reflexology, 782
  of Reiki, 436-437
  of relaxation therapies, 117-120
  of Rolfing Structural Integration, 446
  of Rosen Method, 457-458
  of Shamanism, 303-304
  of spiritual healing and prayer, 131-132
  of Tai Chi, 221
  of therapeutic touch, 464
  of traditional Chinese herbal medicine, 208-209
  of Trager Approach, 474
  of yoga, 144-145
Thistle, blessed, use, interactions, adverse effects, and
    contraindications of, 556t
Thixotropy of connective tissue, 409
Tivy, Desmond, in myotherapy history, 418
Tongue diagnosis in traditional Chinese medicine, 206-207, 208t
Touch, aromatherapy by, 657-658
Touch-based healing, energy in, exploring concept of, 483-493;
    see also Bioenergy therapies
Toxicity of mercury amalgam, 667-668
Trace minerals, 577
Traditional Chinese medicine (TCM)
  acupuncture in, 194
  herbal, 203-218
    actions of, 212
    adverse reactions to, 213
    applications of, 210-211
    associations for, 216
    barriers to, 216
    basic substances in, 204-205
    credentialing in, 215
    demographics in, 209
    diagnostic approaches in, 206-207
    disharmony in, 205-206
    drug interactions with, 212-213
    druglike information on, 212-214
    efficacy of, 212
    forms of, 208
    history of, 203
    issues in, key, 216
    in lactation, 213
    mechanisms of action of, 203-208

Traditional Chinese medicine (TCM)—Cont.
    organ systems in, 205
    origins of, 203
    pharmacokinetics of, 212
    in pregnancy, 213
    provider selection in, 216
    referral for, 209-210
    research on, 211-212
    risks in, 211
    safety of, 211
    self-help versus professional approach to, 214
    trade products in, 213-214
    training in, 215
    treatment principles of, 207
    visiting professional in, 214-215
    warnings on, 212
  Qi Gong in, 231-244; see also Qi Gong
Tragacanth, use, interactions, adverse effects, and
    contraindications of, 556t
Trager, Milton, in Trager Approach history, 472
Trager Approach
  applications of, 476-477
  associations for, 481
  barriers to, 480-481
  contraindications to, 478
  credentialing in, 479
  demographics of, 474-475
  druglike information on, 477-478
  forms of, 474
  history of, 472
  issues in, key, 480-481
  mechanisms of action of, 472-474
  origins of, 472
  precautions with, 478
  provider selection in, 479-480
  referral for, 475-476
  research on, 477
  training in, 479
  visiting professional in, 478-479
Training
  in acupressure, 187
  in acupuncture, 200
  in Alexander technique, 356
  in applied kinesiology, 646-647
  in art therapy, 27
  in Aston-Patterning, 369
  in Ayurveda, 255
  in biofeedback, 37-38
  in biologic dentistry, 675
  in Bonnie Prudden myotherapy, 421
  in Bowen technique, 377-378
  in chelation therapy, 513
  in chiropractic, 320-321
  in colon hydrotherapy, 687
  in color therapy, 698

Training—Cont.
in CranioSacral therapy, 389-390
in dance/movement therapy, 48
in detoxification therapy, 714
in environmental medicine, 725
in enzyme therapy, 528-529
in fasting, 737-738
in Feldendrais Method, 402
in flower essence therapy, 542-543
in Hellerwork Structural Integration, 414
in homeopathy, 268-269
in hypnotherapy, 60
in interactive guided imagery, 69
in iridology, 765-766
in light therapy, 160-161
in macronutrients, 573
in magnetic field therapy, 173
in massage therapy, 346
in meditation, 80-81
in micronutrients, 591
in music therapy, 93
in Native American medicine, 298-299
in naturopathic medicine, 280-281
in neuro linguistic programming, 102
in orthomolecular medicine, 613
in osteopathic medicine, 334-335
in poetry therapy, 111
in Polarity Therapy, 431
in prayer/spiritual healing, 138
in Qi Gong, 240-241
in quartz crystal therapy, 776-777
in reflexology, 787
in Reiki, 441
in relaxation therapies, 125
in Rolfing Structural Integration, 450
in Rosen Method bodywork, 459-460
in shamanism, 306-307
in Tai Chi, 227-228
in Therapeutic Touch, 469
in traditional Chinese medicine, 215
in Trager Approach, 479
in Yoga, 149
Transcendental meditation, 73
Transcutaneous nerve stimulation (TENS), 183
Trauma
efficacy of enzyme therapy for, research on, 523
sports, aromatherapy for, 656
Travell, Janet, in myotherapy history, 417-418
Trigger points Bowen technique, 373
Triple energizer in traditional Chinese medicine, 205t
Trypsin in enzyme therapy, 520
Tumeric, use, interactions, adverse effects, and contraindications of, 562t
Twisted Hairs Blessed Beauty Way of Shamanic Healing, 301-308; see also Shamanism

U

Ulcers, decubitus, aromatherapy for, 656
Ultraviolet therapies, 158
Upadhatus in Ayurveda, 248
Upledger, John E., in CranioSacral Therapy history, 381
Urinary disorders, essential oils and, indications and applications methods for, 654t
Usui, Mikao, in Reiki history, 435

V

Vaginal infections, aromatherapy for, 655-656
Valerian, use, interactions, adverse effects, and contraindications of, 562t
Valner, Jean, in aromatherapy history, 651
van Helmont, Jan Baptista, in hypnotherapy history, 53
Vascular system, magnets and, 165
Vata dosha in Ayurveda, 247
foods and herbs for, 250t
Vegetables, seasonal, 704
Vietnamese traditions, acupuncture in, 195
Viniyoga, 145
Virally mediated diseases, efficacy of enzyme therapy for, research on, 524
Viscerosomatic spinal reflexes, segmental, in Bowen technique, 373
Vishnu-devananda in Yoga history, 142
Visiting professional
in acupuncture, 199
in Alexander Technique, 355
in antineoplastons, 504-505
in applied kinesiology, 645-646
in aromatherapy, 663
in art therapy, 26-27
in Aston-Patterning, 368-369
in Ayurveda, 255
in biofeedback, 37
in biologic dentistry, 673-674
in Bonnie Prudden Myotherapy, 420
in Bowen Technique, 377
in chelation therapy, 513
in chiropractic, 318-319
in colon hydrotherapy, 686-687
in color therapy, 698
in CranioSacral therapy, 389
in dance/movement therapy, 47
in detoxification therapy, 713
in environmental medicine, 724-725
in fasting, 736-737
in Feldenkrais Method, 401-402
in flower essences, 542
in Hellerwork Structural Integration, 413-414
in homeopathy, 267-268
in hypnotherapy, 59-60
in interactive guided imagery, 69
in iridology, 764

Visiting professional—Cont.
   in Latin American traditional medicine, 290
   in light therapy, 160
   in macronutrients, 573
   in massage therapy, 345
   in meditation, 80
   in micronutrients, 590
   in music therapy, 92-93
   in Native American medicine, 298
   in naturopathic medicine, 280
   in neuro linguistic programming, 101
   in orthomolecular medicine, 613
   in osteopathic medicine, 334
   in poetry therapy, 109-110
   in Polarity Therapy, 431
   in Qi Gong, 239-240
   in quartz crystal therapy, 775-776
   in reflexology, 786
   in Reiki, 440-441
   in relaxation therapies, 125
   in Rolfing Structural Integration, 449
   in Rosen Method, 459
   in Shamanism, 306
   in spiritual healing and prayer, 137
   in Tai Chi, 227
   in therapeutic touch, 468
   in traditional Chinese herbal medicine, 214-215
   in Trager Approach, 478-479
   in Yoga, 149
Visualization, active, interactive guided imagery in, 67
Vital force in homeopathy, 260
Vitamin(s), 576-594; see also Micronutrients
   antioxidant, 602
   deficiencies of, marginal, effects of, 579t
Vitamin A compounds, supplemental, 624
Vitamin C
   actions of, 597t
   clinical conclusions on, 603
Vitamin C challenge in oxidant stress assessment, 601
Vitamin E
   actions of, 597t
   Alzheimer's disease and, 610
   supplemental, 624
Vitex, use, interactions, adverse effects, and contraindications
      of, 562t
Volition, passive, 33
von Goethe, Johann Wolfgang, in color therapy history, 690
Von Peczely, Ignatz, in iridology history, 756

                         W
Wang Zongyue in Tai Chi history, 219
Warnings/contraindications/precautions
   on acupressure, 185-186
   on acupuncture, 198

Warnings/contraindications/precautions—Cont.
   on antineoplastons, 502-503
   on aromatherapy, 660-661
   on art therapy, 24, 25
   on Aston-Patterning, 367
   on biologic dentistry, 672-673
   on Bonnie Prudden Myotherapy, 419
   on chelation therapy, 513
   on color therapy, 697
   on CranioSacral therapy, 388
   on dance/movement therapy, 46
   on detoxification therapy, 712-713
   on enzyme therapy, 526-527
   on fasting, 735-736
   on flower essences, 540
   on homeopathy, 266
   on hypnotherapy, 59
   on juice therapy, 749-751
   on macronutrients, 571-572
   on magnetic field therapy, 171
   on massage therapy, 344
   on micronutrients, 587-588
   on music therapy, 92
   on Native American medicine, 297
   on neuro linguistic programming, 100
   on orthomolecular medicine, 611
   on reflexology, 785
   on relaxation therapies, 124
   on Tai Chi, 226
   on therapeutic touch, 467
   on traditional Chinese medicine, 212
   on Trager Approach, 478
   on Yoga, 148
Water, intake of, 571
Weight control, neuro linguistic programming for, 98
Wheat grass juice, 747
White, Ann, in poetry therapy history, 106
White light therapy for seasonal affective disorder, 157, 158
Whitehouse in dance/movement therapy history, 42
Wiltsie, James A, in colon hydrotherapy history, 680
Wolf, Max, in enzyme therapy history, 517
Wu Tai Chi, 221
Wudang Tai Chi, 221
Wuhao Tai Chi, 221

                         X
Xenobiotics, 571

                         Y
Yang Tai Chi, 221
Yin/yang principle
   in acupressure, 180
   in Qi Gong, 232
   in Tai Chi, 219-220

Yoga, 141-151
    applications of, 145-146
    associations for, 150
    Ayurveda and, 251
    barriers to, 150
    credentialing in, 149
    demographics of, 145
    druglike information on, 148
    efficacy of, 148
    forms of, 144-145
    history of, 142
    issues in, key, 150
    in lactation, 148
    mechanisms of action of, 143-144
    origins of, 141-142
    polarity, 423
    in pregnancy, 148

Yoga—Cont.
    provider selection in, 149-150
    referral for, 145
    research on, 146-148
    risks in, 148
    safety of, 148
    self-help versus professional approach to, 148
    training in, 149
    visiting professional in, 149
    warnings on, 148
Yohimbe, sources and uses of, 555t

Z

Zarlino in music therapy history, 86
Zero balancing, 340
Zhang Sanfeng in Tai Chi history, 219